Current Therapy of Diabetes Mellitus

CURRENT THERAPY SERIES

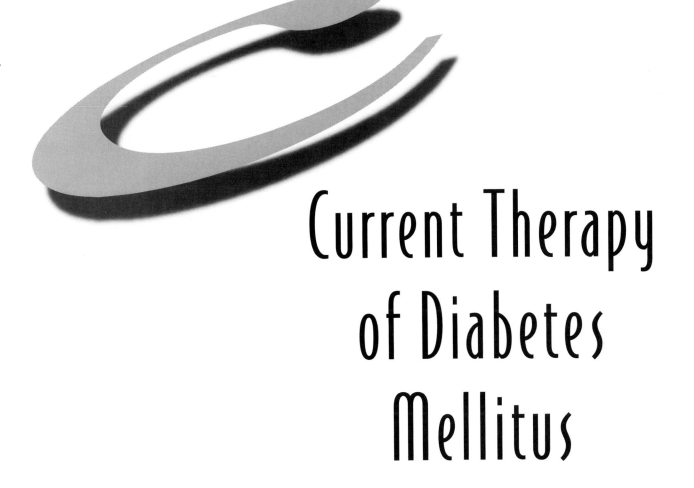

Current Therapy of Diabetes Mellitus

Ralph A. DeFronzo, M.D.

Professor of Medicine
Chief, Diabetes Division
University of Texas Health Science Center at San Antonio
Deputy Director,
Texas Diabetes Institute
San Antonio, Texas

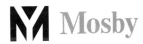 Mosby

St. Louis Baltimore Boston Carlsbad Chicago Minneapolis New York Philadelphia Portland
London Milan Sydney Tokyo Toronto

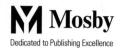

Mosby
Dedicated to Publishing Excellence

A Times Mirror
Company

Vice President and Publisher: Anne S. Patterson
Senior Managing Editor: Lynne Gery
Project Manager: Linda Clarke
Production Editor: Jennifer Harper
Composition Specialist: Christine Boles
Manufacturing Supervisor: William A.Winneberger, Jr.
Design Manager: Nancy J. McDonald

Printed in the United States of America
Composition by Mosby Electronic Production, Philadelphia
Printing/binding by R.R. Donnelley & Sons

Mosby–Year Book, Inc.
11830 Westline Industrial Drive
St. Louis, Missouri 63146

ISBN 0-8151-2757-X

98 99 00 01 02 / 9 8 7 6 5 4 3 2

I would like to dedicate this book to my wife, Toni, who has added new inspiration to my life.

Contributors

K. George M.M. Alberti, D Phil
Professor of Medicine, University of Newcastle upon Tyne, Newcastle upon Tyne, United Kingdom
Hyperosmolar Hyperglycemic Nonketotic Coma

Barbara J. Anderson, Ph.D.
Associate Professor of Psychology, Department of Psychiatry, Harvard Medical School; Senior Psychologist, Joslin Diabetes Center, Boston, Massachusetts
Psychosocial Problems in Children

Janet Blodgett, M.D.
Clinical Faculty, University of Texas Health Science Center; Private Practice, San Antonio, Texas
Alpha-Glucosidase Inhibitors

Geremia B. Bolli, M.D.
Professor of Metabolism, Department of Internal Medicine and Endocrine and Metabolic Science, University of Perugia, Perugia, Italy
Hypoglycemia in Type 1 Diabetic Patients

Jean L. Bolognia, M.D.
Associate Professor of Dermatology, Yale University School of Medicine; Attending Physician, Yale-New Haven Hospital, New Haven, Connecticut
Skin and Subcutaneous Tissues

Andrew J.M. Boulton, M.D., F.R.C.P.
Professor of Medicine, Manchester University; Consultant Physician, Manchester Royal Infirmary, Manchester, United Kingdom
The Diabetic Foot

Irwin Braverman, M.D.
Professor of Dermatology, Yale University School of Medicine; Attending Physician, Yale New Haven Medical Center, New Haven, Connecticut
Skin and Subcutaneous Tissues

Scott E. Buchalter, M.D.
Associate Professor of Medicine, Division of Pulmonary and Critical Care, University of Alabama School of Medicine; Chief of Staff, University of Alabama Hospital, University of Alabama Health System, Birmingham, Alabama
Therapeutic Considerations for Lactic Acidosis

Marshall W. Carpenter, M.D.
Associate Professor, Brown University School of Medicine; Director of Maternal-Fetal Medicine, Women and Infants Hospital of Rhode Island, Providence, Rhode Island
Gestational Diabetes

Agostino Consoli, M.D.
Associate Professor of Endocrinology, University of Chieti, Chieti, Italy
Metformin

Anne Daly, R.D., M.S., C.D.E.
Instructor, St. John's Hospital School of Diabetes; Director of Nutrition and Diabetes Education, Springfield Diabetes and Endocrine Center, Springfield, Illinois
Medical Nutrition Therapy in Type 1 Diabetes Mellitus

Ralph A. DeFronzo, M.D.
Professor of Medicine, and Chief, Diabetes Division, University of Texas Health Science Center at San Antonio and Audie L. Murphy Memorial VA Hospital; Deputy Director, Texas Diabetes Institute, San Antonio, Texas
Classification and Diagnosis of Diabetes Mellitus
Goals of Diabetes Management
Combination Therapy: Insulin-Sulfonylurea and Insulin-Metformin
Troglitazone (Rezulin)
Diabetic Nephropathy: Diagnostic and Therapeutic Approach
Diabetic Retinopathy
Sulfonylureas

John T. Devlin, M.D.
Associate Professor, University of Vermont College of Medicine, Burlington, Vermont; Medical Director, Maine Medical Center Diabetes Center, Portland, Maine
Exercise in the Management of Type 1 Diabetes Mellitus

Robert DiBianco, M.D.
Associate Clinical Professor of Medicine, Georgetown University School of Medicine, Washington, D.C.; Director, Cardiology Research, Heart Failure and Risk Factor Reduction Clinic, Washington Adventist Hospital, Takoma Park, Maryland
Heart Failure

David A. Escalante, M.D.
Assistant Professor of Medicine, Division of
Endocrinology and Molecular Metabolism, University
of Kentucky School of Medicine, Lexington, Kentucky
Atherosclerotic Cardiovascular Disease

Eva L. Feldman, M.D., Ph.D.
Associate Professor of Neurology, University of
Michigan, Ann Arbor, Michigan
Diabetic Peripheral Neuropathy

S. Edwin Fineberg, M.D., F.A.C.P.
Professor of Medicine, Division of Endocrinology and
Metabolism, Indiana University School of Medicine,
Indianapolis, Indiana
*Hypersensitivity Reactions to Insulin and Insulin
Resistance*

Eli A. Friedman, M.D.
Distinguished Teaching Professor of Medicine and
Chief, Renal Disease Division, Department of
Medicine, State University of New York Health
Science Center at Brooklyn College of Medicine;
Attending Physician, University Hospital of Brooklyn,
Brooklyn, New York
Diabetic Nephropathy: End Stage

Alan J. Garber, M.D., Ph.D.
Professor of Medicine, Biochemistry and Cell Biology,
Baylor College of Medicine; Chief of Endocrinology,
Diabetes and Metabolism, The Methodist Hospital,
Houston, Texas
Atherosclerotic Cardiovascular Disease

Carrie Garber, M.S.
formerly Genetics Counselor, Division of Medical
Genetics, Cedars-Sinai Medical Center, Los Angeles,
California
Genetic Counseling

Laurence A. Gavin, M.D., F.R.C.P., F.A.C.P.
Clinical Professor of Medicine, University of California
at San Francisco School of Medicine, San Francisco;
Private Practice, Comprehensive Diabetes-Endocrine
Medical Associates, Daly City, California
Type 1 Diabetes Mellitus in Pregnancy

Henry N. Ginsberg, M.D.
Irving Professor of Medicine, Columbia University
College of Physicians and Surgeons, New York,
New York
Dyslipidemia

John R. Graybill, M.D.
Professor of Medicine, and Chief, Infectious
Diseases, University of Texas Health Science Center
at San Antonio and Audie Murphy VA Hospital,
San Antonio, Texas
Infections and Diabetes Mellitus

Douglas A. Greene, M.D.
Professor of Internal Medicine, University of Michigan
Medical School; Chief, Division of Endocrinology and
Metabolism, Department of Internal Medicine,
University of Michigan Medical Center, Ann Arbor,
Michigan
Diabetic Peripheral Neuropathy

Kay Griver, R.D.
Metabolic Research/Diabetes Dietitian, VA San Diego
Health Care System, San Diego, California
Diet Therapy of Type 2 Diabetes Mellitus

Leif C. Groop, M.D.
Professor of Medicine, Department of Endocrinology,
University of Lund; Chief Physician, University Hospital
MAS, Malmoe, Sweden
Sulfonylureas

Lawrence B. Harkless, D.P.M.
Professor, Department of Orthopaedic Surgery;
Professor and Director, Podiatry Residency Training
Program, University of Texas Health Science Center,
San Antonio, San Antonio, Texas
The Diabetic Foot

Kristin Story Held, M.D.
Clinical Associate Professor, University of Texas Health
Science Center at San Antonio, San Antonio, Texas
Cataract in the Diabetic Patient

Robert R. Henry, M.D., F.R.C.P.(C.)
Professor of Medicine, University of California, San
Diego, School of Medicine; Director, Endocrinology,
Metabolism and Diabetes Clinics, VA Medical Center,
San Diego, California
Diet Therapy of Type 2 Diabetes Mellitus

Irl B. Hirsch, M.D.
Associate Professor of Medicine, University of
Washington School of Medicine; Medical Director,
Diabetes Care Center, University of Washington
Medical Center, Seattle, Washington
Surgery and Diabetes Mellitus

Barry S. Horowitz, M.D.
formerly Division of Preventive Medicine and
Nutrition, Department of Medicine, Columbia
University College of Physicians and Surgeons, New
York, New York
Dyslipidemia

Alan M. Jacobson, M.D.
Professor of Psychiatry, Harvard Medical School;
Medical Director, Joslin Diabetes Center, Boston,
Massachusetts
Psychosocial Problems in Children

Norman M. Kaplan, M.D.
Professor of Internal Medicine and Head, Hypertension
Division, University of Texas Southwestern Medical
Center at Dallas Southwestern Medical School, Dallas,
Texas
Hypertension in Patients with Diabetes

Michael S. Katz, M.D.
Professor and Chief, Division of Geriatrics and
Gerontology, Department of Medicine, University of
Texas Health Science Center at San Antonio;
Director, Geriatric Research Education and Clinical
Centers, South Texas Veterans Health Care Center,
Audie L. Murphy Division, San Antonio, Texas
Geriatrics and Diabetes Mellitus

Duk Kyu Kim, M.D., Ph.D.
Associate Professor, Dong-A University Medical
College; Chief, Division of Endocrinology, Dong-A
University Hospital, Pusan, Korea
Atherosclerotic Cardiovascular Disease

John L. Kitzmiller, M.D.
Director, Maternal-Fetal Medicine, Good Samaritan
Hospital, San Jose, California
Type 1 Diabetes Mellitus in Pregnancy

Robert A. Kreisberg, M.D.
Clinical Professor of Medicine, University of Alabama;
Director, Internal Medicine Education, Baptist Health
System, Birmingham, Alabama
Diabetic Ketoacidosis in Adults
Therapeutic Considerations for Lactic Acidosis

Marvin E. Levin, M.D.
Professor of Clinical Medicine and Associate Director,
Endocrinology, Diabetes and Metabolism Clinic,
Washington University School of Medicine, St. Louis,
Missouri
Peripheral Vascular Disease

Lynne Lyons, M.P.H., R.D., C.D.E.
Assistant Manager, Perinatal Services, Columbia
Good Samaritan Hospital, San Jose, California
Type 1 Diabetes Mellitus in Pregnancy

Mariana S. Markell, M.D.
Associate Professor of Medicine, State University of
New York Health Science Center at Brooklyn College
of Medicine; Director, Transplant Nephrology,
University Hospital of Brooklyn, Brooklyn, New York
Diabetic Nephropathy: End Stage

Jennifer B. Marks, M.D.
Associate Professor of Medicine, Division of
Endocrinology, and Assistant Director, Behavioral
Medicine Research Center, University of Miami
School of Medicine, Miami, Florida
Surgery and Diabetes Mellitus

**Sally M. Marshall, B.Sc., M.B., Ch.B., M.D.,
F.R.C.P. (Lon), F.R.C.P. (Glas)**
Reader in Diabetes Medicine, University of Newcastle
upon Tyne, Honorary Consultant Physician, Royal
Victoria Infirmary, Newcastle upon Tyne,
United Kingdom
Hyperosmolar Hyperglycemic Nonketotic Coma

Ram K. Menon, M.D.
Associate Professor of Pediatrics, Division of
Endocrinology, Department of Pediatrics, University
of Pittsburgh School of Medicine, Pittsburgh,
Pennsylvania
Infant of the Diabetic Mother

Julie S. Meyer, M.S.N., R.N., C.D.E.
Associate Professor, University of Texas Health Science
Center School of Nursing; Diabetes Clinical Nurse
Specialist, University Health System, San Antonio,
Texas
The Diabetes Nurse Educator

Antonio Morgado, M.D.
Associate Professor of Medicine, Seton Hall School of
Graduate Medical Education, South Orange; Chief of
Endocrinology, Jersey City Medical Center, Jersey City,
New Jersey
Exercise in the Management of Type 2 Diabetes Mellitus

Merri Pendergrass, M.D., Ph.D.
Instructor of Medicine, University of Texas Health
Science Center at San Antonio, San Antonio, Texas
Infections and Diabetes Mellitus

Jacqueline A. Pugh, M.D.
Associate Professor, University of Texas Health
Science Center at San Antonio; Ambulatory Care
Staff Physician, Central Texas Veterans Health Care
System, San Antonio, Texas
Geriatrics and Diabetes Mellitus

Leslie J. Raffel, M.D.
Assistant Professor of Pediatrics and Medicine, UCLA
School of Medicine; Associate Director, Common
Disease Genetics, Division of Medical Genetics,
Cedars-Sinai Medical Center, Los Angeles California
Genetic Counseling

Matthew C. Riddle, M.D.
Professor of Medicine and Head, Section of Diabetes,
Oregon Health Sciences University, Portland, Oregon
*Combination Therapy: Insulin-Sulfonylurea and
     Insulin-Metformin*

Jerome I. Rotter, M.D.
Professor of Medicine and Pediatrics, UCLA School of
Medicine; Director, Division of Medical Genetics, and
Cedars-Sinai Board of Governors' Chair in Medical
Genetics, Cedars Sinai Medical Center, Los Angeles,
California
Genetic Counseling

Julio V. Santiago, M.D.
Professor of Pediatrics and Medicine, Washington
University School of Medicine; Physician and
Pediatrician, Barnes-Jewish Christian Health System,
St. Louis, Missouri
Diabetic Ketoacidosis in Children

Stephen H. Schneider, M.D.
Professor of Medicine, University of Medicine and
Dentistry of New Jersey Robert Wood Johnson
Medical School, New Brunswick, New Jersey
Exercise in the Management of Type 2 Diabetes Mellitus

Gregorio A. Sicard, M.D.
Professor of Surgery, Washington University School of
Medicine; Director, Vascular Service, Barnes-Jewish
Hospital, St. Louis, Missouri
Peripheral Vascular Disease

Jay S. Skyler, M.D.
Professor of Medicine, Pediatrics and Psychology,
University of Miami, Miami, Florida
*Insulin Therapy in Type 1 Diabetes Mellitus
Monitoring of Type 1 Diabetes Mellitus
Insulin Therapy in Type 2 Diabetes Mellitus*

Mark A. Sperling, M.D.
Vira I. Heinz Professor and Chairman, Department of
Pediatrics, University of Pittsburgh School of
Medicine, and Children's Hospital of Pittsburgh,
Pittsburgh, Pennsylvania
Infant of the Diabetic Mother

Martin J. Stevens, M.D.
Assistant Professor of Internal Medicine, Division of
Endocrinology and Metabolism, University of
Michigan, Ann Arbor, Michigan
Diabetic Peripheral Neuropathy

Sompongse Suwanwalaikorn, M.D.
formerly Division of Endocrinology and Metabolism,
University of Massachusetts Medical Center,
Worcester, Massachusetts
Autonomic Neuropathy

W.A.J. van Heuven, M.D.
Professor and Herbert F. Mueller Chair of
Ophthalmology, University of Texas Health Science
Center, San Antonio, Texas
Diabetic Retinopathy

Aaron I. Vinik, M.D., Ph.D., F.C.P., F.A.C.P.
Professor of Medicine, Vice Chairman for Research and
Director, Diabetes Research Institute, The Diabetes
Institutes, Eastern Virginia Medical School of the
Medical College of Hampton Roads, Norfolk, Virginia
Autonomic Neuropathy

Neil H. White, M.D., C.D.E.
Associate Professor, Department of Pediatrics,
Washington University School of Medicine, St. Louis,
Missouri
Diabetic Ketoacidosis in Children

Rena R. Wing, Ph.D.
Professor of Psychiatry, Psychology and Epidemiology,
University of Pittsburgh School of Medicine,
Pittsburgh, Pennsylvania
Behavioral Weight Control

Preface

Diabetes mellitus is a common disorder that affects approximately 17 million individuals in the United States. Type 2 diabetes mellitus, which accounts for the great majority of patients with diabetes, is growing at an epidemic rate, not only in the United States; but throughout the world. The health care cost for the treatment of diabetes and its associated microvascular and macrovascular complications currently exceeds 100 billion dollars per year. Although the complications of diabetes are largely preventable by the appropriate treatment of hyperglycemia, dyslipidemia, hypertension, and microalbuminuria, in combination with patient/physician education, morbidity and mortality in diabetic patients remains unacceptably high because of inadequate control of these metabolic and cardiovascular abnormalities. Despite the availability of a wide variety of medications that are capable of normalizing plasma glucose and lipid levels, blood pressure, and microalbuminuria, the great majority of diabetic patients remain poorly controlled. Interventional strategies for the prevention of ophthalmologic and foot complications also are well established.

In the present treatise, we provide a simple and pragmatic approach to the treatment of patients with diabetes mellitus and its associated complications. In each chapter a leading national/international authority presents a brief overview about the background/pathophysiology of his/her topic and this is followed by a concise, yet comprehensive discussion of the clinical manifestations and therapy. Specific recommendations and medication doses are provided to assist the primary care physician in the management of the diabetic patient. By combining these guidelines with patient/physician education programs and with the involvement of other members of the diabetes care team (nurse educator, dietitian, social worker, exercise therapist, ophthalmologist, podiatrist) when indicated, it is anticipated that the complications of diabetes can be eliminated and that the quality of life for all diabetic patients will be improved.

Ralph A. DeFronzo

Contents

SPECIAL PROBLEMS

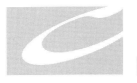

INTRODUCTION

CLASSIFICATION AND DIAGNOSIS OF DIABETES MELLITUS

Ralph A. DeFronzo, M.D.

In 1979, the National Diabetes Data Group (NDDG), working under the sponsorship of the National Institutes of Health, developed a system for the classification and diagnosis of diabetes mellitus and related disorders. The draft document developed by this international work group was widely distributed throughout the diabetes community to incorporate the comments and suggestions of the many reviewers. The World Health Organization (WHO) Expert Committee on Diabetes, the WHO Study Group on Diabetes Mellitus, and the American Diabetes Association (ADA) endorsed the primary components of the recommendations of the NDDG.

The classification scheme that emerged represented a hybrid system based in part on etiology, but more so on the pharmacologic treatment that was employed to manage the disease. The NDDG subdivided diabetes into two major forms: insulin-dependent diabetes mellitus (IDDM), or type 1 diabetes, and non–insulin-dependent diabetes mellitus (NIDDM), or type 2 diabetes. Patients with NIDDM were further subdivided into those who were lean and those who were obese. Within this broad classification the work group also provided evidence that diabetes is a heterogeneous group of disorders with distinct clinical presentations that shared the biochemical characteristic of hyperglycemia. In addition to the two broad categories of IDDM and NIDDM, the NDDG classification recognized two further groups: gestational diabetes mellitus (GDM) and other types of diabetes mellitus. The latter included a wide variety of conditions and syndromes. This classification scheme also included a fifth category, termed "impaired glucose tolerance" (IGT), which was defined on the basis of the oral glucose tolerance test (OGTT). The IGT category was composed of individuals whose OGTT did not satisfy the diagnostic criteria for diabetes mellitus, but whose plasma glucose levels were significantly above those considered to be normal.

The diabetes classification published in 1979 was based upon a combination of treatment requirements (i.e., IDDM versus NIDDM) and pathogenesis (other types). Except for a few disorders included under other types, a definite etiology had not been established for most of the subclasses of diabetes.

■ UPDATED CLASSIFICATION OF DIABETES MELLITUS

In May of 1995, the ADA convened an expert committee to re-examine the classification and diagnosis of diabetes mellitus, and this work group proposed a revised classification scheme based on the etiology of diabetes mellitus. This new etiologic classification is consistent with the original tenets of the NDDG, which recognized that as knowledge about diabetes expanded the classification would have to be revised. With recent advances in immunology and molecular biology a number of distinct etiologic causes of diabetes mellitus have been defined, and it is anticipated that in the near future many other etiologic causes of diabetes mellitus will be recognized. The primary features of the new classification of diabetes mellitus (Table 1) are as follows:

1. The terms "insulin-dependent diabetes mellitus" and "non–insulin-dependent diabetes mellitus" and their abbreviated designations, IDDM and NIDDM, have been dropped, while the terms type 1 diabetes mellitus and type 2 diabetes mellitus have been retained. The terms IDDM and NIDDM represent a classification based on treatment rather than etiology and present a confusing picture to primary care physicians who do not understand the need and/or importance of treating NIDDM patients with insulin.
2. The category of diabetes referred to as "type 1 diabetes mellitus" encompasses all causes of diabetes that result from destruction of the pancreatic beta cells.
3. The category of diabetes referred to as "type 2 diabetes mellitus" encompasses all forms of diabetes that are characterized by the combination of insulin resistance and deficient secretion of insulin. The circulating plasma insulin levels may be increased in absolute terms but are deficient relative to the severity of insulin resistance. This category of diabetes represents the majority of diabetic patients who are seen in everyday practice by primary care physicians.

4. The category of GDM has been retained as defined by the NDDG. The diagnostic criteria for GDM remain unchanged from those originally proposed by the NDDG, although these criteria currently are being re-examined by an international work group.
5. The term "impaired glucose tolerance" (IGT) has been retained to denote a metabolic state that is intermediate between normal and diabetic based upon the OGTT, because it is unusual for normal individuals to have a fasting plasma glucose concentration above 110 mg per deciliter.

Type 1 Diabetes Mellitus

This type of diabetes is subdivided into two major categories: (1) immune-mediated diabetes mellitus and (2) idiopathic diabetes mellitus. "Immune-mediated type 1 diabetes mellitus" (previously referred to as "insulin-dependent diabetes mellitus," "type I diabetes mellitus," or "juvenile-onset diabetes") is caused by an autoimmune cell-mediated destruction of the pancreatic beta cells. Islet cell autoantibodies, insulin autoantibodies, and autoantibodies to glutamic acid decarboxylase (GAD_{65}) are found in more than 90 percent of individuals at the time of diagnosis but disappear after the beta cells have been completely destroyed. At least 12 distinct genetic loci on 9 chromosomes have been linked to the development of type 1 diabetes mellitus. The major disease locus, IDDM1 in the major histocompatibility complex (MHC) on chromosome 6p21, accounts for 35 percent of observed familial clustering and involves polymorphic residues of class II molecules in T-cell–mediated autoimmunity. Environmental factors also have been implicated in the development of type 1 diabetes mellitus but their precise role has yet to be defined. The peak onset of type 1 diabetes is during childhood and adolescence, with the majority of patients (approximately 75 percent) presenting before age 30. It is now recognized that approximately 10 percent of Caucasian diabetics of European descent have slowly evolving type 1 diabetes mellitus. These patients present clinically as type 2 diabetics who eventually fail on oral agents and progress to insulin dependency.

"Idiopathic type 1 diabetes mellitus" refers to forms of type 1 diabetes characterized by insulinopenia and lack of immunologic evidence of autoimmune beta-cell destruction. Insulin sensitivity, when measured, is normal. This form of diabetes has been described most commonly in African Americans, although its frequency, even in this population, appears to be low.

Type 2 Diabetes Mellitus

Individuals with type 2 diabetes mellitus (previously termed "non–insulin-dependent diabetes mellitus," "type II diabetes mellitus," or "adult-onset diabetes") are characterized by insulin resistance and relative or absolute insulin deficiency and represent the majority of patients seen by physicians in everyday practice. This type of diabetes has a strong genetic disposition, typically has its onset later in life, and is associated with features of the insulin resistance syndrome (dyslipidemia, hypertension, atherosclerotic cardiovascular disease). The majority of individuals are obese, with a preponderance of intra-abdominal fat distribution. It is anticipated that the number of diabetic individuals in this category will decrease progressively as specific genetic defects are defined to allow a more precise etiologic classification.

Other Specific Types of Diabetes Mellitus

This category of diabetes includes a wide variety of unrelated disorders, many with well-defined etiologies, that can not be categorized as either type 1 or type 2 diabetes mellitus.

Gestational Diabetes Mellitus

"Gestational diabetes mellitus" refers to the onset or first recognition of diabetes mellitus during pregnancy, most commonly during the third trimester. Women with GDM are characterized by insulin resistance and impaired insulin secretion, and approximately three-fourths have a family history of type 2 diabetes mellitus. Most of these women probably have typical type 2 diabetes mellitus that was unmasked by the stress of pregnancy. Women with GDM should be reclassified on the basis of the fasting plasma glucose concentration obtained 6 or more weeks after delivery. They are at very high risk to develop overt type 2 diabetes mellitus within a 10-year period and require frequent long-term follow-up.

Impaired Glucose Tolerance and Impaired Fasting Glucose

The diagnosis of IGT is reserved for individuals whose glucose tolerance is intermediate between normal and diabetic as defined by a 2-hour postprandial glucose concentration of at least 140 mg per deciliter and less than 200 mg per deciliter. These people typically have normal or only modestly elevated fasting plasma glucose concentrations and manifest hyperglycemia only when challenged with an oral glucose load. Approximately one-third of individuals with IGT develop overt type 2 diabetes mellitus after 10 years. IGT also is part of the insulin-resistance syndrome (syndrome X or the metabolic syndrome) and is a risk factor for atherosclerotic cardiovascular disease.

The diagnosis of diabetes mellitus is made when the fasting plasma glucose concentration is ≥ 126 mg per deciliter.

Table 1 Classification of Diabetes Mellitus

PRESENT CLASSIFICATION	NEW CLASSIFICATION
I. Type I diabetes mellitus or Insulin-dependent diabetes mellitus (IDDM)*	I. Type 1 diabetes mellitus A. Autoimmune B. Idiopathic
II. Type II diabetes mellitus or Non–insulin-dependent diabetes mellitus (NIDDM)* A. Nonobese B. Obese	II. Type 2 diabetes mellitus A. Nonobese B. Obese
III. Other types of diabetes	III. Other specific types of diabetes
IV. Impaired glucose tolerance (IGT)	IV. Gestational diabetes mellitus (GDM)
V. Gestational diabetes mellitus (GDM)	V. Impaired glucose tolerance (IGT) and impaired fasting glucose (IFG)

*Deleted in the revised classification.

Nonetheless, in the normal population fasting glucose levels of 110 mg per deciliter or more are uncommon. Moreover, fasting glucose levels ≥ 110 mg per deciliter are associated with the loss of first-phase insulin secretion and an increased risk of developing both microvascular and macrovascular complications. Therefore, a new diagnostic category called "impaired fasting glucose" (IFG) has been created to identify a metabolic state that is intermediate between normal glucose homeostasis and diabetes. Individuals with IFG have fasting glucose levels of at least 110 mg per deciliter, but less than 126 mg per deciliter.

■ DIAGNOSIS OF DIABETES MELLITUS

Presently the diagnosis of diabetes can be made by one of three measures (Table 2):

1. Symptoms of diabetes plus a random plasma glucose of 200 mg per deciliter (11.1 mmol per liter) or higher. Random glucose can be obtained anytime during the day, irrespective of meals. Symptoms of diabetes include any of the following: polyuria, polydipsia, or unexplained weight loss with glucosuria and ketonuria.
2. Fasting plasma glucose of 140 mg per deciliter (7.8 mmol per liter) or higher, where the fasting glucose value is determined in the morning after abstinence from caloric intake for 10 to 12 hours.
3. Plasma glucose of 200 mg per deciliter (11.1 mmol per liter) or higher at 2 hours during a 75-g OGTT *plus* one other plasma glucose value of 200 mg per deciliter or higher taken between administration of the oral glucose load and the 2-hour time point.

The ADA has recommended that the above criteria be altered and the following diagnostic criteria be adopted.

1. Symptoms of diabetes plus a random plasma glucose of 200 mg per deciliter (11.1 mmol per liter) or higher. Criterion #1 remains unchanged.
2. Fasting plasma glucose of 126 mg per deciliter (7.0 mmol per liter) or higher. This represents a significant

reduction in level of fasting hyperglycemia needed to establish the diagnosis of diabetes mellitus.
3. Plasma glucose of 200 mg per deciliter (11.1 mmol per liter) or higher at 2 hours during the OGTT. This represents a significant change in that only the 2-hour value is required to establish the diagnosis of diabetes mellitus.

Whatever test is employed to establish the diagnosis of diabetes, if unequivocal hyperglycemia is not present, one of the three diagnostic tests described above should be repeated to confirm the presence of diabetes mellitus.

The scientific basis underlying the new diagnostic criteria is as follows: (1) analysis of glucose distributions in populations with a high prevalence of diabetes demonstrates bimodality with a separation point of 200 mg per deciliter for the 2-hour time point during an OGTT; (2) the prevalence of microvascular disease (retinopathy and proteinuria) increases sharply when the 2-hour postprandial plasma glucose concentration during the OGTT exceeds 200 mg per deciliter; (3) a fasting plasma glucose concentration of 125 mg per deciliter is equivalent to a 2-hour postprandial glucose concentration of 200 mg per deciliter in predicting future microvascular complica-

Table 3 Diagnostic Criteria for Impaired Glucose Tolerance

NEW CRITERIA	PRESENT CRITERIA
Fasting plasma glucose <126 mg/dl (7.0 mmol/L) plus 2-hr plasma glucose during the OGTT <200 mg/dl (11.1 mmol/L) but ≥140 mg/dl	Fasting plasma glucose <140 mg/dl (7.8 mmol/L) plus 2-hr plasma glucose during the OGTT ≥ 140 mg/dl (7.8 mmol/ L) but <200 mg/dl (11.1 mmol/L) plus ½-hr or 1-hr or 1½-hr plasma glucose during the OGTT ≥200 mg/dl

OGTT = Oral glucose tolerance test.

Table 4 Diagnostic Criteria for Impaired Fasting Glucose

NEW CRITERIA	PRESENT CRITERIA
Fasting plasma glucose ≥110mg/dl (6.1 mmol/L) but <126 mg/dl (7.0 mmol/L)	None

Table 2 Diagnostic Criteria For Diabetes Mellitus

NEW CRITERIA	PRESENT CRITERIA
Symptoms* of diabetes plus a random plasma glucose ≥200 mg/dl (11.1 mmol/L)	Symptoms* of diabetes plus a random plasma glucose ≥200 mg/dl (11.1 mmol/L)
or	or
Fasting plasma glucose ≥126 mg/dl (7.0 mmol/L)	Fasting plasma glucose ≥140 mg/dl (7.8 mmol/L)
or	or
2-hr plasma glucose during the oral glucose tolerance test ≥200 mg/dl	2-hr plasma glucose plus one other glucose value during the oral glucose tolerance test ≥200 mg/dl

*Symptoms include polyuria, polydipsia, and unexplained weight loss with glucosuria and ketonuria.

Table 5 Diagnostic Criteria for Gestational Diabetes Mellitus

	VENOUS PLASMA	
	mg/dl	(mmol/L)
Fasting	105	(5.8)
1 hr	190	(10.6)
2 hr	165	(9.2)
3 hr	145	(8.1)

*If two or more values are exceeded during a 100-g OGTT, the diagnosis of GDM is established.

tions and discriminating bimodality; (4) a number of recently completed epidemiologic studies have demonstrated that the ability of the 2-hour postprandial and fasting plasma glucose concentrations to predict microvascular complications and to discriminate bimodal glucose distributions are equivalent. Because of these considerations and the ADA's desire to make the fasting and 2-hour postprandial glucose values equivalent in their ability to predict diabetes, the fasting glucose concentration needed to make the diagnosis of diabetes has been lowered to 126 mg per deciliter. These new diagnostic criteria also will be consistent with the revised criteria of the WHO.

Impaired Glucose Tolerance and Impaired Fasting Glucose

At present the diagnosis of IGT requires that each of the following three criteria be satisfied: (1) a fasting plasma glucose concentration less than 140 mg per deciliter (7.8 mmol per liter); (2) 2-hour postprandial plasma glucose concentration during the OGTT greater than or equal to 140 mg per deciliter and less than 200 mg per deciliter (11.1 mmol per liter); (3) ½ hour or 1 hour or 1½ hour plasma glucose concentration greater than or equal to 200 mg per deciliter (11.1 mmol per liter) (Table 3).

According to the new diagnostic criteria, the diagnosis of IGT is made if the fasting plasma glucose concentration is less than 126 mg per deciliter (7.0 mmol per liter) and the 2-hour plasma glucose concentration during the OGTT is greater than or equal to 140 mg per deciliter (7.8 mmol per liter) and less than 200 mg per deciliter (11.1 mmol per liter) (Table 3).

Impaired fasting glucose (IFG) is a new diagnostic category. It is defined by a fasting plasma glucose greater than or equal to 110 mg per deciliter (6.1 mmol/L) but less than 126 mg per deciliter (7.0 mmol/L). The addition of IFG recognizes that a fasting plasma glucose concentration at 110 mg per deciliter or more is uncommon in the general population.

Gestational Diabetes Mellitus

The criteria for the diagnosis of GDM remain unchanged. All pregnant women should be screened during weeks 24 to 28 of gestation with a 50-g oral glucose load followed by determination of the plasma glucose concentration 1 hour later. The screening test can be administered any time during the day or in relation to the previous meal. If the 1-hour postprandial glucose concentration is greater than or equal to 140 mg per deciliter (7.8 mmol per liter), a 3-hour 100-g OGTT should be performed. Cutoff values are shown in Table 5. If two or more values are exceeded, the diagnosis of GDM is made.

Suggested Reading

American Diabetes Association. Standards of medical care for patients with diabetes mellitus. Diabetes Care 1996; 19(suppl 1):S3–S118.

Summary of the ADA's present criteria for the diagnosis of diabetes mellitus and related disorders.

Harris MI, Couric CC, Reiber G, et al. Diabetes in America. 2nd ed. Washington, DC: U.S. Government Printing Office, 1995.

Exhaustive, up-to-date review of the epidemiology of diabetes and its complications. This reference source contains a wealth of statistics on all aspects of diabetes mellitus.

National Diabetes Data Group. Classification and diagnosis of diabetes mellitus and other categories of diabetes mellitus. Diabetes 1979; 28:1039–1057.

Detailed summary of the original classification system and diagnostic criteria for diabetes mellitus and related disorders. This classification system and diagnostic criteria for diabetes mellitus, IGT, and GDM currently represents the "gold standard" in the United States. However, the ADA has proposed a new classification system based upon etiology and a new set of diagnostic criteria for diabetes mellitus and IGT.

Report of the Expert Committee on the Diagnosis and Classification of Diabetes Mellitus. Diabetes Care, July 1997 (in press).

This publication presents the new ADA diagnostic and classification scheme.

World Health Organization. Diabetes mellitus: Report of a WHO study group. Technical Report Series No. 727. Geneva: WHO, 1985.

Summary of the WHO classification system and diagnostic criteria for diabetes mellitus and related disorders.

GOALS OF DIABETES MANAGEMENT

Ralph A. DeFronzo, M.D.

Diabetes mellitus, both insulin-dependent (type 1, or IDDM) and non–insulin-dependent (type 2, or NIDDM), is a metabolic disorder characterized by disturbances in carbohydrate, lipid, and protein metabolism. These metabolic derangements result from a combination of insulin deficiency and/or insulin resistance and lead to a variety of acute and chronic complications. The acute complications include symptomatic hyperglycemia, hypoglycemic hyperosmolar nonketotic coma, and diabetic ketoacidosis. Chronic complications usually occur 10 to 15 years after the onset of diabetes and include microvascular (nephropathy, retinopathy, neuropathy); macrovascular (stroke, myocardial infarction); and peripheral vascular (amputation) disease. An abundance of epidemiologic evidence, experimental animal and human data, and human intervention studies clearly have linked eye, kidney, and neurologic complications in IDDM and NIDDM to poor glycemic control. The results of the Diabetes Control and Complications Trial (DCCT), carried out in 1,441 type 1 diabetic patients, and the Japanese Intervention Trial, carried out in 110 type 2 diabetic patients, have shown that tight glycemic control markedly reduces the incidence of diabetic retinopathy, nephropathy, and neuropathy. In the DCCT, eye, kidney, and neurologic complications decreased by 76 percent, 54 percent, and 60 percent, respectively (Fig. 1). Hyperglycemia also contributes to the increased incidence of macrovascular complications, but dyslipidemia and hypertension, as well as obesity (especially central) and smoking,

also play major roles in the accelerated rate of coronary artery and cerebrovascular disease (Fig. 2). Importantly, these cardiovascular risk factors have been shown to be additive or even synergistic in diabetic patients. Although all of these metabolic cardiovascular abnormalities contribute to the high rate of macrovascular complications, dyslipidemia represents the single most important risk factor for coronary artery disease (see Fig. 2).

Comprehensive treatment of the diabetic patient includes meticulous attention to the achievement of normoglycemia, correction of hypertension and dyslipidemia, attainment of ideal body weight, and an increase in physical activity.

The management objectives for both IDDM and NIDDM patients are similar and include the following: (1) prevention of acute complications; (2) prevention of chronic microvascular and neuropathic complications; (3) prevention of premature atherosclerotic cardiovascular and peripheral vascular complications; and (4) attainment of normal quality of life without symptoms referable to diabetes.

Epidemiologic studies have demonstrated that diabetic retinopathy and nephropathy are distinctly uncommon if the postprandial plasma glucose concentration is less than 200 mg per deciliter and the fasting plasma glucose concentration is below 140 mg per deciliter. This level of glycemic control corresponds to a hemoglobin A_{1c} level of 7.0 percent. Consequently, these values have been established as acceptable end points of therapy in all diabetic patients. However, it is desirable to have the fasting and postprandial plasma glucose concentrations and HbA_{1c} levels as close to normal as possible (Table 1). It should be noted, however, that the results of several recent, large prospective epidemiologic studies indicate that the incidence of diabetic microvascular complications (retinopathy and albuminuria) begins to increase when the fasting plasma glucose concentration increases to about 126 mg per deciliter. On the basis of these observations the American Diabetes Association (ADA) and the World Health Organization (WHO) have agreed to lower the cutoff value (fasting plasma glucose concentration) for the diagnosis of diabetes mellitus to about 126 mg per deciliter. It follows logically that the acceptable goal for therapy (fasting plasma glu-

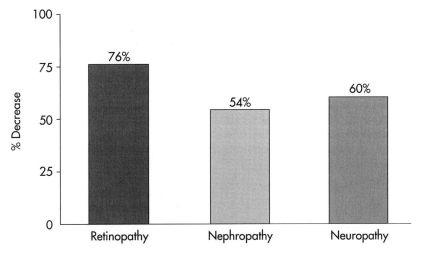

Figure 1
Effect of glycemic control on microvascular complications (DCCT).

cose concentration) will decline to less than 126 mg per deciliter. No change in the 2-hour postprandial plasma glucose concentration (200 mg per deciliter) was recommended by the ADA and the WHO.

Hypertriglyceridemia invariably occurs in association with a reduction in high-density lipoprotein (HDL) cholesterol, and both of these dyslipidemias represent major and independent cardiovascular risk factors in both diabetic and nondiabetic individuals. An acceptable level for the plasma triglyceride concentration is 200 mg per deciliter, while the normal value is less than 150 mg per deciliter (see Table 1). The HDL cholesterol should be as high as possible. Exercise and, to a lesser extent, weight loss can increase the HDL cholesterol, but drug therapy generally is ineffective. An elevated low-density lipoprotein (LDL) cholesterol level needs to be treated aggressively in diabetic patients because of its additive, perhaps even synergistic, effect of accelerating coronary artery disease (see Fig. 2). Even if the LDL cholesterol level is nor-

mal, the presence of hypertriglyceridemia favors the formation of a small, dense LDL particle (subphenotype B) that is highly atherogenic. This represents another reason for reducing the plasma triglyceride concentration below 150 to 200 mg per deciliter.

Because hypertension represents a major risk factor for both cardiovascular disease and diabetic nephropathy, even a modest elevation in the blood pressure requires prompt attention. Systolic hypertension is as ominous as diastolic blood pressure. Ideally, one should reduce the blood pressure to the level that was present before the onset of hypertension or renal impairment. Unfortunately, for many diabetic patients this is not known. In this instance, an acceptable value is less than 130 to 140/85 mm Hg but further reduction is desirable as long as there are no untoward side effects (see Table 1). Microalbuminuria (30 to 300 mg per day) increases the likelihood of clinically overt albuminuria (>300 mg per day) within a 10-year period ten- to twentyfold in IDDM

Table 1 Biochemical and Cardiovascular End Points of Diabetes Management

	NORMAL	ACCEPTABLE
Fasting plasma glucose (mg/dl)*	< 110	< 140**
Postprandial (2h) plasma glucose (mg/dl)	< 140	< 200
HbA$_{1c}$ (%)	< 6.0	< 7.0
Plasma low-density lipoprotein (LDL) cholesterol (mg/dl)	< 100	< 130
Plasma triglyceride (mg/dl)	< 150	< 200
Blood pressure (mm Hg)	< 120/80	< 130–140/85
Microalbuminuria (mg/day)	< 30	< 300†
Ideal body weight (%)	< 100	< 120

*In IDDM patients premeal plasma glucose concentrations should be less than 140 mg/dl and ideally less than 110 mg/dl.
†As low as possible.
**Will decrease to <126 mg/dl with new diagnostic criteria for diabetes mellitus.

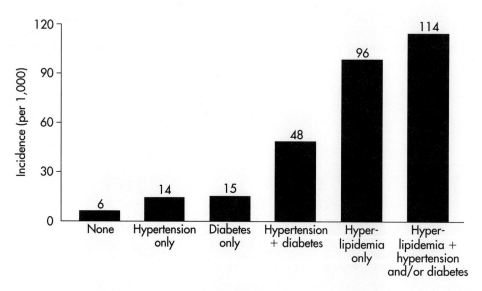

Figure 2

PROCAM (Prospective Coronary Artery Munster) Study: Incidence of myocardial infarction in 2,754 men, ages 40 to 65, over 4 years. (Adapted from Assmann G, Schulte H. The Prospective Cardiovascular Munster (PROCAM) Study: Prevalence of hyperlipidemia in persons with hypertension and/or diabetes mellitus and the relationship to coronary heart disease. Am Heart J 1988; 116:1713–1724; with permission.)

patients and five- to eightfold in NIDDM patients. Therefore, microalbuminuria should be treated aggressively (see Table 1). If microalbuminuria is present in the absence of hypertension or after the hypertension has been successfully treated, the dose of antihypertensive medication (angiotensin-converting enzyme inhibitor or calcium channel blocker) should be increased progressively until the microalbuminuria disappears completely, declines to a stable unchanging level, or untoward side effects occur.

Obesity, especially central adiposity, physical inactivity, and smoking all represent major cardiovascular risk factors. Obesity, sedentary life-style, and smoking also are associated with insulin resistance and impaired glucose tolerance. Therefore, a major effort should be made to achieve and maintain ideal body weight in all diabetic patients, to increase the level of physical activity, and to encourage the cessation of smoking.

All of the above goals are desirable, but they must be achieved without a significant deterioration in the patient's quality of life. It is important for the physician to individualize goals in each diabetic patient. For instance, in the patient with advanced diabetic complications, less stringent glycemic control may be indicated to prevent serious hypoglycemic reactions.

Patient education also is an essential goal of the treatment regimen. If the patient does not understand why it is desirable to achieve specific end points, it is unlikely that he or she will be willing or able to follow an intensive management regimen.

Suggested Reading

American Diabetes Association. Standards of medical care for patients with diabetes mellitus. Diabetes Care 1994; 17:616–623.

This article, written by the American Diabetes Association, defines the standards of good medical care for patients with diabetes mellitus and is essential reading for all primary care physicians and general internists.

American Diabetes Association. Clinical practice recommendations 1996. Diabetes Care 1996; 18(suppl 1):S1–S118.

This comprehensive treatise gathers all of the clinical practice guidelines published by the ADA into one easy read-able source. It covers every aspect of the treatment of diabetes mellitus and its many complications.

Assmann G, Schulte H. The Prospective Cardiovascular Munster (PROCAM) Study: Prevalence of hyperlipidemia in persons with hypertension and/or diabetes mellitus and the relationship to coronary heart disease. Am Heart J 1988; 116:1713–1724.

Prospective population-based epidemioloic study that documents the synergistic interaction between hypertension, hyperlipidemia, and diabetes mellitus in the development of coronary artery disease.

DeFronzo RA. Diabetic nephropathy: Etiologic and therapeutic considerations. Diabetes Rev 1995; 3:510–564.

Exhaustive review of the etiology, clinical manifestations, and therapy of renal disease in type 1 and type 2 diabetic patients.

The Diabetes Control and Complications Trial Research Group. The effect of intensive treatment of diabetes on the development and progression of long term complications. N Engl J Med 1993; 329:977–986.

The largest, most definitive study documenting that tight glycemic control with insulin prevents/delays microvascular complications (retinopathy, nephropathy, neuropathy) in patients with type 1 (insulin-dependent) diabetes mellitus.

Garg A, Grundy SM. Treatment of dyslipidemia in patients with NIDDM. Diabetes Rev 1995; 3:433–445.

Well-written clinical review on the treatment of lipid disorders in individuals with diabetes mellitus.

Ohkubo Y, Kishikawa H, Araki E, et al. Intensive insulin therapy prevents the progression of diabetic microvascular complications in Japanese patients with non-insulin dependent diabetes mellitus: A randomized prospective six-year study. Diabetes Res Clin Pract 1995; 28:103–117.

Well-designed prospective study demonstrating that tight glycemic control with insulin prevents microvascular complications in type 2 (non–insulin-dependent) diabetes mellitus.

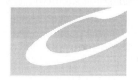

TYPE 1 DIABETES MELLITUS

PSYCHOSOCIAL PROBLEMS IN CHILDREN

Alan M. Jacobson, M.D.
Barbara J. Anderson, Ph.D.

As any other chronic illness that affects children and adolescents, insulin-dependent diabetes mellitus (IDDM) poses a wide range of challenges and problems for patients and family members. These may include physical pain, hospitalization, change in life-style, altered vocational plans, physical disabilities, and threatened survival. The demands of diabetes are influenced by the age, developmental stage, and situation of the child, but they also have commonalities for all patients and their families. For example, dietary restrictions can be problems for children of any age, but challenges also differ for families of toddlers and adolescents. Because these issues are pervasive, concerns have often been raised about the psychological or psychiatric consequences of having diabetes mellitus during childhood. Strikingly, most research has indicated that the presence of IDDM in children and adolescents does not lead to changes in personality, an increased prevalence of psychiatric illness, or major deviations from normal psychological development. However, a growing body of studies indicates that psychological and social issues can have profound influences on the success diabetic patients and their families have in caring for their diabetes. This chapter examines the clinical implications for health care providers of this research on the relationship between psychosocial issues and diabetes mellitus. It also presents an approach for the health care provider to develop an optimal therapeutic relationship with the patient and family.

Supported in part by NIH Grants AM-27845 and DK-42315.

■ PSYCHOSOCIAL EFFECTS OF DIABETES

There is currently a controversy over the extent and nature of psychological problems that are caused by IDDM. The onset of IDDM in young adolescents may lead to transient adjustment reactions best described as a period of bereavement such as might occur after any major loss. From this perspective the child experiencing the onset of IDDM must adjust to the changes in his or her life. Longitudinal studies have indicated that adjustment reactions at onset of IDDM are common. It is not clear whether early adjustment problems foretell later development of more serious psychiatric illness. Indeed, many children and families are able to acknowledge the losses brought on by the new illness, pull together, identify new and even positive consequences to their lives, and then take on the challenge of IDDM. There are some recent suggestions that IDDM may be associated with an increased likelihood of clinical eating disorders, such as anorexia nervosa and bulimia, as well as subclinical eating problems among adolescent girls and young women. However, definitive conclusions about the prevalence of eating disorders in girls and women with diabetes have not yet been drawn.

In a related area, recent research suggests that IDDM may cause alterations in cognitive or intellectual functioning. These studies indicate that some patients with IDDM with an onset before the age of 5 may be at special risk for subtle problems in their intellectual development. These studies do not suggest that patients with later onset are at risk for similar problems. It is important to note that most of these studies were conducted before the widespread use of self-monitoring of blood glucose levels in very young children with IDDM and that the studies do not definitely indicate that clinically meaningful problems in cognitive functioning actually occur in children with early onset before age 5.

While the underlying cause of these cognitive changes is not well understood, an increased frequency of severe insulin reactions in younger children may be critical. Although hypoglycemia causes reversible cognitive problems, no studies have systematically examined the effects of recurrent hypoglycemia on permanent changes in cognitive functioning. Intensive treatment strategies designed to lower patient blood glucose levels to the range of persons who do not have diabetes increase the risk of hypoglycemia. If used in treating young children, they could increase the risk of cognitive deficits. The Diabetes Control and Complications Trial (DCCT) included an extensive neuropsychological test battery to compare the effects of standard versus tight-control treatment strategies. However, no significant differences were reported in neuropsychological performance between the intensively treated group and the standard care group in the DCCT. This study included IDDM patients as young as age 13 and did not include any preadolescents or very young children.

Although much further research is required to better understand the impact of IDDM on the development of major personality problems, psychiatric illness, and cognitive deficits, there are well-recognized, important personal responses to its diagnosis, life-style requirements, and threatened complications. These responses can include changes in the pattern of family interactions as well as in the focus of patient and family concerns. Parents of younger children with diabetes often re-evaluate the need to protect their children from anticipated dangers. This can influence family values around the promotion of independence and can lead to overt worries of parents and children about separation. For example, among parents of diabetic children, there may be increased worry about allowing the child greater independence because of the risk of hypoglycemic episodes. This can make the parents reluctant to let their child take on age-appropriate activities such as bicycling or driving. Similarly, children and parents may develop a heightened awareness of possible diabetic complications, leading to increased fear or concern about the future and heightened familial tension about blood glucose control. Such concerns and changes in family environment may also lead to difficulties accepting the diagnosis and facing the daily demands of the illness. When patients and their families respond differently to stresses from diabetes, conflicts among them may develop. For example, parents of an adolescent with IDDM may worry more than their child about future complications, leading to nagging and disagreements when self-care routines are not followed "perfectly" by the patient.

Changes in family attitudes following the onset of IDDM do not necessarily represent pathologic processes requiring intervention. For example, past research suggested that diabetic children were more dependent than children without chronic illness. However, more recent studies indicate that increased parent-child involvement represents an appropriate shift in the family, important to healthy emotional development of the child in the face of a chronic illness, rather than pathologic dependence. Indeed, the failure of families to increase involvement may be far more problematic than so-called "overprotectiveness." Thus, identifiable differences in diabetic patients and their families can reflect healthy and necessary changes as well as psychosocial problems. Assessments of families of children with IDDM need to take such issues into account. Furthermore, studies of normal development suggest that promotion of secure child attachment to parental figures provides the most important basis for future independence. Thus, parental attempts to prematurely push their diabetic children toward independence may be counterproductive. Accepting the extra involvement needed by a diabetic child is more likely to promote greater security and better adjustment. In essence, the parents of a child with diabetes have to promote autonomy in their developing child while maintaining an involvement in the diabetes treatment plan. Thus, full independence, especially with respect to diabetes management, is not an appropriate goal, and acceptance of this parental involvement is likely to favor better long-term adaptation.

Clearly, the age and developmental stage of the child affect the specific issues posed by diabetes. Table 1 summarizes the

---

Table 1 Challenges Facing Parents and/or Children with Diabetes

PARENTS OF INFANTS AND TODDLERS (0–3 YEARS OLD)
Monitoring diabetes control and avoiding hypoglycemia
Establishing a meal schedule despite the child's normally irregular eating patterns
Coping with the very young child's inability to understand the need for injections
Managing the conflicts with older siblings that result from unequal sharing of parental attention

PRESCHOOLERS AND EARLY ELEMENTARY SCHOOLCHILDREN (4–7 YEARS OLD)
Mastering separation from the family and adapting to the expectations of teachers
Blaming self for having diabetes; regarding injections and restrictions as punishments
Educating school personnel, coaches, and scout leaders about diabetes (parents)

LATER ELEMENTARY SCHOOLCHILDREN (8–11 YEARS OLD)
Engaging in wide range of activities with peers
Understanding long-term benefits of diabetes care
Becoming involved in diabetes self-care tasks (selecting snacks, selecting and cleaning injection sites, and identifying symptoms of low blood glucose)

EARLY ADOLESCENCE (12–15 YEARS OLD)
Integrating physical changes into the self-image
Acknowledging that the young teenager is on the threshold of becoming an adult (parents)
Continuing to share increased responsibility for diabetes management with parents in the face of physiologic changes in insulin resistance and sensitivity caused by puberty
Fitting in with the peer group
Maintaining good glycemic control while remaining concerned about possible weight gain

LATER ADOLESCENCE (16–19 YEARS OLD)
Making decisions regarding post–high school plans
Living more independently of parents
Strengthening relationships with fewer friends
Assuming more independent responsibility for health and health care

From Anderson B, Wolfsdorf J, Jacobson AM. Psychosocial adjustment in children with type 1 diabetes. In Lebovitz H, ed. Therapy for diabetes mellitus and related disorders. Alexandria, Va: ADA Press, 1994.

major developmental challenges for parents and their children with diabetes. Recognition of the normal developmental challenges at each stage is a critical starting point for treating the pediatric patient and the family. The clinician can use these milestones as a basis for evaluating patients and families as well as customizing their approach to the developmental stage of the patient.

There is now ample evidence in patients with IDDM that several psychosocial issues influence self-care behaviors. These include psychiatric problems, stressful life events, social support, attitudes and beliefs about medical care, and the health care provider's approach to medical care. For example, patients undergoing more stressful life experiences are at risk for worsened glucose control. Stressful experiences may affect glycemic control by influencing patient self-care behaviors or through more direct impact on stress-related hormones such as adrenaline. Extremely brittle diabetes, recurrent severe hypoglycemia, diabetic ketoacidosis, hyperosmolar states, misuse of insulin, and very high levels of glycosylated hemoglobin may be markers of underlying psychosocial difficulties. Diabetes control problems can also reflect health or medical care attitudes. Patients anticipating an early cure, those who believe the regimen too difficult to adapt to their lives, and those who believe that medical care is unlikely to change their medical problems are less likely to take care of their diabetes. Children frightened by the effects of a nighttime insulin reaction may become fearful of falling asleep and as a result may overeat during their bedtime snack. Health care providers provide a critical part of the educational as well as emotional support of child patients and their families. A positive therapeutic relationship is the centerpiece of this support.

■ BUILDING A SUCCESSFUL THERAPEUTIC RELATIONSHIP

Certain general principles can guide the health care provider to maximize the patient's and family's ready participation in their care and alleviate psychosocial problems that may impair adjustment to diabetes. Even if psychological problems are not prevented, these principles may lead to early identification, referral, and treatment of problems.

The point of departure for successful care of the diabetic patient and his or her family is through the establishment of agreeable treatment goals and a "therapeutic alliance." The establishment of a working alliance relies on the identification of the patient's and family's true goals as opposed to idealized objectives. As a basis for discussion in establishing realistic goals of treatment, the patient and family must be encouraged to identify their expectations. This can be done with even young children by talking with them in ways appropriate to their age. This may involve drawings or playing out stories with puppets or games. By eliciting the child's concerns and wishes, diabetes treatment and education can be modified. These goals should be redefined and discussed at regular intervals. The parents or patient should not be forced to set goals they are not prepared to meet. It is important to work in collaboration with the family to set treatment goals. It is also helpful to broaden the goals of treatment to include improved quality of life or adjustment of the family as well as better metabolic control. Families are likely to be very respon-

sive to improved quality of life as a goal even if there are no changes in diabetes control. Later, this approach might lead to better control when barriers to care are better understood. In any case, the better the therapeutic alliance, the more likely that parents and children will reveal their inner concerns, which in turn leads to improved detection of problems.

Empathic listening is the cornerstone method for eliciting patient and family goals, concerns, and hidden issues relevant to formation of an effective therapeutic alliance. As described by Bellet and Maloney, "empathy is the capacity to understand what another person is experiencing from within the other person's frame of reference, i.e., the capacity to place oneself in another's shoes." Empathy is the basis for the patient-provider relationship. The interview is the time and method for eliciting information that leads to understanding of the parents and children. This involves willingness to ask open-ended questions and to keep the conversation oriented toward the patient's or family's concerns.

For example, within days of diagnosis of IDDM in her 12-year-old son, a mother brought the boy for admission into a diabetes treatment unit. While the providers initially tried to focus on teaching this mother how to care for her son's diabetes, she was very distracted. Her entire focus at this point was on making sure that the referring physician had correctly diagnosed the problem as diabetes. She was convinced that her son's symptoms were caused by another disease that had gone unrecognized so treatment would be misdirected. Initial attempts at careful explanation of the logic of the diagnosis and the need to learn about diabetes were met with insistence for a more complete workup including further blood tests and radiography. Because treatment had reached an impasse, the physician redirected attention to her concerns. By answering open-ended questions about her son and her worries, she began discussing other illnesses in the family, especially her own mother's fatal cancer. She believed that this illness had been misdiagnosed when medical intervention was first sought. Now the mother was, to her way of thinking, quite logically trying to avoid a second failure. Only by knowing about and acknowledging this set of concerns could the physician address the differences between the two situations and negotiate a process of care that would take into account the mother's goals for the admission and the physician's plan.

This leads to another critical step in facilitating the therapeutic alliance: negotiation. In many instances, during the course of treatment of a chronic condition like diabetes, differences between health care providers and families and/or patients will arise. Once identified, the patient or family may be able to acknowledge the underlying concerns and negotiate with the physician's recommendations. This negotiation is critical in setting goals for the next phase of treatment.

An approach that emphasizes the identification of patient goals, empathic listening, and negotiation will lead to more actively engaged families, i.e., families who take a large role in directing their own medical care. Health care research has suggested that actively engaged patients are more adherent and responsive to health care provider suggestions than more passive patients who look to the provider for direction.

Sometimes specific questions about presumably taboo subjects are useful to promote discussions. These questions let the family or patient know you are willing to listen to even embarrassing problems. Such problems may involve sexuality among adolescents. Adolescent boys may have heard that impotence is a possible complication of diabetes but fear any discussion. Making such areas of inquiry "normal" and not forcing the adolescent to answer questions may open the door for later discussions. With adolescent patients, such discussions are often most effective when the health care provider is of the same sex as the patient. Different health professionals in the office may be helpful in conducting such discussions.

Cultural, family, and personal barriers may affect family readiness to follow suggested treatment. For example, patients may fail to follow diets for many reasons. These may include cultural beliefs about weight that don't match the health care provider's. Adolescent and young adult women are at special risk for bulimic behaviors, including withholding insulin because of cultural attitudes about acceptable weight and body types and because most patients lose weight at diagnosis prior to starting insulin.

Table 2 summarizes areas for possible inquiry in trying to elicit issues affecting patient and family behaviors and attitudes that might impede successful care of diabetes.

In all situations, it is important to be nonjudgmental about patient and family attitudes. Trying to comprehend patient views of personal experiences can help the provider retain a sense of neutrality when their behaviors place patients at risk for problems from diabetes. This will decrease the possibility of taking a patient's refusal to follow recommendations as a personal affront. Counterproductive anger at the family may ensue when differences in viewpoint are taken as personal rejections.

■ EATING DISORDERS AND DIABETES CONTROL

As discussed earlier, young women with type 1 diabetes may be at high risk for serious eating disorders. Recent studies have reported a relationship between subclinical eating disorders and glycemic control in IDDM females. Thus, even if patients with diabetes do not experience a greater prevalence of clinical eating disorders (bulimia and anorexia nervosa), these less severe eating problems frequently cause poor glycemic control. Of particular concern, young women with type 1 diabetes may use insulin manipulation (i.e., omission) as a means of postbinge purging. Insulin omission is a particularly effective method of caloric purging and therefore has the potential for becoming quite addictive. These patients also find that restarting insulin is associated with water retention. This sudden weight gain is frightening and contributes to further avoidance of insulin. Studies of eating disorders in women with diabetes have established that insulin manipulation is linked to poor glycemic control and the onset of serious microvascular complications.

Where weight is a concern, attitudes toward insulin management may be very influential in determining adherence to the insulin regimen. Among adolescent and adult women with IDDM, nearly half may fear that getting blood glucose under control will cause weight gain and believe that taking insulin causes weight gain. This suggests that young women with IDDM, especially those with poor diabetes control, may have a fear of normoglycemia that can translate into the avoidance of insulin in order to avoid weight gain.

Disordered eating behaviors are often well hidden, but in the context of a physician-patient relationship characterized by a high degree of acceptance, patients can be encouraged to bring up and discuss issues such as their current level of satisfaction with their weight, weight goals, and—though less often—experiences with bingeing. Physicians can also play an important role in helping to prevent these disordered eating behaviors by (1) preparing newly diagnosed patients that starting insulin will be associated with weight gain (primarily fluid gain) and that the physician will work closely with the patient to see that this gain is not excessive, and (2) making a commitment to the patient to pay attention to patient's satisfaction with weight as well as to metabolic goals. When

---

Table 2 Areas of Inquiry

Ask patients periodically at regular medical visits about the following:

COMMON REACTIONS TO AND CONCERNS ABOUT DIABETES
Fears of future complications
Lack of acceptance of being diabetic or the need to care for diabetes
Concerns about the dangers of hypoglycemic episodes
Barriers to following recommended self-care activities because of school, work, or family activities

HEALTH/MEDICAL CARE BELIEFS AND ATTITUDES
A cure will be found, so the patient doesn't have to care for himself or herself.
Necessary self-care behaviors are impossible to institute.
Luck accounts for outcomes of diabetes.
Measuring blood glucose is not useful in caring for diabetes.
Careful diabetes management can't help a patient avoid complications.
Only perfect blood glucose levels are worth achieving and are worth the cost of severe insulin reactions.
Changes in diet are not worth the effort.
The doctor only cares about the patient's "numbers."

Finances make medical visits impossible.
The doctor will be angry if the patient reveals negative information about diabetes care, e.g., diet.

LIFE STRESSES
Include questions about changes in job, school, living situation, immediate family.

PSYCHIATRIC PROBLEMS
Include questions about mood, anxiety level, sense of well-being.
Among adolescent girls include questions about bingeing, vomiting, skipped insulin doses, and excessive dieting.

SOCIAL AND FAMILY SUPPORT
Include questions about whom the patient can turn to for help in diabetes care or for support when upset about diabetes.
Does immediate family and/or best friend know what is happening with diabetes care?

CAPACITY TO USE INFORMATION
Periodically, reassess the patient's and parents' actual ability to retain diabetes knowledge and process new information.

problem eating behavior is identified, referral for mental health treatment is indicated. This treatment often combines group therapy, individual and family counseling, and in some patients with coexisting depression or clear binges, antidepressants. Furthermore, some patients may require hospitalization in units designed to treat eating disorders with psychological and medical treatments.

■ SURREPTITIOUS INSULIN ADMINISTRATION AND/OR REPEATED EPISODES OF HYPOGLYCEMIA

Along the continuum of adherence difficulties and regimen manipulation in diabetes, the secretive use of extra insulin by IDDM patients represents one of the most frightening and potentially life-threatening examples of "noncompliance." Surreptitious overuse of insulin is often extremely difficult to diagnose because patients try to hide the overdoses at all costs. The dynamics behind the overdosing are quite variable. Excess insulin use, even though it may cause serious medical problems, may not be a suicide attempt. Children may inject insulin in secret to lower their blood sugar before a regular blood sugar monitoring by the parents in order to try to convince them that they no longer have diabetes. Adolescent patients with type 1 diabetes, desperate to escape from stressful living situations, have been known to surreptitiously take extra insulin in order to cause a predictable medical emergency and hospitalization with a severe hypoglycemic reaction. Less frequently, a severe personality disorder may trigger surreptitious insulin use.

The documented number of cases of surreptitious insulin administration among type 1 patients thought to be brittle has forced many in-patient hospital units for diabetic patients to insist that all insulin be administered to patients by the nursing staff and to keep all insulin bottles and syringes away from the bedside. Unexplained "good" or "normal" blood sugars or predictable low–blood sugar reactions should be "red flags" for consideration of surreptitious insulin misuse.

■ PARENT/CHILD ALIENATION

One of the most predictable crises of diabetes in families with children with IDDM is prolonged diabetes-related conflict and eventual alienation that may occur between some parents and children. The origin of this deterioration in the relationship between parent and child is eroding of self-esteem in both parent and child or adolescent because of frustration over the child's inability to adhere "perfectly" to the diabetes treatment regimen or to consistently achieve "perfect" blood sugar levels. Frequently the child is held solely responsible for blood sugar levels that the parent or health care team find unacceptable or unsafe. Although the developing youngster may be blamed for cheating, it is important to keep in mind that high or fluctuating blood sugars may, in fact, at some times be due to causes other than the child's eating behavior, such as an insufficient insulin dose in the context of recent physical growth, puberty, stress, or infectious illness. Anger and resentment toward diabetes as well as toward parents can build up inside the child who is chronically accused. The child or adolescent may begin

to label himself or herself as a "bad diabetic" and feel a deteriorating sense of self-worth. Even when parents are not overly critical of the young diabetic patient, the child's obvious inability to meet treatment expectations can leave him or her with a profound sense of failure, hopelessness, and fear about the future. Furthermore, when a parent is trying everything within his or her power to help the child achieve blood sugar levels that are stable and acceptable and does not succeed, the parent may feel to blame for this failure. Parents may blame themselves for not having a more disciplined child or for not being able to provide the food or family schedule needed to achieve more acceptable blood sugar readings. Parents who have been blamed by health care providers at some point during the course of their child's diabetes sometimes carry this sense of blame for years, while also feeling frightened by the devastating complications of diabetes. Unfortunately, in many families years of conflicts and accusations as well as low self-esteem of the child and parents caused by difficulties in adherence to treatment requirements can contribute to a profound alienation between parent and child.

Repeated family conflicts over nonadherence to treatment or severe parental or child distress or depression over blood sugar readings should be red flags for referral to a child or family therapist for parent-child counseling focused on family communication about diabetes and on sharing responsibility for diabetes management.

Suggested Reading

Anderson BJ, Auslander WF, Jung KC, et al. Assessing family sharing of diabetes responsibilities. J Pediatr Psychol 1990; 15:477–492.

Presents a new instrument for measuring how families share the responsibilities of diabetes management and the relationships between different patterns of responsibility-sharing and metabolic control.

Anderson B, Wolfsdorf J, Jacobson AM. Psychological adjustment in children with type I diabetes. In: Lebovitz H, ed. Therapy for diabetes mellitus and related disorders, Alexandria, Va: American Diabetes Association, 1994:53.

This chapter reviews the major developmental tasks at different stages of child development and their implications for the family's response to diabetes management expectations.

Bellet PS, Maloney MJ. The importance of empathy as an interviewing skill in medicine. JAMA 1991; 266: 1831–1832.

Discusses the role of empathic listening in clinical practice. It is a practical introduction to one important aspect of interview skills.

DCCT Research Group, prepared by Jacobson A, Cleary P, Baker L. The effect of intensive treatment on quality of life outcomes in the diabetes control and complications trial. Diabetes Care 1995; 19:195–203.

DCCT Research Group, prepared by Lan S, Ryan C, Adams K, Grant I, Jacobson A, Cleary P. The effects of intensive treatment on neuropsychological functions in adults in the DCCT. Ann Intern Med 1996; 124:379–388.

The above two studies present the neuropsychological results of the DCCT.

Hamburg BA, Inoff GE. Coping with predictable crisis of diabetes. Diabetes Care 1983; 6:409–416

Provides a conceptual framework for anticipating difficult problems faced by patients with diabetes based on normal developmental tasks and the normal progression of the disease. The authors argue persuasively that "anticipatory coping" should be encouraged in all patients with diabetes.

Hauser S, Jacobson A, Lavori P, et al. Adherence among children and adolescents with IDDM over a four-year longitudinal follow up: II. Immediate and long-term linkages with the family milieu. J Pediatr Psychol 1990; 15:527–542.

This article examines the effect of family environment on adherence in children with diabetes. It shows that the family's supportiveness, involvement, and organization influence long-term adaptation of child patients.

Jacobson AM, Hauser S, Anderson B, Polonsky W. Psychosocial aspects of diabetes. In: Kahn C, Weir G, eds. Joslin's diabetes mellitus. 13th ed. Philadelphia: Lea & Febiger, 1994:431.

This chapter introduces the reader to a broad range of issues relevant to patients with diabetes. It includes a scholarly review of topics such as stress and diabetes, cognitive and psychiatric effects of diabetes, and family life.

Jacobson AM, Hauser S, Lavori P, et al. Adherence among children and adolescents with IDDM over a four-year longitudinal follow up. I. The influence of patient coping and adjustment. J Pediatr Psychol 1990; 15:511–526.

Demonstrates the influence of child psychological functioning on adherence to diabetes care.

Polonsky W, Anderson B, Lohrer P, et al. Insulin omission in women with IDDM. Diabetes Care 1994; 17:1178–1185.

Examines psychological and medical aspects of insulin misuse, eating and weight concerns, other bulimic behaviors in women with diabetes.

DIABETIC KETOACIDOSIS IN CHILDREN

Neil H. White, M.D., C.D.E.
Julio V. Santiago, M.D.

Diabetic ketoacidosis (DKA) is the most serious metabolic disturbance of insulin-dependent (type 1) diabetes mellitus (IDDM). Identified in approximately 40 percent of children with newly diagnosed IDDM, DKA is responsible for more than 160,000 hospital admissions each year in the United States. The highest rates of DKA are found in teenagers and in the elderly. The mortality rate from DKA has been reported to be as high as 19 percent in the elderly, but is much lower in children. Nevertheless, DKA accounts for about 50 percent of the deaths of diabetic subjects younger than 24 years of age and is the most common cause of death in diabetic children. The majority of the morbidity and mortality associated with DKA during childhood is preventable by appropriate treatment and careful monitoring. In this chapter, we review the pathophysiology of DKA in children and summarize its treatment.

■ PATHOPHYSIOLOGY

Ketoacidosis is a state of severe metabolic decompensation manifested by the overproduction of ketoacids, resulting in metabolic acidosis. Specifically, DKA refers to the occurrence of ketoacidosis, usually accompanied by hyperglycemia, as a result of diabetes mellitus. During DKA, disturbances of protein, fat, and carbohydrate metabolism are present. Diabetic ketoacidosis represents a state of absolute or relative insulin deficiency and occurs in association with counter-regulatory or stress hormone excess. Elevations of the counter-regulatory hormones (glucagon, catecholamines, cortisol, and growth hormone) antagonize the effect of insulin. In the absence of a compensatory increase in insulin secretion, the elevated counter-regulatory hormones stimulate lipolysis and ketogenesis. The increased levels of counter-regulatory hormones (primarily catecholamines and growth hormone) enhance lipolysis, thus increasing circulating free fatty acids. These free fatty acids are taken up by the liver where they are esterified to triglycerides and oxidized to ketone bodies. Glucagon, which is usually elevated during the evolution of DKA, enhances hepatic ketogenesis. Hyperglucagonemia plays an important, perhaps essential, role in the development of DKA. Diabetic ketoacidosis is best defined by the presence of metabolic acidosis secondary to ketosis and not simply by hyperglycemia. The hallmark features of DKA are ketosis and ketonuria, metabolic acidosis (low serum bicarbonate and elevated anion gap), and dehydration. The ketosis and metabolic acidosis contribute to electrolyte disturbances and vomiting, which are frequent occurrences in severe DKA.

Since elevated counterregulatory hormones also stimulate hepatic glucose production from glycogenolysis and gluconeogenesis, the blood glucose concentration is usually elevated (>250 mg per deciliter) in subjects with DKA. As blood glucose rises, the amount of glucose appearing in the glomerular ultrafiltrate exceeds the ability of the proximal tubule to reabsorb glucose, and glucosuria occurs. The glucosuria increases until the rate of glucose loss in the urine equals the rate of hepatic glucose production. The blood glucose concentration often stabilizes in the range of 400 to 600

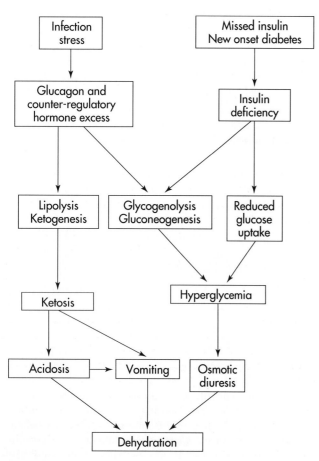

Figure 1
Pathophysiology of diabetic ketoacidosis.

mg per deciliter, and this results in an osmotic diuresis. Along with reduced fluid intake and vomiting (secondary to acidosis and ketosis), this leads to depletion of the extracellular volume. Once volume depletion worsens to the point that the glomerular filtration rate (GFR) is reduced, the quantity of filtered glucose falls. This diminishes urinary glucose losses, and blood glucose rises further to reach a new steady state that can exceed 600 to 800 mg per deciliter. Marked hyperglycemia suggests either severe volume depletion with declining GFR or recent ingestion or infusion of large quantities of carbohydrate or glucose without adequate insulin coverage.

Ketoacidosis can occur in association with conditions other than diabetes. If a patient, not known to have diabetes, presents with ketoacidosis without hyperglycemia, other diagnoses may need to be considered. These include alcoholic ketoacidosis, starvation ketosis, and certain inborn errors of metabolism. However, diabetes is by far the most common cause of ketoacidosis. Diabetic ketoacidosis is almost always associated with hyperglycemia (plasma glucose >250 mg per deciliter), although normoglycemia does not rule out DKA. Diabetic ketoacidosis without severe hyperglycemia can be seen during pregnancy, in partially treated cases of DKA where supplemental insulin and oral non–carbohydrate-containing fluids have already been given, or in individuals with prolonged vomiting and little carbohydrate intake for a long period of time before presentation.

Electrolyte abnormalities are nearly universal in DKA. The glucose-induced osmotic diuresis of DKA causes reduced sodium and water resorption by the kidney and excessive urinary losses of both water and sodium. In addition, sodium and potassium are excreted along with the excess ketoacids. During DKA, serum sodium is usually low as a result of the hyperglycemia-induced osmotic shift of intracellular water to the extracellular compartment. This dilutional reduction in serum sodium approximates 1.6 mEq per liter for each 100 mg per deciliter rise in blood glucose concentration above the normal range. This means that for a blood glucose of 800 mg per deciliter (700 mg per deciliter above the normal range) the serum sodium concentration would be expected to be reduced by 11.2 mEq per liter ($7 \times 1.6 = 11.2$) to about 125 to 130 mEq per liter. Potassium losses during DKA can be substantial, and potassium depletion is common. The potassium losses are due to the urinary excretion of potassium along with ketoacids, the glucose-induced osmotic diuresis, and the effects of increased aldosterone levels that occur secondarily to volume contraction. Because both acidosis and hypertonicity enhance the shift of potassium into the extracellular space from within the cells, the serum potassium concentration is often elevated or normal on presentation. The serum potassium concentration is an unreliable indicator of the body's potassium status. Urinary phosphate losses also are high during DKA as a result of acidosis and the osmotic diuresis.

The acid-base disturbances of DKA are typical for those of a metabolic acidosis. In the absence of central nervous system (CNS) or pulmonary impairment, respiratory compensation will occur. The ketone bodies (beta-hydroxybutyrate and acetoacetate) and hydrogen ion stimulate chemoreceptors in the CNS to cause hyperventilation. Early in the course of DKA, the result is a reduction of pCO_2, and a metabolic acidosis with respiratory compensation and near normal pH. However, as the DKA progresses to more severe stages, more significant acidemia occurs, and blood pH falls.

■ DIAGNOSIS

Any diabetic patient with either symptoms of hyperglycemia (polyuria, polydipsia) or measured hyperglycemia along with urinary ketones should be considered to be in DKA. Mild forms of DKA may require no more attention than oral fluids, supplemental insulin, and attention to sick-day guidelines for diabetes management. The condition should be considered severe, however, if there is abdominal pain, vomiting, dehydration, rapid or deep breathing (Kussmaul respiration), or altered mental status. Diabetic ketoacidosis should also be considered in any child with new onset of these symptoms, especially if the classic symptoms of diabetes (polyuria, polydipsia, nocturia, polyphagia, and weight loss) are present. Because abdominal pain and vomiting are common in severe DKA, the presentation often is confused with other medical conditions, including gastroenteritis, appendicitis, pancreatitis, urinary tract infection or pyelonephritis, pneumonitis, and asthma.

Events precipitating DKA include the new diagnosis of IDDM, deliberate or inadvertent omission of insulin, infection (pneumonia, gastroenteritis, influenza, otitis media, meningitis, appendicitis, and so on), pancreatitis, trauma, psychological and emotional stresses (especially in adolescents), myocardial infarction or stroke (in older patients), or the initiation of drugs that cause insulin resistance or suppress insulin secretion (e.g., corticosteroids, diuretics). In each case of DKA, a search for precipitating factors should be initiated, and if any are found the patient should be treated for them. DKA is a life-threatening condition, and if episodes are recurrent a search for their cause and interventions aimed at their prevention should be aggressive.

The classical signs and symptoms of DKA include polyuria, polydipsia, hyperventilation, and intravascular volume depletion. The latter is manifested as dry mucous membranes, absent tearing, poor skin turgor, weight loss, poor tissue perfusion, and orthostatic hypotension. The breath may have a sweet odor as a result of exhaled ketone bodies. Abdominal pain, which can be severe enough to suggest gastroenteritis or an acute surgical abdomen, is common. Tenderness to palpation, guarding, diminished or absent bowel sounds, and ileus can be seen as a result of DKA alone. Extreme thirst, tachycardia, nausea, vomiting, hypotension, weakness, anorexia, volume depletion, warm dry skin, visual disturbances, hyperventilation, somnolence, hypothermia, hyporeflexia, and impaired consciousness can all be present in DKA. Shock or coma are uncommon in children with DKA unless it is unusually severe or cerebral edema is present. In children, shock usually is the result of hypovolemia and is corrected by fluid resuscitation. Cardiogenic shock, as a result of myocardial dysfunction, myocardial infarction, or cardiac dysrhythmias, is uncommon in children, but can occur.

The common laboratory findings in DKA include metabolic acidosis (low serum HCO_3, pCO_2, and pH), ketonemia and ketouria, elevated anion gap from ketone bodies (beta-hydroxybutyrate and acetoacetate), hyperglycemia, leukocytosis, hyponatremia, hypophosphatemia, hyperosmolality, and elevated amylase. In mild cases of DKA, the serum bicarbonate and pH may be only slightly reduced, but in severe cases, the arterial pH is usually less than 7.2, plasma bicarbonate is less than 15 mEq per liter, and ketones are present in both blood and urine. Although the blood glucose concentration is usually elevated to 400 to 600 mg per deciliter, a blood glucose level below 300 mg per deciliter and even one within the normal range does not exclude DKA. In the presence of hyperglycemia, marked hyponatremia can be seen. The serum sodium concentration can be expected to decrease by 1.6 mEq per liter for each 100 mg per deciliter glucose increase above a plasma glucose concentration of 100 mg per deciliter. Serum potassium concentration can be normal, elevated, or decreased. Regardless of the serum potassium, however, total body potassium depletion is nearly always present as a result of urinary or gastrointestinal losses. An elevation of the peripheral white blood cell count is often seen in DKA and cannot be used as a reliable indicator of infection. However, the white blood cell count normalizes quickly with treatment, and persistent elevations or marked granulocytosis may indicate underlying infection, which should be considered in any patient with DKA of unidentified etiology. An electrocardiogram (ECG) should be obtained for all adult patients with DKA to rule out myocardial infarction. Although an ECG may not be necessary in all cases of DKA in children, we routinely obtain one if there is hypotension, arrhythmia, severe hyperkalemia or hypokalemia, or evidence of congestive heart failure. The ECG can be used for rapid assessment of a critically low or high potassium level. Hypokalemia results in flattened or inverted T waves, depressed ST segment, prolonged QT interval, and the presence of U waves. Hyperkalemia results in peaked T waves, widened QRS interval, depressed P waves, and AV dissociation.

■ THERAPY

Initial evaluation and treatment of children with DKA should be aimed at ensuring adequate ventilation and cardiovascular function, restoring intravascular volume depletion and tissue perfusion, and assessing mental status. Patients with severe DKA should be cared for in an environment equipped to provide skilled nursing care and to perform frequent monitoring of vital signs, bedside blood glucose determination, and serum electrolyte and blood gas analyses around the clock. In cases of severe DKA, hospitalization is necessary, and access to a pediatric or medical intensive care unit is essential. Milder cases of DKA can sometimes be managed at home or with very short stays in the emergency room setting.

The general goals in the treatment of DKA are to (1) establish and maintain adequate ventilatory and cardiovascular function, (2) correct fluid deficits and electrolyte imbalance, (3) correct the metabolic acidosis, (4) provide adequate insulin to stop ongoing ketogenesis and lower the plasma glucose concentration, (5) determine and treat the underlying etiology and precipitating cause of DKA, and (6) monitor for and prevent complications of treatment. Initial therapy of severe DKA should be directed at correcting life-threatening abnormalities and stabilizing the patient. Adequate ventilation should be established, if necessary. Intravenous (IV) access should be established as soon as possible. Shock or poor tissue perfusion should be corrected with vigorous fluid resuscitation. This is best accomplished with isotonic saline. Even if shock is not present, IV access should be established as quickly as possible. Laboratory studies should be sent to confirm the diagnosis of DKA and to determine the severity of electrolyte abnormalities, acidosis, and azotemia. A medical history, physical examination, and additional laboratory studies should be performed to rule out any precipitating causes and underlying medical conditions. Comatose patients should have a carefully placed and maintained nasogastric tube to prevent aspiration. After initial stabilization and evaluation, the mainstay of therapy for DKA are correction of intravascular volume depletion, ketoacidosis, and hyperglycemia. This can be accomplished with IV fluid therapy and insulin administration, as described in the following sections.

Fluids and Electrolytes

In patients with mild DKA and no vomiting, oral administration of fluids may be all that is required. In these cases, 3 to 8 oz each hour (often taken as smaller quantities every 20 to 30 minutes) is usually adequate. While blood glucose is high (>250 to 300 mg per deciliter), these fluids should be carbohydrate free; after the glucose falls, carbohydrate-containing fluids should be used. For cases of severe DKA, or if vomiting prevents oral hydration in milder cases, IV fluids are essential and should be initiated as soon as possible.

Initially, IV fluids should be administered as rapidly as necessary to expand the intravascular volume and restore tissue perfusion. Thereafter fluids are given at a rate necessary to provide maintenance fluids and to replace ongoing losses. However, there are certain considerations that are unique to the management of DKA, especially in children.

The initial volume expansion phase should be started immediately and usually is given as 10 to 20 ml per kilogram of isotonic (0.9 percent) saline over 30 to 60 minutes. Normal saline has the advantage of being isotonic, and this prevents a rapid drop in serum osmolality. Some authorities prefer lactated Ringer's solution. The lactate can be metabolized to bicarbonate to aid in correcting severe acidosis, and the reduced chloride may help prevent the subsequent development of hyperchloremic acidosis. If peripheral perfusion continues to be poor, additional fluid boluses of 10 ml per kilogram should be given until pulse and blood pressure are stable and extremities are warm, with capillary refill of less than 2 to 3 seconds. If tissue perfusion is poor, part of the anion gap may be attributable to the production of lactic acid. In this situation, the administration of lactated Ringer's solution is not advised since the administered lactate will not be converted to bicarbonate and will serve only to increase the anion gap although the metabolic acidosis per se will not be affected. After expansion of the intravascular fluid volume has been achieved, hypotonic fluid replacement should be started to correct hypertonicity and water deficits.

During the hydration phase, fluid therapy must correct water and electrolyte deficits and replace ongoing excessive fluid losses (through vomiting, osmotic diuresis); individualized maintenance requirements must be taken into consideration. Ongoing fluid losses should be minimized by reducing the blood glucose to limit the osmotic diuresis. However, ongoing losses from vomiting, diarrhea, or nasogastric drainage need to be taken into consideration, if these are excessive. Maintenance fluid needs can be calculated as 1,500 to 2,000 ml/m^2 per day or higher if fever is present. Hyperventilation increases insensible losses. Fluid deficits may be estimated based on recent weight loss, and this information can be used to help calculate replacement needs. The usual clinical signs of extracellular volume depletion, however, often underestimate the degree of volume depletion in DKA. If fluid deficits are not known, an estimated fluid deficit of 10 to 15 percent should be assumed and used as an initial guide to treatment. After the initial volume expansion phase with isotonic saline, fluid replacement usually can be accomplished using 0.45 percent saline. If severe hyponatremia (serum sodium below what can be accounted for by hyperglycemia), extreme hyperosmolality (serum sodium normal despite marked hyperglycemia), hypotension, or shock is present, it may be appropriate to continue hydration with 0.9 percent saline. In these patients, it is essential to accurately monitor intake and output. Bladder catheterization may be indicated in very severe cases, especially if documentation of urine output is difficult and if hydration status is uncertain.

Contrary to general pediatric teachings for fluid replacement in simple dehydration due to gastroenteritis, it is generally recommended that fluid replacement during therapy of DKA in children be administered evenly over 24 to 36 hours. This can be accomplished by using a rate of 3 to 3.6 L/m^2 per day. For those with severe hyperosmolality (marked hyperglycemia with a normal or elevated serum sodium), replacement should be given more slowly (2.5 to 3 L/m^2 per day) over 36 to 48 hours. In addition, the corrected serum sodium (Na_{corr} = serum Na $- 1.6 \times$ [(glucose -100)/100]) should be monitored to prevent too rapid hydration. Na_{corr} should gradually rise (or, if elevated, should fall) toward the normal range as blood glucose falls and rehydration occurs. A Na_{corr} below normal and falling suggests overhydration, and indicates the need for reducing the IV fluid rate (perhaps to no more than 2.5 L/m^2 per day) and increasing vigilance for possible cerebral edema. If clinical status permits, the final stages of rehydration can be accomplished via oral administration.

In nearly all cases of DKA, total body potassium depletion exists despite a normal or even elevated serum potassium concentration. Potassium replacement should begin immediately after the initial fluid bolus is administered unless renal failure is suspected. If the serum potassium early in the course is so low as to endanger the patient (serum potassium <3.0 to 3.5 mEq per liter, or ECG changes indicate hypokalemia), potassium should be started during the volume expansion phase. If renal failure (acute or chronic) is suspected or if potassium is high (>5.5 mEq/L), potassium administration should be delayed until urine output is established and the serum potassium begins to fall. Generally, the potassium concentration in the IV fluid should be 30 to 40 mEq per liter or 0.1 to 0.5 mEq per kilogram per hour and can be given as potassium chloride, potassium acetate, or potassium phosphate. We routinely use some potassium phosphate in therapy. Phosphate should be given if serum phosphate is low to prevent worsening of hypophosphatemia and depletion of red blood cell 2,3-DPG. However, administration of potassium phosphate should not exceed 1.5 mEq per kilogram per day because of the danger of hypocalcemia and hypomagnesemia. Furthermore, there is no conclusive evidence that phosphate replacement substantially affects clinical outcome in the treatment of DKA. We believe that the exclusive use of potassium chloride should be avoided. A mild component of hyperchloremic acidosis often occurs in children in DKA, and overzealous administration of chloride-containing solutions can worsen this. Thus, we prefer to use a combination of potassium phosphate and potassium acetate. The latter is metabolized by the liver to form bicarbonate.

Serum potassium levels need to be monitored closely (every 1 to 2 hours) until stable, and then every 4 to 6 hours while IV fluid and insulin therapy continue. The rate of potassium administration should be adjusted as necessary, based on the serum potassium concentration. If serum potassium continues to fall and reaches the hypokalemic range, a higher rate of potassium administration may be needed. This may require solutions containing 40 to 60 mEq per liter. In these cases, ECG monitoring is certainly indicated to serve as a guide to potassium status.

Insulin

All patients with DKA have an absolute or relative deficiency of insulin. Therefore, exogenous insulin must be provided. Insulin reverses protein breakdown and lipolysis and suppresses ketone body and ketoacid formation, thus interrupting the production of excess acid. Once excess acid formation is halted, ketone bodies are removed by urinary excretion and oxidation in muscle, leading to correction of the acidosis. Insulin also lowers the blood glucose concentration by inhibiting hepatic glycogenolysis and gluconeogenesis and stimulating muscle glucose uptake and oxidation.

Insulin is effective regardless of its route of administration. The choice of the route depends upon the clinical situation. For mild DKA, especially that in which IV fluids may not be necessary, subcutaneous insulin (0.25 U per kilogram every 3 to 4 hours) can be used. In cases of severe DKA, continuous IV insulin infusion is the preferred route of administration, although subcutaneous or intramuscular insulin can also be effective. In cases complicated by shock, hypotension, or poor tissue perfusion, only IV insulin should be used because, in the face of poor peripheral perfusion, absorption of insulin given subcutaneously or even intramuscularly may be reduced or delayed. Regular (fast-acting) insulin is the primary insulin preparation used in the management of DKA and is the only insulin that should be given intravenously or intramuscularly.

Continuous IV insulin infusion is begun with a bolus of Regular insulin, 0.1 U per kilogram (rarely are more than 5 to 7 U necessary), followed by an infusion of Regular insulin at 0.1 U per kilogram per hour (rarely are more than 5 to 7 U per hour necessary). Although some authorities believe that the bolus is not necessary since steady state hyperinsulinemia is achieved within 30 minutes, we routinely use a bolus. Insulin can be mixed in normal saline at a concentration of 0.1 to 1.0 U per milliliter in order that the fluid delivery rate necessary to administer 0.1 U per kilogram per hour is about 10 to 20 milliliters per hour. Alternatively, the weight of the patient in kilograms is used to calculate the units of Regular insulin that must be added per 100 ml of saline, and this solution is then given at a fixed rate of 10 ml per hour; this will administer 0.1 U per kilogram per hour. For example, for a 40-kg child, add 40 U of Regular insulin to 100 ml of saline (or 200 U to 500 ml), and infuse this solution at 10 ml per hour. The insulin infusion should be "piggy-backed" into the existing IV line and should be controlled by an electronic infusion pump. We do not recommend mixing the insulin with the hydration fluid because the insulin infusion rate and the fluid rate and composition often require independent adjustments. Some centers recommend adding albumin or several milliliters of the patient's own plasma to the insulin solution to reduce adherence to the plastic tubing. Alternatively, the IV tubing can be flushed with 50 ml of insulin solution to saturate binding sites on the tubing before administration. Failure to do this can result in diminished insulin delivery over the first few hours. If no improvement in blood pH, anion gap, plasma bicarbonate, or plasma glucose is seen by 1 to 2 hours after initiation of IV insulin therapy, the insulin infusion rate can be doubled. However, in our experience, this is rarely necessary.

Blood Glucose and Dextrose Administration During Treatment of Diabetic Ketoacidosis

Blood glucose concentration should decline at about 75 to 125 mg per deciliter per hour during the treatment of DKA as a result of both volume expansion and insulin administration. Volume expansion lowers blood glucose by increasing the extracellular fluid space and by restoring GFR, thus increasing renal glucose losses. During the volume expansion phase, blood glucose concentration can fall especially rapidly, often by 200 to 400 mg per deciliter per hour down to 300 to 400 mg per deciliter. After the volume expansion phase, insulin is required to lower the plasma glucose further.

Insulin lowers blood glucose by inhibiting hepatic glucose production from both glycogenolysis and gluconeo-genesis and by enhancing glucose uptake and oxidation.

The blood glucose concentration usually normalizes more quickly than the ketosis and acidosis. An attempt should be made to stabilize the plasma glucose concentration near the renal threshold, i.e., about 200 mg per deciliter. This will minimize urinary fluid losses from osmotic diuresis and avoid the occurrence of hypoglycemia, which could trigger a counterregulatory hormone response with worsening of the ketosis. Therefore, when the blood glucose approaches 250 mg per deciliter, a 5 percent dextrose solution should be started at the rate designed to deliver 3 to 5 mg per kilogram per minute of dextrose. This usually is adequate to stabilize the blood sugar at the desired goal, i.e., about 200 mg per deciliter. If this fails to stabilize the blood glucose, higher concentrations of dextrose can be used or the insulin infusion rate can be reduced if the anion gap has decreased concomitantly with a rise in serum bicarbonate concentration. However, the insulin infusion rate should not be reduced if acidosis is not correcting and should not be reduced to below 0.05 U per kilogram per hour in absolute terms. In general, IV insulin should be continued until the patient can tolerate oral fluids well, electrolyte abnormalities are largely corrected, serum bicarbonate is greater than 15 mEq per liter, and acidosis has resolved. Because of the short half-life of circulating insulin (about 5 to 7 minutes), the IV insulin infusion should not be discontinued until approximately 30 minutes after regular subcutaneous insulin has been given. In patients known to have IDDM, the usual insulin dosage can be resumed. In patients with new onset of IDDM, subcutaneous insulin should be started as discussed in the chapter *Insulin Therapy in Type 1 Diabetes Mellitus.*

Bicarbonate Administration in Diabetic Ketoacidosis

The need for bicarbonate administration during the treatment of DKA in children remains controversial. We rarely find it necessary to use bicarbonate unless the initial blood pH is below 7.0 to 7.1. It has been our experience that severely ketoacidotic children usually recover well without bicarbonate use. The potential risks include rebound alkalosis, hypokalemia, and hypernatremia. Bolus doses of bicarbonate should be avoided and when bicarbonate is used it should be given as an infusion of 1 to 2 mEq per kilogram over 2 hours. This is best accomplished by adding 50 to 100 mEq (1 to 2 ampules) of sodium bicarbonate per liter of rehydration fluid and administering it at the rehydration fluid rate. If sodium bicarbonate is to be added to the rehydration fluid, it is advisable to use 0.2 percent saline as the primary rehydration fluid (instead of 0.45 percent saline) in order to avoid administration of excessive quantities of sodium or chloride. Bicarbonate administration rarely needs to be continued beyond the first 2 to 3 hours, and should certainly be discontinued when the blood pH rises to above 7.1 to 7.2 or the venous bicarbonate concentration rises to above 10 to 12 mEq per liter.

Monitoring During Treatment of Diabetic Ketoacidosis

Following patients with DKA requires careful and frequent monitoring. Clinical status, including neurologic condition, should be assessed frequently (at least every 0.5 to 2 hours) for the first 6 to 12 hours. An accurate record of intake and output should be maintained, and blood glucose should be measured hourly using bedside monitoring. Serum electrolytes should be determined at least every 2 to 6 hours, with serum potassium, bicarbonate, and pH measured more frequently in severe cases. Unexpected changes in clinical status, mental status, or laboratory results should be promptly investigated, and therapy should be changed appropriately. As noted above, a low and falling corrected serum sodium (Na_{corr}) should trigger a reduction of fluid administration rate and an increase in monitoring for possible cerebral edema. The vast majority of children with DKA do quite well, unless the situation is complicated by significant underlying medical or surgical conditions.

Fever in a subject with DKA warrants evaluation and treatment for possible underlying infection. Blood, urine, and throat cultures, and a chest radiograph should be obtained for febrile DKA patients. Lumbar puncture is performed only if meningitis is suspected. Gastric decompression and nasogastric drainage is recommended in severe cases, especially if there is persistent vomiting or if there is a reduced level of consciousness. Aspiration of gastric contents is a common complication in any comatose subject. If appendicitis or another acute surgical condition is suspected, surgical consultation should be obtained early. However, if possible, surgical exploration should be delayed for several hours until severe acidosis is corrected.

Complications of Diabetic Ketoacidosis and Its Treatment

Complications associated with treatment of DKA include hypoglycemia, aspiration of gastric contents, fluid overload with congestive heart failure, and cerebral edema. The first three of these usually can be avoided by careful attention to all aspects of the therapy. Hypoglycemia is avoided by frequent bedside glucose monitoring and the use of dextrose-containing fluids when blood glucose falls to about 250 mg per deciliter. Aspiration is prevented by the judicious placement and maintenance of nasogastric drainage for patients who have an altered mental status or neurologic compromise. Fluid overload is prevented by careful attention to the guidelines of fluid therapy and close monitoring. However, even when careful attention is paid to all of these details, children treated for severe DKA occasionally die as a result of rapid and unexpected neurologic deterioration secondary to the development of cerebral edema. Occasionally, thrombosis, infarct, or hemorrhage within the brain can occur.

Cerebral edema, as a complication of DKA and its treatment, occurs primarily in children. Although the incidence of clinically significant cerebral edema is low (probably about 1 to 2 percent), the outcome after its development is poor, and cerebral edema remains a leading cause of death in diabetic children, accounting for 31 percent of deaths associated with DKA and 20 percent of the overall mortality in children with diabetes. Radiologic evidence of cerebral edema may be present at initial presentation of DKA, even though there is no obvious clinical evidence of increased intracranial pressure. Delayed diagnosis is the main factor that contributes to death from cerebral edema in children with DKA.

There is no single accepted explanation for cerebral edema or why it seems to occur more commonly in children than in adults. Four explanations have been proposed: (1) rapid shifts in extracellular and intracellular osmolality; (2) CNS acidosis; (3) cerebral hypoxia; and (4) excessive fluid administration. Although each of these explanations has some experimental support, none is a completely satisfactory explanation for the occurrence of cerebral edema, and controlled clinical studies to support these hypotheses are, in general, lacking.

The most commonly cited explanation is that cerebral edema results from a rapid decline in extracellular osmolality during the treatment of DKA. During the development of DKA hyperglycemia and hypertonicity cause fluid to shift out of the brain. In an attempt to prevent volume loss, the brain accumulates osmotically active substances. The majority of these accumulated "osmoles" can be accounted for by glucose, polyols, low–molecular-weight peptides, and amino acids, primarily taurine and glycine. These osmotically active particles, previously referred to as "idiogenic osmoles," prevent volume loss, thus preventing shrinkage and hemorrhage that might occur if the brain mass were to contract and tear away from the cranial vault. During the treatment of DKA, serum osmolality falls acutely as dehydration is corrected. Water moves down its osmotic gradient into the brain cells that have an increased osmolality, and modest degrees of cerebral swelling can occur. This course of events is likely to occur in many subjects during treatment of DKA. Insulin also appears to play an important role in the development of cerebral edema, through its effect to stimulate brain uptake of electrolytes, water, and amino acids.

Excessive fluid administration contributes to the development of cerebral edema. Brain swelling has been associated with initial rates of rehydration that exceed 4.0 L/m^2 body surface area per day. However, other investigators point out that in many cases of cerebral edema there is no evidence of excessive fluid replacement or rapid decrements in serum osmolality. Furthermore, higher rates of fluid replacement in some patients simply may have reflected a more severe or more prolonged period of dehydration and ketoacidosis and the cerebral edema may have occurred more likely because of the greater severity of metabolic derangement at the time of presentation.

It is likely that the etiology of cerebral edema is multifactorial, including components of more than one of the explanations discussed in the previous paragraphs or others not yet considered. Fluid administration rates currently recommended for the treatment of DKA during the first 12 to 18 hours are generally slower than those recommended to correct childhood nonketoacidotic dehydration secondary to diarrhea, vomiting, and gastroenteritis where cerebral edema is an uncommon problem.

There is evidence to suggest that some degree of cerebral edema is common in children with DKA and that early intervention may reduce its severity. The use of computed tomography (CT) scan and intracranial pressure monitors (in severe cases) to assess cerebral edema may help in its management. More helpful are very close monitoring of the patient for the presence or development of early signs of cerebral edema and prompt initiation of treatment in suspect cases. Cerebral edema should be considered if any of the following occur: (1) coma, or declining or fluctuating mental status; (2) dilated, unresponsive, sluggish, or unequal pupils; (3) papilledema (this is a late finding); (4) sudden development of hypertension that was not present at time of presentation; or (5) development of hypotension or bradycardia.

Treatment of cerebral edema involves use of IV mannitol, reduction in the rates of fluid administration, and possibly mechanical hyperventilation to help reduce brain swelling. Dexamethasone and furosemide are frequently administered but have no proven benefit. Early consultation with a neurologist and/or neurosurgeon is indicated. Although relatively large doses (1 g per kilogram body weight) of mannitol have been used, we prefer relatively smaller doses (0.2 g per kilogram over 30 minutes) with repeated doses at hourly intervals as indicated by the clinical response. Supportive measures and intensive monitoring in an intensive care unit setting are essential. Patients who present with evidence of brain herniation, papilledema, and/or diabetes insipidus due to acute cerebral edema seldom recover completely, and many die.

■ PREVENTION OF DIABETIC KETOACIDOSIS

The treatment of severe DKA in children requires timely, aggressive, and often expensive in-hospital intervention, and very close follow-up. Although the majority of patients do quite well, despite our best efforts, a small percentage of children with severe DKA develop significant complications, and some of these children will die. Therefore, prevention clearly is the best approach.

Educated families who seek advice early in the course of an intercurrent illness rarely develop severe DKA. All diabetic patients and their families should be taught how to deal with sick days. The primary goal for the management of diabetes during any illness is to prevent the need for hospitalization. Guidelines for the management of sick days should be established and discussed early in the relationship between the patient and health care team (Table 1). General guidelines that all diabetic subjects should follow as a part of sick day management include: (1) monitor blood glucose at least every 2 to 4 hours; (2) monitor urinary ketones, regardless of blood glucose level; (3) never omit insulin; (4) drink plenty of fluids; and (5) use supplemental insulin, if necessary, to break ketosis.

Close monitoring is an essential part of the management of diabetes, and this is even more important during an intercurrent illness. Whenever a diabetic patient is ill, regardless of the symptoms or the blood sugar, urine ketones should be monitored. Likewise, whenever the blood sugar is unexpectedly high (>240 mg per deciliter), urine ketones should be monitored regardless of whether there are any symptoms. Ketones in the urine indicate insulin deficiency and/or stress-related insulin resistance. In the presence of ketonuria, supplemental doses of insulin are required. During an illness, supplemental insulin often is given as subcutaneous Regular insulin in a dose equivalent to approximately 10 percent of the total daily dose; this may be repeated every 2 to 4 hours until the ketosis clears. When hyperglycemia is absent or minimal in the face of significant ketones, supplemental insulin should be given anyway, and additional sugar, in the form of carbohydrate-containing beverages, should be used to prevent hypoglycemia.

Table 1 Sick Day Management Guidelines
Monitor blood glucose every 2 to 4 hours.
Monitor urinary ketones, regardless of blood glucose.
Do not omit insulin.
Drink plenty of fluids.
Use supplemental doses of insulin to break ketosis.

Table 2 Sick Day Management
Seek medical assistance *immediately* if any of the following occur:
Shortness of breath or respiratory difficulty
Severe abdominal pain
Persistent vomiting (three or more times in the same day)
Severe dehydration
Acute visual loss
Seek medical attention if any of the following *persist*:
Unexplained hyperglycemia that is not responding to therapy
Ketonuria not responding to therapy
Persistent diarrhea
Other unexplained symptoms
Fever above 100°F

Fluids are an essential part of managing diabetes during a sick day. It is recommended that a teenager or young adult attempt to take in 6 to 8 oz of fluid each hour. Young children should take proportionately less (perhaps 3 to 6 oz every hour). In people with gastrointestinal illness, more-frequent ingestion of smaller quantities of fluid is usually better tolerated than less-frequent ingestion of larger quantities. Ingestion of food is not essential during the course of a brief intercurrent illness, but the inability to take in fluids is an indication for IV therapy. For those who are unable to eat, carbohydrate-containing fluids should be taken to replace the carbohydrate content of the meal plan. Additional fluids should be carbohydrate free while hyperglycemia is present, but carbohydrate-containing as necessary to maintain blood glucose in the 150 to 200 mg per deciliter range.

If ketosis or vomiting persists despite implementation of these guidelines, or if symptoms of severe DKA or their medical illness occur, the patient or family should seek medical attention as soon as possible (Table 2). Early intervention is the best way to eliminate significant morbidity and mortality associated with the occurrence of severe DKA and its treatment.

Suggested Reading
General Reviews

Duck SC, Wyatt DT. Factors associated with brain herniation in the treatment of diabetic ketoacidosis. J Pediatrics 1988; 113:10–14.

This original article examines nine new cases and 33 prior reports of cerebral edema in DKA to determine the relationship of excessive fluids.

Ellis EN. Concepts of fluid therapy in diabetic ketoacidosis and hyperosmolar hyperglycemic nonketotic coma. Ped Clin North Am 1987; 37:313–321.

This is a brief but excellent review (with 36 references) of the pathophysiology and treatment of fluid losses in DKA.

Foster DW, McGarry JD. The metabolic derangement and treatment of diabetic ketoacidosis. N Engl J Med 1983; 309:159–169.

This is a frequently cited review (with 91 references) of the metabolic derangements seen in DKA and their implications in developing treatment protocols.

Krane EJ. Diabetic ketoacidosis: Biochemistry, physiology, treatment, and prevention. Ped Clin North Am 1987; 34:935–960.

This is a good general review (with 105 references) of the biochemistry, physiology, and treatment of DKA.

Krane EJ, Rockoff MA, Wallman JK, Wolfsdorf JI. Subclinical brain swelling in children during treatment of diabetic ketoacidosis. N Engl J Med 1985; 312:1147–1151.

This important report demonstrates that some degree of brain swelling seen on CT scan is common in children with DKA, even if no clinical manifestations of cerebral edema are present.

Kreisberg RA. Diabetic ketoacidosis: New concepts and trends in pathogenesis and treatment. Ann Intern Med 1978; 88:681–695.

This is an excellent and frequently cited review (with 137 references) of the pathogenesis and treatment of DKA.

Levandoski LA, White NH, Santiago JV. How to weather the sick-day season. Diabetes Forecast 1983; 36:30–33.

This is a summary written for patients about how to handle a sick day in order to prevent DKA.

Rosenbloom AL: Intracerebral crisis during treatment of diabetic ketoacidosis. Diabetes Care 1990; 13:22–33.

This is a retrospective review of 69 cases of DKA with intracerebral complications examining predictive factors and effects of interventions on the development of cerebral edema.

DIABETIC KETOACIDOSIS IN ADULTS

Robert A. Kreisberg, M.D.

Diabetic ketoacidosis (DKA) is an acute, often life-threatening complication of poorly controlled diabetes and occurs in patients with both type 1 or insulin-dependent and type 2 or non–insulin-dependent diabetes mellitus (IDDM and NIDDM). Despite a better understanding of predisposing factors and improved educational programs, episodes of DKA and death from DKA continue to be important problems. Although DKA easily can be prevented, it is still responsible for 2 to 14 percent of all hospitalizations related to diabetes. Based upon a frequency of 5 to 13 episodes per 1,000 diabetic patients per year, it can be estimated that there are 100,000 to 150,000 episodes of DKA per year in the United States.

■ MISCONCEPTIONS

There are several important misconceptions concerning DKA.

Misconception #1: Diabetic ketoacidosis is a disease of the young. The average age of patients with DKA is 43 years. Approximately 85 percent of the episodes occur in adults. It has been estimated that patients with adult-onset diabetes (most of whom have NIDDM) account for 97 percent and patients with juvenile-onset diabetes mellitus (IDDM) account for 3 percent of all hospital admissions for diabetes. Diabetic ketoacidosis occurs in 3 percent of adult patients with diabetes and in 30 percent of patients with juvenile-onset diabetes. Consequently, it can be calculated that 76 percent of DKA episodes occur in adult patients with diabetes and 24 percent occur in young patients with diabetes. This information was obtained before the terms "juvenile-onset" and "adult-onset" diabetes were discarded in favor of IDDM and NIDDM. Most of the adult patients had NIDDM.

Misconception #2: Diabetic ketoacidosis occurs only in thin or normal-weight patients. Obesity is present in approximately 20 percent of patients who have DKA, again emphasizing the importance of older patients with NIDDM.

Misconception #3: Diabetic ketoacidosis is encountered most frequently at the onset of diabetes. Approximately 80 percent of episodes of DKA occur in patients previously known to have diabetes mellitus, while in 20 percent it occurs as the presenting manifestation of diabetes mellitus. Therefore, DKA represents the presenting manifestation of diabetes in no more than 20 percent of patients with diabetes mellitus.

Misconception #4: The mortality rate in DKA is low. Diabetic ketoacidosis accounts for approximately 5 percent of all deaths directly attributable to diabetes and is responsible for 40 percent of deaths in diabetic patients less than 24 years of age. Although DKA decreases in importance as a cause of death in older diabetics, the absolute number of deaths due to DKA increases, and 78 percent of DKA deaths occur in patients over the age of 45 years. The likelihood that an episode of DKA will end fatally increases with increasing age; 15 to 28 percent of all episodes of DKA occurring in individuals above the age of 65 are fatal.

■ PATHOPHYSIOLOGY

Diabetic ketoacidosis is due to a relative or absolute deficiency of insulin. The concentrations of the insulin counter-regulatory hormones (glucagon, epinephrine, growth hormone, and cortisol) are increased in patients with DKA. The release of counter-regulatory hormones is provoked by illness, as well as physical and emotional stress, and is accentuated in patients with poorly controlled diabetes. The biologic response to counter-regulatory hormones also is exaggerated in patients with poorly controlled diabetes. In addition to differences in the release and biologic response to the counter-regulatory hormones, there is a synergistic interaction between these hormones that accentuates both the hyperglycemic and ketonemic responses in the presence of insulin deficiency. It is now reasonably clear that an imbalance between insulin and the insulin counter-regulatory hormones is the principal cause of DKA. Although insulin concentrations within the normal range (≥ 5 to 15 µ/ml) usually are encountered in patients with DKA, they are inappropriately low for the prevailing blood glucose concentration.

The relative or absolute deficiency of insulin leads to overproduction of glucose by the liver and underutilization of glucose by peripheral tissues and increases the conversion free fatty acids to ketoacids in the liver. Insulin deficiency and glucagon excess increase the rate of ketogenesis in the liver by activating acylcarnitine transferase and facilitating transfer of fatty acids into the mitochondrion. Underutilization of ketoacids in peripheral tissues accentuates ketonemia and ketoacidosis. Thus, overproduction and underutilization of both glucose and ketoacids in DKA contribute to the hyperglycemia and ketosis.

The overproduction of ketoacids leads to a reduction in body buffer stores and a decrease in the serum bicarbonate concentration. For each millimole of ketoacid formed, 1 mmole of hydrogen ion will be produced. This hydrogen titrates 1 mmole of bicarbonate or buffer, thereby reducing the plasma bicarbonate concentration. The increment in ketoacid anion concentration quantitatively reflects the decrement in plasma bicarbonate concentration, since each ketoanion that is produced is accompanied by a hydrogen ion. When the DKA is reversed by insulin therapy, the metabolism of each ketoanion that has been retained within the body generates a bicarbonate ion. To the extent that the ketoacids produced during DKA are excreted in the urine, there will be a deficit of potential bicarbonate, and successful treatment of the DKA will result in the development of a hyperchloremic metabolic acidosis (retained chloride replaces the ketoanion lost in the urine).

The osmotic gradient created by hyperglycemia causes water to shift out of the intracellular compartment into the extracellular compartment and, at least initially, to expand the size of the vascular compartment. This leads to increased glomerular filtration and an osmotic diuresis. The latter is responsible for the polyuria that is characteristic of uncontrolled diabetes. While water is lost in excess of solute, that is not reflected in the serum sodium concentration, which almost invariably is reduced owing to expansion of the extracellular fluid compartment with water. The combined concentrations of sodium and potassium in the urine are approximately 80 mEq per liter, emphasizing that water is lost in excess of solute. Magnesium and phosphate also are excreted in the urine at increased rates, but this is seldom of any clinical consequence.

In general, there is only a weak relationship between the severity of hyperglycemia and acidosis in DKA because the intake of water and the prevailing glomerular filtration rate (GFR) play a major role in urinary excretion of glucose.

■ PRECIPITATING FACTORS

The major cause of DKA is the development of an intercurrent medical illness. This accounts for approximately 50 to 60 percent of all patients who present with DKA. The omission of insulin, which would be considered by many to be the most likely explanation for the development of DKA, occurs in only 20 to 30 percent of episodes. Although many believe that emotional factors and stress can precipitate the development of DKA, there are relatively few experimental data to support this concept. The risk of DKA is 50 percent higher among women than among men. In children with DKA, emotional factors contribute, totally or in part, to approximately 50 percent of the episodes. DKA also can be encountered in surgical, obstetric, and psychiatric settings.

■ DIAGNOSIS

The diagnosis of DKA is relatively easy. It should be considered in patients not previously known to have diabetes who present with coma, shock, dehydration, unexplained tachypnea, or infection. In addition, nausea, vomiting, and abdominal pain are common presenting complaints in patients with DKA. The diagnosis is established by the finding of a large anion gap, presence of ketonemia or ketonuria, and a blood glucose concentration of greater than 250 mg per deciliter. The physical examination frequently reveals hypertension, dehydration, and tachypnea with a Kussmaul respiratory pattern. A careful search for precipitating factors should be undertaken, and a careful pelvic and rectal examination should be performed because appendicitis, diverticulitis, cholecystitis, and pelvic inflammatory disease may be present as precipitating factors in such individuals. It should be remembered that many patients with acute metabolic acidosis have acute abdominal pain. In most patients with DKA this pain resolves as their metabolic disturbance is controlled. However, in many situations the underlying precipitating medical illness may be an intra-abdominal process and the abdominal pain may be an important sign of primary disease. An extensive search should be undertaken for infection even if the temperature of the patient is normal. In the older patient, a silent myocardial infarction or stroke may present as DKA.

■ LABORATORY FINDINGS

The cardinal laboratory features of DKA are hyperglycemia and anion-gap metabolic acidosis. The average blood-glucose concentration is usually 500 to 600 mg per deciliter, but in 15 percent of episodes it may be less than 350 mg per deciliter.

Greater hyperglycemia can be seen in patients with DKA if there is severe volume contraction. There is a poor correlation between the degree of hyperglycemia and the severity of the metabolic acidosis. Hyperglycemia is influenced by the state of hydration as well as the hormonal milieu. Glucose concentrations tend to be disproportionately low in DKA associated with pregnancy and with alcoholism. The continued utilization of glucose by the fetoplacental unit in the absence of insulin leads to a lower glucose concentration for any degree of metabolic acidosis, while the inhibitory effect of ethanol on gluconeogenesis leads to a disproportionately low glucose concentration relative to the bicarbonate concentration and the degree of acidosis.

Patients with DKA typically have an anion-gap metabolic acidosis. In this condition the increase in the anion gap (the difference between the patient's anion gap and the normal anion gap, where the normal anion gap is 10 to 12 mEq per liter) should be equivalent to the decrease in the serum bicarbonate concentration (between normal bicarbonate and the patient's bicarbonate). When the increase in the anion gap matches the decrease in serum bicarbonate concentration within 2 to 3 mEq per liter, it is reasonable to assume that metabolic acidosis is due exclusively to the accumulation of an unmeasured anion. Some patients have a combined anion-gap and hyperchloremic metabolic acidosis. This can be recognized by an increase in the serum chloride concentration in patients in whom the increase in anion gap is significantly less than the decrease in serum bicarbonate concentration. Rare patients with DKA have a predominant hyperchloremic metabolic acidosis.

The type of metabolic acidosis is related to the magnitude of the fluid deficit. The more severe the volume contraction, the more likely it is that the increment in the anion gap will be equivalent to the decrement in the bicarbonate concentration, since the ketoanions are not excreted in the urine. If the intravascular volume is well maintained by patients during the development of ketoacidosis, a combined anion-gap and hyperchloremic metabolic acidosis or a predominant hyperchloremic metabolic acidosis is not uncommon, because the chloride anion replaces the ketoanion that has been lost in the urine.

· The serum sodium concentration commonly is reduced in DKA. This is the result of both sodium depletion and a shift of water from the intracellular to the extracellular space secondary to hyperglycemia (hyperosmolality) and increased osmotic gradient. For each 100 mg per deciliter increment in the glucose concentration, the serum sodium falls by 1.5 to 2.0 mEq per liter. When the serum sodium concentration is normal, water loss is extreme. Hypertriglyceridemia also can spuriously reduce the serum sodium concentration; for each 1,000 mg per deciliter increase in the serum triglyceride concentration, the serum sodium decreases by 1.5 to 2.0 mEq per liter. If significant hypertriglyceridemia is present, as it often is in patients with DKA, the degree of hyponatremia will be greater than can be accounted for by the hyperglycemia. As the hyperglycemia and hypertriglyceridemia clear in response to therapy, the patient may become hypernatremic. The total body deficit of sodium (primarily the result of the osmotic diuresis) has been estimated to range from 7 to 10 mEq per kilogram of body weight in patients with advanced DKA.

The mean serum potassium concentration in DKA is approximately 5.2 mEq per liter. Hyperkalemia is the rule in patients with DKA despite a total body potassium deficit on the order of 3 to 5 mEq per kilogram of body weight. The primary cause of the hyperkalemia is insulin deficiency per se. Insulin promotes potassium entry into the cellular compartment. The development of metabolic acidosis with the intracellular entry of hydrogen ion in exchange for potassium also contributes to the development of hyperkalemia.

The water deficit in DKA varies and in extreme cases may reach 10 to 12 percent of body weight (approximately 100 ml per kilogram of body weight). However, these estimates are derived from balance studies conducted in metabolic units in the late 1930s and early 1940s as patients recovered from DKA. The likelihood of such extreme water deficits in today's climate of education and awareness is relatively low, but they may happen occasionally.

The serum magnesium and phosphate concentrations are frequently elevated in patients with DKA, but with therapy they fall into the normal range or, in the majority of patients, to lower than normal levels. The deficiencies of magnesium and phosphate that exist in patients with DKA generally are of no clinical importance but on rare occasions supplementation may be required (discussed later in this chapter).

The serum creatinine concentration may be spuriously elevated due to interference of acetoacetate with the measurement of creatinine by automated techniques. In this situation, the blood urea nitrogen (BUN) may be a better indicator of renal function than the serum creatinine concentration.

The nitroprusside reaction (Acetest) detects acetoacetate and acetone but not beta-hydroxybutyric acid. If beta-hydroxybutyrate is the predominant ketone body in DKA, the serum Acetest result will be spuriously low. This situation occurs commonly in alcoholic ketoacidosis or when oxygen delivery is inadequate.

Hyperamylasemia commonly is encountered in patients with DKA. This is important because abdominal pain is also common in DKA. Some patients with pain have normal amylase, some patients with elevated amylase have no abdominal pain, and some patients have both pain and hyperamylasemia. Most patients do not have pancreatitis. However, these patients must be followed carefully because of the possibility of intra-abdominal pathology. The pain should resolve during treatment if it is related to the DKA. The amylase often is of salivary origin, and elevations of pancreatic amylase levels do not correlate with clinical symptoms.

■ THERAPY

The cornerstone of therapy in DKA involves the appropriate use of insulin, correction of fluid deficits, and replacement of potassium. Meticulous attention should be paid to identification of precipitating factors such as infection, silent myocardial infarction, and intra-abdominal pathology. If an adynamic ileus is present or develops during the course of DKA, a nasogastric tube should be inserted to empty the dilated stomach of its contents. Failure to do so may result in aspiration of gastric contents with respiratory arrest and even death, despite an improving metabolic picture.

Insulin (Table 1)

Although the hyperglycemia in DKA often improves with replacement alone, insulin is absolutely necessary to inhibit hepatic glucose and ketone production, suppress lipolysis (free fatty acids are the precursor of ketone bodies), and reverse the metabolic acidosis. Insulin also improves ketone body utilization by peripheral tissues and consequently regeneration of bicarbonate. It is generally accepted that "low" doses of insulin (5 to 10 U per dose) can be successfully used to correct ketoacidosis in the majority of patients. It should be noted that these "low" doses of insulin produce plasma insulin concentrations in the high physiologic/pharmacologic range, that is, more than 150 to 200 μU per milliliter. Although a minority of patients (5 to 10 percent) may require larger doses of insulin, there are no clinical or laboratory features that permit these patients to be identified early. Consequently, it is important to follow patients with DKA very carefully so that patients who fail to respond to "low" doses of insulin can be quickly identified and larger doses of insulin used. Regular insulin (0.1 U per kilogram or 5 to 10 U total) is recommended as an intravenous priming dose, to be followed by continuous insulin infusion at a rate of 0.1 U per kilogram per hour (or 5 to 10 U per hour). Although the intravenous route is preferred, the intramuscular route is acceptable, except when volume contraction is severe. The blood glucose concentration should decrease at a rate of approximately 75 to 100 mg per deciliter per hour. On average, the glucose concentration reaches 250 to 300 mg per deciliter after approximately 5 to 6 hours of therapy, but the bicarbonate level increases more slowly, reaching a target of 15 to 18 mEq/L in approximately 10 to 12 hours. It has been estimated that 75 percent of the reduction that occurs in the glucose concentration during treatment of DKA is due to the excretion of glucose in the urine and/or volume re-expansion and dilution of glucose in the extracellular compartment. If there is no reduction in the blood glucose concentration after 1 to 2 hours of therapy, the dose of insulin should be increased to 20 to 50 U per hour. The major risk of larger doses of insulin is not a more rapid decrease in the plasma glucose concentration, but a more protracted hypoglycemia when the blood glucose concentration has reached its nadir and a greater likelihood of the development of hypokalemia and hypophosphatemia. Insulin should be continued at 0.1 U per kilogram per hour (or 5 to 10 U per hour) even when the glucose concentration reaches 250 to 300 mg per deciliter. Further reduction in the glucose concentration is prevented by adding glucose to the parenteral fluids. This allows continued administration of insulin to correct the acidosis, while protecting against hypoglycemia. One of the more common therapeutic mistakes is to reduce the rate of insulin infusion when the glucose concentration reaches 250 to 300 mg per deciliter. The correction of the acidosis "lags" by many hours behind the correction of hyperglycemia. Consequently, premature reduction in the rate of insulin administration leads to prolonged recovery from ketoacidosis. When the bicarbonate concentration reaches 15 to 18 mEq per liter or the blood pH reaches 7.30, the insulin infusion rate should be reduced to 1 to 3 U per hour. Despite the success of "low-dose" insulin therapy, patients with DKA are resistant to insulin (the average individual would require 150 to 200 U every 24 hours). Insulin clamp studies have demonstrated that a patient with DKA is only 10 to 15 percent as sensitive as a normal subject to a given rate of administration of insulin.

Fluid Replacement (Table 2)

Despite hyponatremia, water has been lost in excess of solute (urinary loss of sodium and potassium is equivalent to approximately 0.5 normal saline). Correction of hypovolemia is critical to the management of DKA, since hypovolemia is a potent stimulus for the release of counter-regulatory hormones. The failure of patients to respond to insulin should suggest the possibility of persistent hypovolemia. In general,

---

Table 1 Insulin Administration

Administer a 5–10 U bolus of Regular insulin intravenously as a priming dose.

Administer Regular insulin at a rate of 0.1 U/kg body weight per hour (or 5–10 U/hr) by continuous intravenous infusion (dilute 50 U of insulin in 250 ml of 0.9% saline; insulin concentration = 10 U/50 ml; run approximately 50 ml of insulin solution through intravenous tubing "piggyback" into intravenous infusion line to coat surfaces of plastic tubing).

When the plasma glucose reaches the "target" value of 250–300 mg/dl, continue insulin infusion rate at 0.1 U/kg body weight per hour. Incorporate sufficient glucose into parenteral fluids to prevent a further decrease in the glucose concentration (see Table 2).

If there is no decrease in the plasma glucose 1–2 hr after the start of therapy, increase the rate of insulin to 20–50 U/hr.

When both the glucose and bicarbonate concentrations reach their "target" values, reduce rate of insulin administration to 1–3 U/hr.

Table 2 Fluid Replacement

1. Infuse 0.9% saline at a rate of approximately 1 L/hr for the initial 1–3 hours of therapy.
2. Infuse 0.9% saline at a rate of 500 ml/hr for 4–8 hours. Plan to administer approximately 50% of the estimated fluid deficit in first 8 hr.
3. Infuse 0.45 or 0.9% saline as indicated by serum sodium and chloride concentrations; replace approximately 80% of the estimated deficit by 24 hr.
4. When the plasma glucose reaches 250–300 mg/dl, change to 5% or 10% dextrose in 0.45% or 0.90% saline.
5. If the fluid deficit is judged to be mild to moderate, less aggressive replacement should be considered (500 ml per hour for the first 3–4 hours followed by 250 ml/hr thereafter). The plasma bicarbonate concentration increases more rapidly in patients with mild to moderate fluid deficits who receive slower rates of fluid administration. Aggressive fluid replacement is important in patients judged to have severe fluid deficits.
6. The decision to switch to 0.45% saline depends on the plasma sodium and chloride concentrations and the calculated serum tonicity. Hyperchloremia is common during recovery from DKA (the anion-gap acidosis is replaced by a non–anion-gap hyperchloremic metabolic acidosis; see text for explanation).

2 to 3 L of normal saline are administered intravenously over the first 2 to 3 hours. If the patient is hypotensive despite the administration of normal saline, colloid should be used. Some individuals may require larger amounts of normal saline (and/or colloid) to restore euvolemia. The ultimate goal is to achieve a normal blood pressure and restore tissue perfusion to normal. This may require 4 to 5 L or more of normal saline within the initial 2 to 3 hours of therapy. Once the intravascular volume has been repleted, normal saline may be continued at a much slower rate. Some experts prefer the use of 0.5 normal saline to replace the remainder of the fluid deficit. When the glucose level reaches 250 to 300 mg per deciliter, glucose should be incorporated into the parenteral fluids (5 percent or 10 percent dextrose in normal saline should be used).

Potassium (Table 3)

In advanced DKA the potassium deficit is 3 to 5 mEq per kilogram of body weight. In the presence of persistent nausea and vomiting, diarrhea, or the use of diuretics, the potassium deficit may be larger. During therapy, the potassium concentration falls dramatically, usually reaching a nadir at 4 to 6 hours. Replacement of potassium during this early phase is crucial to avoid the consequences of severe hypokalemia. The serum potassium concentration decreases during therapy because of insulin's effect on transmembrane movement of potassium, correction of acidosis, and continuing urinary potassium losses. Potassium, usually as the chloride salt, should be incorporated into fluids from the outset of therapy for DKA unless the patient is oliguric or significantly hyperkalemic (>5.0 to 5.5 mEq/L). Others have suggested that the incorporation of potassium be delayed until urine flow is established. In the absence of any major problem in potassium homeostasis, 20 mEq of potassium chloride should be incorporated into each liter of fluid replacement. The serum potas-

sium should be maintained above 3.5 mEq per liter. As much as 40 to 80 mEq of potassium chloride can be added to each liter of administered fluid, if necessary, to maintain the serum potassium concentration in an acceptable range. If the patient becomes hyperkalemic, the potassium supplement should be discontinued. Since approximately 50 percent of the potassium administered during therapy is excreted in the urine, the amount of potassium supplement should be markedly reduced or even curtailed in the presence of oliguria or renal failure. If oliguria or renal failure is present, the serum potassium concentration must be followed closely (every 1 to 2 hours) to judge the need for potassium supplementation. Some experts have suggested that potassium phosphate should be substituted for potassium chloride if patients have concomitant hypophosphatemia (see subsequent discussion).

Bicarbonate (Table 4)

There is considerable controversy over whether bicarbonate should be used in the treatment of DKA. Both prospective and retrospective studies have failed to demonstrate that bicarbonate supplementation is of any benefit. Consequently, bicarbonate is not usually recommended unless the blood pH is less than 7.1, the serum bicarbonate concentration is less than 5 mEq per liter, and pCO_2 is at the limit of compensation (approximately 10 to 12 mm Hg). Given these parameters, when severe acidosis exists in a patient with maximum hyperventilation and a pCO_2 of 10 to 12 mm Hg, any further change in the bicarbonate concentration will be associated with a rapid worsening of pH. These patients should receive limited bicarbonate replacement to increase the serum bicarbonate concentration to 10 to 12 mEq per liter. The bicarbonate space of distribution is approximately 40 percent of body weight or 28 L in a 70-kg person. To raise the serum bicarbonate concentration from 5 to 10 mEq per liter in such a person requires 140 mEq of bicarbonate (5 mEq/L × 28 L). If bicarbonate is to be used, it should be administered in 250 to 1,000 ml of 0.5 normal saline and infused over 30 to 60 minutes.

Table 3 Potassium Replacement

1. The serum potassium is increased in most patients with DKA at the time of presentation. A low serum potassium at presentation indicates a severe deficit in body potassium stores and requires immediate correction.
2. The average potassium deficit is 3–5 mEq/kg body weight.
3. Potassium chloride (20–30 mEq) should be added to each liter of administered fluid, if the serum potassium concentration is not >5.0–5.5 mEq/L and the patient has a good urine output. In patients with hyperkalemia (>5.5 mEq/L), addition of potassium chloride to the intravenous fluids can be delayed until the potassium concentration decreases to 4–5 mEq/L. The potassium level should be kept above 3.5 mEq/L.
4. The rate of potassium administration depends upon the serum potassium level:

>6 mEq/L	No potassium
5–6 mEq/L	10 mEq/hr
4–5 mEq/L	20 mEq/hr
3–4 mEq/L	30–40 mEq/hr
<3 mEq/L	40–80 mEq/hr

5. Increase the frequency of serum potassium measurement if the change in serum potassium requires more aggressive potassium supplement.
6. The serum potassium usually reaches its nadir at 4–6 hours after therapy.

Table 4 Bicarbonate, Magnesium, and Phosphate Replacement

1. Bicarbonate is not indicated in the routine management of DKA. If the pH is <7.1, pCO_2 = 10–12 mm Hg, and the bicarbonate ≤5 mEq/L, bicarbonate should be administered in 0.45% saline over 30–60 minutes to raise the serum bicarbonate concentration to 10–12 mEq/L.
2. Magnesium parenteral administration is not necessary in most cases despite total body deficits of approximately 1 mEq/kg. Magnesium administration may be necessary if phosphate replacement produces hypocalcemia and tetany.
3. Phosphate replacement is not routinely advocated. The total body deficit is 0.5 mmol/kg. If the plasma phosphate concentration decreases to <1.0 mg/dl, phosphate replacement should be considered. Potassium phosphate (20 mEq potassium per 12 mmol phosphate) is preferred over potassium chloride and should be given with parenteral fluid therapy. Approximately 0.5 mmol/kg body weight of potassium phosphate should be given over 24 hr. The serum calcium and phosphate concentrations should be monitored closely if phosphate replacement is initiated. The plasma phosphate concentration reaches a nadir at 4–6 hours after the initiation of therapy for DKA (similar to potassium).

Phosphate (Table 4)

Although hyperphosphatemia usually is present at the outset of therapy of DKA, hypophosphatemia invariably develops. In most patients, the body deficit of phosphate is relatively small, averaging 0.5 mmol per kilogram of body weight. The total body pool of phosphate is approximately 6,000 mmol. Prospective studies have not demonstrated any clinical benefit of phosphate supplementation in patients with DKA. Consequently, it can not be recommended routinely. If the hypophosphatemia is severe (<1.0 mmol/L), phosphate replacement can be given as long as the serum calcium concentration is normal.

Magnesium (Table 4)

Although magnesium deficiency exists in patients with DKA, the deficit is not large and rarely is associated with signs or symptoms. It almost never is corrected during active therapy but corrects spontaneously when a regular diet is resumed. Because magnesium deficiency impairs both the secretion and action of parathyroid hormone, patients may develop symptomatic hypocalcemia if they receive phosphate supplements. Under these circumstances correction of magnesium deficits may be necessary.

Patient Monitoring (Table 5)

Proper management of DKA requires fastidious monitoring and follow-up by physicians and nurses. The glucose concentration should be measured hourly and the serum potassium should be measured at intervals of 1 to 2 hours as indicated clinically. Other electrolytes can be measured at 4-hour intervals. Hourly intake and output should be recorded. If frequent measurement of the serum potassium concentration can not be obtained, the height of the T wave on the electrocardiogram can be used as an index of the change in serum potassium concentration.

Patients commonly develop a hyperchloremic metabolic acidosis during successful treatment of DKA. There are no adverse clinical consequences of this mild acid-base disturbance. As a general rule, the bicarbonate concentration will increase during therapy of DKA to approximately 15 to 18 mEq per liter and the pH to 7.30. At this point the typical anion-gap metabolic acidosis is replaced by a hyperchloremic metabolic acidosis that resolves slowly over the next several days as the kidney excretes the excess hydrogen ion load as NH_4Cl. The hyperchloremia results from a deficit of buffer (i.e., ketone bodies lost in the urine), which is needed to regenerate the bicarbonate that was titrated by the production of hydrogen ion (1 mEq of hydrogen ion accompanies the production of each milliequivalent of ketone anion). During the development of DKA the decrease in serum bicarbonate concentration (that results from the production of metabolic acid) is substantially greater than the quantity of ketone bodies retained in the body (there is significant excretion of ketone anions in the urine) even though there is a close relationship between the increase in the anion gap and the reduction in bicarbonate. During the correction of hypovolemia with the rapid administration of fluids, the increase in GFR results in a further loss of ketone bodies, and this accentuates the discrepancy between the base deficit and the number of ketoanions available to regenerate base. Consequently, the ability to reverse the loss of bicarbonate and correct the pH is limited by the availability of substrate bicarbonate equivalents (ketoanions). In the face of decreased capacity to restore bicarbonate, the kidney reabsorbs the most plentiful ion, chloride, as it increases its resorption of sodium and potassium. Consequently, the development of a mild hyperchloremic metabolic acidosis in the recovery phase from DKA should be anticipated. It should be remembered that, when the glucose concentration reaches 250 to 300 and the bicarbonate concentration increases to 18 mEq per liter and the pH to 7.30, the rate of administration of insulin can be reduced.

■ CHILDREN

The principles of management of DKA in children are similar to those described for adults (see the chapter *Diabetic Ketoacidosis in Children*). However, the doses of insulin, fluids, and electrolyte supplements must be adjusted for size. It is particularly important to avoid excessive administration of hypotonic fluids because of their potential to lead to the development of cerebral edema.

Table 5 Patient Monitoring

		HOURS*											
PARAMETER	**ADMISSION**	**1**	**2**	**3**	**4**	**5**	**6**	**7**	**8**	**9**	**10**	**11**	**12**
CBC	X												
Urinalysis	X												
Glucose	X	X	X	X	X	X	X		X		X		X
Potassium	X		X		X		X						X
Sodium chloride/ bicarbonate	X						X						X
Phosphate	X						X						
Calcium	X												
Magnesium	X												
BUN/Cr	X												
Chest x-ray	X												
ECG	X												
Intake and Output	X	X	X	X	X	X	X	X	X	X	X	X	X

*Suggested frequency of measurement; to be modified as indicated clinically.

■ COMPLICATIONS

Cerebral edema is a dreaded and devastating complication of the treatment of DKA. It usually is encountered in young children in whom DKA is the presenting manifestation of their disease. Signs and symptoms of cerebral edema develop over several hours, paradoxically, while laboratory indices indicate improvement in the metabolic disturbance. These signs and symptoms include headache, altered level of consciousness, bradycardia, papilledema, and fixed dilated pupils. Development of headaches during the course of therapy is an ominous symptom and should suggest the development of cerebral edema. Although there are no randomized prospective studies about its efficacy, intravenous mannitol at a rate of 10 to 20 g per square meter every 2 to 4 hours is recommended. The rate of parenteral fluid administration should be reduced, and controlled hyperventilation should be considered (hypocapnia reduces cerebral blood flow).

Virtually all patients treated for DKA develop cerebral edema. However, it is unusual for them to develop symptoms. Those patients who develop life-threatening cerebral edema during therapy of DKA differ quantitatively but not qualitatively from those who do not develop symptoms. The cause of cerebral edema is unknown and can not be related to the infusion rate or the osmolality or volume of fluids administered.

It is extremely important to continue to monitor the patient closely for underlying medical conditions that precipitated the DKA or that may develop during the treatment of DKA. These include silent myocardial infarction, stroke, pancreatitis, infection, sepsis, aspiration, venous thrombosis, and pulmonary embolus.

Suggested Reading

Androgue HJ, Barrero J, Eknoyan G. Salutory effects of modest fluid replacement in the treatment of diabetic ketoacidosis. JAMA 1989; 262:2108–2113.

Demonstrates that modest fluid replacement with saline in patients without extreme volume deficit leads to the development of hyperchloremia.

Adrogue HJ, Wilson H, Boyd AE, Suki WN, Eknoyan G. Plasma acid-base patterns in diabetic ketoacidosis. N Engl J Med 1982; 307:1603–1610.

Discusses anion-gap and non–anion-gap acidosis patterns in DKA as well as the mechanisms that lead to the development of hyperchloremia during successful therapy.

DeFronzo RA, Matsuda M. Diabetic ketoacidosis: A combined metabolic-nephrologic approach to therapy. Diabetes Rev 1994; 2:209–238.

The most recent, updated review of the pathogenesis and treatment of DKA.

Fisher JSN, Kitabchi A. A randomized study of phosphate therapy in the treatment of diabetic ketoacidosis. J Clin Endocrinol Metab 1983; 57:177–180.

Demonstrates that routine use of phosphate during treatment of DKA is without benefit.

Foster DW, McGarry JD. The metabolic derangements and treatment of diabetic ketoacidosis. N Engl J Med 1983; 309:159–169.

The definitive article on the biochemistry of DKA by highly respected investigators in this area.

Kreisberg RA. Diabetic ketoacidosis: New concepts and trends in pathogenesis and treatment. Ann Intern Med 1978; 88:681–695.

A comprehensive clinical review. Concepts are relevant despite being 20 years old. Specific guidance is given for use of "low" dose insulin therapy, correction of volume deficits, and replacement of potassium.

Lever E, Jaspan JB. Sodium bicarbonate therapy in severe diabetic ketoacidosis. Am J Med 1983; 75:263–268.

Routine use of bicarbonate does not alter the rate of recovery from DKA.

Rosenbloom AL. Intracerebral crises during treatment of diabetic ketoacidosis. Diabetes Care 1990; 13:22–33.

A comprehensive review of all reported cases of cerebral edema during treatment of DKA. The author demonstrates that there are no clinical features that identify children at risk, nor is there a unifying explanation about its etiology.

HYPEROSMOLAR HYPERGLYCEMIC NONKETOTIC COMA

Sally M. Marshall, M.D
K. George M.M. Alberti, D Phil

Hyperosmolar hyperglycemic nonketotic coma (HHNC) represents one end of a metabolic spectrum, at the other end of which is diabetic ketoacidosis (DKA). The cardinal features of extreme hyperglycemia, hyperosmolarity, and dehydration often are more marked than in DKA, but ketosis and acidosis are absent or minimal. Elderly patients with type 1 or non–insulin-dependent diabetes mellitus (NIDDM) are most commonly affected, although the metabolic disturbance may occur at any age and in patients with type 2 or insulin-dependent diabetes mellitus (IDDM). The condition is relatively common, occurring with an incidence that is one-sixth that of DKA. It affects about 1 of 500 diabetic patients. Mortality remains high (17 to 50 percent), reflecting the older age of most patients and the presence of intercurrent illness, as well as the severity of the metabolic abnormalities. Mortality correlates most closely with age and osmolarity and is about threefold greater than in DKA.

■ ETIOLOGY AND PATHOGENESIS

Up to 50 percent of episodes occur in patients not previously known to have diabetes. Precipitating factors are similar to those in DKA. Any acute illness, particularly infection, myocardial infarction, and cerebrovascular events, may precipitate HHNC. In addition, HHNC is associated with the use of certain drugs, such as thiazides and steroids. Patients at highest risk are elderly, female, and socially isolated. Most of those with known diabetes have NIDDM and are being treated with dietary modifications with or without oral hypoglycemic agents.

The underlying cause of the extreme hyperglycemia without ketoacidosis is related to the presence of relative insulin deficiency in association with elevated levels of glucagon and other counter-regulatory hormones that depress glucose utilization by peripheral tissues and stimulate hepatic glycogenolysis and gluconeogenesis. The resultant hyperglycemia induces an osmotic diuresis. If the diabetic individual fails to maintain a sufficient oral intake, owing to defective thirst mechanisms in the elderly or a concomitant gastrointestinal disorder, depletion of the extracellular fluid volume and declining renal perfusion ensue. Serum urea and creatinine concentrations rise, and the kidneys are unable to excrete the glucose load, further exacerbating the hyperglycemia. There often is pre-existing renal impairment, which raises the renal threshold for glucose and helps to sustain the hyperglycemia. The failure of ketosis to develop may be explained by the presence of circulating levels of insulin sufficient to inhibit lipolysis by peripheral tissues and to suppresses beta oxidation of fatty acids in the liver. In addition, hyperosmolarity per se suppresses lipolysis. Decreased glucose excretion by the kidney probably is the most important factor that allows the development of severe hyperglycemia without ketoacidosis.

■ DIAGNOSIS

Most patients give a classic history of polyuria, thirst, and polydipsia, with lethargy progressing to drowsiness and coma. However, a high index of suspicion is necessary since many patients present with nonspecific symptoms and signs (Table 1). Often, the features of the precipitating illness are paramount. Nausea, vomiting, Kussmaul's respiration, and mild hypothermia—hallmarks of DKA—are absent, but extracellular volume depletion is severe and hypotension is common. Neurologic syndromes, including seizures and transient hemiparesis, are not uncommon. Urine testing shows marked glycosuria with minimal or no ketonuria, and test-strip measurement of capillary blood glucose concentration reveals marked hyperglycemia. The diagnosis is easily confirmed by laboratory blood glucose determination and measurement of the serum osmolarity (greater than 350 mOsm per liter). Metabolic acidosis is either absent or mild. The elevated anion gap is explained by a combination of lactate and ketones. The plasma sodium concentration often is elevated, reflecting severe water loss. However, low serum sodium concentration also is a common finding due to the dilutional effect of hyperglycemia (each 100 mg per deciliter rise in plasma glucose decreases the serum sodium by about 1.6 mEq per liter). After correction for the osmotic shift of water, the great majority of patients with HHNC will have a normal, or more commonly an elevated serum sodium concentration. In all patients it is important to calculate the plasma osmolality to gauge the severity of hypertonicity and to assist in fluid repletion. Plasma osmolality can be calculated as follows:

$$2(Na^+ + K^+) + \frac{BUN}{2.8} + \frac{Glucose}{18}$$

Blood urea nitrogen (BUN) is markedly elevated and will contribute to the hyperosmolarity. The hematocrit is predictably high, and triglycerides may also be markedly elevated.

Table 1 Clinical Features of Hyperosmolar Hyperglycemic Nonketotic Coma

Elderly
More likely to occur in women than in men
No previous history of diabetes
Nonspecific symptoms and signs
Marked dehydration
Tachycardia
Hypotension
Mental dysfunction
Signs of precipitating illness

■ MANAGEMENT

The goals of management are to correct the fluid and electrolyte deficits, particularly sodium and potassium, to lower the blood glucose toward normal with insulin, and to identify and treat the underlying precipitating cause, if one can be identified. In elderly patients with underlying vascular disease, monitoring of central venous pressure or, ideally, pulmonary capillary wedge pressure is important to ensure adequate rehydration without fluid overload (Table 2).

Fluid Replacement

Patients are both volume contracted (loss of isotonic saline) and dehydrated (pure water loss). The former is reflected by tachycardia and reduced blood pressure, while the latter is reflected by hypertonicity. The average fluid deficit is about 9 L. Opinion is divided about the choice of fluid for replacement. On the grounds that water loss has exceeded electrolyte loss and that the serum osmolality is very high, many authorities have advocated the use of hypotonic fluid such as half normal (0.45 percent) NaCl. Others have raised concern that infusion of hypotonic solutions causes a rapid reduction in serum osmolality, osmotic disequilibrium across the cell membrane, and large fluxes of hypotonic fluid into cells, including those of the brain. The cornerstone of therapy is to restore tissue perfusion and to stabilize the cardiovascular system. This is best accomplished by infusion of isotonic (0.9 percent) saline. It should be remembered that the tonicity of isotonic saline (308 mOsm per liter) always will be hypotonic to the patient's tonicity. In subjects in whom the initial sodium concentration is normal or low (<140 mEq per liter), isotonic saline should be started at a rate (usually 1 L per hour) that is sufficient to restore normal blood pressure, heart rate, and organ perfusion. In individuals with an elevated serum sodium concentration (>145 to 150 mEq per liter) on admission, some combination of isotonic saline (to correct volume deficits) and hypotonic fluids (to correct hypertonicity and water deficits) will be necessary to prevent hypernatremia. There is a small, but serious risk that cerebral edema (see chapter on *Diabetic Ketoacidosis in Children and in Adults*) and adult respiratory distress syndrome (ARDS) will develop during treatment. These complications have been associated with the use of hypotonic fluids and crystalloids in DKA but are rare in HHNC.

As stated above, the initial objective of fluid replacement is to restore circulating volume. Therefore, it is our current practice to begin resuscitation with isotonic (0.9 percent) NaCl before laboratory results are available. The small, temporary rise in plasma sodium during such therapy may be beneficial, acting as a buffer to the rapid fall in osmolality as blood glucose declines. If serum sodium concentration exceeds 150 mEq per liter, it is advisable to switch to half-normal (0.45 percent) saline. This is obligatory at serum sodium levels greater than 155 mEq per liter. If hypotension persists (systolic blood pressure less than 80 to 100 mm Hg), 1 to 2 L of plasma expander (blood or albumin) should be given. A recent report suggests that dopamine may improve survival in patients with HHNC who are in shock.

One liter of isotonic saline should be infused over the first hour, followed by a second liter over the next 2 hours. This should ensure rapid expansion of the intravascular compartment and a rise in blood pressure and tissue perfusion. In some cases with severe extracellular volume depletion, more aggressive therapy with normal saline may be required. Urine output will increase, allowing excretion of glucose, while improved peripheral circulation will enhance tissue

---

Table 2 Main Features of Management of Hyperosmolar Hyperglycemic Nonketotic Coma

FLUID REPLACEMENT*

Normal (0.9%) saline:	1 L in first hr
	1 L in next 2 hr
	2 L in next 8 hr
	1 L every 8 hr
Half normal (0.45%) saline if serum Na+ >150–155 mEq/L	
1–2 L colloid/blood if persistently hypotensive	

POTASSIUM†

20 mEq KCl per hour initially	
Adjust according to serum K+:	60 mEq/hr if K+<3.0 mEq/L
	40 mEq/hr if 3.0> K+ <3.5 mEq/L
	20 mEq/hr if 3.5> K+ <5.0 mEq/L
	0–10 mEq/hr if 5.0> K+ <6.0 mEq/L
	0 if K+>6.0 mEq/L

INSULIN

3–4 U/hr IV infusion initially
When glucose <300 mg/dl, give 2 U/hr and add
    10% dextrose at 80 ml/hr.
Continue saline if signs of volume depletion persist.

ANTICOAGULATION

Low-dose subcutaneous heparin in all patients (5000 IU every 6 hr)
Full-dose IV heparin if high risk

*Use central venous pressure line, if indicated, to guide rate of fluid replacement.
†Monitor with continuous electrocardiographic record.

metabolism of glucose. Thereafter, the rate and tonicity of fluid administration must be governed by the clinical state of the patient. A useful guideline is to infuse 2 L of fluid (either 0.45 percent or 0.9 percent saline) over the next 8 hours, followed by 1 L every 8 hours, thereafter. Elderly patients or patients with known heart disease are particularly prone to develop cardiac failure if rehydration is too rapid. In such individuals fluid replacement should be somewhat slower and close monitoring is essential. Intravenous (IV) fluids should be continued until the patient is fully rehydrated and able to maintain fluid balance orally. This will require continuation of IV fluids along with the glucose and insulin infusion until the blood glucose level has returned to normal (see below).

Insulin

Rehydration per se will lower the blood glucose concentration significantly by allowing renal excretion of glucose, enhancing glucose utilization by peripheral tissues, and by expansion of extracellular compartments. Nonetheless, all patients require insulin therapy, even though they are said to be less insulin resistant than patients with ketoacidosis. All authors now recommend "low-dose" insulin therapy to reduce the incidence and risk of hypokalemia and delayed hypoglycemia. We use continuous infusion of Regular insulin, by syringe pump, initially at the rate of 3 to 4 U per hour, aiming to lower the blood glucose concentration by 60 to 100 mg per deciliter per hour. Some authorities have recommended even lower insulin infusion rates of 1 to 2 U per hour. An initial bolus dose of insulin has been recommended by some clinicians, but it is our practice to simply start the continuous insulin infusion. It is unnecessary to add a small amount of albumin or colloid to the infusate to prevent insulin absorption to the tubing. If the blood glucose level does not fall in the first 1 to 2 hours, the fluid replacement regimen, pump function, and integrity of the system should be checked before the insulin rate is doubled. In our experience, this is uncommon, even in patients in shock. When the blood glucose level falls to around 250 mg per deciliter, the insulin fusion rate should be reduced to 1 to 2 U per hour and infusion of 10 percent dextrose in water containing 20 mEq potassium at the rate of 80 ml per hour begun. If blood glucose is reduced below 250 mg per deciliter too quickly, the risk of cerebral edema is said to be increased. Although this is still controversial, there is little to be gained by aiming for normoglycemia. Therefore, a conservative approach is warranted. We maintain the blood glucose concentration between 180 and 250 mg per deciliter for 24 hours by adjusting the insulin infusion rate on the basis of hourly bedside blood glucose determinations, while continuing the dextrose infusion at a constant rate. After 24 hours, blood glucose levels are lowered to 90 to 180 mg per deciliter. As stated previously, it is necessary to continue the saline infusion to correct salt and water losses in almost all cases.

Hourly intramuscular (IM) injection of insulin is a satisfactory alternative, giving a loading dose of 10 to 20 U initially, followed by 4 to 6 U per hour.

Potassium

The average potassium deficit is large, often exceeding 800 to 1,000 mEq. This deficit is greater than that usually seen in DKA patients, presumably because of the more prolonged diuresis and greater contraction of the intracellular volume.

Extreme hyperkalemia is rare, and the serum potassium concentration falls as soon as the renal output improves and insulin therapy is started. The majority of the early fall is due to continued renal potassium loss plus expansion of the intracellular space. For these reasons, we begin potassium infusion immediately at the rate of 20 mEq per hour. The infusion rate is adjusted thereafter on the basis of frequent measurements of the serum potassium concentration. Since up to 75 percent of the infused potassium is excreted in the urine, patients may require as much as 80 mEq per hour. If the serum potassium rises to more than 6.0 mEq per liter, potassium infusion should be stopped. Continuous electrocardiographic monitoring is a useful guide to potassium status. It is probably wise to continue potassium replacement orally for several days after the acute episode. During potassium replacement therapy, urine output and renal function (serum creatinine and urea nitrogen) should be monitored closely. If renal failure develops, potassium replacement should be stopped or appropriately reduced.

Many authorities administer up to half the potassium as the dihydrogen phosphate salt since all patients are phosphate depleted and become hypophosphatemic during treatment. From a theoretic standpoint, hypophosphatemia can lead to impaired oxyhemoglobin dissociation and neurologic and muscular dysfunction. From the clinical standpoint, however, controlled trials in DKA have shown no benefit of phosphate replacement. As long as the serum calcium concentration is normal, some of the potassium replacement can be achieved with phosphate, although our standard practice is to give only potassium chloride. Magnesium and calcium are lost in the urine during the osmotic diuresis. However, we normally do not replace these ions with IV therapy since deficits are rapidly corrected when the patient resumes a normal dietary intake.

Anticoagulation

Thromboembolism accounts for up to 33 percent of deaths in comatose patients with HHNC. This can occur up to 1 week after the acute event. Hyperosmolality, hyperviscosity, and low blood flow all contribute to produce a hypercoagulable state. Diffuse intravascular coagulation also can occur. We, therefore, routinely use low-dose heparin, 5,000 U subcutaneously every 6 hours, in all patients with HHNC. In patients with extreme hyperosmolarity and in those who are comatose or have other recognized risk factors for thrombosis, we use full dose IV heparin. It is important to rule out intracranial bleeding in patients with focal neurologic signs before heparin therapy.

Antibiotics

Some authors recommend routine use of broad-spectrum antibiotics in all patients with HHNC. We prefer to search for objective evidence of infection by obtaining a chest x-ray, blood cultures, microscopy and cultures of sputum and urine. Antibiotics are administered only if there is reasonable suspicion of infection. Low-grade fever and elevation of the neutrophil count are common and may be attributable to the hyperosmolar state per se and elevated circulating catecholamine levels. Leukocyte counts can rise to as high as 20×10^9 per liter in the absence of infection owing to catecholamine-induced margination of the peripheral leukocyte pool.

Search for Precipitating Cause

Many patients die from the underlying precipitating cause of HHNC. Therefore, it is imperative that any associated medical illness be identified and, if possible, treated vigorously. Thorough physical examination, chest x-ray, electrocardiogram, search for infection, and other investigations as indicated are essential.

■ GENERAL MANAGEMENT

The prerequisite of successful management is attention to detail (Table 3). Pulse, blood pressure, urine output, central venous pressure, and capillary blood glucose should be monitored hourly. Laboratory analysis of blood glucose, urea, creatinine, and electrolytes should be performed at presentation and at 2, 5, and 12 hours and every 12 hours thereafter. If significant abnormalities in the serum sodium or potassium concentrations are present, more frequent measurement may be needed. It is essential to record all results on a flowsheet, so that trends in parameters can be spotted easily. If the patient is semicomatose or comatose, a nasogastric tube should be inserted to prevent aspiration of gastric content. Urinary catheterization is important if the patient is comatose, uncooperative, or unable to void spontaneously, or has passed no urine the first 3 hours of treatment. In comatose patients a thorough search for toxins and central nervous system catastrophes should be undertaken. However, it is worth noting that it may take a fully comatose HHNC patient up to 72 hours to reach full consciousness despite prompt normalization of all biochemical and metabolic abnormalities.

■ LATE MANAGEMENT

When the patient is able to eat and drink normally, IV therapy should be stopped and subcutaneous insulin begun, generally as twice daily injections of Regular and intermediate-acting insulin. Oral potassium replacement also may be useful. It is our policy to continue insulin therapy until full recovery from the acute event has taken place. After some days, or weeks, it may be possible to stop insulin therapy and switch the patient to oral agents or dietary treatment alone. However, this should be done under careful supervision.

■ COMPLICATIONS AND PITFALLS IN MANAGEMENT

Fluid overload is the most common complication of therapy and can be avoided by close monitoring of fluid balance and physical examination of the patient. Cerebral edema is much more rare in HHNC than in DKA and can be minimized by allowing the blood glucose concentration to fall slowly during the first 24 hours of therapy to levels that are not below 250 mg per deciliter. Localizing neurologic signs and grand mal seizures may resolve completely on correction of the metabolic state. Hypernatremia is the most common metabolic complication and can result in a deterioration of the neurologic state after some initial recovery has been noted. It is prevented by careful attention to fluid replace-

Table 3 Monitoring of Initial Therapy	
Pulse, blood pressure, central venous pressure, urine output	Hourly
Capillary blood glucose	Hourly
Laboratory biochemistry: sodium, potassium, chloride, BUN, creatinine	At presentation; 2, 5, 12 hr

ment and appropriate infusion of hypotonic saline or 5 percent dextrose (as described earlier).

■ MORTALITY

Death rates as high as 30 to 45 percent commonly have been reported in HHNC, although a large recent series reported only 17 percent mortality. Advanced age and the severity of hypertonicity on admission are the main indicators of poor outcome. In some series, increased BUN and serum sodium concentrations also have been shown to be associated with increased morbidity and mortality. Mortality in HHNC has not changed significantly over the last 20 years. This is most likely due both to the advanced age of the patients and to the serious conditions that precipitate HHNC. Given the high mortality of HHNC, prevention is paramount. Since much of the mortality is related to the underlying precipitating cause, early identification of associated medical disorders and careful attention to the details of management are essential.

Suggested Reading

Alberti KG. Diabetic emergencies. Br Med Bull 1989; 45:242–250.
Proponent of isotonic fluid replacement.

Ennis ED, Stahl EJ von B, Kreisberg RA. The hyperosmolar hyperglycemic syndrome. Diabetes Rev 1994; 1:115–126.
An overview.

Gehab MA. Clinical approach to the hyperosmolar patient. Critical Care Clinics 1987; 5:797–805.
Discuss hyperosmolarity in general, and in HHNC.

Gerich JE, Martin MM, Recant L. Clinical and metabolic characteristics of hyperosmolar nonketotic coma. Diabetes 1971; 20:228–238.
Description of large series and discussion of metabolic state.

Kitabchi AE, Murphy MB. Diabetic ketoacidosis and hyperosmolar hyperglycemic nonketotic coma. Med Clin North Am 1988; 72:1545–1563.
Lively discussion of the therapeutic controversies. The author is a proponent of hypotonic fluid replacement.

Marshall SM, Alberti KG. Hyperosmolar nonketotic diabetic coma. In: KG Alberti, LP Krall, eds. The Diabetes annual. 4th ed. Amsterdam: Elsevier Science Publishers, 1988:235.
A detailed overview covering all aspects.

Matz R. Hyperosmolar nonacidotic diabetes (HNAD). In: H Rifkin, D Porte Jr, eds. Diabetes mellitus, Theory and practice. 4th ed. New York: Elsevier, 1990:604.
A thoughtful review, particularly of pathogenesis.

THERAPEUTIC CONSIDERATIONS FOR LACTIC ACIDOSIS

Scott E. Buchalter, M.D.
Robert A. Kreisberg, M.D.

Lactic acidosis (LA), now recognized as the most common cause of metabolic acidosis in hospitalized patients, was brought into perspective by Huckabee in 1961, when he demonstrated that the association of lactate and metabolic acidosis occurred both in situations of tissue hypoxia and, less commonly (and less well understood), with certain disorders such as liver disease, malignancies, diabetes mellitus, and rare enzymic deficiencies and with exposure to or ingestion of various drugs and toxins. Though most often seen in situations of abnormal tissue perfusion or oxygenation in critically ill patients, the occurrence of LA in situations where reduced oxygen delivery is not apparent suggests that this disorder is biochemically and pathophysiologically heterogeneous.

Regardless of causes, an accumulation of lactate with an associated acidosis indicates that normal pathways of lactate production and utilization have been disrupted. The poor prognosis of critically ill patients with LA underscores the need for improved understanding of the pathogenesis and therapy of this disorder. Although specific therapy remains unsatisfying, better understanding of the biochemistry and metabolic fate of lactate has provided insight for re-evaluating currently accepted modes of therapy and examining new ones.

Several recent reviews provide comprehensive discussions of the regulatory aspects of lactate biochemistry. In this chapter, a brief summary of key aspects of lactate metabolism provides a basis for a more in-depth discussion of the therapy of LA.

■ METABOLIC BASIS FOR THERAPY OF LACTIC ACIDOSIS

Lactate is a metabolic end product, capable of being consumed or produced only through conversion to or from pyruvate. Thus, understanding the control mechanisms of glycolysis and the metabolic fate of pyruvate is central to understanding events leading to the generation of a clinical lactic acidosis.

Occurring in virtually all tissues, glycolysis is the cytosolic pathway that oxidizes glucose to pyruvate and is the predominant mechanism providing substrate for subsequent formation of adenosine triphosphate (ATP). The predominant mechanisms for control of oxidation of glucose to pyruvate are related to enzymatic activity and the reduction/oxidation

(or redox) state in the cytosol of the cell. Therefore, further understanding of the pathogenesis of LA can be simplified by concentrating on a limited number of key biochemical reactions (Fig. 1).

The phosphofructokinase (PFK) reaction, one of the major rate-limiting steps in glycolysis, is inhibited both by ATP and by a decrease in intracellular pH. Conversely, its activity (and thus glycolytic flux) is enhanced by increased concentrations of ADP, AMP, and phosphate, as well as alkalosis. Thus, conditions that increase cellular metabolic demands or decrease production of ATP, such as hypoxia, serve to stimulate PFK and the formation of pyruvate.

Another pivotal step in glycolysis is the oxidation of glyceraldehyde-3-phosphate. NAD⁺ serves as a cofactor and is converted to NADH by the transfer of hydrogen. Thus, for glycolysis to continue, NAD⁺ must be regenerated. Aerobic tissues, under normal circumstances, regenerate NAD⁺ through oxidative reactions that occur in the mitochondria. Thus, under normal circumstances, both the energy state (ATP level) and the redox state (NADH-NAD⁺ ratio) of the cell are determined by mitochondrial oxidative reactions. During aerobic conditions, the bulk of pyruvate formed through glycolysis enters the mitochondria and serves as substrate for these oxidative processes in the tricarboxylic acid (TCA) cycle and, ultimately, the electron transport chain.

The production or utilization of lactate is regulated by a reversible cytosolic reaction, catalyzed by the enzyme lactate dehydrogenase (LDH):

$$\text{Pyruvate} + \text{NADH} + \text{H}^+ \xleftrightarrow{\text{LDH}} \text{Lactate} + \text{NAD}^+$$

The equilibrium constant (k) for this reaction strongly favors the formation of lactate. Under aerobic conditions, some lactate is formed from pyruvate, with an expected lactate-pyruvate (L-P) ratio of approximately ten to one. Rearranging the previous equation yields the following:

$$\text{Lactate} = k\ \frac{(\text{pyruvate})\ (\text{NADH})\ (\text{H}^+)}{\text{NAD}^+}$$

where k is the equilibrium constant for the reaction catalyzed by LDH; H⁺ is the cytosolic hydrogen ion concentration; and NADH and NAD⁺ are the concentration of free (unbound) reduced and oxidized pyridine nucleotides, respectively. It can be seen that the concentration of lactate in the cell is determined by the concentration of pyruvate, the redox state of the cytosol, and the intracellular hydrogen ion concentration.

Thus, lactate is produced normally in small amounts through glycolysis, along with stoichiometric amounts of hydrogen ion, and yet, under aerobic circumstances, complete oxidation of glucose to carbon dioxide and water is not acidifying. The final key concept in understanding LA lies in understanding the metabolic fate of lactate. As pointed out by Krebs and others, the overall reaction for glycolysis occurring in the cytosol ("aerobic" glycolysis) is likely:

$$\text{Glucose} + 2\text{ADP}^{3-} + 2\text{P}^{2-} \longrightarrow 2\ \text{Lactate}^{1-} + 2\text{ATP}^{4-}$$

Thus lactate, not lactic acid, is the end product. It appears that the hydrogen ion produced is related to subsequent hydrolysis of ATP, in the following manner:

$$ATP^{4-} \longrightarrow ADP^{3-} + P^{2-} + H^{+}$$

Under normal circumstances, this hydrogen ion is initially neutralized by intracellular buffers (bicarbonate). As a metabolic end product, lactate must be metabolized, either through oxidation in the TCA cycle or through conversion to glucose, which together constitute the Cori cycle, a pivotal pathway in liver and kidney by which lactate is salvaged and efficiently reutilized. Both of these processes consume hydrogen ion (or regenerate body pools of buffer) (Fig. 2). Thus, under normal conditions, glucose is oxidized to pyruvate, the bulk of which enters the mitochondria, leading to oxidative phosphorylation and efficient production of ATP. In the process, NAD^{+} is regenerated, ATP levels are adequate, glycolysis proceeds at a rate required for maintenance of homeostasis, and the efficient reutilization of lactate formed from pyruvate in the cytosol allows for consumption of hydrogen ion generated by the normal process of hydrolysis of ATP, thus maintaining acid-base balance.

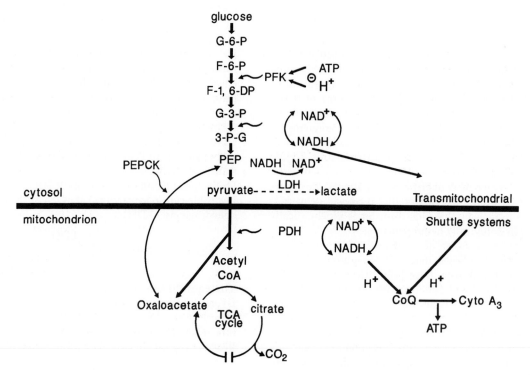

Figure 1

During aerobic conditions and normal mitochondrial function, glycolytic flux and the formation of pyruvate depend upon mitochondrial oxidative reactions to regenerate NAD^{+} and balanced concentrations of ATP and hydrogen ion. Small amounts of lactate are formed and reutilized.

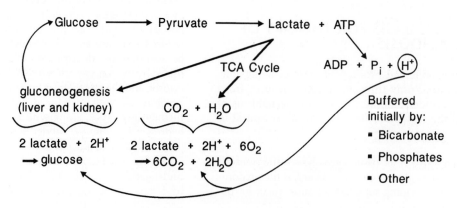

Figure 2

The Cori cycle and metabolic fate of lactate and hydrogen ion.

The abnormalities that occur in situations of hypoxia alter glycolysis and the delicate balance between the production and utilization of pyruvate, lactate, and hydrogen ion, resulting in LA. With impaired mitochondrial function, as occurs most commonly with reduced oxygen delivery, synthesis of ATP is impaired, and the reoxidation of NADH to NAD^+ is inhibited. Cellular stores of ATP and NAD^+ are markedly diminished. The development of LA in this setting can be understood by examining several important processes that are altered.

First, a reduction in ATP both stimulates glycolysis (through the PFK reaction) and the formation of pyruvate and inhibits the reutilization of pyruvate in gluconeogenesis through conversion to oxaloacetate, the obligatory first step in gluconeogenesis.

Second, a reduction in NAD^+ inhibits mitochondrial conversion of pyruvate to acetyl-CoA through the enzyme pyruvate dehydrogenase but stimulates the conversion of pyruvate to lactate. This process regenerates NAD^+, allowing the conversion of glyceraldehyde-3-phosphate to 3-phosphoglycerate and glycolysis to continue and providing, however inefficiently, critically needed ATP, which is in turn rapidly hydrolyzed to ADP and hydrogen ion. Since reutilization of lactate through gluconeogenesis or in the TCA cycle is markedly impaired in this setting, neither lactate nor hydrogen ion can be reutilized. Thus, hyperlactatemia and a metabolic acidosis ensue, with a reduction in the body pool of buffer, and with L-P ratios much greater than ten to one. If mechanisms that reutilize lactate are intact in situations where pyruvate concentration is increased, such as in hypermetabolic states like sepsis, burns, or trauma, one may see a modest hyperlactatemia (serum lactate levels 2.0 to 5.0 mEq per liter), with a normal L-P ratio, and no acidosis. Though sometimes very difficult to distinguish clinically from an elevated lactate related to reduced tissue oxygenation, the difference may be very important clinically and serves now as further basis for discussion of issues related to diagnosis and therapy of LA, which must of necessity be examined together.

■ CLASSIFICATION OF LACTIC ACIDOSIS

A modest elevation in blood lactate concentration (usually no greater than 5.0 mEq per liter) may occur with hypermetabolic states without changes in blood pH, and may represent an increased "setpoint" for lactate. In contrast, true LA, in which an elevated blood lactate (usually greater or equal to 5.0 mEq per liter) is associated with significant hemodynamic and metabolic decompensation, usually has a lowered blood pH. The most widely used classification of LA was devised in 1976 by Cohen and Woods, who divided LA into two broad categories: type A is LA associated with disorders in which there exists clinical evidence of reduced oxygen delivery (DO_2); type B is LA not associated with clinical evidence for reduced DO_2 (Table 1).

Type A LA is much more common than type B and forms the basis for most of our understanding of the biochemistry of LA. Obviously, for oxidative metabolism to continue, oxygen supply and demand must be matched. Type A LA occurs when systemic DO_2 (the product of cardiac output, concentration, and percent oxygen saturation of hemoglobin, plus a small amount of oxygen carried dissolved in blood) is inadequate to meet the metabolic demands of tissues, resulting in anaerobic glycolysis. Systemic shock; regional hypoperfusion, hypoxemia, and/or anemia severe enough to reduce DO_2; and carbon monoxide intoxication are all examples of LA related to decreased oxygen delivery. Vigorous exercise, seizures, and severe asthma are examples of type A LA where tissue oxygen demand outstrips supply. The hemodynamic abnormalities of mismatched supply and demand with type A LA precede and lead to the LA.

Type B LA develops in settings in which there is no clinical evidence for reduced DO_2 to tissues, and has been further divided into subcategories related to underlying disease (type B_1), drugs or toxins (type B_2), and inborn errors of metabolism (type B_3). The mechanisms by which LA develops in this large group of disorders are not clear, and the diversity of settings in which LA occurs supports the concept

---

Table 1 Some Causes of Lactic Acidosis

TYPE A (CLINICAL EVIDENCE OF INADEQUATE OXYGEN DELIVERY)
  Shock (septic, cardiogenic, hypovolemic)
  Severe hypoxemia or anemia
  Carbon monoxide poisoning
TYPE B (NO CLINICAL EVIDENCE OF INADEQUATE OXYGEN DELIVERY)
  B_1 (LA associated with underlying disease)
  Diabetes mellitus
  Malignancy
  Liver disease
  Sepsis
  B_2 (LA due to drugs or toxins)
  Biguanides
  Ethanol or methanol
  Acetaminophen
  Salicylates
  Cyanide
  Nitroprusside

B_3 (LA due to congenital defects in gluconeogenesis or pyruvate oxidation)
  Deficiency of:
  Glucose-6-phosphatase
  Pyruvate carboxylase
  Fructose 1,6-diphosphatase
  Pyruvate dehydrogenase
  Oxidative phosphorylation

that these disorders are biochemically and pathophysiologically heterogeneous.

■ DIAGNOSIS OF LACTIC ACIDOSIS

Determination of serum lactate concentrations in the setting of obvious clinical shock with acidemia may be unnecessary, at least diagnostically. However, in the absence of clinical signs of hypoperfusion, or when an unexplained anion-gap acidosis exists, the demonstration of an elevated blood lactate concentration allows for a diagnosis of LA to be made and prompts a search for occult tissue hypoperfusion.

In the past, significant controversy has existed regarding the diagnostic criteria used to define LA. Recent prospective data suggest that a blood lactate concentration greater than or equal to 5.0 mEq per liter and a blood pH of less than 7.35 constitute the criteria for defining LA in which false-positive and false-negative diagnoses would be minimized. Though these criteria are generally accepted, it should be emphasized that LA frequently occurs in association with disorders in which other acid-base disturbances are common and dynamic in nature, such as the metabolic alkalosis of liver disease, or hyperventilation related to early sepsis or mechanical ventilation which may result in a normal or near-normal pH and mask a significant LA.

Interpretation of blood lactate concentrations less than 5 mEq per liter becomes somewhat problematic, since it is intuitive that, despite specific criteria, the range of "significant" hyperlactatemia should be considered with knowledge of underlying clinical disorders. Most authors agree that a lactate concentration of less than 2.0 mEq per liter is normal, suggesting no underlying derangement of lactate metabolism or oxygen delivery. Blood lactate concentrations between 2.0 and 5.0 mEq per liter represent a "gray zone," the clinical significance of which is not clear, and critically ill patients with lactate levels in this range, especially without an associated acidosis, are particularly challenging.

Under normal physiologic circumstances (i.e., in patients with intact autoregulatory mechanisms), oxidative metabolism is under close control through metabolic, neural, and hormonal feedbacks systems, such that systemic and regional blood flow and DO_2 are adjusted for tissue needs. The specific mechanisms responsible for the autoregulation are in part speculative and will not be discussed here. However, this autoregulatory capacity allows for increasing systemic extraction of oxygen to meet tissue requirements in the setting of reduced DO_2. Thus, systemic oxygen consumption (VO_2; the product of cardiac output and arterial-venous oxygen difference), a measure of oxidative metabolism, remains normal and is independent of supply of oxygen over a wide range of changing values for DO_2). Ultimately, beyond the point of maximal tissue oxygen extraction, a further reduction in DO_2 fails to serve systemic oxidative metabolic needs, and anaerobic glycolysis and lactic acidosis ensue, represented clinically by a falling DO_2. Below this critical DO_2, VO_2 becomes dependent upon delivery, and a state of "supply-dependency" exists. A rise in DO_2 (such as with administration of volume, blood, vasodilators, or possibly inotropes) associated with a concomitant increase in VO_2 and a subsequent fall in blood lactate concentration would suggest the existence of tissue hypoperfusion and would support continued therapy to augment DO_2. In patients who are critically ill with LA, but with presumably normal autoregulatory mechanisms (such as uncomplicated hypovolemic, hemorrhagic, or cardiogenic shock), one should continue to augment DO_2 until VO_2 reaches a plateau, during which time the lactate levels should return toward normal.

In contrast, in many patients with sepsis, the adult respiratory distress syndrome, trauma, or fulminant hepatic failure, tissue autoregulatory capacity is deranged, resulting in an inability to increase systemic oxygen extraction in the face of increasing tissue needs. This extraction defect, which in essence "fixes" maximal oxygen extraction at an abnormally low level, creates the situation whereby VO_2 and oxidative metabolism are dependent upon DO_2 over a much greater range of delivery than would be expected.

This pathologic supply dependency of oxygen consumption is usually associated with markers of lost autoregulation (reduced systemic vascular resistance) and reduced systemic oxygen extraction (increased PvO_2). In contrast to the normal state with intact autoregulation, a rising or normal PvO_2 in this circumstance may not be an indication of adequate tissue oxygenation, and may in fact be associated with a severe lactic acidosis. The preponderance of data suggests that this disordered autoregulation and extraction defect is related to microcirculatory abnormalities, with maldistribution of flow among organ systems and within tissues of organs with varying needs.

The existence of supply-dependent oxygen consumption is very useful in the diagnosis and treatment of patients with hyperlactatemia of uncertain significance, such as those with lactate levels in the 2.0 to 5.0 mEq per liter range and/or with disorders associated with acid-base disturbances that mask underlying acidemia. In these settings with only mild to moderate hyperlactatemia, the demonstration of supply-dependent VO_2 (i.e., an increase in VO_2 associated with augmented DO_2), accompanied by reduction in lactate levels, is consistent with occult tissue hypoperfusion and an oxygen debt and would support continued efforts to further augment DO_2.

In contrast, some patients with sepsis or other disorders, particularly after initial resuscitation, will not have obvious systemic hypoperfusion and may demonstrate hyperlactatemia, usually in the 2.0 to 5.0 mEq per liter range, with an increased cardiac output and no acidosis. In response to augmentation of DO_2, VO_2 and lactate levels may remain constant, indicating that the patient is likely not supply dependent, implying a metabolic cause for the modest hyperlactatemia. In this regard, major abnormalities in glucose metabolism have been shown to exist with sepsis and trauma, including insulin resistance in skeletal muscle, impaired pyruvate dehydrogenase (PDH) activity and reduced utilization of pyruvate in the TCA cycle, and increased oxidation of branched-chain amino acids in skeletal muscle. These processes favor the formation of lactate and alanine, which are converted subsequently to glucose, thus fueling glycolysis and increasing pyruvate concentrations, such that the cycle is repeated. In these hypercatabolic states, the gray-zone hyperlactatemia of 2.0 to 5.0 mEq per liter might be viewed as an alteration in the normal setpoint for blood lactate concentration. It is not clear in this setting that further attempts to increase DO_2 or reduce lactate are beneficial.

In summary, the demonstration of supply dependency in the setting of initially increased lactate concentrations and concomitant lactate reduction with augmentation in DO_2, regardless of underlying mechanisms for hyperlactatemia, suggests that inadequate DO_2 and tissue hypoperfusion exists and should be corrected. This finding is particularly important in patients with gray-zone hyperlactatemia, because failure to recognize perfusion defects could lead to inadequate hemodynamic resuscitation. These patients should be managed by increasing DO_2 (fluids, blood, possibly inotropic agents), until VO_2 reaches a plateau, as long as lactate is elevated and decreasing with treatment.

It is important to recognize that in addition to metabolic alkalosis, other situations could exist which could mask LA, either by altering the magnitude of the expected anion gap, which would be higher than expected for a given level of hyperlactatemia with unmeasured cations (phosphate), or anions (beta-hydroxybutyrate, D (−) lactate); and lower than expected with hypoalbuminemia or hyperglobulinemia. Additionally, in patients with significant depletion of glycogen stores not receiving nutritional support, the elevation in lactate and the associated acidosis may be spuriously low and therefore misleading in a situation of hypoperfusion.

■ MANAGEMENT OF LACTIC ACIDOSIS

It must be remembered that the cornerstone for treatment of LA is treatment of the underlying disorders and factors that predispose to lactic acidosis. The high mortality in cases of LA relates both to the severity of associated primary disorders and to our inability to specifically treat the LA itself.

In addition to therapy of the underlying disorder, DO_2 must be optimized. Clinically obvious shock should be dealt with swiftly and aggressively. Critically ill patients who have mild to moderate hyperlactatemia (2.0 to 5.0 mEq per liter), with or without an associated acidosis, should have a trial to determine whether an occult perfusion defect and supply dependency exist.

Beyond these approaches, treatment for LA is empiric, supportive, and often unsuccessful. Perhaps the most controversial question regards the use of bicarbonate therapy in patients with severe acidosis. The use of bicarbonate as a buffering agent would seem rational and important for improvement in DO_2, providing time for treatment of the underlying disorder. Unfortunately, the use of bicarbonate is not without adverse effects, and its use has undergone intense scrutiny. The development of electrolyte disturbances (hypokalemia or hypocalcemia) and paradoxical cerebrospinal fluid acidosis have been reported in association with bicarbonate administration, but are rare and probably of little clinical significance. Because of the large quantities of bicarbonate required, hypernatremia, hyperosmolality, and volume overload can become significant problems, especially in the setting of already reduced flow, poor renal perfusion, and reduced renal excretion of sodium and water. Further, a leftward shift in the oxyhemoglobin dissociation curve can occur, especially with overshoot alkalosis. These problems may be manageable by careful attention to volume status and acid base balance.

However, there are some adverse effects related to bicarbonate therapy that may be of great clinical importance, and largely unmanageable. In this regard, recent animal and human data suggest that the administration of sodium bicarbonate can significantly worsen myocardial function. The administration of bicarbonate likely leads to increased quantities of carbon dioxide (CO_2), which can rapidly gain access to the interior of the myocardial cell, causing a fall in intracellular pH and worsened myocardial cell function. The existence of this proposed mechanism is supported by the finding that carbicarb, which buffers in the same way as bicarbonate but does not generate CO_2, can improve cardiac output compared with bicarbonate. The reduced contractility and cardiac output just described might be especially important in clinical settings with LA where CO_2 removal is a problem, such as ventilatory failure or during cardiopulmonary resuscitation.

Further, bicarbonate may have a detrimental effect on lactate production, likely related to the effect of pH on PFK activity, which increases dramatically as pH rises from 6.80 to 7.20. Thus, bicarbonate administration might be expected to increase PFK activity, stimulating glycolysis and lactate production and possibly nullifying any potential benefit.

Finally, some animal data exist that suggest that bicarbonate might adversely affect survival. All these observations explain the current re-evaluation of the use of bicarbonate in the therapy of LA. Though adverse effects clearly may exist when bicarbonate is administered to patients with LA, data are not conclusive, and most clinicians would agree that administration of sodium bicarbonate should continue in severely acidotic patients with cardiovascular compromise to correct the systemic pH to 7.20 or greater and the serum bicarbonate level to 12 mEq per liter or greater, with careful attention to volume status and cardiac output. Some authors have suggested administering bicarbonate as a continuous infusion, since bolus administration has been noted to cause a transient drop in systemic vascular resistance and blood pressure.

Recent data have suggested that dichloroacetate (DCA) may be useful in the treatment of lactic acidosis. DCA has been shown to have a beneficial effect on LA production and utilization, in both animal and human studies of types A and B LA. Dichloroacetate activates PDH and augments both oxidation of pyruvate and aerobic lactate utilization. Probably related to increased ATP content, DCA exerts positive inotropic effects on myocardium and appears to increase cardiac output and produce peripheral vasodilatation. Animal and human data demonstrate that DCA markedly reduces lactate concentrations while increasing pH and bicarbonate levels. Some animal data suggest improved survival with DCA therapy compared with bicarbonate or saline therapy in some types of experimentally induced LA. Additionally, recent human studies demonstrate that many patients with LA, even those who fail to respond to bicarbonate, respond to DCA administration with a significant fall in lactate levels and an improvement in acidosis. Despite these findings, at least in these small studies, no clear improvement in survival was demonstrated. Nevertheless, DCA may be useful in the future treatment of LA, and data comparing DCA with standard (bicarbonate) therapy in a large series of patients with LA will likely be available in the near future.

Suggested Reading

Buchalter SE, Crain MR, Kreisberg R. Regulation of lactate metabolism in vivo. Diabetes Metab Rev 1989; 5:379–391.

Cohen RD, Woods HF. Clinical and biochemical aspects of lactic acidosis. Boston: Blackwell Scientific Publications, 1976.

Kreisberg RA. Lactic acidosis: An update. J Intensive Care Med 1987; 2:76–84.

Kreisberg RA. Pathogenesis and management of lactic acidosis. Annu Rev Med 1984; 35:181–193.

Madias NE. Lactic acidosis. Kidney Int 1986; 29:752–774.

Mizock BA. Controversies in lactic acidosis: Implications in critically ill patients. JAMA 1987; 258:497–501.

Mizock BA. Lactic acidosis. Disease-a-Month 35:235–300, 1989.

Narins RG, Cohen JJ. Bicarbonate therapy of organic acidosis: The case for its continued use. Ann Intern Med 1987; 106:615–618.

Stacpoole PW. Lactic acidosis: The case against bicarbonate therapy. Ann Intern Med 1986; 105:276–279.

INSULIN THERAPY IN TYPE 1 DIABETES MELLITUS

Jay S. Skyler, M.D.

Insulin was isolated and became available for clinical use in the early 1920s. It revolutionized the treatment of diabetes mellitus. Today, insulin therapy is required by essentially all patients with type 1 and many patients with type 2 diabetes. Although insulin has been available for 75 years, over the past two decades major advances have been made in the way insulin therapy is used in clinical practice. Much of the progress is a consequence of three factors: (1) the introduction of self-monitoring of blood glucose (SMBG) into routine practice; (2) a change in philosophy of diabetes management such that patient self-management and flexibility in life-style have come to drive contemporary treatment approaches; and (3) the demonstration that meticulous glycemic control reduces the risk of chronic complications. This chapter emphasizes these changing practices and treatment strategies for insulin therapy of type 1 diabetes mellitus.

■ INSULIN PHARMACOLOGY

Insulin was first isolated in 1921 by Banting and Best. Pancreatic extracts were found to lower blood glucose. These were first used in therapy in 1922. Soon thereafter, processes were developed for isolation and commercial production of insulin from beef and pork pancreas glands. Insulin was purified from acid-ethanol extracts of pancreas and crystallized-with zinc. The initial insulin preparations were relatively impure. The blood glucose lowering effect lasted a few hours, necessitating that injections be given several times daily.

Since that time, a number of modifications in the insulin production procedure have resulted in insulin preparations of improved purity, of varying action profiles (short acting, intermediate acting, prolonged), and with structure identical to native human insulin. Most recently, tailored genetically engineered alterations in the insulin molecule have resulted in insulin analogues with planned action profiles—either rapid onset or prolonged acting.

The major characteristics distinguishing insulin preparations today are degree of purity, species of origin, time course of action, concentration of insulin, and stability and miscibility.

It is also important to consider factors influencing the pharmacokinetics of insulin absorption, such as the site of injection.

Degree of Purity

Purity of insulin preparations generally is reflected by the amount of non–insulin-pancreatic proteins in the preparation. Proinsulin content is usually used to reflect purity. Insulins are defined as "purified" when they contain less than 10 parts per million (ppm) of proinsulin. This is true of all insulin preparations sold in the United States and is increasingly true in most other western countries.

Clinical problems related to impurity of insulin preparations include: (1) local and systemic insulin allergies; (2) lipodystrophy at injection sites; (3) immunologic insulin resistance; and (4) altered time course of action due to antibodies. These problems have been virtually eliminated by improvements in purification and by the advent of human insulin (see later discussion).

Improved purification over the past two decades has resulted in marked improvement in purity of commercially available insulin. Insulin formulated by recrystallization according to old U.S. Pharmacopoeia (USP) criteria was only 92 percent pure, containing 8 percent noninsulin substances. "Standard" (i.e., non-"purified") insulin preparations in the United States prior to the early 1970s contained more than 20,000 ppm of proinsulin, and even chromatographically purified "single-peak" insulin contained up to 10,000 ppm of proinsulin when first introduced in 1972. Improvements in

Supported by NIH Grant HL-36588, U.S. Public Health Service.

the production process throughout the 1970s progressively lowered that to less than 100 ppm by the end of the decade and nominally less than 10 ppm (actually <5 ppm) in standard insulin preparations now sold in the United States. Simultaneously, the purified "monocomponent" or "single-component" insulins have also undergone improvement such that the purity of these preparations now is usually less than 1 ppm of proinsulin. Although proinsulin is used as the marker for noninsulin proteins in pancreatic insulin preparations, other proteins are found as well, including pancreatic polypeptide, somatostatin, glucagon, and vasoactive intestinal peptide. These, too, have largely been eliminated by contemporary production processes.

Current preparations of Regular insulin are packaged at neutral pH. Initially, however, Regular insulin was prepared and marketed at acid pH, which was necessary both to solubilize other proteins in the extract and to protect the insulin from degradation by pancreatic enzymes contaminating the preparation.

Species of Origin

Until the early 1980s, commercial insulin preparations were derived by extraction from beef and pork pancreas. Most commercial preparations contained mixtures of beef and pork insulin, while others were of single-species origin. Purified insulin preparations generally were marketed as monospecies pork or beef. Over the past decade, insulin of the same amino acid sequence as native human insulin has been commercially produced both by recombinant DNA technology and by enzymatic conversion of pork insulin to the human sequence. Human insulin preparations are less immunogenic than animal preparations and are rapidly becoming the predominant species in the marketplace in western countries.

The recognition that human insulin differs in structure from that in animal preparations suggests that some of the immunogenicity of commercial preparations might be due as much to differences between species of insulin as to the impurities in the commercial products. The insulin molecule consists of two amino acids chains: an A chain of 21 amino acids and a B chain of 30 amino acids. Although relatively well conserved in nature, there are differences in amino acid sequences of insulin among different species. Those for beef and pork insulin, the commercial sources, are contrasted to human insulin in Table 1. Beef insulin differs from human insulin at three amino acid positions, whereas pork insulin differs from human insulin only at the terminal amino acid of the B chain. Because of the greater disparity between human insulin and beef insulin than between human insulin and pork insulin, pork insulin is less immunogenic than beef insulin. These differences in primary structure (along with impurities in preparations) are responsible for the immuno-

genicity of commerical insulin, which may lead to (1) local and systemic insulin allergies; (2) lipodystrophy at injection sites; (3) immunologic insulin resistance; and (4) formation of anti-insulin antibodies.

The use of human insulin obviates most of the immunogenicity of commercial preparations. Human insulin has been prepared in four ways: (1) extraction from pancreases of human cadavers; (2) full chemical peptide synthesis from the constituent amino acids; (3) semisynthetic production through enzymatic conversion of pork insulin to human insulin by transpeptidation, in which there is replacement of the B-30 alanine in pork insulin with threonine, resulting in a sequence identical to native human insulin; and (4) biosynthetic production through recombinant deoxyribonucleic acid (DNA) technologies. Several recombinant DNA processes have been used: (1) biosynthesis of A and B chains of human insulin in two separate clones of *Escherichia coli*, followed by chain purification and combination into insulin; (2) biosynthesis in *E. coli* of human proinsulin, the insulin precursor, followed by cleavage of the proinsulin into insulin and C-peptide, the connecting sequence which links the A and B chains; and (3) biosynthesis in *Saccharomyces cerevisiae* (a yeast) of an insulin precursor, in which a few amino acids link the A and B chains, followed by liberation of insulin from the precursor. All three of these recombinant " biosynthetic" processes have been found suitable for commercial insulin preparation, also has the "semisynthetic" enzymatic conversion method.

Human insulin has both reduced immunogenicity (i.e., fewer patients have the induction of insulin antibodies) and reduced antigenicity (i.e., there is a lowering of titer of anti-insulin antibody on substitution of human insulin for animal insulin) when compared with animal insulins. Therefore, only human insulin should be used in patients being exposed to insulin for the first time or in whom insulin use is anticipated as temporary (since starting and stopping insulin therapy increases the antigenic potential). Human insulin is the preferred insulin for patients having any of the immunologic side effects of animal insulin therapy. There is no obvious circumstance in which human insulin is contraindicated. Progressively, patients with stable diabetes on animal insulins are being converted to human insulin, which is now the predominant species in the marketplace. I am of the bias that animal insulins can be removed from production and eliminated from the marketplace.

Time Course of Insulin Action

The time course of action of insulin preparations can be divided into three general categories—rapid-onset short-acting (e.g., Regular [soluble] insulin and the analogue insulin lispro); intermediate-acting (e.g., NPH [isophane] and Lente [insulin zinc suspension]); and long-acting (e.g., Ultralente

Table 1 Species Differences of Insulins				
AMINO ACID POSITION				
	A CHAIN			**B CHAIN**
	8	9	10	30
Human	Threonine	Serine	Isoleucine	Threonine
Pork	Threonine	Serine	Isoleucine	Alanine
Beef	Alanine	Serine	Valine	Alanine

[extended insulin zinc suspension]). Table 2 summarizes the generally reported time action profiles—time to peak action and duration of action—of insulin preparations. A general principle is that the longer the time to peak, the broader the peak will be and the longer will be the duration of action. Another principle is that the breadth of the peak and the duration of action will be lengthened by increasing the insulin dose. The values included in Table 2 are for adult doses of 10 to 15 U, or 0.1 to 0.2 U per kilogram.

Regular Insulin

Regular (also known as soluble or unmodified) insulin has relatively rapid onset and short duration of action. It may be given intravenously (IV), intramuscularly (IM), or subcutaneously (SC). When given IV, it has almost immediate onset of action and a circulating half-life of approximately 6 minutes. Peak blood glucose lowering effect is seen 20 to 30 minutes after an IV bolus of Regular insulin, and the effect is fully dissipated within 2 to 3 hours. Continuous IV infusions are useful for the treatment of diabetic ketoacidosis (DKA); during surgery or labor and delivery; and in acutely ill patients. After IM injections of Regular insulin, a blood glucose nadir is reached in 60 to 90 minutes, and some activity continues for 3 to 4 hours. Regular insulin, given IM on an hourly basis, has been used to treat DKA. The usual route is to give Regular insulin subcutaneously, which results in an onset of action in 30 to 60 minutes, a peak effect approximately 2 to 4 hours after administration, and a duration of action of 4 to 6 hours. The duration of action may be longer when large doses are used or when patients have insulin antibodies.

Rapidly Absorbed Analogues

Genetic engineering has led to the design of insulin analogues with rapid onset of action and shorter duration of action than human Regular insulin, when given subcutaneously. The basis for speeding the biologic availability of insulin is to accelerate insulin absorption, by making either monomeric preparations or ones that break down into monomers more rapidly than Regular insulin. One of these analogues, insulin lispro, has now reached clinical availability. Insulin lispro, or [Lys(B28), Pro(B29)]-human insulin, an insulin analogue in which the amino acid sequence of the B chain at positions 28 and 29 is inverted, has the most rapid onset and shortest duration of action of any currently available insulin preparation, i.e., onset of action in 15 to 30 minutes, a peak effect approximately 1 to 2 hours after administration, and a duration of action of 3 to 5 hours. This permits the administration of insulin lispro immediately before meals rather than the 20 to 40 minutes before meals needed for optimal administration of Regular insulin. It also may be given IV or IM. Its IV action profile is identical to that of Regular insulin. Studies have demonstrated that even meals of high caloric content can be accommodated without loss of glycemic control. Clinical trials have shown that insulin lispro used as preprandial insulin seems to permit greater freedom of life-style, to reduce early postprandial hyperglycemia, and to reduce late postprandial hypoglycemia, without alteration in overall glycemic control as measured by HbA_{1c}. Studies using insulin lispro in infusion pumps have demonstrated its use in this approach, provided that there is not extended interruption of insulin delivery.

Modified Insulins

Shortly after the introduction of insulin therapy in the 1920s, attempts began to develop insulin preparation with prolonged biologic availability. The basis for prolonging the biologic availability of insulin was to retard insulin absorption. This was done by either complexing insulin with various substances (e.g., basic proteins) or otherwise varying the physical form of the insulin (e.g., by altering the zinc content in acetate buffer) in order to delay its absorption. Although

Table 2 Time Course of Action of Insulin Preparations

INSULIN PREPARATION	ONSET OF ACTION (HR)	PEAK ACTION (HR)	DURATION OF ACTION (HR)
Rapid onset Regular (crystalline; soluble)	½–1	2–4	4–6
Rapid onset Lispro (analogue)	¼–½	1–2	3–5
Intermediate acting NPH (isophane)	1–4	8–10	12–20
Intermediate acting Lente (insulin zinc suspension)	2–4	8–12	12–20
Long acting Ultralente (extended insulin zinc suspension)	3–5	10–16	18–24
Combinations 70/30–70% NPH, 30% Regular	½–1	Dual	12–20
Combinations 50/50–50% NPH, 50% Regular	½–1	Dual	12–20

Based on doses of 0.1–0.2 U/kg, in the abdomen, for human insulin.

many variations on the theme were attempted, two procedures endured. One was the production of neutral protamine Hagedorn (NPH) insulin, where absorption is retarded by protamine. The other was the development of the "Lente" series by the use of zinc-insulin complexes.

Neutral Protamine Hagedorn Insulin.
Neutral protamine Hagedorn insulin, also called "isophane insulin", was introduced in Europe in 1946 and in North America in 1949. This compound is produced by mixing insulin and protamine in a stoichiometric ratio, at neutral pH, in the presence of a small amount of zinc and phenol. This set of conditions was called "isophane" (Greek *iso* [equal] + *phane* [appearance]), as the insulin and protamine are present in controlled quantities so that there is no excess of either one. With an onset of action 1 to 4 hours after administration, NPH human insulin has a peak effect of 8 to 10 hours after administration and a duration of action of 12 to 20 hours.

Lente Insulins.
Insulin zinc suspensions were introduced in the early 1950s as the "*Lente*" (slow-acting) series of insulins. In these formulations, the time course of action is altered by creating relatively insoluble zinc-insulin complexes, in acetate buffer at physiologic pH. There are two physical forms of these insulins; crystalline and amorphous. The amorphous form is more rapidly absorbed and is called "Semilente insulin". The more insoluble crystalline form, "Ultralente insulin", is very long acting. "Lente insulin" is approximately 30 percent amorphous and 70 percent crystalline zinc insulin suspension (although it is not made in this way). The Lente series of insulins have time courses of action such that Lente human insulin is similar to NPH human insulin (for Lente: onset in 2 to 4 hours, peak in 8 to 12 hours, duration of 12 to 20 hours); Ultralente human insulin is of longer duration (onset in 3 to 5 hours, peak in 10 to 16 hours, duration of 18 to 24 hours). Semilente human insulin is not available.

Mixtures
Preparations of mixtures of Regular and NPH insulins are sold in the marketplace. In the United States, mixtures containing 70 percent NPH and 30 percent Regular insulin (called "70/30") and mixtures containing 50 percent NPH and 50 percent Regular insulin (called "50/50") are available. In Europe, a series of insulin mixtures are available, containing 10 percent, 20 percent, 30 percent, 40 percent, or 50 percent Regular, with the balance as NPH.

Premixed insulins are helpful with the treatment of infants, elderly patients, and blind patients, all of whom may have difficulty mixing insulin in the syringe. However, these mixtures limit flexibility and are not useful for most patients using flexible or intensive insulin programs.

Insulin Concentration
Insulin was initially prepared at a concentration of 5 U per milliliter. This was rapidly increased to 10 and 20 U per milliliter. By 1924 and 1925, preparations of 40 and 80 U per milliliter, known as U-40 and U-80 insulin, were introduced and remained the basic concentrations marketed for the next half century. In 1972 and 1973, preparations of 100 U per milliliter, known as U-100 insulin, were introduced. Subsequently, in the United States (and many other countries), the other concentrations have been withdrawn, U-80 in 1980 (in

the United States), and U-40 in 1991 (in the United States). For special circumstances, highly concentrated U-500 Regular insulin (500 U per milliliter) is available.

Stability and Miscibility
Insulin is stable for long periods of time if refrigerated. However, insulin is generally stable at room temperature for several weeks and does not need to be stored in the refrigerator after the bottle is opened. On the other hand, it should not be exposed to extremes of temperature, such as might occur in a car, near a window, or next to a heating or air-conditioning vent. It should not be exposed to direct sunlight or heat (including temperatures above 25° C or 75° F). Also, insulin should not be frozen.

Only Regular insulin and insulin lispro are in solution. Other insulin preparations are in suspension. Vials containing insulin suspensions must be gently rolled, in order to assure a uniform suspension, before the insulin is withdrawn from the vial.

Mixtures of two types of insulin vary in their degree of stability in vitro. Regular and NPH insulins are freely miscible in all proportions. These insulins may be mixed in the same syringe and their action profiles maintained. On the other hand, mixtures of Regular insulin and insulins of the Lente series may not be stable in vitro. When Regular insulin is mixed with Lente insulins (either Lente or Ultralente), the rapid onset of the Regular insulin may be blunted if the insulin remains in the syringe for more than a few minutes. There may be loss of rapid activity in as few as 2 to 10 minutes. However, most or all of the rapid action is retained if mixing is done in a syringe immediately before injection. Full action is retained if separate syringes are used to inject the insulin through a single needle. Loss of soluble material from such mixtures increases over time (at least up to 24 hours) and with increased proportions of Lente in the mixture.

Regular insulin preparations containing phosphate buffer (e.g., Velosulin-BR) can not be mixed with the Lente series, as the phosphate causes precipitation and insulin activity will be lost.

For reproducibility and to assure equivalent dosing of insulin, it is important for patients to follow routinely from day to day the same technique for measuring insulin dose, mixing insulins, and administering insulin. If a patient is having significant glycemic excursions surrounding meals, and needs a more rapid insulin effect, consider that there may be some loss of rapid insulin activity. This can be tested by temporarily switching to separate injections. For patients who have their insulin premixed in the syringe by health care personnel or family and saved for one or more days before use, it is desirable to be sure that an exception is not made on the day the mixing is actually done. Namely, a visiting nurse premixing insulin for a week should mix the insulin for the day she or he will next visit, so that all syringes have been stored for at least 24 hours prior to use.

Pharmacokinetics of Insulin Absorption
A critical determinant of insulin availability is its absorption characteristics from subcutaneous tissue. Subcutaneous insulin regimens are based on the assumption that insulin absorption and availability are predictable and reproducible. Yet, many factors may influence insulin absorption and alter insulin availability. Indeed, intraindividual variation in

insulin absorption from day to day is approximately 25 percent, and between patients is up to 50 percent. Although this variation is approximately the same (in percentage terms) for all insulin preparations, in absolute terms (minutes or hours) there will be much less variation in absorption of rapidly absorbed insulins (Regular of lispro) and greater variation in absorption of longer acting insulins. As a consequence, insulin programs that emphasize rapid-onset insulin are more reproducible in their effects on blood glucose.

Injection Site

There are regional differences in insulin absorption, especially for rapidly absorbed insulin. Absorption is fastest from the abdomen, followed by the arm, buttocks, and thigh. Differences in absorption rate among these areas are likely due to variation in blood flow. The variation is sufficiently great that random rotation of injection sites, once routinely taught to diabetic patients, should be avoided. It is desirable to rotate injection sites within regions rather than among regions. Any particular injection (e.g., prebreakfast) should be administered in the same region to decrease day-to-day variability. Since the abdomen ordinarily is the region with the most rapid insulin absorption (in the absence of exercise), it may be the preferred injection region for preprandial injections. Some patients are willing to use the abdomen for all preprandial injections, rotating sites within that region. Others will use the abdomen for the prebreakfast injection, another region for the prelunch or presupper injection, and so on.

Selection of the injection site can be used to influence the time course of action of any insulin formulation. The choice of injection sites also depends on the insulin program prescribed and the patient's life-style. This is particularly the case for intermediate- or long-acting insulins. Thus, if an intermediate-acting insulin is used to provide basal insulin for a long period of the day (15 hours or more), it is desirable to inject into a site from which absorption is slow, e.g., the thigh. On the other hand, if the intermediate-acting insulin is used to provide basal insulin for a shorter period of the day (e.g., 8 to 10 hours), any injection site may be used. However, if empirically the duration of action of any insulin preparation is longer or shorter than desired, a site may be chosen that provides faster or slower insulin absorption.

Timing of Premeal Insulin Injections

In order to match insulinemia with glycemic excursions after meals, timing of preprandial insulin injections is crucial. For Regular insulin, rather than injection just prior to eating, the desired injection time optimally is 30 to 60 minutes before eating, with 20 to 30 minutes being a practical alternative. In contrast, with insulin lispro, injection should immediately precede meal consumption.

However, the timing of injections should be altered depending on the level of premeal glycemia. Thus, in the face of blood glucose levels above a patient's target range, it may be desirable to increase the interval between insulin administration and meal consumption, to permit the insulin to begin to have its effect. If premeal blood glucose levels are below a patient's target range, it is desirable to delay the administration of Regular insulin until immediately prior to meal consumption and to either decrease the dose of insulin

lispro or delay its administration until after the initiation of meal consumption.

Factors Increasing Insulin Absorption Rate

Blood flow and skin thickness influence insulin absorption. Physical exercise increases blood flow to an exercising part and thus accelerates absorption of insulin in that region. Sporadic exercise may induce variability in insulin absorption. One should try to avoid injections in a region that will be exercised while that injection is absorbed. For example, when planning exercise (e.g., jogging) shortly after injection, one should avoid giving that injection into a limb that will be undergoing that exercise (in the case of jogging, the thighs). When exercise is contemplated, one might use the abdomen preferentially, since this is the least likely region to have significant increases in absorption (unless the exercise includes sit-ups).

Other factors influencing absorption of Regular insulin are ambient temperature (e.g., a hot bath or sauna), smoking, and local massage of the injection site.

In very thin patients, there may be little subcutaneous tissue, resulting in insulin being injected intramuscularly rather than subcutaneously. This will result in more rapid absorption of any given preparation. It may mean that a different formulation should be selected. For example, human Ultralente insulin may be used as an intermediate-acting insulin in such patients. Or, the interval between injection of preprandial Regular insulin and meal consumption may need to be shortened. Insufficient information is available about insulin lispro in such circumstances.

■ PRINCIPLES OF THERAPY

Patients with type 1 diabetes do not produce insulin and thus are dependent on exogenous insulin for survival. As a consequence of insulin deficiency, hyperglycemia ensues, and the diabetic state develops.

Physiologic insulin secretion includes both continuous basal insulin secretion and substrate-related incremental insulin secretion following meal consumption. Basal insulin secretion modulates hepatic glucose production and metabolic homeostasis in the postabsorptive period. Thus, basal insulinemia restrains hepatic glucose production and keeps it in equilibrium with basal glucose utilization by the brain and other tissues that are obligate glucose consumers. After meals, substrate-related incremental insulin secretion stimulates glucose utilization and storage, while inhibiting hepatic glucose output. Figure 1 depicts hypothetical glucose and insulin profiles in a nondiabetic individual.

Insulin is essential for the physiologic utilization of all substrates, and thus is the primary regulator of energy metabolism. Therefore, underlying the management of type 1 diabetes is the necessity to balance energy availability (food intake) with energy expenditure (activity) and insulin dosage. From this framework, three components of therapy emerge: (1) the nutritional plan, (2) exercise, and (3) insulin dosage. Successful treatment of diabetes then, by definition, involves the balancing of these three components and careful monitoring of that balance (by patient SMBG). The attainment of balance among food, activity, and insulin assumes that neither physical nor emotional stress is altering this balance, by stress-induced secretion of glucose counter-regulatory hormones (e.g., catecholamines, glucagon, cortisol, growth hormone).

Since the patient must be engaged in this balancing on a daily basis, there are two additional critical principles: (1) patient education is essential to successful therapy, and (2) the treatment program must be sufficiently flexible and dynamic to allow for highly varied and changing life-styles without sacrificing careful metabolic control.

■ THERAPEUTIC STRATEGIES

There are a number of different therapeutic strategies for the management of type 1 insulin-dependent diabetes mellitus. For the past two decades, several new strategies have been evolving.

The term "conventional insulin therapy" has been used to describe an approach that provides global insulin replacement (one or two injections of primarily intermediate-acting insulin), a defined prescribed meal plan, periodic monitoring of therapy, and modest treatment goals (e.g., avoidance of both ketoacidosis and of frequent or severe hypoglycemia); yet, few, if any, diabetes experts recommend this strategy today. Thus, "conventional" therapy is not conventional. Rather, it is obsolete. Perhaps a better term would be "global insulin therapy".

I have used the term "intensive insulin therapy" (or more accurately, "intensive therapy of type 1 diabetes") to describe a system of management that includes a number of important therapeutic elements described in more detail in Table 3. In general, this approach involves multiple insulin components for different time periods of the day, balancing of food intake with activity and insulin dosage, frequent monitoring of therapy, and variable (but defined) treatment goals which often involve achievement of near-normal glycemia.

I use the term "flexible insulin therapy" to modify the description "intensive insulin therapy" to specifically emphasize the need for preprandial insulin before each meal, separate from basal insulin, and to allow more liberal food choices (particularly in terms of size, timing, and potential omission of meals), while balancing food intake with activity and insulin dosage, and including even more frequent monitoring of therapy, in order to promote a more normal life-style. Thus, "flexible insulin therapy" is a variant of "intensive insulin therapy" which is becoming increasingly popular among experts. (The term "functional insulin therapy" has been used by Howorka to describe a specific program of "flexible insulin therapy").

Critical to both intensive and flexible insulin therapy is a multiple-component insulin program designed to provide effective insulinemia coinciding with each major meal and continuous basal insulinemia throughout the 24-hour day. Equally important is a careful balance of food intake, activity, and insulin dosage. The meal plan should be flexible and adapted to the patient's activity program. Instrumental to the overall plan is SMBG several times daily. The patient should take action on the basis of SMBG results, which are used to help make appropriate changes in insulin dosage, food intake, and activity profile. The changes are made according to a predetermined plan—set of algorithms—provided by the physician to the patient. Each patient should have defined blood glucose targets, individualized for their needs.

Implementation requires frequent contact between the patient and diabetes management team. Patient education is essential. Success depends on patient motivation. All patients also can benefit from psychological support, to deal with the stress created by the burdens imposed by the therapeutic program, the consequences of therapeutic errors, and the threat of devastating complications.

Assessment is made by independent (laboratory) determination of glycated hemoglobin, not by patient determination of SMBG. Self-monitoring of blood glucose is considered a part of therapy and not a means of assessment.

Alternative Definitions

In contrast to the way it is used here, the term "intensive insulin therapy" has had several different connotations in the literature and in clinical practice. Some authors and practitioners have based the definition on the tools of therapy used (e.g., SMBG; or use of either continuous subcutaneous insulin infusion [CSII] or multiple daily insulin injections [MDII]—defined as three or more per day); while others have based the definition on the goals of therapy used (e.g., near-normal levels of glycemia and of glycated hemoglobin); while still others have based the definition on the total system of therapy employed, as has been done herein.

It is limiting to base the definition on the tools of therapy used. Shortly after the introduction of SMBG, use of SMBG was equated by some to be intensive therapy. Yet, the mere measurement of blood glucose does not necessarily intensify therapy at all. On the other hand, intensive therapy does not require frequent blood glucose monitoring. The real issue,

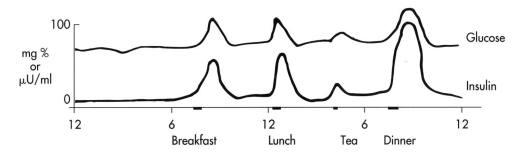

Figure 1
Schematic representation of 24-hour plasma glucose and insulin profiles in a hypothetical nondiabetic individual.

however, is what one does with the blood glucose information. Likewise, although MDDII and CSII may be important methods of insulin delivery, they are merely ways of delivering the insulin and do not of themselves necessarily intensify therapy.

To base information on the goals of therapy, i.e., the blood glucose targets that are sought, is also limiting. The assumption in such a definition is that meticulous glycemic control is the central theme of intensive management. However, it must be noted that attempts at meticulous control are not warranted in all patients, e.g., those who have either hypoglycemic unawareness or counter-regulatory unresponsiveness. In fact, meticulous control is contraindicated in such circumstances. Nevertheless, intensive therapy is not only useful, but probably is essential, in such patients.

Therefore, all of these are important components of intensive therapy. Therefore, it is best defined as an overall system of diabetes management involving all of the elements listed in Table 3.

Flexible Insulin Programs—General Points

Patients with type 1 diabetes lack both basal and prandial insulin secretion. Contemporary insulin programs for type 1 diabetes (both intensive and flexible) have multiple components that attempt to mimic these two normal types of endogenous physiologic insulin secretion by providing com-

ponents that give prandial insulin coinciding with each meal, and separate components that provide basal insulinemia overnight and between meals. Flexible insulin programs specifically emphasize the need for preprandial insulin before each meal.

Prandial Insulin Therapy

Prandial incremental insulin secretion is best duplicated by giving preprandial injections of rapid-onset insulin (Regular or lispro) prior to each meal, by a syringe, by pen, or by pump. Each preprandial insulin dose is adjusted individually to provide meal insulinemia appropriate to the size of the meal. In addition, the timing of meals need not be fixed, and meals may be omitted along with the accompanying preprandial insulin dose. The use of preprandial insulin doses permits total flexibility in meal timing.

Regular insulin administered subcutaneously is relatively rapid in its onset of action, but not immediate. Therefore, as noted earlier, it is best to give prandial injections at least 20 to 30 minutes (or longer) prior to eating a given meal in an attempt to have prandial insulinemia parallel meal related glycemic excursions. Insulin lispro has more rapid onset and may be given immediately before eating a given meal.

Basal Insulin Therapy

Basal insulinemia is given either as (1) intermediate-acting insulin (NPH or Lente) at bedtime and in a small morning dose; (2) one or two daily injections of long-acting Ultralente insulin, which in most patients is relatively peakless after steady state has been attained; or (3) as the basal component of a CSII program.

Specific Flexible Insulin Programs
Multiple Dose Program with Premeal Rapid-Onset and Basal Intermediate-Acting Insulin

This program, schematically depicted in Figure 2, uses three preprandial injections of rapid-onset insulin (Regular or lispro), and intermediate-acting insulin (NPH or Lente) given at bedtime to provide overnight basal insulinemia with peak serum insulin levels prior to breakfast (a time of rela-

---

Table 3 Elements of a System of Intensive Therapy of Type 1 Diabetes

A multiple component insulin program
Careful balance of food intake, activity, and insulin dosage
Daily SMBG
An action plan for patient adjustment of food intake and/or insulin dosage, and the use of insulin supplements
Defined target blood glucose levels (individualized)
Frequent contact between patient and staff
Patient education and motivation
Psychological support
Assessment (glycated hemoglobin)

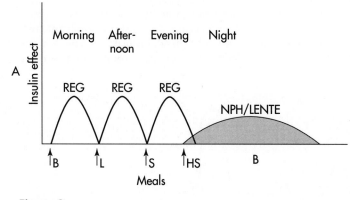
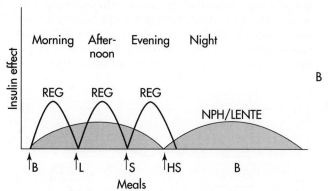

Figure 2

A, Schematic representation of idealized insulin effect provided by multiple dose regimen providing preprandial injections of Regular (REG) insulin before meals, and basal intermediate-acting insulin (*NPH* or *LENTE*) at bedtime. **B,** Schematic representation of idealized insulin effect provided by multiple dose regimen providing preprandial injections of Regular (REG) insulin before meals, and basal regimen consisting of two daily injections of intermediate-acting insulin (*NPH* or *LENTE*). B = Breakfast; *L* = Lunch; *S* = Supper; *HS* = bedtime snack. Arrows indicate time of insulin injection, 30 minutes before meals.

tive insulin resistance known as the "dawn phenom-enon"). Bedtime administration of intermediate-acting insulin also eliminates nocturnal peaks of insulin action, therefore reducing the risk of nocturnal hypoglycemia. A small, morning dose of intermediate-acting insulin (perhaps 20 to 40 percent of the bedtime dose) provides daytime basal insulinemia and is used in most patients, and is essential in patients using lispro in order to avoid gaps in attaining adequate insulinemia. (Some patients on lispro may require a third basal injection of intermediate-acting insulin at supper time, in order to avoid insulin deficiency at bedtime.) The intermediate-acting insulins are used this way quite effectively, as they have their onset of action about 2 hours after injection and produce peak insulin levels approximately 8 to 10 hours after injection.

Rapid-onset insulin is given before each meal, by syringe or by pen. Each of the doses is adjusted individually. The premeal doses permit total flexibility in meal timing. The size of meals may be altered, and the size of the accompanying premeal insulin dose may be altered proportionately. Meals may be omitted along with the accompanying premeal insulin dose, provided the morning dose of intermediate-acting insulin is included in the program.

The multiple dose program with premeal rapid onset and bedtime intermediate has become increasingly popular in recent years for a variety of reasons. It offers flexibility in meal size and timing. It is straightforward and easy to both understand and implement, since each meal and each time period of the day has a well-defined insulin component providing primary insulin action. Moreover, the introduction of insulin pens has stimulated its popularity.

Multiple Dose Program with Premeal Rapid-Onset and Basal Ultralente Insulin

This program, schematically depicted in Figure 3, uses three preprandial injections of rapid-onset insulin (Regular or lispro) and uses long-acting Ultralente insulin to provide basal insulinemia. The Ultralente insulin in most patients is relatively peakless after a steady state has been attained.

Rapid-onset insulin (Regular or lispro) is given before each meal, by syringe or by pen. Each of the doses is adjusted individually. The premeal doses permit total flexibility in meal timing. The size of meals may be altered, the size of the accompanying premeal insulin dose may be altered proportionately, and meals may be omitted along with the accompanying premeal insulin dose.

This program was originally developed with beef or mixed beef-pork Ultralente insulin preparations, which have a sluggish onset and an essentially flat action profile extending more than 36 hours. Even with these insulins, many authorities divide the Ultralente into two injections, administering half with the prebreakfast insulin and half with the presupper insulin. This takes advantage of the small peak in action seen in some patients 12 to 15 hours after administration, and also limits the total volume of injection.

Human Ultralente insulin has a broad peak about 10 to 16 hours after injection and sustains its action up to 24 hours and sometimes beyond. In most patients the peak of human Ultralente is sufficiently blunted at steady state to use as a "peakless" basal insulin. As a consequence of waning insulin effect around 24 hours, there may be a rise in fasting glucose

if human Ultralente insulin is administered in a single morning dose. Therefore, it probably is best to divide Ultralente insulin into two doses (or give it all in the evening, either before supper or at bedtime). There are some patients (usually thin individuals) who appear to be fast absorbers of human insulin (both Ultralente and intermediate-acting), in whom it may be desirable to use human Ultralente as if it were an intermediate-acting insulin preparation.

Continuous Subcutaneous Insulin Infusion

The most precise way to mimic normal insulin secretion clinically is the use of an insulin pump in a program of CSII, schematically shown in Figure 4. The pump delivers microliter amounts of rapid-onset insulin (Regular or lispro) on a continual basis, therefore replicating basal insulin secretion. Indeed, in many pumps the basal rate may be programmed to vary at times of diurnal variation in insulin sensitivity, if this

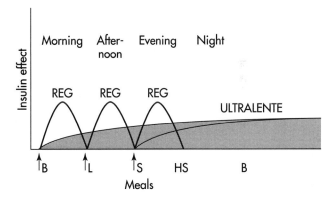

Figure 3
Schematic representation of idealized insulin effect provided by multiple dose regimen providing preprandial injections of Regular (*REG*) insulin before meals and basal long-acting (*ULTRALENTE*) insulin. *B* = Breakfast; *L* = Lunch; *S* = Supper; *HS* = bedtime snack. Arrows indicate time of insulin injection, 30 minutes before meals.

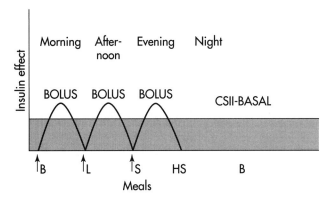

Figure 4
Schematic representation of idealized insulin effect provided by continuous subcutaneous insulin infusion. *B* = Breakfast; *L* = Lunch; *S* = Supper; *HS* = bedtime snack. Arrows indicate time of Bolus insulin, 30 minutes before meals.

results in disruption of glycemic control. Thus, the basal infusion rate may be programmed either to be decreased overnight in order to avert nocturnal hypoglycemia or to be increased to counteract the dawn phenomenon that often results in hyperglycemia on awakening.

The pump may be activated before meals to provide increments of insulin as meal *boluses* or *boosts* whenever that meal is consumed. This allows total flexibility in meal timing. If Regular insulin is used, the meal boluses are given about 20 to 30 minutes before a meal. If insulin lispro is used, the meal boluses are given immediately before eating a meal. If a meal is skipped, the insulin bolus is omitted. If a meal is larger or smaller than usual, a larger or smaller insulin bolus is selected.

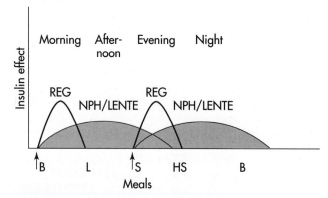

Figure 5
Schematic representation of idealized insulin effect provided by insulin regimen consisting of two daily injections of Regular (*REG*) insulin and intermediate-acting insulin (*NPH* or *LENTE*). B = Breakfast; L = Lunch; S = Supper; HS = bedtime snack. Arrows indicate time of insulin injection, 30 minutes before meals.

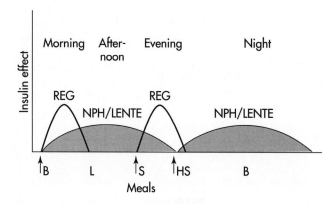

Figure 6
Schematic representation of idealized insulin effect provided by insulin regimen consisting of a morning injection of Regular (*REG*) insulin and intermediate-acting insulin (*NPH* or *LENTE*), a presupper injection of Regular insulin, and a bedtime injection of intermediate-acting insulin. B = Breakfast; L = Lunch; S = Supper; HS = bedtime snack. Arrows indicate time of insulin injection, 30 minutes before meals.

Therefore, CSII patients have the potential of easily varying meal size and meal timing, as well as omitting meals, without sabotaging glycemic control

Programmability also extends to the ability to suspend insulin delivery with increased physical activity, which serves to reduce the risk of exercise-related hypoglycemia. Caution should be used in "suspending" delivery of insulin lispro, as hyperglycemia may rapidly supervene if insulin delivery is interrupted for more than 1 hour. With Regular insulin, insulin delivery usually may be interrupted for 2 to 3 hours without significant hyperglycemia emerging.

Patients should have syringes or pens available for use any time there is an interruption of insulin delivery, both in emergencies and during times that they may find the pump inconvenient (e.g., a day at the beach).

Other Intensive (But Less Flexible) Insulin Programs
Separately considering prandial and basal insulin needs permits flexibility in eating and activity. Yet, such an approach requires a motivated, educated patient who carefully monitors blood glucose several (4 or more) times per day. In the absence of either motivation, education, or frequent blood glucose monitoring, an alternative approach is to maintain day-to-day relative consistency both of activity and of timing and quantity of food intake, and therefore permit prescription of a relatively constant insulin dose.

Split-and-Mixed Insulin Program
This program, schematically depicted in Figure 5, uses twice-daily administration of mixtures of rapid-onset insulin (Regular or lispro) and intermediate-acting insulin (NPH or Lente). Despite the development of more sophisticated and physiologic insulin programs, the twice-daily split-and-mixed insulin schedule continues to be popular among doctors and patients and receives much emphasis in the training of physicians and medical students.

The advantage of this program is that it requires only two injections. Also, the doses of Regular insulin before breakfast and supper may be increased or decreased for meals that are larger or smaller than average. Nevertheless, there are potential disadvantages that often preclude this program from being used in patients in whom the therapeutic goal is meticulous glycemic control. These disadvantages relate to the time-action profile of intermediate-acting insulin.

One problem concerns the daytime intermediate-acting insulin, given before breakfast to provide both daytime basal insulinemia and meal-related insulinemia for lunch. Because the intermediate-acting insulin has a broad peak, lunch and supper must be eaten on time to avoid hypoglycemia. Also, the peak effect of the insulin occurs 8 to 10 hours after administration, too late to provide optimal insulin availability for lunch. Moreover, recent studies suggest that afternoon glycemia may be more dependent on morning Regular than morning intermediate-acting insulin, contrary to traditional wisdom. Finally, because the intermediate-acting insulin is given before breakfast, it is difficult for the patient to make changes in the size or timing of lunch.

Another difficulty is that intermediate-acting preparations have an onset of action about 2 hours after injection and produce peak insulin levels approximately 8 to 10 hours after injection. Thus, if intermediate-acting insulin is administered before supper, it often does not sustain its effect throughout the night, resulting in morning hyperglycemia, a time of relative insulin resistance—the dawn phenomenon. Attempts to correct this fasting hyperglycemia by increasing the dose often are complicated by nocturnal hypoglycemia when insulin action peaks.

Split-and-Mixed Program with Bedtime Intermediate Insulin

This program, schematically depicted in Figure 6, uses morning administration of a mixture of rapid-onset insulin (Regular or lispro) and intermediate-acting insulin, with presupper rapid-onset insulin (Regular or lispro) and bedtime intermediate-acting insulin, an approach used to minimize nocturnal hypoglycemia and to counteract the dawn phenomenon. It has been shown that taking intermediate-acting insulin at bedtime instead of before supper results in lower fasting and after-breakfast blood glucose levels.

The disadvantage of this program is that the patient still has little flexibility in meal schedule, and the above problems related to daytime intermediate-acting insulin. In addition, some patients are not willing to administer three injections each day.

Other (Nonintensive) Insulin Programs

Generally, it is not possible to adequately control glycemia in type 1 diabetes using one or two injections of intermediate-acting insulin alone. The exception may be early in the course of the disease when some endogenous insulin secretion remains.

Insulin Dose and Distribution
Initial Insulin Doses

In typical patients with type 1 diabetes who are within 20 percent of their ideal body weight, in the absence of intercurrent infections or other periods of instability, the total daily insulin dose required for meticulous glycemic control is 0.5 to 1.0 U per kilogram of body weight per day.

The needed dose is lower during the honeymoon period of relative remission early in the course of the disease (e.g., 0.2 to 0.6 U per kilogram per day). Moreover, during the honeymoon period, because there is some continuing endogenous insulin secretion, it may be relatively easy to achieve glycemic control with virtually any rational insulin program. Some patients may find it easier to use twice-daily premixed insulin for a few months, while learning the overall principles of diabetes management. Then, they can switch to a flexible or other intensive program prior to the end of their honeymoon period.

During periods of intercurrent illness, insulin requirement may increase markedly (even double). Doses show progressive increases during pregnancy, increasing in units per kilogram, and since kilograms also increase, the total dose may even triple. Doses also are increased during the adolescent growth spurt, and some adolescents have a sustained increased dose requirement.

Insulin Dose Distribution

About 40 to 50 percent of the total daily insulin dose is used to provide basal insulinemia. The remainder is divided among the meals either empirically, proportionate to the relative carbohydrate content of the meals, or by initially giving (in adults) approximately 0.8 to 1.2 U insulin for every 10 g carbohydrate consumed. Breakfast generally requires a slightly larger amount of insulin per 10 g of carbohydrate than does other meals.

Alternatively, a starting point for the initial distribution of insulin is: basal 40 to 50 percent of total daily dose, prebreakfast rapid-onset insulin 15 to 25 percent of total daily dose, prelunch rapid-onset insulin about 15 percent of total daily dose, presupper rapid-onset insulin 15 to 20 percent of total daily dose. Some patients desire or require a small dose of rapid-onset insulin to cover a bedtime snack (0 to 10 percent of daily total). Obviously, unusual meal distributions dictate a deviation from this scheme. Moreover, this dosage distribution is arbitrary and designed for an idealized average patient. Clearly, it must be individualized for any given patient, which is why it is best to base the premeal rapid-onset insulin on meal content.

Blood Glucose Targets

Instrumental to the management of type 1 diabetes is the choice of blood glucose targets. The selection of appropriate blood glucose targets is one of the most important aspects of management and one that should be quite explicit. Each patient should have defined blood glucose targets. These must be individualized for the needs of each patient. The targets must be explicitly defined, in order to avoid confusion and for the patient to understand his or her management goal.

Often the goal of therapy is meticulous glycemic control with near-normal glycemic targets. Table 4 shows an example of meticulous control targets for a young otherwise healthy patient who recognizes hypoglycemic symptoms and spon-

Table 4 Representative Target Blood Glucose Levels Suitable for a Young Otherwise Healthy Patient		
	IDEAL mg/dl mmol/L	**ACCEPTABLE** mg/dl mmol/L
Preprandial	70–105 (3.9–5.8)	70–130 (3.9–7.2)
1-hr postprandial	100–160 (5.6–8.9)	100–180 (5.6–10.0)
2-hr postprandial	80–120 (4.4–6.7)	80–150 (4.4–8.3)
2:00 to 4:00 AM	70–100 (3.9–5.6)	70–120 (3.9–6.7)

Ideal values approximate those seen in nondiabetic individuals; they are included for illustrative purposes. *Acceptable* values are attainable in a reasonable number of patients without creating an undue frequency of hypoglycemia; they are provided to appropriate patients.

taneously recovers from hypoglycemia. In this example, the preprandial blood glucose targets are 70 to 130 mg per deciliter (3.9 to 7.2 mmol per liter). These targets need to be lower during pregnancy. Table 5 shows an example of the even more stringent targets appropriate for a pregnant woman with type 1 diabetes. In this example, the preprandial blood glucose targets are 60 to 90 mg per deciliter (3.3 to 5.0 mmol per liter).

Yet, such meticulous targets are inappropriate in patients who have difficulty perceiving hypoglycemic symptoms (hypoglycemia unawareness), patients who do not spontaneously recover from hypoglycemia (e.g., those with counter-regulatory insufficiency or who are using beta-blockers), patients in whom hypoglycemia might be particularly dangerous (e.g., patients with angina pectoris or transient ischemic attacks), or patients with other complicating features. Such patients might require higher preprandial blood glucose targets, for example, 150 to 250 mg per deciliter (8.3 to 13.9 mmol per liter).

Targets may also vary with age. A wider range may be desirable in toddlers or young children with diabetes, who may not readily recognize or report hypoglycemic symptoms and who have active and varied life-styles. Here, preprandial blood glucose targets might be 80 to 180 mg per deciliter (4.4 to 10.0 mmol per liter). Likewise, in an elderly person there may be a greater desire to avoid hypoglycemia and greater tolerance of modest hyperglycemia. Here, for example, preprandial blood glucose targets might be 100 to 220 mg per deciliter (5.6 to 11.1 mmol per liter).

Targets may also be changed with time. For example, when initiating flexible or intensive therapy, even if the ultimate goal is meticulous glycemic control, the initial targets might be preprandial blood glucose targets might be 100 to 220 mg per deciliter (5.6 to 12.2 mmol per liter). Sequential changes might then be introduced, until the ultimate target is achieved.

It should be appreciated that the target range should be wide enough to be realistically achievable. A preprandial blood glucose target range of 90 to 110 mg per deciliter (5.0 to 6.1 mmol per liter) is unrealistically narrow and will lead to frustration, since it is not likely to be achieved on a regular basis. In motivated patients, realistic targets are achievable 70 to 80 percent of the time. (It is unrealistic to expect targets to be achieved 100 percent of the time, and patients should appreciate this fact.) If targets are not being regularly achieved, and the patient is adhering to his or her management program, then one should consider changing the targets to ones that are achievable.

The overall system of therapy applies no matter what targets are selected.

Selection of Patients for Meticulous Control

A system of flexible or intensive therapy is appropriate for all patients with type 1 diabetes. The ideal candidate for meticulous glycemic control is the patient who is otherwise healthy and does not yet have signs of diabetic complications. Patient motivation is crucial and perhaps the determining factor in treatment success or failure. Other criteria for assessing patients for implementation of a meticulous control program are:

- Motivation to pursue meticulous glycemic control
- Suboptimal glycemic control with existing treatment plan
- Ability and willingness to perform frequent SMBG
- Sufficient education and technical ability to follow treatment program
- Psychological stability adequate to manage treatment program
- Availability of trained and skilled medical staff to direct treatment program and provide necessary attention

A preliminary program of counseling, education, and training is desirable. Success in achieving meticulous glycemic control depends on daily SMBG and careful adherence to diet. It is desirable to have most patients demonstrate that they can do these things well. There should be ongoing surveillance to ensure that the patient is following the treatment plan.

Risks of Meticulous Control

The major danger of meticulous glycemic control is hypoglycemia. There are several hypoglycemic risks related to attempts to achieve meticulous glycemic control. These are:

- Increased frequency of hypoglycemia
- Increased frequency of severe hypoglycemic events (those that require the assistance of another person for treatment)
- Increased frequency of very severe hypoglycemic events resulting in hypoglycemic coma or seizures
- Nocturnal hypoglycemia, which may be difficult to recognize and may lead to severe hypoglycemia
- Increased risks if patients have the syndrome of hypoglycemic unresponsiveness and/or the syndrome of counter-regulatory insufficiency
- The potential that attainment of near-normal hypoglycemic control per se may reduce the counter-regu-

Table 5 Representative Target Blood Glucose Levels Suitable for a Pregnant Woman with Type 1 Diabetes		
	mg/dl	**mmol/L**
Fasting	60–90	(3.3–5.0)
Preprandial	60–105	(3.3–5.8)
1-hr postprandial	70–140	(3.9–7.8)
2-hr postprandial	60–120	(3.3–6.7)
2:00 to 4:00 AM	Above 60	(Above 3.3)

latory response to hypoglycemia, thus impairing both symptom recognition and ability to spontaneously recover from hypoglycemia

The Diabetes Control and Complications Trial (DCCT) reported a threefold increased risk of severe hypoglycemia and of very severe hypoglycemia (with coma or seizures) in the experimental group (which aimed for meticulous glycemic control) versus the standard treatment group. The data suggest that meticulous glycemic control may pose an increased risk of severe hypoglycemic events. Therefore, it is clear that one must exercise increased vigilance in detecting and preventing hypoglycemia in patients being meticulously controlled.

Nocturnal hypoglycemia poses the most dangerous threat to diabetic patients, since sleep may impair recognition of the event. In the DCCT, more than 50 percent of severe hypoglycemia occurred at night.

It is clear that the greatest risk from hypoglycemia occurs in individuals who fail to detect symptoms of hypoglycemia—hypoglycemia awareness—and in those who fail to spontaneously recover from hypoglycemia—counter-regulatory insufficiency. Obviously, hypoglycemia is more dangerous in individuals with hypoglycemia unawareness or with counter-regulatory unresponsiveness than in those who are fully intact in their ability to detect and/or spontaneously recover from hypoglycemia.

Of additional concern is that hypoglycemia itself begets hypoglycemia unawareness and may reduce counter-regulatory hormone responses to hypoglycemia, apparently by lowering the plasma glucose threshold required for counter-regulatory hormone release. Therefore, scrupulous avoidance of hypoglycemia is necessary to permit recovery from hypoglycemia awareness.

When meticulous control is desired, the real issues in terms of hypoglycemic risk are appropriate selection of blood glucose treatment targets and constant vigilance to prevent, detect, and treat hypoglycemia. Hypoglycemic episodes are often precipitated by delayed or decreased food intake or by increased physical exercise. These represent circumstances of preventable hypoglycemia. Patients need to be familiar with their own symptom cluster associated with hypoglycemia. They need to frequently measure blood glucose to detect trends towards a lowering of glycemia to a potentially dangerous level. When patients exert such vigilance, and when gly-cemic targets are appropriately modified depending on individual circumstances, meticulous glycemic control can be sought and attained without significant danger.

Hypoglycemia is discussed in greater detail in the chapter *Hypoglycemia in Type 1 Diabetic Patients*.

Education and Action

Patients are provided with an action plan to alter their therapy to achieve their individual defined blood glucose targets. These actions are guided by SMBG determinations and daily records. The actions are a sequence of responses, predetermined by the physician. The system used for this purpose is that of "algorithms." The algorithms dictate that the patient intervene as necessary by altering the insulin dosage, changing the timing of insulin injections in relation to meals, or changing the size or content of food to be consumed.

Two general types of algorithms are used: Preprandial Algorithms and Pattern Adjustment Algorithms. The Preprandial Algorithms (also called "Supplements") provide an action plan that permits immediate action to be taken in response to current circumstances. The Pattern Adjustment Algorithms (also called "Adjustments") provide an action plan that permits corrective action to be taken when a recurrent pattern is seen in blood-glucose fluctuations. Attainment of therapeutic goals requires that both types of algorithms be used.

Preprandial Algorithms

The Preprandial Algorithm Action Plan has also been called a "Scheme of Insulin Supplements" and a "Sliding Scale". Many experts prefer to avoid the use of the term "sliding scale" because the traditional sliding scale used in many hospitals did not recognize the ongoing (basal and prandial) insulin requirements and would prescribe no insulin when the blood glucose was in the target range. The concept of "supplements" was introduced to emphasize that these changes in insulin dosage were supplemental to the ongoing insulin requirements. Thus, insulin supplements are dosage variations to prevent or correct momentary deviations of blood glucose outside the target range. They may be used when there is variation in the quantity or pattern of meals or activities, when there is intercurrent illness or other stress, or to correct variations in glycemia. Supplements, then, are temporary insulin doses. Conceptually, there are two types of supplements: (1) anticipatory supplements, given to limit expected hyperglycemia (e.g., before a large meal) are used prospectively; and (2) compensatory supplements, given in response to glycemic levels outside the target range, are used retrospectively. Supplements may actually be decrements ("negative supplements"), e.g., a lowering of preprandial Regular insulin in anticipation of an usually small meal or in the face of prevailing blood glucose levels lower than the preprandial target.

Because the actions taken may include changes in food intake and in timing of insulin administration, as well as changes in insulin dosage, the term "Preprandial Algorithm Action Plan" is preferable to "Scheme of Insulin Supplements".

The Preprandial Algorithms provide an action plan for the patient. The actions are guided by SMBG determinations and daily records. The action taken depends on the answers to several questions the patient needs to ask at the time of any premeal insulin injection. These include:

(1) What is my blood glucose now?
(2) What do I plan to eat now (i.e., usual size meal, large meal, or small meal; how much carbohydrate)?
(3) What do I plan to do after eating (i.e., usual activity, increased activity, decreased activity)?
(4) What has happened under these circumstances previously?

The answers dictate treatment response and become sensible routine decisions. The intervention actions dictated by the plan include: food intake (altering the size or content of food), activity, insulin dosage, and timing of injections in relation to meals. An example of a Preprandial Algorithm Action Plan is shown in Table 6. The illustrative plan assumes

Table 6 Sample Preprandial Action Plan

This Action Plan assumes that the Preprandial Blood Glucose Targets are 70–130 mg/dl (3.9–7.2 mmol/L).
Plans should be individualized for each patient.
Once insulin dosage is stable, use the following scheme for premeal alteration of dosage of Regular insulin:

IF BLOOD GLUCOSE IS BELOW 50 MG/DL:
Reduce premeal Regular insulin by 2–3 U.
Delay injection until immediately before eating.
Include at least 10 g of rapidly available carbohydrate in the meal.

IF BLOOD GLUCOSE IS 50–70 MG/DL:
Reduce premeal Regular insulin by 1–2 U.
Delay injection until immediately before eating.

IF BLOOD GLUCOSE IS 70–130 MG/DL:
Take prescribed premeal dose of Regular insulin.

IF BLOOD GLUCOSE IS 130–150 MG/DL:
Increase premeal dose of Regular insulin by 1 U.

IF BLOOD GLUCOSE IS 150–200 MG/DL:
Increase premeal dose of Regular insulin by 2 U.

IF BLOOD GLUCOSE IS 200–250 MG/DL:
Increase premeal dose of Regular insulin by 3 U.
Consider delaying meal an extra 15 min (to 45 min after injection

IF BLOOD GLUCOSE IS 250–300 MG/DL:
Increase premeal dosage of Regular insulin by 4 U.
Consider delaying meal an extra 20–30 min (to 40–60 min after injection).

IF BLOOD GLUCOSE IS 300–350 MG/DL:
Increase premeal dosage of Regular insulin by 5 U.
Delay meal an extra 20–30 min (to 40–60 min after injection).
Check urine ketones. If moderate to large, increase fluid intake, consider extra insulin (1–2 U). Recheck blood glucose and urine ketones in 2–3 hr.

IF BLOOD GLUCOSE IS 350–400 MG/DL:
Increase premeal dosage of Regular insulin by 6 U.
Delay meal an extra 20–30 min (to 40–60 min after injection).
Check urine ketones. If moderate to large, increase fluid intake, consider extra insulin (1–2 U). Recheck blood glucose and urine ketones in 2–3 hr.

IF BLOOD GLUCOSE IS MORE THAN 400 MG/DL:
Increase premeal dosage of Regular insulin by 7 U.
Delay meal an extra 30 min (to 50–60 min after injection).
Check urine ketones. If moderate to large, increase fluid intake, consider extra insulin (1–2 U). Recheck blood glucose and urine ketones in 2–3 hr.

IF PLANNED MEAL IS LARGER THAN USUAL:
Increase Regular insulin by 1–2 U.

IF PLANNED MEAL IS SMALLER THAN USUAL:
Decrease Regular insulin by 1–2 U.

IF UNUSUALLY INCREASED ACTIVITY IS PLANNED AFTER EATING:
Eat extra carbohydrate and/or decrease Regular insulin by 1–2 U.

IF UNUSUALLY SEDENTARY ACTIVITY IS PLANNED AFTER EATING:
Consider increasing Regular insulin by 1–2 U.

If insulin lispro is used as the preprandial insulin, the alterations in insulin timing do not apply.

that the preprandial and bedtime blood glucose target is 70 to 130 mg per deciliter (3.9 to 7.2 mmol per liter).

Pattern Adjustment Algorithms

There should be a separate action plan used in response to a pattern of glycemia occurring over several days. These Pattern Adjustment Algorithms are small empiric changes made in the usual or basic insulin dosage, designed to gradually tailor, model, or shape the insulin dosage to the patient's usual or basic needs. In this sense, these algorithms are an ongoing iterative titration process based on experience.

The actions taken in the Pattern Adjustment Algorithms have been termed "insulin adjustments". Thus, insulin adjustments are modifications in the usual or basic insulin dose, made in response to a pattern of glycemia. Adjustments are actions that presuppose that the patient has a relatively stable pattern of meals and activities, has no intercurrent illness, and is free from unusual stress.

Pattern Adjustment Algorithms provide that when the blood glucose is consistently above or below the target range at a particular time of the day, a pattern has been established and action must be taken. The action is that the insulin dose (of the relevant insulin component most likely responsible) must be either increased or decreased to correct the pattern of glycemia outside the target range. The continuing need for Preprandial Actions (e.g., compensatory insulin supplements) to correct unexplained ambient glycemia outside the target range at a particular time of the day indicates that an

adjustment should be made in the relevant insulin component covering the time period leading up to the time that compensatory supplements were required. Pattern Adjustment Algorithms provide for prospective changes based on retrospective data. They are not dependent on the blood glucose at the moment when they are implemented. Rather they anticipate insulin need for the next time period. An example of a Pattern Adjustment Algorithm Plan is shown in Table 7 for an insulin program involving preprandial rapid-onset insulin combined with bedtime and morning intermediate-acting insulin.

In order to implement the management plan, considerable patient education is required. Moreover, the patient needs continued access to and interaction with a specialized diabetes management team, if successful management is to be achieved. Thus, the management of type 1 diabetes with a contemporary flexible or intensive insulin program mandates management by an expert multidisciplinary diabetes team.

Successful participation in a demanding management program requires a committed, motivated patient. The management team often must take extra effort to help maintain motivation. This is often the most difficult component of treatment. Patients and families with new-onset type 1 diabetes need psychological support to adjust to having diabetes. Additional support is required to aid in the management program. To this end, some psychological support, e.g., routine diabetes support group meetings, may be desirable for all patients with type 1 diabetes.

Table 7 Sample Pattern Adjustment Action Plan

This Action Plan assumes that the Preprandial Blood Glucose Targets are 70–130 mg/dl (3.9–7.2 mmol/L). Plans should be individualized for each patient.

ASSUMPTIONS

Basal insulin (bedtime intermediate-acting NPH insulin Ultralente insulin, or basal rate of insulin pump) is the major insulin acting overnight. Its effect is reflected in the results of blood glucose tests during the middle of the night and on arising the next morning.

Prebreakfast rapid-acting insulin (Regular or lispro) has major action between breakfast and lunch. Its effect is primarily reflected in the results of blood glucose tests before lunch.

Prelunch rapid-acting insulin (Regular or lispro) has major action between lunch and supper. Its effect is primarily reflected in the results of blood glucose tests before supper.

Presupper rapid-acting insulin (Regular or lispro) has major action between supper and bedtime. Its effect is primarily reflected in the results of blood glucose tests at bedtime.

HYPERGLYCEMIA NOT EXPLAINED BY UNUSUAL DIET, EXERCISE, OR INSULIN

If prebreakfast blood glucose is greater than 130 mg/dl for 3–5 days in a row, increase basal insulin (bedtime NPH or Ultralente) by 1 or 2 U (0.05–0.1 U/hr for CSII). (Before making such changes, verify that the blood glucose nadir, usually around 3–4 am, is not below 70 mg/dl.)

If prelunch blood glucose is greater than 130 mg/dl for 3–5 days in a row, increase prebreakfast rapid-acting insulin (Regular or lispro) by 1 or 2 U.

If presupper blood glucose is greater than 130 mg/dl for 3–5 days in a row, increase prelunch rapid-acting insulin (Regular or lispro) by 1 or 2 U.

If bedtime blood glucose is greater than 130 mg/dl for 3–5 days in a row, increase presupper rapid-acting insulin (Regular or lispro) by 1 or 2 U.

Only increase one insulin component at a time, starting with the one affecting the earliest blood glucose during the day.

HYPOGLYCEMIA NOT EXPLAINED BY UNUSUAL DIET, EXERCISE, OR INSULIN

If prebreakfast blood glucose is less than 70 mg/dl, or if there is evidence of hypoglycemic reactions occurring during the night, reduce basal insulin (bedtime NPH or by 1 or 2 U (0.05–0.1 U/hr for CSII).

If prelunch blood glucose is less than 70 mg/dl, or if you have a hypoglycemic reaction between breakfast and lunch, reduce prebreakfast rapid-acting insulin (Regular or lispro) by 1 or 2 U.

If presupper blood glucose is less than 70 mg/dl, or if you have a hypoglycemic reaction between lunch and supper, reduce prelunch rapid-acting insulin, (Regular or lispro) by 1 or 2 U.

If bedtime blood glucose is less than 70 mg/dl, or if you have a hypoglycemic reaction between supper and bedtime, reduce presupper rapid-acting insulin (Regular or lispro) by 1 or 2 U.

Verify hypoglycemic symptoms with blood glucose measurements. Treat hypoglycemic reaction with 10–15 g of rapidly absorbed simple sugar.

Suggested Reading

Albisser AM, Sperlich M. Adjusting insulins. Diabetes Educator 1992; 18:211–222.

Reviews the variables to be considered in changing insulin doses, with particular emphasis on changing injection sites.

Schade DS, Santiago JV, Skyler JS, Rizza R. Intensive insulin therapy. Princeton, NJ: Excerpta Medica, 1983.

Provides details for implementation of insulin programs.

Hirsch RF, ed. Intensive diabetes management. Alexandria, Va: American Diabetes Association, 1995.

Howorka K. Functional insulin treatment. Berlin: Springer-Verlag, 1990.

The two preceding monographs provide details for implementation of contemporary insulin programs.

Skyler JS, Skyler DL, Seigler DE, O'Sullivan MJ. Algorithms for adjustment of insulin dosage by patients who monitor blood glucose. Diabetes Care 1981; 4:311–318.

Skyler JS. Insulin-dependent diabetes mellitus. In: Kohler PO, ed. Clinical endocrinology. New York: John Wiley, 1986:491.

Skyler JS. Insulin-dependent diabetes mellitus: Flexibility in contemporary management. Postgraduate Medicine 1987; 81(6):163–174.

Hirsch IB, Farkas-Hirsch R, Skyler JS. Intensive insulin therapy for treatment of type 1 diabetes. Diabetes Care 1990; 13:1265–1283.

Skyler JS. Current concepts: Insulin therapy for type 1 diabetes mellitus. Kalamazoo, Mich: The Upjohn Company, 1991.

The five preceding references provide successive iterations of the author's approach to insulin therapy.

DCCT Research Group. Implementation of treatment protocols in the diabetes control and complications trial.

Discusses intensive therapy as used in the Diabetes Control and Complications Trial.

Nolte MS. Insulin therapy in insulin-dependent (type 1) diabetes mellitus. Endocrinol Metab Clin North Am 1992; 21:281–312.

A review of implementation of contemporary insulin therapy.

Lebovitz H, ed. Therapy for diabetes mellitus and related disorders. 2nd ed. Alexandria, Va: American Diabetes Association, 1994.

An ADA monograph.

Santiago JV, ed. Medical management of insulin-dependent (type 1) diabetes mellitus. 2nd ed. Alexandria, Va: American Diabetes Association, 1994.

An ADA monograph.

American Diabetes Association. Clinical practice recommendations: 1996. Diabetes Care 1996; 19(suppl 1):S1–S118.

The American Diabetes Association's annually updated clinical practice recommendations.

MONITORING OF TYPE 1 DIABETES MELLITUS

Jay S. Skyler, M.D.

Patients with type 1 diabetes who are stable should be followed approximately every 3 months. An independent measure of integrated glycemic control, glycated (glycosylated) hemoglobin, is used for metabolic assessment. At each visit, glycated hemoglobin (HbA_1 or HbA_{1c}) is determined to monitor long-term glycemic control. In patients in whom the target is near-normal glycemia, glycated hemoglobin values should be within 120 percent of the upper limit of normal of the assay being used. Patient-determined blood glucose values are part of treatment, not assessment (but should be compared with the glycated hemoglobin value). Urine ketone measurements complement patient blood glucose monitoring. In addition, patient compliance and responsibility for diabetes management should be assessed on a regular basis.

At each visit, weight, height (if a child or adolescent), and blood pressure also are measured. At least annually, the patient should have a complete physical examination, including funduscopic examination through dilated pupils; determination of creatinine clearance and urinary albumin excretion; determination of plasma lipids; and obtaining of an electrocardiogram in adults over age 30.

◼ SELF-MONITORING OF BLOOD GLUCOSE

Patient self-monitoring of blood glucose (SMBG) was introduced in the late 1970s as a tool to facilitate assessment of diabetes control on an ambulatory basis. As it has evolved, it has become an important component of treatment, rather than an assessment tool. This is a subtle but, in my view, important distinction. Properly used, SMBG values are considered by the patient to make immediate treatment decisions. The decisions are based on a predetermined action plan that consists of actions designed to achieve blood glucose values within a given target range. The use of such action plans is discussed in detail in the preceding chapter. The use of SMBG as the basis for alteration of therapy is the cornerstone of contemporary programs of diabetes management. The value of such in achieving meticulous glycemic control was clearly established by the Diabetes Control and Complications Trial (DCCT).

A major advantage of SMBG is that it enables therapeutic goals to be clearly defined and permits assessment of glycemic control during ordinary life. In this regard, it complements glycated hemoglobin measurements. Self-monitoring of blood glucose defines the extent of glycemic excursions, while glycated hemoglobin documents average glycemic control. More importantly, SMBG determinations are used on an ongoing basis by patients, to aid in the adjustment of the therapeutic regimen. Thus, in the context of a flexible or intensive program of diabetes management, SMBG is an integral component of treatment, facilitating the attainment of improved glycemic control, rather than an assessment tool.

Technique

This involves patient measurement of blood glucose on capillary samples, obtained by using an automated device for pricking the finger, with the drop placed on a test strip, read in a meter or sensor. A variety of strips and meters or sensors are available for blood glucose testing. Some strips may be interpreted visually (without a meter), although this practice is not recommended. Two of the most important technologic advances that facilitated the widespread use of SMBG were (1) the introduction of single-pronged narrow-gauge sharp-pointed lancets; and (2) the availability of automated, spring-operated devices that make the finger-pricking process simple and virtually painless.

Frequency of Monitoring

The frequency of monitoring depends on the treatment program of any individual patient. As a general principle, unstable labile diabetes requires more frequent monitoring than stable diabetes. As a second principle, fasting and preprandial glucose measurements alone underestimate the extent of postprandial glucose excursions and are inadequate as the sole monitoring times if excellent control is desired.

According to a study from Montreal, patients with type 1 diabetes who had attained excellent control (near-normal glycated hemoglobin values) demonstrated that such control deteriorated if SMBG was reduced to less than four determinations per day (Fig. 1). Moreover, this prompted the investigators to institute a subsequent crossover study in which they demonstrated that better control was attained with four or more daily blood glucose determinations than with fewer measurements. This demonstrates the necessity for frequent daily blood glucose self-monitoring and for taking action on the information, if excellent control is desired. These findings are congruent with other observations. For example, it has been shown that lower glycated hemoglobin values are correlated with the number of blood-glucose values charted per week.

The DCCT investigators also noted the importance of frequent SMBG measurements. They recommended four or more daily determinations, with an overnight value at least once weekly. At least quarterly, profiles were obtained that included postprandial values as well. During the entire study, for which subjects were followed for a mean of 6.5 years, on 86 to 92 percent of days there was compliance with at least three of the recommended four daily measurements. In addition, overnight values were obtained over 70 percent of the time. The DCCT study group noted the importance of frequent monitoring, careful record keeping, and actions taken upon the results, if meticulous control was to be achieved. Indeed, adjustment of insulin dosage based on SMBG was reported by 94 to 98 percent of intensive patients throughout the DCCT.

Supported by NIH Grant HL-36588, U.S. Public Health Service.

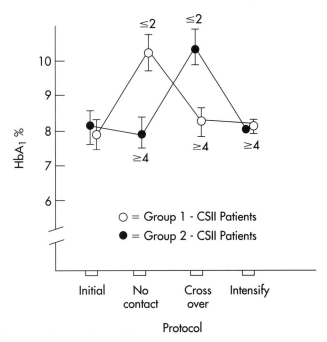

Figure 1
Glycemic control, assessed by glycated hemoglobin, in relation to number of daily blood glucose measurements. The initial HbA$_1$ was obtained after 1 year of intensive therapy. After 6 months of "no contact," some subjects maintained near-normal HbA$_1$ values and had continued to measure blood glucose four or more times daily; others had higher HbA$_1$ values and had measured blood glucose an average of two or fewer times daily. The next 3-month period (crossover), they changed the frequency of blood glucose monitoring, and the last 3-month period (intensify), they all resumed blood glucose measurement four or more times daily. (*Adapted from Schiffrin A, Belmonte M. Mutiple daily self-glucose control in insulin-dependent diabetic patients treated with pump and multiple subcutaneous injections. Diabetes Care 1982; 5:479–484.*)

Knowledge of preprandial, bedtime, and nocturnal blood glucose concentrations is required to determine the appropriate basal and preprandial insulin doses. Therefore, in type 1 diabetes in a program of intensive therapy, the author recommends that blood glucose be determined four times per day most days (before meals and at bedtime), with additional samples obtained in the middle of the night (2:00 AM to 4:00 AM) once every 1 to 2 weeks and anytime the overnight insulin dosage is to be altered. Additional samples are obtained any time hypoglycemia is suspected and to measure the impact of alterations in food, activity, or the insulin program. Periodically, postprandial samples are obtained as well. Certainly, there should be a minimum of one measurement per insulin component. Dosage decisions can then be based on a measured value rather than an unknown value.

During initiation of a program of intensive therapy aimed at meticulous control, more frequent sampling is recommended, i.e., seven to nine determinations daily: prebreakfast, postprandial breakfast, prelunch, postprandial lunch, presupper, postprandial supper, bedtime, midnight,

and 2:00 to 4:00 AM. When a relatively stable pattern is obtained, the frequency of monitoring is reduced to four daily samples as described above. If glycemic control deteriorates, it is necessary to increase the frequency of monitoring. Frequent sampling is also necessary during intercurrent illness and for problem assessment. Finally, more frequent sampling, including routine postprandial measurements, is essential during pregnancy.

Records

Quite clearly, record keeping is essential to successful treatment, particularly if one is to consider the impact of previous responses. The patient should keep a careful diary of daily blood glucose measurements, insulin doses, hypoglycemic episodes, and departures from daily routine (e.g., unusually large meals, increased physical activity, intercurrent illness). Careful recording, critical review by patient and health professional, and intelligent interpretation become important elements in successful management. The patient record is the focus of discussion at each follow-up visit. In particular, it is desirable to determine if the patient has followed the action plans and made appropriate changes in insulin dose or meals in response to prevailing blood glucose, meals, and activity. Explanation of hypoglycemic episodes and unusual hyperglycemia is sought.

Unfortunately, some patients and physicians suffer from "data overload" when faced with blood glucose monitoring data. This can be crippling. To that end, a number of systems have been developed to handle the data and to provide graphic display and even advice according to customized action plans. These systems can greatly facilitate the management of both the data and the patient.

■ GLYCATED HEMOGLOBIN

The most important clinical tool in the assessment of chronic glycemic control is the measurement of glycated (glycosylated) hemoglobin (HbA$_1$ or HbA$_{1c}$). It has become the "gold standard" in assessment. It correlates with integrated plasma-glucose levels over a period of several weeks, by virtue of the fact that glucose becomes covalently linked to hemoglobin through a nonenzymatic reaction that is proportionate to the concentration of the reactants, i.e., glucose and hemoglobin. Thus, with a single random blood sample, the physician can make a quantitative assessment of overall patient progress.

Glycated hemoglobin values reflect integrated glycemic control during the life span of the hemoglobin molecule. The correlation is strongest for glycemic control 4 to 8 weeks before glycated hemoglobin determination. Values appear to be more sensitive to deterioration in control than improvement in control, presumably because of the irreversibility of the Amadori rearrangement forming the ketoamine. Measurement of the ketoamine component of glycated hemoglobin provides an accurate assessment of mean level of glycemia over a period of several weeks, using a single sample, and only minimally influenced by acute changes in glycemic control.

Glycated hemoglobin measurements are used to document glycemic control and confirm that the patient blood glucose record is an accurate reflection of events. To this end, determinations of glycated hemoglobin are made every 1 to 2 months

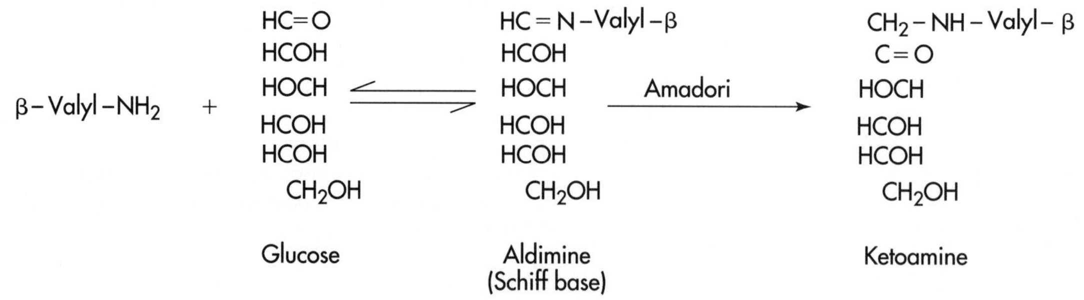

$$\beta-Valyl-NH_2 \quad + \quad
\begin{array}{c} HC=O \\ HCOH \\ HOCH \\ HCOH \\ HCOH \\ CH_2OH \end{array}
\quad \rightleftharpoons \quad
\begin{array}{c} HC=N-Valyl-\beta \\ HCOH \\ HOCH \\ HCOH \\ HCOH \\ CH_2OH \end{array}
\quad \xrightarrow{Amadori} \quad
\begin{array}{c} CH_2-NH-Valyl-\beta \\ C=O \\ HOCH \\ HCOH \\ HCOH \\ CH_2OH \end{array}$$

Glucose   Aldimine   Ketoamine
        (Schiff base)

Figure 2

Schematic representation of the process of nonenzymatic glycosylation of hemoglobin at the terminal amino group of the hemoglobin beta chain. *(Adapted from Bunn H. Evaluation of glycosylated hemoglobin in diabetic patients. Diabetes 1981; 30:613–617.)*

during stabilization, to document progress, and approximately every 2 to 4 months when glycemia appears stable.

In patients in whom meticulous glycemic control is sought, the target is normalization or near normalization of glycated hemoglobin, or the lowest value attainable without inducing an unacceptable frequency of hypoglycemia. However, this is not often attainable. Realistically, in patients in whom the target is near-normal glycemia, it is possible to attain glycated hemoglobin values within 125 percent of the upper limit of normal of the assay being used.

Discrepancies between glycated hemoglobin determinations and patient reports of blood glucose measurements indicate a need to review the management program. The patient may not be accurately measuring blood glucose and therefore may be missing wide fluctuations, or he or she may be providing fraudulent results.

Chemistry

The formation of glycated hemoglobin occurs by the process of nonenzymatic glycosylation. Nonenzymatic glycosylation of proteins occurs at both N-terminal amino groups and at epsilon amino groups of intrachain amino acids (e.g., lysine). It involves the addition of glucose to protein by a slow continuous reaction that is a function of the duration of contact between the reactants and the integrated glucose concentration during the time of contact. The reaction scheme is depicted in Figure 2. The first product is an aldimine (or Schiff base), which then undergoes an internal rearrangement of the double bond (an Amadori rearrangement) to form a ketoamine. The kinetics of this latter reaction are such that it is essentially irreversible (or more accurately, occurs at a rate such that the reversibility is not readily appreciated owing to the short life span of erythrocytes). Thus, although the reaction occurs slowly, the ketoamine is a stable product and reflects integrated glycemic control during the life span of the hemoglobin molecule. In contrast, the formation of the aldimine is both relatively rapid and more easily reversible.

The most abundant glycated hemoglobin is HbA_{1c}, which is the ketoamine formed by the addition of glucose to the terminal valine groups on the beta chains of hemoglobin HbA. This is also known as "stable HbA_{1c}," while "total HbA_{1c}" includes both the stable ketoamine and the labile aldimine, also known as "pre-A_{1c}." Other minor glycated hemoglobins include HbA_{1a1}, HbA_{1a2}, and HbA_{1b}, which are formed by the addition of sugar phosphates to the terminal

valine of the beta chains of HbA or by a further modification of HbA_{1c}. Collectively, these components involving modification of the terminal valine of the beta chain have been referred to as HbA_1, which is $(HbA_{1a1}+_{a2} +_b+_c)$. (This too may be "stable HbA_1" or "total HbA_1" depending on whether or not the labile pre-A_{1c} has been removed.) In addition, as noted, there are non-HbA_1 glycated hemoglobins (HbA-G1c) formed by the addition of glucose either to the N-terminus of alpha chains or to epsilon amino groups on lysine residues. These latter glycated components can be measured in chemical assays, but not in cation exchange chromatographic or electrophoretic methods.

A number of different assays have been developed to measure glycated hemoglobin. All of the methods should be carefully standardized with appropriate quality control. Clinicians should be familiar with the method used by their local laboratory and its pitfalls. All of the methods show excellent correlation with one another. The absolute numbers obtained by one or another method, or between laboratories, cannot be directly compared, however.

Each method has its own pitfalls. For example, the chromatographic methods are influenced by a number of circumstances. For example, carbamylated hemoglobin, formed in uremia, and HbAA (formed by acetaldehyde addition to hemoglobin in alcoholics) coelute with $HbA_{1a}+_b$, while fetal hemoglobin (HbF) (elevated in pregnancy, thalessemia, and certain hemoglobinopathies) coelutes with HbA_{1c}. These have the potential for creating falsely elevated glycated hemoglobin determinations. In contrast, slowly migrating hemoglobins (e.g., sickle hemoglobin, HbS; and HbC) although also glycated will not be measured by the chromatographic techniques, therefore leading to falsely low glycated hemoglobin determinations.

◼ OTHER GLYCATED PROTEINS

The process of nonenzymatic glycosylation occurs with all proteins. Thus, in addition to the measurement of glycated hemoglobin, it is possible to use measurement of other glycated proteins to reflect glycemic control over a period related to the life span of that protein. Clinically, assays of glycated serum albumin and of serum fructosamine (reflecting glycation of serum proteins generally) have been used. These reflect glycemic control over a shorter period than glycated hemoglobin, approximately 2 to 4 weeks. As a consequence, some clinicians have used one of these measures, in conjunction with glycated hemoglobin, in order to infer the time period over which changes in glycemic control have occurred. I have not found such measurements useful and therefore do not employ them.

■ URINE GLUCOSE

Historically, urine glucose was commonly used to reflect glycemic control. However, urine glucose is a second order reflection of blood glucose and does not always accurately reflect blood glucose. Urine glucose measurements are influenced not only by the amount of glucose present but also by fluid intake, urine flow, and urine concentration. The presence of glycosuria indicates that the renal threshold was exeeded sometime after the previous urination, but does not indicate when during that interval that occurred. Thus, the interval since the previous urination influences results. The renal threshold for glucose varies between individuals and is altered by changes in kidney function. Moreover, negative urine-glucose tests do not distinguish among hypoglycemia, euglycemia, and moderate hyperglycemia. In addition, some medications may interfere with urine glucose determinations. All of these factors contribute to the inaccuracy of urine glucose measurements in monitoring of diabetes. As a consequence, the American Diabetes Association (ADA) recommends that all patients treated with insulin monitor blood glucose rather than urine glucose. Urine glucose measurements are used only in patients who are unable or unwilling to perform regular blood glucose measurements.

■ URINE KETONES

Urine-ketone determinations continue to be an important measurement in the management of diabetes. Urine-ketone determinations help patients detect decompensation of their diabetes. Patients with type 1 diabetes should measure urinary ketones whenever there is significant hyperglycemia, i.e., greater than 240 mg per deciliter (13.4 mmol per liter), to detect uncontrolled diabetes and potential impending ketoacidosis. Measurements should be made during intercurrent illness or when there are medical symptoms of uncontrolled diabetes (e.g., polyuria, polydipsia) or of potential ketocidosis (e.g., nausea, vomiting, abdominal pain). Their presence dictates the need for actions to prevent ketoacidosis. A sample action plan for illness is shown in Table 1.

Ketonuria may occur for reasons other than insulin deficiency. Ketosis and ketonuria may arise as a consequence of four conditions: (1) insulin deficiency and uncontrolled diabetes; (2) starvation (insufficient calorie intake); (3) posthypoglycemia in response to secretion of counter-regulatory hormones (catecholamines, glucagon, growth hormone, and cortisol) which are lipolytic; and (4) stress with attendant hormonal secretion (again, of catecholamines, glucagon, growth hormone, and cortisol), be that stress physical (e.g., illness, infection, vomiting) or emotional. Ketone production rate also increases during exercise, but ketosis and ketonuria generally occur only if there is concomitant insulin deficiency.

Table 1 Sample Action Plan for Illness.

DURING ILLNESS:
Check blood glucose every 3–4 hr.
Check urine ketones at time of each blood-glucose measurement.
If urine ketones are large and blood glucose is 300 mg/dl or more, double the amount of extra insulin taken.
Drink plenty of fluids—more than you think you need.
If blood gluose is higher than 200 mg/dl, the fluids should be free of sugar.
If blood glucose is lower than 200 mg/dl, the fluids should contain sugar.
Contact your physician or diabetes clinical specialist if:
You have taken two to three insulin supplements—to let them know you are having a problem.
You are unable to keep food down or are vomiting.
Your blood glucose does not seem to be responding to the supplements you have taken.
You have large ketones two to three times in a row.
You are having to breathe fast or hard.
You have any questions.

Ketosis is to be particularly avoided during pregnancy, where it may have an adverse effect on fetal development. Starvation ketosis and/or posthypoglycemia ketosis both may occur only during pregnancy. Therefore, urine ketones should be routinely measured during pregnancy, especially in the morning.

Morning urine ketone determinations may also be used to detect suspected nocturnal hypoglycemia. Some physicians recommend routine testing for this purpose. Others recommend testing only if nocturnal hypoglycemia is otherwise detected.

Commercial methods for urine ketone determination are based on the nitroprusside reaction in which acetoacetate and acetone (but not beta-hydroxybutyrate) produce a purple color, the intensity of which provides a qualitative estimate of the degree of ketosis. It should be appreciated that beta-hydroxybutyrate is the largest fraction of ketones, and yet is not included in the measurement. This may confuse interpretation of results, which should be used only as a relative indicator. Humidity adversely affects the reagent such that false-negative readings may occur.

■ LIPIDS

Abnormalities in plasma lipids and lipoproteins have been correlated with inadequacy of diabetic control. Thus, increased concentrations of cholesterol and triglyceride and decreased levels of HDL cholesterol may be indicative of inadequate metabolic control. These values often can be corrected, albeit slowly over weeks, with the attainment of improved diabetic control. Extent of lipid abnormality has been shown to correlate with glycated hemoglobin level and may be an additional indicator of long-term diabetic control.

Suggested Reading
American Diabetes Association. Consensus statement on self-monitoring of blood glucose. Diabetes Care 1987; 10:93–99.

American Diabetes Association Consensus Statement. Self-monitoring of blood glucose. Diabetes Care 1994; 17:81–86.

American Diabetes Association. Position statement, urine glucose and ketone determinations. Diabetes Care 1996; 18(suppl 1):S35.

American Diabetes Association. Clinical practice recommendations: 1996. Diabetes Care 1996; 19(suppl 1):S1–S118.

The four preceding references are American Diabetes Association clinical practice recommendations dealing with monitoring.

Bunn HF. Evaluation of glycosylated hemoglobin in diabetic patients. Diabetes 1981; 30:613–617.

Reviews the clinical utility of glycated hemoglobin.

de Veciana M, Major CA, Morgan MA, et al. Postprandial versus preprandial blood glucose monitoring in women with gestational diabetes mellitus requiring insulin therapy. N Engl J Med 1995; 333:1237–1241.

Discusses number of daily blood glucose measurements needed to attain excellent control in gestational diabetes mellitus.

Diabetes Control and Complications Trial Research Group. The effect of intensive treatment of diabetes on the development and progression of long-term complications in insulin-dependent diabetes mellitus. N Engl J Med 1993; 329:683–689.

Diabetes Control and Complications Trial Research Group. Implementation of treatment protocols in the diabetes control and complications trial. Diabetes Care 1995; 18:361–376.

The DCCT established the importance of meticulous glycemic control and emphasized the role of self-monitoring in achieving it.

Goldstein DE, Little RR, Lorenz RA, et al. Tests of glycemia in diabetes. Diabetes Care 1995; 18:896–909.

Provides an overview of the clinical utility of contemporary glucose-monitoring approaches.

Goldstein DE, Parker KM, England JD, et al. Clinical application of glycosylated hemoglobin measurements. Diabetes 1982; 31(suppl 3):70–78.

Reviews the clinical usefulness of glycated hemoglobin.

Nathan DM, McKitrick C, Larkin M, et al. Glycemic control in diabetes mellitus: Have changes in therapy made a difference? Am J Med 1996; 100:157–163.

Provides an overview of the clinical usefulness of contemporary glucose-monitoring approaches.

Nathan DM, Singer DE, Hurxthal K, Goodson JD. The clinical information value of the glycosylated hemoglobin assay. N Engl J Med 1984; 310:341–346.

Reviews the clinical usefulness of glycated hemoglobin.

Pernick NL, Rodbard D. Personal computer programs to assist with self-monitoring of blood glucose and self-adjustment of insulin dosage. Diabetes Care 1986; 9:61–69.

Description of a computer program to facilitate self-monitoring and self-adjustment.

Peterson CM, Jovanovic L, Chanoch LH. Randomized trial of computer-assisted insulin delivery in patients with type 1 diabetes beginning pump therapy. Am J Med 1988; 81:69–72.

Discusses the number of daily glucose measurements needed to attain excellent control.

Schade DS, Santiago JV, Skyler JS, Rizza R. Intensive insulin therapy. Princeton, NJ: Excerpta Medica, 1983.

This monograph provides details for management of type 1 diabetes.

Schiffrin A, Belmonte M. Multiple daily self-glucose monitoring: Its essential role in long-term glucose control in insulin-dependent diabetic patients treated with pump and multiple subcutaneous injections. Diabetes Care 1982; 5:479–484.

Discusses number of daily blood glucose measurements needed to attain excellent control.

Skyler JS. Patient self-monitoring of blood glucose. Med Clin North Am 1982; 66:1227–1250.

A review of self-monitoring of blood glucose.

Skyler JS. Monitoring diabetes mellitus. In: Galloway JA, Potvin JH, Shuman CR (eds), 9th ed. Diabetes mellitus. Indianapolis, Ind: Lilly, 1988:160.

A review of the monitoring of diabetes.

Tattersall RB. Home blood glucose monitoring. Diabetologia 1979; 16:71–74.

A review of self-monitoring of blood glucose.

HYPOGLYCEMIA IN TYPE 1 DIABETIC PATIENTS

Geremia B. Bolli, M.D.

Hypoglycemia is an integral part of daily life for people with type 1 diabetes mellitus. Mild, asymptomatic episodes occur once or twice a week in insulin-treated diabetic subjects. Nocturnal, asymptomatic hypoglycemia occurs in about 25 percent of diabetic subjects treated with either conventional or intensive insulin therapy. In the Diabetes Control and Complications Trial (DCCT), the frequency of severe hypoglycemia, i.e., coma or the need for external assistance (intramuscular [IM] glucagon or intravenous [IV] glucose injection), increased threefold in diabetic subjects treated with intensive therapy as compared with subjects receiving conventional therapy.

Even brief hypoglycemia can cause profound dysfunction of the brain. Prolonged, severe hypoglycemia can cause permanent neurologic sequelae. In addition, it is possible that hypoglycemia accelerates the vascular complications of diabetes by increasing platelet aggregation. Finally, hypoglycemia may be fatal. If data in the literature are pooled, at least 4 percent of deaths in nearly 1,000 patients with type 1 diabetes mellitus were the result of hypoglycemia. Moreover, it is likely that this figure is an underestimation. Familiarity with the causes and mechanism of insulin-induced hypoglycemia is highly desirable if the frequency and the consequences of hypoglycemia among insulin-treated diabetic patients are to be reduced.

■ DEFINITION OF HYPOGLYCEMIA GLYCEMIC THRESHOLDS

Hypoglycemia is defined as a plasma glucose concentration below 50 mg per deciliter (2.8 mmol per liter). However, this level is low, if one considers that counter-regulatory hormonal responses are elicited at plasma glucose levels of approximately 65 mg per deciliter (approximately 3.6 mmol per liter). Extensive clinical investigation has established the glycemic thresholds, not only for the secretion of counter-regulatory hormones, but also for the appearance of symptoms of hypoglycemia and deterioration of cognitive function.

In response to a fall in blood glucose, increased secretion of glucagon, epinephrine, cortisol, and growth hormone occurs at a glycemic level of approximately 65 mg per deciliter (approximately 3.6 mmol per liter). At this glycemic threshold subjects do not experience any symptoms of hypoglycemia, either autonomic or neuroglycopenic (see later). Thus, in this early phase of hypoglycemia, nondiabetic healthy subjects are unaware that the counter-regulatory response has been activated. Only when the plasma glucose concentration falls below approximately 58 mg per deciliter (3.2 mmol per liter) do the symptoms of hypoglycemia appear. These symptoms include those due to activation of the sympathetic system (e.g., sweating, heart pounding, tremor, hunger), as well as the symptoms of glucose deprivation in the brain (neuroglycopenic symptoms, e.g., difficulty thinking, dizziness, tingling). The appearance of autonomic and/or neuroglycopenic symptoms testifies that hypoglycemia has progressed from a mild, asymptomatic stage to a more severe, symptomatic phase.

■ GLUCOSE HOMEOSTASIS AND THE CENTRAL NERVOUS SYSTEM

The glycemic threshold for activation of hormonal counter-regulation (approximately 65 mg per deciliter or 3.6 mmol per liter) lies just below the normal postabsorptive plasma glucose concentration, 80 mg per deciliter (4.5 mmol per liter). This emphasizes the importance for the human body to recognize and prevent a fall in blood glucose to protect brain metabolism and function. The brain has a high energy requirement, approximately 1 mg per kilogram per minute of glucose, or approximately 100 g per 24 hours in an adult. Under normal conditions, the brain can not oxidize substrates other than glucose. Since the brain can not synthesize glucose and has reserves sufficient for only a few minutes, its function is almost totally dependent on an uninterrupted supply of glucose by the circulation.

■ PHYSIOLOGY OF THE GLUCOSE COUNTER-REGULATORY SYSTEM

Glucose counter-regulation is essential for survival and serves to protect the brain from hypoglycemia under physiological circumstances, such as prolonged fasting, as well as during the treatment of diabetic patients with oral or parenteral administration of hypoglycemic drugs or insulin. The glucose counter-regulatory system consists of several intergrated parts: (1) the brain, which "senses" a decrease in glucose delivery from circulation and initiates neurogenic stimulation of the hypothalamus and pituitary gland to augment the secretion of growth hormone and adrenocorticotrophin; (2) the adrenal medulla and adrenergic nervous system, which release catecholamines; (3) the pancreatic islets, which respond directly to the low blood glucose concentration and also to central neurogenic signals to reduce insulin and augment glucagon secretion; and (4) autoregulation of hepatic glucose production. This complex system maintains the plasma glucose concentration above a critical threshold, which is essential to ensure sufficient blood glucose delivery to the brain.

The acute response to hypoglycemia is exemplified by changes in glucose production and utilization and the counter-regulatory hormone response following injection of insulin in healthy nondiabetic individuals (Fig. 1). Insulin enhances glucose utilization by peripheral tissues and suppresses hepatic glucose release, leading to a decline in the plasma glucose concentration. Recovery from acute hypoglycemia is related to an increase in the rate of hepatic glucose

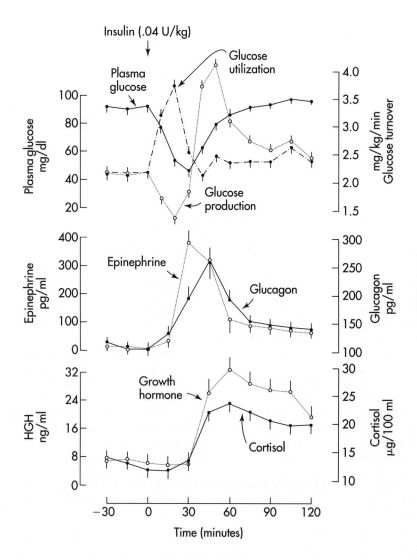

Figure 1
Glucose metabolic (*upper panel*) and counter-regulatory hormonal (*middle and lower panels*) responses to insulin-induced hypoglycemia. (*From Gerich J, et. al. Metabolism 1980; 29: 1164–1175; with permission.*)

production, which is coincident with the stimulation of all counter-regulatory hormones. Glucagon, by increasing hepatic glucose production, is the primary hormone responsible for the recovery from acute hypoglycemia. In many longstanding, poorly controlled diabetics, glucagon secretion is deficient and epinephrine replaces glucagon as the critical counter-regulatory hormone in the defense against acute hypoglycemia. Neither growth hormone nor cortisol plays an important role in recovery from acute insulin-induced hypoglycemia.

The response to hypoglycemia in type 1 diabetic patients given subcutaneous (SC) insulin differs significantly from that described earlier for acute hyperglycemia: (1) clinical hypoglycemia usually has a gradual onset, lasts for several hours, and is reversed slowly; and (2) the mechanisms of counter-regulation during prolonged hypoglycemia differ from those of acute hypoglycemia. When prolonged hypoglycemia is induced by low-dose insulin administration, suppression of endogenous insulin secretion represents an important defense mechanism and contributes both to the increase in hepatic glucose production and suppression of peripheral glucose uti-

lization in the muscle. Glucagon and epinephrine increase hepatic glucose production both acutely and in the long term. In contrast to glucagon, which does not possess extrahepatic effects, epinephrine also reduces the uptake of glucose in the muscle and stimulates lipolysis. The resultant increase in plasma free fatty acid concentration stimulates hepatic gluconeogenesis and suppresses glucose utilization in the muscle (Randle's cycle). Growth hormone and cortisol represent "slow" counter-regulatory hormones because it takes 2 to 3 hours to observe their insulin-antagonistic effects. Both growth hormone and cortisol increase glucose production from the liver, suppress glucose utilization in the muscle, and stimulate lipolysis.

The response to the "rapid" counter-regulatory hormones (glucagon and epinephrine) are more important than those of the slow hormones (growth hormone and cortisol) because they exert their counter-regulatory effects quickly in the early phase of recovery from hypoglycemia. In diabetic patients with severe sustained hypoglycemia, hepatic autoregulation (i.e., an increase in hepatic glucose production in response to hypoglycemia per se) is activated.

CAUSES OF HYPOGLYCEMIA IN TYPE 1 DIABETES MELLITUS

In clinical practice, hypoglycemia usually is observed in one of three clinical situations: (1) injection of an excessive amount of insulin, (2) a missed meal after an insulin injection, and (3) physical exercise. The latter is discussed in the chapter *Exercise in the Management of Insulin-Dependent Diabetes Mellitus*. It is important to recognize that all diabetic subjects are at risk to develop hypoglycemia for two reasons: (1) insulin is administered subcutaneously, creating peripheral hyperinsulinemia and increased muscle glucose utilization, and (2) many diabetics have impaired glucose counter-regulatory hormonal responses.

Although peripheral hyperinsulinemia of diabetes mellitus is the initiating factor responsible for hypoglycemia, it does not explain why hypoglycemia is more prolonged and more severe in some diabetic patients. This is explained by an impaired counter-regulatory hormonal response. Patients with type 1 diabetes mellitus are unable to reduce circulating insulin levels during hypoglycemia because of lack of pancreatic beta cells and continued absorption of insulin from the SC depot after an injection. In addition, the secretion of counter-regulatory hormones in response to hypoglycemia is impaired in type 1 diabetes mellitus. In longstanding diabetics, there is a reduced or absent glucagon response to hypoglycemia and this leads to a blunted increase in hepatic glucose production. Type 1 diabetic individuals also commonly manifest an impaired epinephrine response to hypoglycemia. The loss of epinephrine secretion usually follows rather than precedes that of glucagon. If the response of both glucagon and epinephrine to hypoglycemia is impaired, hypoglycemia is more severe and prolonged and is not preceded by any of the typical adrenergic warning symptoms. If hypoglycemic episodes are common and the diabetic subject's blood glucose level is too tightly controlled, there may be an iatrogenic down regulation in the release of all counter-regulatory hormones even though the intrinsic ability to secrete epinephrine and glucagon is intact. Chronic overinsulinization also impairs the perception of the autonomic symptoms of hypoglycemia.

THE SOMOGYI PHENOMENON

Excessive glucose counter-regulation may cause hyperglycemia in type 1 diabetes mellitus by inducing insulin resistance after hypoglycemia, the so-called "Somogyi phenomenon." This is due primarily to secretion of epinephrine, growth hormone, and cortisol. However, nocturnal hypoglycemia may not result in fasting hyperglycemia if overnight plasma insulin concentrations are high, i.e., after the injection of a large dose of intermediate-acting insulin before supper or at bedtime. Since the hypoglycemia occurs during the sleeping hours, the patients may not experience any symptoms of hypoglycemia. The post-hypoglycemic insulin resistance is typically prolonged for several hours and may cause important postmeal hyperglycemia even though the fasting hyperglycemia is modest. Patients who awake with wet undergarments and/or are hungry or who complain of nightmares should be suspected of having nocturnal hypoglycemia. The presence of urinary ketones in the first voided morning specimen (due to epinephrine release) also should raise suspicion about nocturnal hypoglycemia. A normal fasting glucose concentration when the diabetic patient goes to sleep also should heighten the suspicion about nocturnal hypoglycemia.

TREATMENT OF HYPOGLYCEMIA

Minor Episodes

Standard treatment is to advise the patient to rest and to take 10 to 20 g of carbohydrate orally. It is important to stress the need for both short-acting and longer-acting carbohydrates, e.g., the regimen might be half a glass of orange juice and two biscuits. Many patients often overtreat hypoglycemia, leading to wide swings in the blood sugar level. When circumstances permit, the diagnosis of hypoglycemia should be confirmed by measuring the blood glucose level. This helps the patient to correctly interpret the subjective feelings of hypoglycemia and avoids unnecessary treatment.

Hypoglycemic Coma

Most individuals who experience episodes of hypoglycemic coma recover spontaneously (if the patient is alone or asleep) or with the help of glucose forced into the mouth by friends or relatives. If teeth are clenched, glucose tablets may be of little use. Moreover, the mouth often is dry, and the glucose tablets may not dissolve normally. Glucose solutions or gels delivered into the cheek space are effective. If the administration of oral glucose fails, the helpers should give an IM injection of glucagon. Glucagon (1 mg) is supplied as a powder that must be dissolved before injection. If glucagon is not available, the emergency service should be contacted or the patient brought to the hospital or clinic and given 25 g of glucose IV.

This conventionally is given as a bolus dose of 50 ml of 50 percent glucose (25 g). However, half of this dose is preferable to avoid rebound hyperglycemia. If the patient does not respond immediately, the blood glucose level should be measured and, if indicated, a second bolus of IV glucose administered.

PREVENTION OF HYPOGLYCEMIA

With appropriate preventive measures hypoglycemic coma and excessive less-serious hypoglycemic episodes can be minimized in diabetic patients, even in those receiving intensive insulin therapy. The following points should be taken into consideration.

First, the therapeutic insulin regimen should mimic insulin dynamics of normal, nondiabetic individuals as closely as possible. Thus, there should be some baseline input of insulin throughout the day and sleeping hours to prevent the excessive production of glucose by the liver and a bolus injection of a short-acting insulin 20 to 30 minutes before each meal. Insulin regimens that meet these objectives are described in the chapter *Insulin Therapy in Type 1 Diabetes Mellitus*.

Second, the glycemic targets must be individualized for each diabetic patient. In general, the premeal plasma glucose concentration should be kept somewhere above the upper limit of the nondiabetic range (Table 1). Because of the time-to-time variability of insulin absorption from the subcutaneous site of injection, the presently available insulin regimens are rather imprecise in achieving the ideal insulin pharmacokinetics and are not precisely reproducible. All type 1 diabetic individuals, especially those receiving intensive insulin therapy, should perform frequent self-blood glucose monitoring (prior to each insulin injection). If frequent hypoglycemic reactions are encountered, less stringent glycemic control is indicated and the insulin dose and/or regimen must be adjusted appropriately. Data from a 7-year follow-up of diabetic patients treated with intensive insulin therapy in the Oslo, Stockholm, and DCCT studies indicate that it is sufficient to maintain the percent HbA$_{1c}$ below 7.0 percent to prevent significant progression of background retinopathy. This is an important finding, because it implies that "absolute" normoglycemia is not a necessary prerequisite for prevention of late microangiopathy in type 1 diabetes mellitus. Thus, prevention of late diabetic complications can be achieved with near-normal glycemia. Mild hyperglycemia is the best protection against severe hypoglycemia. In patients in whom intensive insulin therapy is contraindicated for whatever reason (e.g., advanced diabetic microvascular complications, severe coronary or cerebrovascular disease, deficient counter-regulation, hypoglycemia unawareness), prevention of hypoglycemia is the primary aim. This is best achieved by setting slightly higher hyperglycemic targets (see Table 1). In non–intensively treated diabetics, it is particularly important to aim for mild to moderate hyperglycemia during the sleeping hours and especially between midnight and 3 AM due to the dawn phenomenon.

Third, candidates for intensive insulin therapy should be carefully screened. Patients with new- or recent-onset type 1 diabetes are the ideal candidates since they are free of complications and are most likely to have intact glucose counter-regulation. Diabetic patients with longer duration of diabetes are potential candidates if they are free of diabetic complications or have early, mild, i.e., reversible, complications and intact counter-regulatory mechanisms. Intensive insulin therapy is a strategy to prevent, not to cure advanced diabetic complications. Diabetic patients with hypoglycemia unawareness and or impaired hypoglycemia are not candidates for intensive insulin therapy. Because recurrent hypoglycemia may of itself blunt the response of counter-regulatory hormones and increase the glycemic thresholds for symptoms, it is important to prevent hypoglycemia and to avoid the vicious cycle leading to hypoglycemia unawareness.

Fourth, and most importantly, patients must receive appropriate education about their disease, and close contact with the medical team is crucial in order to maintain good blood glucose control while minimizing the risk of hypoglycemia. Diabetes education includes emphasis on the timing of meal consumption and the injection of Regular insulin, and advice on the amount of carbohydrate needed to avoid hypoglycemic (as well as hyperglycemic) episodes. Patients should be warned specifically of the dangers of excessive alcohol consumption, particularly if food is omitted. They also should know that there is a danger of delayed hypoglycemia after heavy alcohol intake or prolonged exercise. Peripheral glucose uptake is acutely enhanced during exercise, and insulin absorption is accelerated if the injected

Table 1 Suggested Glycemic Targets to Prevent Hypoglycemia in Insulin-Treated Diabetic Patients

	BLOOD GLUCOSE (PRIOR TO MEALS)	HBA$_{1c}$ (%)*
Intensive therapy	110–140 mg/dl (6.1–7.8 mmol/l)	6.5–7.0
Nonintensive therapy	140–180 mg/dl (7.8–10 mmol/l)	7.0–8.5

*Normal HbA$_{1c}$ (determined by HPLC) in nondiabetics is 3.8–5.5%.

limb is exercised within an hour or two of the injection. Insulin sensitivity may be increased for several hours following sustained exercise, producing a risk of delayed hypoglycemia. Other factors that modify the response to exercise include time of day and degree of glycemic control. Plasma glucose drops rapidly during exercise in the well-insulinized diabetic patient, but relatively little in the hyperglycemic individual with low circulating insulin levels. Advice must therefore be tailored to the needs of each patient.

Anticipatory downward adjustment of insulin dose is mandatory in the diabetic patient who plans to exercise (see chapter *Exercise in the Management of Insulin-Dependent Diabetes Mellitus*). All patients who plan to exercise should carry a rapidly absorbable source of carbohydrate with them.

Suggested Reading

Bolli GB. From physiology of glucose counter-regulation to prevention of hypoglycemia in type 1 diabetes mellitus. Diabetes Nutr Metab 1990; 4:333–349.

Summarizes the physiologic mechanisms of glucose counter-regulation to hypoglycemia in normal humans and its abnormalities in insulin-dependent diabetes mellitus (IDDM). Also describes the most relevant steps to be taken in practice to prevent hypoglycemia in IDDM.

Bolli GB. The pharmacokinetic basis of insulin therapy. Diabetes Res Clin Pract 1989; 6:S3–S16.

Reviews the kinetics and dynamics of short-acting and long-acting insulin injected subcutaneously in IDDM patients and derives models of therapy of IDDM based on these aspects.

Bolli GB, DeFeo P, Perriello G. Nocturnal blood glucose control in type 1 diabetes mellitus. Diabetes Care 1993; 16(suppl 3):71–89.

Deals with the causes of nocturnal hypoglycemia in IDDM and proposes a rational model of insulin therapy to prevent hypoglycemia at night.

Cryer PE. Iatrogenic hypoglycemia as a cause of hypoglycemia-associated autonomic failure in IDDM: A vicious circle. Diabetes 1992; 41:255–260.

Underlines the new concept that recurrent hypoglycemia in IDDM favors further hypoglycemia and responses of counter-regulatory hormones.

Cryer P, Binder C, Bolli G, et al. Hypoglycemia in IDDM. Diabetes 1989; 38:1193–1199.

Reports the epidemiology, the physiopathology, and the rational approach to the problem of hypoglycemia in IDDM.

Cryer PE, Gerich JE. Glucose counter-regulation, hypoglycemia, and intensive insulin therapy. N Engl J Med 1985; 313:232–241.

Reviews in detail the causes of hypoglycemia in IDDM.

Fanelli C, Epifano L, Rambotti AM, et al. Meticulous prevention of hypoglycemia near normalizes magnitude and glycemic thresholds of neuroendocrine responses to, symptoms of, and cognitive function during hypoglycemia in intensively treated patients with IDDM of short duration. Diabetes 1993; 42:1683–1689.

Reports the possibility of reversing hypoglycemia unawareness in IDDM and, most important, maintaining good glycemic control.

HYPERSENSITIVITY REACTIONS TO INSULIN AND INSULIN RESISTANCE

S. Edwin Fineberg, M.D.

Despite the development of recombinant DNA and semisynthetic human insulins, insulin allergy and antibody–mediated-insulin resistance continue to be observed because of the inherent immunogenicity of insulin-injection therapy and the occurrence of autoimmune syndromes. The incidence of insulin allergy in previously insulin-naive individuals treated with highly purified pork or human insulin is about 2 percent. Injection-site lipoatrophy in such individuals is virtually nonexistent whereas with beef-pork or beef insulin, the incidence of lipoatrophy is 4 percent to 5 percent. Even with the most immunogenic insulins of the past (which had an incidence of hypersensitivity responses of 15 percent to 55 percent), the incidence of anaphylaxis was very rare and the current incidence of severe antibody–mediated-insulin resistance is less than 0.1 percent. Local and systemic allergy, injection-site lipoatrophy, and antibody–mediated-insulin resistance are described in this chapter, and therapeutic approaches are suggested. In addition, problems associated with the insulin autoimmune syndrome and type B insulin resistance (secondary to antireceptor antibodies) are discussed briefly.

■ ETIOLOGY AND PATHOPHYSIOLOGY

Insulin allergy may be associated with antibodies directed to insulin itself, non-insulin peptides (in older insulins), insulin degradation products, or antibodies directed to protamine (NPH insulin); zinc; or to contaminants in the insulin diluting fluids (i.e., latex particles in plasticizers from the vial cap). Allergic reactions to insulin are classified and described in Table 1. Generally, allergic reactions to insulin develop within 2 weeks to 2 months after the onset of therapy and are usually confined to the injection site. Remissions within 2 months occur in more than 90 percent of individuals, and most of the remainder remit within 1 year of onset. Local wheal and flare and biphasic reactions, as well as anaphylaxis, are secondary to the cross linking of tissue-fixed IgE antibodies and antigens on the surface of mast cells and basophils with subsequent release of cytokines and histamine. The Arthus reaction involves the formation of complement-fixing immune complexes within the vasculature with a subsequent inflammatory response. Delayed hypersensitivity (tuberculin-like) is mediated by sensitized clones of lymphocytes. The role of allergy in injection-site lipoatrophy is not certain. However, this problem is rarely seen in human or pork-insulin–treated individuals; injection of such lesions with pork or human insulins causes filling in of an atrophied site; and biopsy has shown increased concentrations of insulin-immune complexes in the borders of lesions.

Therapy of insulin hypersensitivity is aimed, if possible, at removal of the offending antigen, alleviation of symptoms, and/or, if necessary, induction of tolerance by desensitization procedures.

Antibody–mediated-insulin resistance may result from excessive binding of insulin prior to receptor binding or interference with the insulin receptor by antireceptor antibodies. In the latter case, the population of receptor antibodies may contain both insulin agonists and antagonists. In the insulin-autoimmune syndrome, hypoglycemia due to release of insulin from anti-insulin antibodies may predominate at times during the patient's course (often occurring postprandially), whereas in type B insulin resistance, the predominant antibody is usually antagonistic, resulting usually in insulin resistance. Severe insulin resistance can be defined in general as an insulin-dose requirement that exceeds 1.5 U per kilogram of body weight in adults or 2.5 U per kilogram in children. Milder degrees of insulin resistance that are seen in clinical diabetes usually can not be attributed to anti-insulin or antireceptor antibodies.

Other etiologies of insulin resistance are outlined in Table 2. Factitious insulin resistance can be eliminated by having a registered nurse or doctor administer insulin dosages in a uniform site. Previous therapy with beef-containing insulins, interrupted therapy, or a history of atopy are common in insulin–antibody-mediated resistance. Such insulin resistance also may be a feature of nondiabetic autoimmune disorders such as lupus erythematosus; an accompaniment of lymphoma; or associated with methimazole or penicillamine

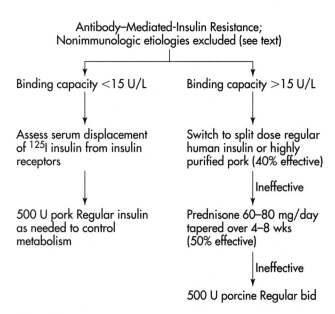

Figure 1
Stepwise approach to the diagnosis and treatment of insulin resistance.

Table 1 Insulin Hypersensitivity Reactions

LOCAL	
Wheal and flare	Immediate onset within 30 min. Duration up to 1 hr. Pruritic, non-painful lesions.
Biphasic	Wheal and flare followed by a late phase of pain and erythema. Peaks at 4–6 hr, lasts 24 hr.
Arthus reaction	Well-defined nodule develops within 8–12 hr and peaks at 24 hr, often pruritic and painful.
Systemic	Most commonly hives, but may result in anaphylaxis. N.B.: Life-threatening anaphylaxis has been most commonly reported in association with reversal of heparinization by protamine in NPH-exposed patients.

therapy. Hirsutism, acanthosis nigricans, and other features consistent with polycystic ovary syndrome are common in individuals with type B insulin resistance. If anti-insulin antibodies are the cause of insulin resistance, the titer of antibodies usually exceeds 15 U per liter and the resistance is primarily related to high-affinity antibodies. In the case of antireceptor antibodies, such antibodies can be shown to displace ^{125}I insulin binding to insulin receptors on cells. Both of these assays are available through many diabetes research laboratories and a few commercial laboratories. A stepwise approach to diagnosis and therapy of insulin resistance is outlined in Figure 1. Subcutaneous (SC) insulin degradation syndrome is associated with a relatively normal IV insulin requirement but greatly increased SC route requirements. Treatment of antibody–mediated-insulin resistance is outlined in Figure 1.

Table 2 Etiologies of Insulin Resistance

ANTIBODY-MEDIATED
Anti-insulin antibodies
Type B insulin-resistance syndrome
OTHER CAUSES
Factitious insulin resistance
Endocrine disorders (hyperthyroidism, hypercortisolism, and acromegaly)
Illness or neoplasia
Subcutaneous insulin resistance
GENETIC SYNDROMES
Lipodystrophy
Type A insulin resistance syndrome
Leprechaunism
Rabson-Mendenhall syndrome

In the case of autoimmune disorders and lymphoma, treatment of the underlying illness will result in a subsidence of insulin resistance. Hypoglycemia is a common feature of insulin autoimmunity secondary to treatment with sulf-hydryl-containing drugs (e.g., methimazole). Spontaneous remission is usually observed. Type B insulin resistance will not respond to insulin switching or steroids and may require massive doses of 500 U insulin daily for therapy in individuals who have developed diabetes (a subset of these individuals). Subcutaneous insulin-resistance syndrome is extremely rare and tends to remit spontaneously. Affected individuals may require prolonged periods of IV insulin therapy.

■ PREFERRED THERAPEUTIC APPROACH

Insulin Hypersensitivity

If insulin hypersensitivity is local and insulin therapy is the only viable therapeutic approach, one must first rule out improper injection techniques or infections. If the patient is on animal insulins, a switch to human insulin is indicated. If symptoms persist for 30 days and do not improve after changing insulin with or without antihistamines, then one should consider skin testing to determine the least reactive insulin. Intradermal injections of 0.02 ml of a 1:1 dilution of 100 U human, pork, and beef insulins in normal saline-phenol, zinc sulfate 700 μg per milliliter in saline-phenol, and 0.1 mg per milliliter of histamine phosphate (positive control) and normal saline-phenol (negative control) should be injected. Patients are observed for a positive wheal and flare reaction within 30 minutes (5 mm > negative control) and for induration (>1 cm) at 6 and 24 hours. The patient should then be switched to the least reactive insulin. Reaction to zinc may be an indication for switching to protamine insulin. Mild persistent allergy should be modified with antihistamines (25 to 50 mg of diphenhydramin every 6 hours). If local allergy is persistent and severe, then divide insulin doses into multiple sites or consider the use of Regular insulin delivered by continuous subcutaneous insulin infusion. Severe delayed or biphasic local reactions may be ameliorated by the addition of 1 μg of dexamethasone per U of insulin administered.

Table 3 Skin Testing and Rapid Desensitization in Severe Systemic Allergy	
SKIN TESTING	**RAPID DESENSITIZATION**
At 20-minute intervals, successively inject 0.02 ml of the following intradermally—0.001, 0.01, 0.1, and 1.0 U of Regular human insulin diluted in normal saline-phenol or neutral insulin dilution fluid. Use saline-phenol or insulin dilution fluid as a negative control. If reaction is 5 mm > negative control, begin again using pork or if necessary beef insulin. If using human or other insulins and all tests are negative, proceed to inject 1 U of insulin intradermally. If no reaction is encountered with 1 U of insulin, suspect that severe hypersensitivity is not present and proceed to treat with the nonreactive insulin. If a positive wheal and flare reaction is encountered, begin rapid desensitization using the least reactive insulin.	Have life-support equipment and a syringe filled with 1 ml of 1:1000 epinephrine available along with adequate assistance. This procedure is best carried out in an intensive care setting. Do not titrate while the patient is being treated with steroids or antihistamines. Prepare serial 1:10 dilutions of the least reactive insulin after initial 1:1 dilution of 100 U insulin (50, 5, 0.5, 0.05, and 0.005 U/ml). If patient reacts to the initial dosage, begin desensitization with 0.005 U/ml. At 30-minute intervals, inject the following intradermally—0.05 U/ml: 0.02, 0.04, and 0.08 ml; 0.5 U/ml: 0.02, 0.04, and 0.08 ml; 5 U/ml: 0.02 ml. Then as subcutaneous injections—5 U/ml: 0.04, 0.08 U/ml; and 50 U/ml: 0.02, 0.04, and 0.08 ml. Reduce by two steps if a wheal and flare plus other symptoms or induration >1 cm is encountered. If no reactions are encountered, double the dosage every 4 hr until metabolic stability is achieved and then add intermediate-duration insulin as needed.

Systemic Allergy

One must first determine if insulin therapy is necessary, i.e. can the patient be managed by diet or oral hypoglycemic agents? Mild systemic allergy manifested only by pruritus and urticaria with or without rhinorrhea can usually be managed by switching to a less-immunogenic insulin and modifying the symptomatology with diphenhydramine. In such individuals skin testing as suggested above may be useful to identify the least reactive insulin preparation. Severe systemic reactions, especially those associated with anaphylaxis, require identification of the least reactive insulin by the skin-testing protocol outlined in Table 3. If the patient is medically stable within 24 hours of the last dose of therapeutic insulin, begin the patient on one-third of the last dose of insulin and increase the dosage every 12 hours until adequate metabolic control is achieved. If the patient develops a hypersensitivity reaction or becomes medically unstable, or if the last dose of insulin was given more than 24 hours previously, then rapid desensitization is indicated as described in Table 3.

■ PROS AND CONS OF THERAPY

Local hypersensitivity reactions seldom require any but the mildest symptomatic therapy. The use of systemic steroids in the treatment of systemic allergy may be associated with dramatic increases in dosage requirements for insulin and rarely the precipitation of diabetic ketoacidosis. Desensitization has been shown to be occasionally followed by a subsequent period of insulin–antibody-mediated severe resistance. Unfor- tunately not all individuals with insulin–antibody-mediated resistance respond to the therapeutic measures outlined previously. Although most individuals spontaneously remit within 1 year without additional therapy, severe insulin resistance persisting for over 5 years has been reported.

Suggested Reading

Davidson JK, DeBra DW. Immunological insulin resistance. Diabetes 1978; 27:307–318.

Drs. Davidson and DeBra treated 35 patients with severe immunologic insulin resistance with sulfated beef insulin.

They studied effects upon insulin-antibody kinetics as well as dose requirements. In 34 of 35 cases substantial improvement was obtained. An excellent review of the older literature is provided.

DeShazo DR, Mather P, Grant W, et al. Evaluation of patients with local reactions to insulin with skin tests and in vitro techniques. Diabetes Care 1987; 10:330–336.

Dr. DeShazo and co-workers sought to better understand the part played by IgE and IgG antibodies to insulin in the production of dermal reactions to insulin. A total of 22 patients with large reactions, 46 patients without reactions, and 22 controls were studied. A simple skin-testing protocol is described along with appropriate therapy and precautions.

Galloway J, DeShazo DR. Insulin chemistry and pharmacology; insulin allergy resistance and lipodystrophy. In: Rifkin H, Porte D, eds. Ellenberg and Rifkin's diabetes mellitus: Theory and practice, 4th ed. New York: Elsevier, 1990:504.

Drs. Galloway and DeShazo provide an encyclopedic chapter that encompasses insulin resistance and allergy and provides detailed protocols for evaluation and therapy. Detailed tables and an extensive bibliography are provided.

Kahn CR, Rosenthal AS. Immunologic reactions to insulin: Insulin allergy, insulin resistance and autoimmune insulin syndrome. Diabetes Care 1979; 2:283–295.

This review concentrates on the common dermal reactions to insulin, the relationship of antibody formation to insulin structure, insulin resistance and the insulin autoimmune syndrome. A review of experimental studies relevant to these topics is included.

Nathan DM, Axelrod L, Flier JS, Carr DB. U500 insulin in the treatment of antibody–mediated-insulin resistance. Ann Intern Med 1981; 94:653–656.

This paper describes the treatment of insulin–antibody-mediated insulin resistance with U 500 insulin.

Soto-Aguilar MS, DeShazo DR, Waring NP. Anaphylaxis. Why it happens and what to do about it. Postgrad Med 1987; 82:154–170.

The pathophysiology and treatment of anaphylaxis from various causes is described in detail. The authors also discuss a more common clinical problem, the anaphylactoid reaction that is not mediated by antibodies.

Taylor SI, Kadowaki T, Kadowaki H, et al. Mutations in insulin-receptor gene in insulin resistant patients. Diabetes Care 1990; 13:257–279.

Dr. Taylor and co-workers review the subject of insulin resistance with emphasis on insulin-receptor abnormalities. They provide a discussion of the differential diagnosis and pathophysiology.

Van Haeften TW. Clinical significance of insulin antibodies in insulin-treated diabetic patients. Diabetes Care 1989; 12:641–648.

Dr. Van Haeften discusses insulin antibodies and their clinical relevance.

Weiler JM, Friedman P, Sharath MD, et al. Serious adverse reactions to protamine sulfate; all alternatives needed? Allergy Clin Immunol 1985; 75:297–303.

A commonly reported complication of reversal of heparin anticoagulation therapy by protamine is anaphylaxis. Such reactions are discussed along with other clinical presentations of adverse reactions to protamine. Also, the relationship of reactions to antibody levels is reported.

EXERCISE IN THE MANAGEMENT OF TYPE 1 DIABETES MELLITUS

John T. Devlin, M.D.

Exercise has been long recognized as an important modulator of insulin requirements in insulin-dependent diabetes mellitus (IDDM). Two major objectives must be considered when prescribing an exercise program for IDDM patients who wish to exercise: (1) optimization of the therapeutic benefit to the individual (i.e., general health and well being), and (2) minimizing the risks (i.e., hypoglycemia, metabolic decompensation, and exacerbation of diabetic complications). The physician who prescribes an exercise regimen must be aware of several important physiologic adaptations to exercise that occur in IDDM and nondiabetic subjects. First, although insulin is not required for contracting skeletal muscle to increase its utilization of glucose, the increment in muscle-glucose metabolism will be enhanced by the presence of insulin. Second, insulin is required to inhibit the excessive production of ketone bodies by the liver, which would occur if insulin deficiency coexisted with the increases in counter-regulatory hormone concentrations (e.g., glucagon, catecholamines) that occur during exercise. Third, in nondiabetic individuals there is a normal decrease in circulating insulin concentrations during exercise. This allows hepatic glucose production to increase and precisely match the augmented rate of skeletal muscle glucose utilization that occurs during exercise. These normal physiologic responses to exercise present a dilemma for people with IDDM who attempt to incorporate an exercise program into their daily schedule. Sufficient insulin must be present to avoid acute metabolic decompensation during exercise (i.e., hyperglycemia and ketoacidosis), while at the same time avoiding excessive hyperinsulinemia (or increasing glucose intake) in order to prevent exercise-induced hypoglycemia.

■ BENEFICIAL EFFECTS OF EXERCISE (Table 1)

A major reason to encourage exercise in IDDM children and adolescents is to reinforce their sense of "normalcy" and well being. With proper advice and education, exercise can be performed safely and successfully, eliminating the stigma of physical limitation. The International Diabetic Athletes Association offers members many benefits, including highly informative annual meetings, opportunities for entering racing competitions, and a good networking system.[*]

From a health professional standpoint, improvements in plasma-lipid profile, blood pressure, and cardiovascular fitness are of great importance to a population that is at increased risk for cardiovascular disease. Exercise also may help to maintain desired body weight, decrease body fat content, preserve muscle mass, and increase strength. In IDDM patients it generally is accepted that improved glycemic control is not a primary goal of physical training, although some type 1 individuals may benefit following the institution of a program of regular physical exercise. This is in contrast to the well-recognized benefits of exercise on glucose control in type 2 diabetes mellitus (see the chapter on this topic). Although physical training will result in improved skeletal-muscle–insulin sensitivity in IDDM, this is usually balanced by either an increase in caloric intake or a reduction in insulin dosage to avoid hypoglycemia during and after exercise. Although the net effect in most type 1 patients is unchanged glycemic control (assessed by HbA$_{1c}$ concentrations), reduced insulin dosage, lowered circulating insulin concentrations, and enhanced insulin sensitivity may be beneficial from the cardiovascular standpoint.

---

[*]The founder and president of the affiliate is Paula Harper, R.N., 1931 East Rovey Avenue, Phoenix, Arizona 85016.

Table 1 Benefits and Risks of Exercise in IDDM

BENEFITS OF EXERCISE	RISKS OF EXERCISE
Improved sense of well-being and enhanced social interactions	Avoid ostracism in children and adolescents
Improvement in cardiovascular risk factors	Metabolic decompensation
Plasma lipids	Hypoglycemia
Blood pressure	Hyperglycemia
Cardiac performance	Ketosis
Platelet hyperaggregability	Aggravation of microvascular complications
Insulin sensitivity	Proliferative retinopathy, vitreous hemorrhage, retinal detachment
Maintenance of desirable body weight	Peripheral neuropathy; foot trauma
Improved glycemic control	Orthostatic hypotension
	Increased albuminuria
	Macrovascular complications
	Myocardial ischemia or infarction
	Cardiac arrhythmia

Table 2 Guidelines for Safe Exercise (ADA)

TELL ALL PATIENTS TO:

Carry an identification card and wear a diabetes medic-alert bracelet at all times.

Be alert for signs of hypoglycemia during exercise and for several hours after.

Have immediate access to a source of readily absorbable carbohydrate (such as glucose tablets) to treat hypoglycemia.

Take sufficient fluids before, after, and, if necessary, during exercise to prevent dehydration.

Measure blood glucose. Take appropriate action if blood glucose is <80 or >240 mg/dl.

■ RISKS OF EXERCISE (Table 1)

Patients with IDDM may suffer acute metabolic decompensation during or after exercise, especially if glycemic control is suboptimal at the onset of exercise. It is well documented that insulin-withdrawn IDDM subjects (blood glucose ≥300 mg per deciliter, plasma ketones ≥2 mmol per liter) develop increasing hyperglycemia and worsening ketosis during moderate exercise. From the clinical standpoint exercise should be avoided when the plasma glucose concentration is above 250 to 300 mg per deciliter. It is important to distinguish between insulin deficiency and increased caloric intake as the cause of hyperglycemia. Urine ketones should be tested prior to exercise whenever the blood-glucose reading is above 250 mg per deciliter. If ketonuria is documented, exercise should be delayed until metabolic control is improved. If there are no urinary ketones and if hyperglycemia is partly the result of an antecedent meal, exercise is permissible, provided adequate fluids are taken, and home blood glucose and urinary-ketone concentrations are monitored after exercise.

Patients with microvascular complications need to use caution when they exercise. Patients with proliferative retinopathy should avoid strenuous exercise, especially those forms that raise intracranial pressure (e.g., Valsalva maneuver during weight lifting), result in a "head low" position, or cause head trauma (e.g., underwater diving).

Patients with sensory loss in the lower extremities should avoid exercise that causes excessive foot trauma (road running) and wear properly fitting and well-supported footwear. Running or walking on hot surfaces (pavement or beach sand) should be avoided. Patients with autonomic neuropathy and orthostatic hypotension must avoid dehydration during exercise, especially during the warmer seasons.

Water aerobics (aquaerobics) may be well tolerated due to the increased hydrostatic pressure under water. Special attention must be given to underlying cardiac autonomic neuropathy and silent coronary ischemia. A stress electrocardiogram should be obtained prior to the start of any exercise program to exclude this possibility.

The urinary albumin excretion rate is increased by exercise. However, the long-term significance, if any, of this on the rate of decline in renal function is unknown. Increases in exercise-associated microalbuminuria have been shown to correlate significantly with the presence and severity of diabetic retinopathy. Whether exercise has any effect on the progression of retinopathy in such individuals is unknown. Although further studies are needed before general recommendations can be made, it seems prudent to advise against strenuous forms of exercise that result in large increases in blood pressure or dehydration in individuals with early diabetic nephropathy and/or retinopathy.

Cardiovascular complications can be minimized by having a thorough medical evaluation prior to beginning an exercise program. This should include an exercise stress test in diabetic individuals over the age of 35 or with a duration of diabetes that exceeds 10 to 15 years. Patients with known cardiovascular disease should enroll in a supervised cardiac rehabilitation program to receive physical training. An exercise program that provides a gradual buildup in duration and intensity, with warm-up and cool-down periods, and uses appropriate pulse-rate targets (see further discussion) is mandatory.

Some general guidelines for safe exercise in IDDM have been provided by the American Diabetes Association (Table 2).

■ TYPES OF EXERCISE PROGRAMS

Beneficial metabolic and cardiovascular effects of a physical training program are best achieved by aerobic exercise. This is defined as exercise that improves the maximal aerobic work capacity (VO_{2max}) by producing increases both in cardiopulmonary function and in the oxidative capacity of skeletal muscles. More recently, resistance weight training types of exercise have also have been shown to offer beneficial metabolic effects. Many exercise programs now use combinations of aerobic and strength training exercise to achieve maximal performance. Cross-training programs (in which the athlete varies the daily exercise regimen, such as running, swimming, cycling) may minimize the risk of overuse syndrome and musculoskeletal injury, in addition to decreasing boredom with a monotonous routine. For individuals with physical limitations, a graded walking program may be the most practical. In those with lower-extremity arthritis, low-back pain, and other medical problems, swimming provides excellent conditioning with minimal physical trauma.

Each patient should discuss the various exercise options with his or her physician or exercise trainer and choose a form that is appealing and enjoyable. For many people, interactive team programs (e.g., aerobics) will enhance compliance by providing useful social interactions. For others, an indoor "home gym" program (e.g., stationary cycle, treadmill, cross-country ski machine), which allows them to exercise year-round despite inclement weather, is preferred. For diabetic individuals it is essential to choose appropriate shoes for each type of exercise program. Getting the advice of a qualified sports trainer or health professional with an interest in sports medicine (e.g., orthopedic surgeon or podiatrist) is highly advisable, especially if foot pathology (neuropathy, callus) already is present.

Aerobic conditioning programs should begin slowly and allow gradual increases in intensity and duration over time. Individuals should estimate their maximal heart rates, unless this has been determined during a maximal-exercise test. Most fitness centers have charts providing the predicted maximum heart rate for each age class, but in their absence a rough approximation is:

Age-predicted maximal heart rate = 220 − Age (years)

Maximal heart rates will be significantly lower than age-predicted values in some IDDM subjects with autonomic neuropathy and in those taking "beta-blocker" medications (i.e., propranolol). To achieve aerobic conditioning, the target heart rate during each exercise bout should be maintained at 60 to 70 percent of the "maximal heart rate reserve" (Table 3).

At the end of the period of initial physical training (8 to 12 weeks), individuals should be exercising for at least 20 to 30 minutes at the target heart rate, three or four times each week. In addition, 10 to 15 minutes should be spent before each exercise session for stretching and warming up, and an additional 10 to 15 minutes after exercise for "cooling down."

Table 3 Pulse Guidelines for the Exercise Prescription

1. Age − predicted maximal heart rate = 220 − Age
2. Estimate maximal heart rate reserve (Max HRR) as:
   Max HRR − (Age = predicted maximal HR) − (Resting HR)
3. For aerobic conditioning, it is recommended to exercise at approximately 60–70 percent of the maximal heart rate reserve (above resting), for 20–30 min each session, 3–4 sessions per week

Example: For a 40-year-old man with a resting heart rate of 60:
Age-predicted maximal heart rate = 220 − 40 = 180
Maximal heart rate reserve = 180 − 60 = 120
Exercise target heart rate = (60 − 70% × 120) + 60 = 132 − 144

■ STRATEGIES TO AVOID METABOLIC DECOMPENSATION DURING EXERCISE

It is important to make appropriate insulin-dose modifications before and after exercise to avoid hypoglycemia or hyperglycemia-ketosis during exercise. Some circulating insulin must be present to prevent worsening of glycemia and ketosis during exercise. In addition, insulin deficiency accelerates protein catabolism, and underinsulinization may limit the ability of a training program to increase strength and result in net protein anabolism. Therefore, education will be required to achieve the optimal insulin regimen for each individual for each type and duration of exercise. IDDM patients who are in poor control (i.e., plasma glucose concentrations above 250 to 300 mg per deciliter) should test their urine for ketones and, if positive, defer exercise until they have achieved better control of their glycemia.

The most common clinical problem encountered by exercising IDDM persons is hypoglycemia during or after exercise. Because insulin sensitivity may be increased for as long as 24 hours after a single bout of intense exercise, insulin-dose reductions may be required long after the exercise has been completed, especially to avoid nocturnal hypoglycemia. General guidelines can be made, but individual differences are great and necessitate the frequent use of home blood-glucose monitoring (HBGM) to make appropriate adjustments in insulin dose and food intake. The preferred time to begin exercise is 1 to 2 hours after a meal, when postprandial elevations in blood glucose are present. Exercising shortly (within 30 minutes) after a meal may be detrimental in those with coronary artery disease and in those with orthostatic hypotension, due to the increased splanchnic blood flow that occurs during digestion and absorption of nutrients. This may place an excessive demand on cardiac output, resulting in coronary ischemia and aggravating an underlying problem with hypotension.

For moderate to strenuous forms of exercise lasting longer than 30 minutes, the usual dose of insulin, which is expected to peak during the exercise session, should be lowered by one-third to one-half. Such a reduction in insulin dosage is sufficient to prevent hypoglycemia in most individuals. Ingestion of 25 to 30 g of glucose can be used to prevent hypoglycemia in the case of unplanned postprandial exercise, in which insulin dosages had not been previously lowered. In IDDM individuals who are using an insulin pump, the premeal bolus should be reduced by half and the basal infusion rate discontinued during exercise to prevent hypoglycemia during exercise. In order to avoid late hypoglycemic reactions after exercise, the basal insulin infusion rate usually needs to be reduced by 25 percent from the usual rate. It should be emphasized that these recommendations must be taken only as approximate guidelines, because there is great interindividual variation. Insulin-dependent diabetes mellitus patients on similar or different insulin regimens must determine for themselves the optimal insulin-dose adjustments before and after exercise in order to prevent hypo- and hyperglycemia.

Many people engaged in prolonged endurance exercise, such as cycling, take small, "permissive" doses of insulin prior to exercise (to avoid ketosis), and ingest frequent small carbohydrate feedings throughout the exercise to prevent hypoglycemia. To facilitate gastric emptying and absorption, consumption of carbohydrates in liquid form (dilute solutions containing glucose or glucose polymers) is preferable, especially during exercise in warm temperatures when prevention of dehydration is critical. Solutions containing glucose polymers (e.g., maltodextrins) offer an advantage over pure glucose solutions because they have a lower osmolarity. Therefore, they are less likely to delay gastric emptying or draw fluids into the intestinal lumen ("dumping"). Glucose solutions should be dilute (10 to 20 percent or 10 to 20 g per 100 ml) for the same reason. Except for very long and arduous competitions, the addition of electrolytes to solutions is unnecessary, because these losses can be replaced by the subsequent meal. The caloric requirement of exercise may be estimated from Table 4, which gives the approximate caloric cost of various activities. The percent of calories utilized from carbohydrate and fat sources varies with the intensity of exer-

cise, with carbohydrate providing a greater percentage of total calories oxidized at higher relative workloads. For the typical workout session, approximately 50 percent of the calories burned may be from carbohydrate sources. Therefore, an individual exercising at a workload of 10 kcal per minute above resting energy expenditure may need approximately 300 carbohydrate calories or 75 g (there are 4 calories per gram) to provide for this requirement. Because these are fairly crude estimates, and because much of the glucose oxidized in muscle is provided by the endogenous glycogen stores in muscle and liver, individual responses need to be determined using HBGM.

Nocturnal hypoglycemia following intense exercise may be much more common than previously recognized. Postexercise late-onset hypoglycemia, typically occurring 6 to 15 hours after the completion of strenuous exercise or play, is

Table 4 Energy Expenditure Associated with Common Exercises

ACTIVITY	CALORIES BURNED EACH MINUTE	CALORIES BURNED IN AN HOUR

Light housework
  Polishing furniture
  Light handwashing
	2–2½	120–150

Golf, using power cart Level walking 2 mph	2½–4	150–240
Cleaning windows, mopping floors, or vacuuming Walking 3 mph Golf, pulling cart Cycling 6 mph Bowling	4–5	240–300
Scrubbing floors Cycling 8 mph Walking 3½ mph Table tennis, badminton, and volleyball Double tennis Golf, carrying clubs Many calisthenics and ballet exercises	5–6	300–360
Walking 4 mph Ice or roller skating Cycling 10 mph	6–7	360–420
Walking 5 mph Cycling 11 mph Water skiing Singles tennis	7–8	420–480
Jogging 5 mph Cycling 12 mph Downhill skiing Paddleball	8–10	480–600
Running 5½ mph Cycling 13 mph Squash or handball (practice session)	10–11	600–660
Running 6 mph or more Competitive handball or squash	11 or more	660 or more

From Physicians Guide to Non–Insulin-Dependent (type 2) Diabetes (ADA Clinical Education Program). 2nd ed. American Diabetes Association 1988:36; with permission.

observed in approximately 15 percent of IDDM individuals. Nocturnal hypoglycemia usually occurs when the exercise takes place between 3:00 PM and 8:00 PM. Nocturnal hypoglycemia often is severe, resulting in stupor, coma and/or seizures, and may require treatment with subcutaneous (SC) glucagon or intravenous glucose. In order to minimize the risk of this occurrence, IDDM patients must be made aware of this possibility and institute adjustments in their management plan in anticipation of unusually strenuous exercise. Such strategies include a reduction in insulin dosage, especially with those insulin preparations that act throughout the night; ingestion of an adequate bedtime snack; and checking the blood-sugar level before going to sleep.

■ VARIABLES AFFECTING INSULIN-DOSE REQUIREMENTS (Table 5)

Type of Insulin
In general, regimens providing more frequent insulin injections or the constant infusion of short-acting (Regular) insulin provide the greatest flexibility for accommodating exercise sessions with the least risk. One-or two-shot per day regimens, which use long-acting insulin, make it more difficult to exercise safely without meticulous attention and planning well in advance of the anticipated exercise sessions. Use of a continuous subcutaneous insulin injection (CSII) device ("open-loop" insulin pump) offers an advantage in providing a relatively small depot of subcutaneous insulin, which may help to avoid inappropriately elevated circulating insulin concentrations and attendant hypoglycemia during exercise. On the other hand, interruptions in insulin delivery by either pump or connecting catheter-tubing malfunction may leave the patient seriously underinsulinized and ketosis-prone during and after exercise.

Site of Injection
Injections in the exercising limb (e.g., the thigh during running or cycling) will result in more rapid absorption of insulin if exercise is performed within 30 to 60 minutes of injection. It is generally recommended that exercise is delayed for at least 1 hour after injection into a limb that will be exer-

cising. Because absorption varies between abdominal, thigh, and arm sites, the individual should attempt to be consistent in the injection sites used before and after exercise to eliminate this possibly complicating variable.

Ambient Temperature
The rate of insulin absorption from a SC depot varies with the ambient temperature (i.e., more rapid in warmer weather). Warm ambient temperature (30° C) and exercise have independent, additive effects to increase the rate of insulin absorption and will result in a lower blood-glucose concentration. Conversely, cool temperature (10° C) and lack of exercise will decrease the rate of insulin absorption, leading to higher blood-glucose levels. Modest adjustments in diet, insulin dose, or both may be required to avoid postprandial hyperglycemia at cool temperatures or hypoglycemia at warm temperatures.

It is especially important to allow the insulin to equilibrate at ambient temperature before use and not to draw up and inject from a recently refrigerated vial.

Time of Day
The effects of exercise on plasma glucose concentrations may vary depending on the time of day at which the exercise is performed. In IDDM patients receiving a long-acting based insulin regimen, moderate-intensity exercise in the afternoon tends to have more of a blood-glucose lowering effect than the same exercise performed in the morning. IDDM patients need to be made aware that the hypoglycemic effect of exercise may vary depending on the time of day that the exercise is performed and the insulin regimen that the patient is taking.

Duration and Intensity of Exercise
Although the usual experience is a decline in blood-glucose concentration during and after exercise, some well-controlled IDDM patients may show increasing glucose concentrations during brief, very intense exercise. This paradoxic hyperglycemic effect is associated with short bursts of very intense exercise, about 80 percent or more VO_{2max}. The exercise-induced rise in blood-glucose level may persist for 2 to 3 hours following cessation of the exercise. This hyperglycemic response has been attributed to the large increase (fourfold) in catecholamines induced by the near-maximal exertion, combined with the brief duration of exercise (10 to 15 minutes) during which skeletal-muscle glucose utilization had not increased sufficiently to match the excess glucose production by the liver. There is a risk of subsequent hypoglycemia if the increase in blood glucose is treated too aggressively with insulin, because the elevation in counter-regulatory hormone concentrations is transient.

■ OPTIMIZING PHYSICAL PERFORMANCE

A major determinant of athletic performance during prolonged high-intensity events, such as distance running or cycling, is the skeletal-muscle glycogen concentration. It has been shown that IDDM patients have normal rates of glycogen synthesis, provided they are well insulinized.

Repletion of muscle glycogen stores after a bout of glycogen-depleting exercise is normally complete within 14 to 16

Table 5 Factors Influencing Insulin-Dose Modifications Before, During, and After Exercise

Food Intake	Insulin Injection
Size	Insulin regimen
Macronutrient composition	CSII, MSI, CIT
Timing in relation to exercise	Site of injection
Rate of gastric emptying	?exercising limb
?gastroparesis	Type/dose of insulin
Exercise	Timing of injection
Time of day	Ambient temperature
Type, intensity, and duration	**Metabolic Control**
Regional muscle groups utilized	Blood-glucose testing
Large vs small groups	
Training status of individual	Urine ketones
Habitual vs sporadic	

CSII = continuous subcutaneous insulin infusion (pump);
MSI = multiple subcutaneous insulin injections (intensive);
CIT = conventional insulin therapy (usual two shots per day).

hours. Many athletes ingest diets containing very high levels of carbohydrates, often in excess of 70 percent of total calories, in order to maintain their muscle glycogen concentrations at maximal ("supercompensated") levels. Approximately 550 g of carbohydrate are required to fully replete muscle glycogen stores after a bout of glycogen-depleting exercise. This can be achieved in IDDM patients using the same general dietary guidelines recommended by the American Diabetes Association. The carbohydrate should be derived primarily from complex, high-fiber food sources such as legumes, pastas, and cereals, rather than from processed or highly refined simple sugars. Provided the proper types of carbohydrates are used to meet the very high total energy and carbohydrate requirements of the competitive athlete with IDDM, there is little risk of the adverse metabolic sequelae (e.g., hypertriglyceridemia) described after the ingestion of diets containing large amounts of simple sugars. The individual must carefully adjust his insulin dose to match the increased caloric intake with the enhanced energy expenditure and prolonged increase in skeletal-muscle insulin sensitivity that occurs following intense exercise. Subjects with IDDM should be cautioned not to follow the traditional method of "carboloading," which uses a low-carbohydrate intake for 3 days following a glycogen-depleting bout of exercise, followed by 3 days of high-carbohydrate intake. A 3-day period of low-carbohydrate intake is not necessary to maximize muscle-glycogen concentrations. Furthermore, this period of low-carbohydrate, high-fat intake may be especially hazardous for IDDM subjects at risk for both hypoglycemia and ketosis.

Suggested Reading

Devlin JT. Effects of exercise on insulin sensitivity in humans. Diabetes Care 1992; 15:1690–1693.

Henriksson J. Effects of physical training on the metabolism of skeletal muscle. Diabetes Care 1992; 15:1701–1711.

Hildebrandt P. Subcutaneous absorption of insulin in insulin-dependent diabetic patients. Influence of species, physico-chemical properties of insulin and physiological factors. Danish Medical Bulletin. 1991; 38:337–346.

Horton ES. Role and management of exercise in diabetes mellitus. Diabetes Care 1988; 11:201–211.

Kemmer FW. Prevention of hypoglycemia during exercise in type 1 diabetes. Diabetes Care 1992; 15:1732–1735.

Laundry GL, Allen DB. Diabetes mellitus and exercise. [review] Clin Sports Med 1992; 11:403–418.

McArdle WD, Katch FI, Katch VL. Exercise physiology, 4th ed. Baltimore: Williams & Wilkins, 1996.

Richter EA, Turcotte L, Hespel P, Kiens B. Metabolic responses to exercise. Effects of endurance training and implications for diabetes. Diabetes Care 1992; 15:1767–1776.

Sonnenberg GE, Kemmer FW, Berger M. Exercise in type 1 (insulin-dependent) diabetic patients treated with continuous subcutaneous insulin infusion: prevention of exercise induced hypoglycemia. Diabetologia 1990; 33:686–703.

Wasserman DH, Zinman B. Exercise in individuals with IDDM. Diabetes Care 1994; 17:924–937.

MEDICAL NUTRITION THERAPY IN TYPE 1 DIABETES MELLITUS

Anne Daly, R.D., M.S., C.D.E.

There are few diseases in which food and nutrition are as important as the management of diabetes. While insulin replacement is the distinguishing feature in treatment of type 1 or insulin-dependent diabetes mellitus (IDDM), optimal therapy includes a careful balance of three modalities: food, insulin, and physical activity.

The primary goals of IDDM treatment are: (1) to promote and maintain day-to-day clinical and psychological well being; (2) to avoid severe hypoglycemia, symptomatic hyperglycemia, and ketoacidosis; and (3) to promote normal growth and development in children. The secondary goals of IDDM treatment are to achieve the best possible glycemic control and to prevent, delay, or arrest micro- and macrovascular complications and excess weight gain. Medical nutrition therapy (MNT) is critical for achieving both these primary and secondary goals.

■ RATIONALE

Insulin-dependent diabetes mellitus and type 2 or non–insulin-dependent diabetes mellitus (NIDDM) are considered to be distinct types of diabetes that require different nutrition-management strategies. Meal-planning strategies can be prioritized according to the type of diabetes (Table 1).

For patients with IDDM, MNT should emphasize the inter-relationships among food, activity, and insulin. Those receiving conventional insulin therapy must maintain consistency in the timing and amount of their food intake. Ideally, the insulin plan should be designed to match the person's preferred eating pattern. Previous recommendations were for total calories to be divided between meals and snacks based on the insulin regimen, using fractions. This is no longer recommended because it does not promote individualization. However, the timing of food intake should be synchronized with the administration of insulin. Because of the limitations of a two-injection insulin regimen, persons on such a regimen may need to alter their usual eating habits. They also need to mon-

Table 1 Diabetes Meal Plan Strategies

STRATEGY	IDDM	NIDDM* OBESE	NIDDM* NONOBESE	GDM	IGT
Regular timing of meals	H	M	M	H	L
Consistency of day-to-day intake	H	M	M	H	L
Meal spacing	M	H	M	M	L
Fat modification†	H	H	H	M	H
Sucrose limitation	M	M	M	M	M
Exercise	M	H	H	M	H
Exercise snack	H	L	L	M	L
Caloric restriction	L	H	L	L$	M¶
Other nutritional variables‡	M	M	M	M	M
Blood glucose monitoring	H	H	H	H	L

H = high priority; *M* = moderate; *L* = low priority; *GDM* = gestational diabetes mellitus; *IDDM* = insulin-dependent diabetes mellitus; *IGT* = impaired glucose tolerance, *NIDDM* = non–insulin-dependent diabetes mellitus.

*Persons taking insulin may need to follow IDDM strategies of timing and consistency more closely. If the person is overweight, weight reduction remains the priority.

†Partially dependent on blood lipid levels.

‡Dependent on other medical conditions (cancer, renal disease, hypertension, food allergies).

§Weight gain should follow weight grid for pregnancy.

¶If overweight, weight reduction is encouraged.

From Powers MA. Handbook of diabetes medical nutrition therapy. Rockville, Md: Aspen Publishers, 1996; with permission.

Table 2 Possible Causes of Growth Deviations in Children with Type 1 Diabetes Mellitus

GROWTH DEVIATION	POSSIBLE CAUSE
Underweight	Inadequate energy intake; poor glycemic control; missed injections; overzealous fat restriction; low income
Overweight	Excessive energy intake; over-insulinized; overtreatment of reactions
Erratic weight	Eating disorders; alcohol/drug abuse; inconsistent self-care

From Connell JE, Thomas-Doberson D. Nutrional management of children and adolescents with insulin-dependent diabetes mellitus: A review by the Diabetes Care and Education Dietetic Practice group. J Am Diet Assoc 1991; 91:1556–1564; with permission.

itor their blood glucose levels and then adjust their short-acting insulin in relation to the amount of food they plan to eat.

Persons receiving intensive insulin therapy—i.e., multiple daily injections or pump infusion—have considerable flexibility in when and what to eat. Nevertheless, they too, need to integrate their insulin regimen with their life-style and adjust the insulin dose when they deviate from their usual eating and exercise patterns. These persons can adjust their premeal insulin dose when they deviate from their meal plan and exercise program. Even with the increase in flexibility, the more consistent they are with their eating and physical activity, the easier overall management is.

As a central feature of diabetes treatment, MNT and meal planning should receive prompt attention from the newly diagnosed patient; insulin dosage should be appropriately adjusted around the patient's diet. At the time of diagnosis, it is critical that all health care team members support and

emphasize the importance of following diabetes nutrition guidelines. Adjustments in both MNT and insulin management will be needed periodically.

■ NUTRITION ASSESSMENT

A thorough nutrition assessment of a child with IDDM is the first and most important step in the nutrition-education process because it provides the database used to make future decisions. The assessment should include the following data:

Pattern of Growth

Growth patterns can be affected by inadequate calories, insufficient insulin, or both. Therefore, assessment of growth pattern is critical to calorie and insulin prescriptions. A child may lose a substantial amount of weight before diagnosis of IDDM owing to metabolic effects of inadequate insulin. Weight and height should be plotted on a standardized growth chart and comparisons made to age-matched controls.

The growth chart is not always an accurate tool for predicting ideal body weight for adolescents. See Table 2 for potential reasons for deviations from a normal growth pattern.

Insulin Regimen

The amount, type, and schedule of insulin injections must be considered when developing a nutrition care plan. On average, children and adolescents require 0.6 to 0.8 U of insulin per kilogram body weight per 24-hour period; adolescents require as much as 1.0 to 1.5 U per kilogram body weight. The dosage is individualized by evaluating blood glucose response to insulin, food, and activity. Children who report taking 2 or more units of insulin per kilogram body weight daily and do not have hypoglycemic reactions are probably not taking all of their insulin.

Blood Glucose Results

Nutrition assessment includes an examination of home blood-glucose test results. The advent of self-monitoring of blood glucose (SMBG) has allowed greater individuality and flexibility of meal planning. The result has been a degree of sophistication and precision that was previously unthinkable. The SMBG has expanded active participation of the patient in self-care management. Blood-glucose test results can be useful to evaluate types of foods being consumed, portion sizes, meal spacing, distribution of food throughout the day, and body-weight changes. For example, high levels of blood glucose before supper may reflect frequent snacking after school, eating the afternoon snack too late, or eating a very late supper (morning insulin is no longer effective). Hypoglycemia before lunch may indicate inadequate or missed breakfast, missed morning snacks, inadequate food intake to cover exercise, or late lunch. Hyperglycemia at breakfast may reflect overconsumption of bedtime snack or rebound hyperglycemia (Somogyi effect) during the night. The goals for IDDM treatment may be characterized in terms of these three levels of treatment—minimal, average, and intensive—each having a typical biochemical and clinical profile (Table 3).

Glycosylated Hemoglobin

Glycosylated hemoglobin provides the best available index of chronic glucose levels. This assay reflects the average blood glucose concentration over the preceding 6 to 10 weeks and can be used to assess the accuracy of blood-glucose records.

Glycosylated hemoglobin is invaluable in identifying patients with relatively high, average, or near-normal levels of chronic glucose control. Normal range for the hemoglobin A_{1c} assay is 4 percent to 6 percent; normal range for hemoglobin A1 and the total hemoglobin assays is 5 percent to 8 percent. A level greater than approximately 15 percent (using hemoglobin A1 and total hemoglobin assays) is usually indicative of more than simple dietary indiscretion (i.e., person may be missing injections or be underinsulinized).

■ FAMILY SITUATION

Diabetes affects the family, and the family situation affects diabetes. The health care team needs to know who the family members are, who the primary caretaker is, what economic resources are available, who shops for and prepares the food, as well as any other social supports that exist. Any special interests, hobbies, or leisure activities of the child with diabetes or other family members should be noted. If care is shared by separate families, or child caretakers, all should be included in the assessment and education. In shared-care situations, it is common for disagreement to arise over diet issues.

■ NUTRITION HISTORY

A nutrition history performed by a registered dietitian, preferably one who is an expert in diabetes and in working with infants, children, or teenagers with IDDM, will be most informative to the health care team. Typically, data is obtained during a personal interview with the child and significant family

Table 3 Levels of Treatment for Type 1 Diabetic Patients

MINIMAL (UNACCEPTABLE UNDER ALL NORMAL CIRCUMSTANCES)
HbA_{1c} 11–13%; glycosylated Hb 13–15%
Many self-monitored blood glucose (SMBG) values ≥300 mg/dl (≥16.7 mM)
Intermittent ketonuria
Mean blood glucose level >300 mg/dl (≥16.7 mM)

AVERAGE (IMPROVEMENT SHOULD BE ATTEMPTED IF THE PATIENT'S CLINICAL AND PERSONAL SITUATION PERMITS)
HbA_{1c} 8–9%; glycosylated Hb 10–11%
Premeal SMBG 160–200 mg/dl (8.8–11.1 mM)
Mean blood glucose level 160–240 mg/dl (8.9–11.1 mM)
Rare ketonuria

INTENSIVE (DESIRED, IF POSSIBLE TO ACHIEVE WITHOUT SIGNIFICANT SERIOUS SIDE EFFECTS)
HbA_{1c} 6–7%; glycosylated Hb 7.0–9.0%
Premeal SMBG 80–120 mg/dl (4.4–6.7 mM)
Bedtime SMBG 100–140 mg/dl (5.6–7.8 mM)
Essentially no ketonuria
Mean blood glucose level 120–160 mg/dl (6.7–8.9 mM)

From American Diabetes Association. Medical management of insulin-dependent (type 1) diabetes, 2nd ed. Alexandria Va: American Diabetes Association, 1994:19; with permission.

members rather than a questionnaire. Basic information about usual nutritional intake and activity is obtained, such as timing and location of meals; types and portion sizes of foods eaten; and food likes and dislikes. Information about frequency of meals eaten away from home is important. Exercise-related questions (type, duration, time of day, frequency, and treatment of hypoglycemia) are generally included. During this interview, the dietitian should assess:

Which stage of education, survival (initial) or in-depth continuing (see next section), is appropriate at this point?

Child/family's expectations and general attitude toward diabetes (How are they coping with diagnosis? Are they ready to learn?)

Style of learning (visual, audio, hands-on) and learning/reading ability.

To whom should education be directed? (Parent, child, significant others?)

Developmental issues (growth, weight control, sports) that are important to them.

Eating difficulties (i.e., binging, eating disorders, eating battles).

■ NUTRIENT RECOMMENDATIONS

The 1994 nutrition recommendations from the American Diabetes Association emphasized that just as no set insulin regimen or exercise program works for all people, no set diet prescription can work for everyone with diabetes. For most people, this means modifying—not abandoning—their usual eating habits.

The only acceptable way to prescribe a diabetic diet is to develop individualized guidelines based on a complete nutrition, medical, and social assessment. No longer are calories arbitrarily distributed according to macronutrient composition. Monitoring outcomes and providing ongoing care are essential.

The goals of MNT are to: (1) achieve blood glucose goals; (2) achieve optimal blood lipid levels; (3) provide appropriate calories for reasonable weight, normal growth and development, pregnancy, and lactation; (4) prevent, delay, or treat nutrition-related complications; and (5) improve health through optimal nutrition.

A summary of nutrition guidelines for children and adolescents with IDDM is given in Table 4. It should be emphasized to children and their families that the meal plan is not a restriction of calories, but a guide to ensure consistency of food intake and a nutritionally balanced diet.

Calories

The determination of a calorie level and a nutrient prescription for a child or adolescent is based on the nutrition assessment. There are various ways to calculate the appropriate calorie needs for a child. Probably the best method is to ascertain what the child usually eats to maintain his or her weight. Adolescents and parents of young children need to learn to adjust insulin intake rather than restrict food to control blood glucose levels. Inappropriate calorie prescriptions can have disastrous consequences. A child who is newly diagnosed with IDDM or who has lost weight is often in negative nitrogen balance and needs additional calories to restore normal body weight. An additional 200 to 700 kcal per day may be needed, depending on appetite and weight loss. The meal plan must then be modified as the child attains an appropriate weight for height. Follow up by the dietitian should be scheduled every 6 to 12 months to monitor the child's growth and appetite and to adjust the meal plan as necessary.

A number of formulas for estimating calorie requirements for children are in common use based on age, weight, sex, or height. The guidelines in Table 5 can be used for the prescription of minimum calorie requirements for children.

Protein

The recommendation for protein intake is similar to that of the general population: 10 percent to 20 percent of total calories. In persons with IDDM and overt diabetic nephropathy, restriction of dietary protein has been shown to retard the progression to renal failure. Therefore, a protein intake of approximately the adult recommended dietary allowance (RDA), 0.8 g per kilogram body weight per day (approximately 10 percent of daily calories), is recommended for persons with evidence of macroalbuminuria. In persons with IDDM and microalbuminuria, there is

---

Table 4 Summary of Nutrition Guidelines for Children and/or Adolescents with Type 1 Diabetes Mellitus

NUTRITION CARE PLAN

Promotes optimal compliance.

Incorporates goals of management: normal growth and development, control of blood glucose, maintenance of optimal nutritional status, and prevention of complications. Uses staged approach.

NUTRIENT RECOMMENDATIONS AND DISTRIBUTION

NUTRIENT	(%) OF CALORIES	RECOMMENDED DAILY INTAKE
Carbohydrate	Will vary	
Fiber	>20 g per day	High fiber, especially soluble fiber; optimal amount unknown
Protein	12–20	
Fat	<30	
Saturated	<10	
Polyunsaturated	6–8	
Monounsaturated	Remainder of fat allowance	
Cholesterol		<300 mg
Sodium		Avoid excessive; limit to 3,000–4,000 mg if hypertensive

ADDITIONAL RECOMMENDATIONS

Energy: If using measured diet, re-evaluate prescribed energy level at least every three months.

Protein: High-protein intakes may contribute to diabetic nephropathy. Low intakes may reverse preclinical nephropathy. Therefore, 12% to 20% of energy is recommended; lower end of range is preferred. In guiding toward the end of the range, a staged approach is useful.

Alcohol: Safe use of moderate alcohol consumption should be taught as routine anticipatory guidance as early as junior high.

Snacks: Snacks vary according to individual needs (generally three snacks per day for children; mid-afternoon and bedtime snacks for junior high children or teens).

Alternative sweeteners: Use of a variety of sweeteners is suggested.

Educational techniques: No single technique is superior. Choice of educational method used should be based on patient needs. Knowledge of a variety of techniques is important. Follow-up education and support are required.

Eating disorders: Best treatment is prevention. Unexplained poor control or severe hypoglycemia may indicate a potential eating disorder.

Exercise: Education is vital to prevent delayed or immediate hypoglycemia and to prevent worsened hyperglycemia and ketosis.

From Connell JE, Thomas-Doberson D. Nutritional management of children and adolescents with insulin-dependent diabetes mellitus: A review by the Diabetes Care and Education Dietetic Practice Group. J Am Diet Assoc 1991; 91:1556–1564; with permission.

inconclusive evidence that a low-protein diet slows the progression of nephropathy.

There is some evidence that the protein source, whether animal or vegetable in origin, may be important in affecting the progression of renal disease. However, the studies are preliminary. If the beneficial renal effects of vegetable proteins are confirmed, less drastic dietary protein restriction may be required in the treatment of diabetic nephropathy. Additional research is needed in this area.

Carbohydrate

The percentage of calories from carbohydrates will vary and is individualized based on a person's eating habits and glucose and lipid goals. The 1994 nutrition recommendations do not specify a specific amount of carbohydrate. Although various carbohydrates produce different glycemic responses, from a clinical perspective, the total amount of carbohydrate consumed is more important than the source of the carbohydrate. Scientific evidence does not support the longtime belief, based on the assumption that sucrose is more rapidly digested and absorbed than starches and thereby aggravates hyperglycemia, that sucrose must be restricted in the diets for people with IDDM. At least twelve studies in which sucrose has been substituted for more complex carbohydrates found no adverse effects on glycemia. Therefore, sucrose can be substituted for other carbohydrates gram for gram in the context of a healthy meal plan. Nevertheless, because good nutrition is a goal of MNT, advising persons with IDDM to be cautious about eating sucrose containing foods is reasonable.

Fiber

The American Diabetes Association recommendations for fiber intake for persons with IDDM are the same as recommendations for the general public: approximately 20 to 35 g per day of dietary fiber from a variety of food sources. Dietary fiber may be beneficial in maintaining normal gastrointestinal (GI) function and in treating or preventing several benign GI disorders and colon cancer. Large amounts of soluble fiber have a beneficial effect on serum lipids. Although selected soluble fibers are capable of delaying glucose absorption, the effect of dietary fiber on glycemia is probably insignificant. American children tend to have low fiber intakes. Following the general recommendations to increase consumption of complex carbohydrates will lead to an increased intake of fruits, vegetables, cereals, and grains. Intake of raw, fresh fruits rather than fruit juices, frequent use of salads and food with edible skins and seeds, bran muffins, and minimal cooking of vegetables, all lead to increased fiber intake.

A practical approach for dietitians is to assess what patients' present average intake of fiber is and counsel them to increase gradually, making sure that fibrous foods are not so filling that they limit other nutrient intakes.

Fat

Adults with IDDM are eleven times more likely to die from cardiovascular disease than their age- and sex-matched peers. Therefore, serious attention to the total amount and type of fat in the diet to minimize or prevent hyperlipidemia is warranted.

An amount for total fat is not specified in the 1994 recommendations. However, to reduce cardiovascular risk, guidelines include: less than 10 percent of calorie intake from saturated fats; and daily cholesterol intake limited to 300 mg or less. Up to 10 percent of calories can be from polyunsaturated fats (PUFAs). This leaves 60 percent to 70 percent of the calories from monounsaturated fats (MUFAs) and carbohydrates. The general recommendation for the U.S. population is to limit total dietary fat to 30 percent or less of total calories, with emphasis on reduction in saturated fat to decrease the risk for developing heart disease. This recommendation continues to apply to people with diabetes who have normal lipid levels and reasonable body weight. However, if obesity and weight-loss

Table 5 Calorie Needs for Children and Young Adults

AGE	KCAL REQUIRED/ LB BODY WT	KCAL REQUIRED/ KG BODY WT
Children		
0–12 mo	55	120
1–10 yr	45–36*	100–80
Young women		
11–15 yr	17	35
≥16 yr	15	30
Young men		
11–15 yr	36–20 (30)	80–50 (65)
16–20 yr		
Average activity	18	40
Very physically active	22	50
Sedentary	15	30

Numbers in parentheses are means.
*Gradual decline in calories per pound as age increases.
From Nutrition guide for professionals: Diabetes education and meal planning. The American Diabetes Association and The American Dietetic Association, 1988; with permission.

are the primary issues, a reduction in dietary fat and increased physical activity should be considered.

Sodium

There is an association between hypertension and IDDM. Sodium intake recommendations for persons with diabetes are the same as for the general population: 3,000 mg per day or less. For persons with hypertension—with or without diabetes—the intake should be reduced to 2,400 mg per day or less.

Alternative Sweeteners

Dietary fructose may not have overall advantage as a sweetening agent, and large amounts of fructose should be avoided in persons with dyslipidemia. Other nutritive sweeteners include corn syrup, fruit juice or fruit juice concentrate, honey, molasses, dextrose and maltose. There is no evidence that these sweeteners have any significant advantage or disadvantage over sucrose in terms of improvement in caloric content or glycemic response. Sorbitol, mannitol, and xylitol are common sugar alcohols (polyols) that contribute some calories and, if used in excessive amounts, have a laxative effect.

Non-nutritive sweeteners currently approved for use in the United States are aspartame, acesulfame K, and saccharin. All have been approved by the U.S. Food and Drug Administration for consumption and can be used safely by a person with diabetes.

Alcohol

With the exception of persons whose blood glucose is out of control, and those who are overweight, have hypertriglyceridemia, or are pregnant, most adults with IDDM may consume alcohol in moderation. Although it is not recommended, teenagers sometimes drink alcoholic beverages with their peers. Diabetes education must include guidelines for safe and moderate use of alcohol.

Guidelines for alcohol use for IDDM include: limit to two drinks per day; drink only with food; do not cut back on food. Hypoglycemic behavior, or loss of consciousness as a result of drinking alcohol, may be misinterpreted as intoxicated behavior, disguising the need for treatment to elevate the blood glucose. Self-monitoring blood glucose before and after alcohol intake, and eating a meal, will help a person to predict potential hypoglycemia and prevent it from occurring.

Sick Days

Because illness can cause blood glucose control to deteriorate rapidly, appropriate education for management of sick days may help prevent hospitalizations. On sick days, frequent, smaller meals may be better tolerated by the person with IDDM. Consuming fluids and taking an adequate dose of insulin are critically important. The person should be encouraged to follow the regular meal pattern as much as possible, but should plan to convert foods from the meal plan to carbohydrate food choices (i.e., regular soda, popsicles, jello) as tolerated. Vomiting and diarrhea cause loss of potassium and sodium. Broth, vegetables, or tomato juice help replace lost sodium. If the blood glucose is 250 mg per deciliter or higher continuously for 24 hours, or if ketones are present, the physician should be contacted.

■ ADOLESCENCE

Adolescence is always a period of both physical and psychosocial transformation. The adolescent seeks independence and often becomes rebellious and resistant to the advice of parents, physicians, and others. Youngsters with diabetes mellitus do not differ from their nondiabetic counterparts. Social pressures often necessitate the creation of greater flexibility in the dietary routine of a diabetic teenager with corresponding variations in the schedule and dosages of insulin. Experience indicates that those insulin-dependent diabetics who have had previous rapport with a dietitian or other members of the medical team, in addition to a supportive family, are most likely to cope successfully with the turmoil of adolescence. Understanding, humor, and flexibility are required of health professionals dealing with the adolescent who requires insulin. In most instances, the most rebellious and resistant patients return to a more compliant and self-caring mode with the onset of adulthood.

■ INSULIN-REQUIRING DIABETES IN THE ELDERLY

Diabetes that requires insulin treatment may develop in individuals during the seventh and eighth decades of life. The clinical presentation and symptoms are similar to those observed in younger diabetic patients. These elderly individuals are of normal weight or underweight and may require some increase in their caloric intake. Because elderly individuals are often set in their eating patterns and food selection, minimal adjustments are advised. Such patients require counseling by a dietitian and family support. Because hypoglycemia is to be avoided in the elderly diabetic patient at all costs, these patients, too, should carry a source of readily available carbohydrate.

■ EATING DISORDERS AND TYPE 1 DIABETES MELLITUS

Bulimia, anorexia nervosa, and subclinical manifestations of these disorders are being recognized in patients with IDDM with increasing frequency. Most of the patients are females. Bulimia is associated with poor metabolic control and should be suspected in young women with otherwise unexplainable severe hyperglycemia. Bulimic diabetics cope with overeating by reducing or omitting their insulin. Ketosis and electrolyte imbalance ensue. Bulimia in diabetic patients is always difficult to treat.

■ THE EDUCATIONAL PROCESS

Once a nutrition assessment has been completed, a nutrition education plan can be developed. All persons should receive an individualized diet, education, and follow-up. Education should proceed in steps small enough to enable patients and family to succeed without feeling overwhelmed with too much information. The American Diabetes Association has defined two stages of education. Initial or survival education—information and skills (which should be presented in simple, concrete terms) that have immediate applicability and will enable the child/family to get through the day without a crisis; and in-depth or continuing education and counseling—a necessary part of long-term diabetes care that includes management skills (information required to make decisions to achieve management goals and enable appropriate self-care) and ideas for improving life-style (problem-solving skills that allow a more flexible self-determined life-style). A record of the educational topics that have been taught to the patient and family should be kept on file. The registered dietitian is the preferred professional for managing nutritional needs and accomplishing fine tuning of persons with IDDM. A dietitian who has had training and experience in working with children and teenagers with IDDM offers an advantage. A dietitian who uses a creative approach with a variety of meal-planning approaches and SMBG records will likely be able to provide the most complete nutrition counseling.

The number of hours that pediatric diabetes nutrition practitioners spend with a patient during the first year after diagnosis of IDDM varies. Table 6 offers a timetable that may be used as a guideline for providing diabetes nutrition education. If time and/or staff are limited in an inpatient setting, referral to an outpatient dietitian can be made. At the time of diagnosis, and periodically throughout the course of the diabetes, the dietitian should assess life-style patterns that may influence time of insulin injections—for example: the beginning and ending of a school year; having gym class at different times; starting or ending a sports season schedule; taking on a part-time job or having irregular sleep patterns that influence meal times; switching to a vegetarian diet. The dietitian is responsible for informing the physician about these situations so that the most reasonable insulin regimen can be implemented.

If the insulin does not coincide with eating, the dietitian must consult with the physician regarding an insulin change. Also, the dietitian is responsible for making recommendations regarding balancing insulin with physical activity.

The ultimate challenge to the dietitian is to capture an interest in the meal plan aimed to establish lifelong healthy eating habits. There is no good age or time to make eating habit changes and there will always be obstacles to change.

■ IMPLEMENTATION OF MEAL PLAN

Although a variety of meal planning approaches are available, persons with IDDM are most often taught the exchange system, or its structural equivalent. The exchange approach is based on the carbohydrate, protein, and fat content of foods. For persons with IDDM, understanding the relation between these three nutrients and blood glucose is critical. Once accomplished, greater flexibility with alternative meal planning approaches, such as carbohydrate counting, is possible. In order to achieve this, several sessions with the diabetes nutrition educator are necessary. The best time to initiate a structured type of meal plan is near the time of diagnosis. Patients will then have a foundation to fall back on as their eating habits and life-style change.

Several key points should be stressed in nutrition education for IDDM:

1. Meals and snacks should be eaten and insulin injections should be given at approximately the same time each day. Chaotic schedules and irregular mealtimes make regulation of blood glucose more difficult. Occasional flexibility in schedules can be obtained by use of planned snacks.
2. Amounts and types of food eaten at each meal or snack should be as consistent as possible from day to day.
3. Food intake should be matched with the anticipated use and fall of insulin levels. Individual schedules must be considered—activity patterns, lunch times, and bus schedules. When children reach junior high school, peer conformance is of utmost importance. Omission of the morning snack is often desirable to the patient, and may be possible by reducing the morning Regular insulin.

Composition of snacks should be individualized according to patient preferences and food accessibility. However, inclusion of fresh fruits and starches for morning and afternoon snacks helps limit protein and fat intake. The best composition of a bedtime snack is not known, however, many dietitians suggest inclusion of a protein source (i.e., a milk or a meat exchange), along with a starch source, to promote a slower and prolonged glycemic effect, thereby avoiding nocturnal hypoglycemia. Bedtime snack can be adjusted based on bedtime glucose reading, and may need to be increased if extra evening physical activity may lower blood glucose during sleep.

■ EVALUATION OF MEAL PLAN

Ongoing evaluation of nutritional care is a necessary step of the education process, although it can easily be overlooked owing to time constraints. Methods of evaluation can include patient's ability to write sample menus, food records, dietary recalls, and practice exercises—i.e., ordering from restaurant menus and food-label reading. Dietary adherence has long been recognized as the most difficult aspect of a diabetes regimen. When poor compliance is noted, a dietitian should be consulted to investigate potential reasons for lack

Table 6 Estimated Timetable for Diabetes Nutrition Education

SURVIVAL INFORMATION		
Interview	1	hr
Basic meal planning	1	hr
Booster snacks for exercise	½	hr
Treating hypoglycemia	½	hr
IN-DEPTH INFORMATION (DISSEMINATED AS NEEDED)		
Pertinent educational video, as needed	½	hr
Exchange system	1	hr
Label reading; supermarket skills	½	hr
Miscellaneous topics	¼ to ½	hr each

From Connell JE, Thomas-Doberson D. Nutritional management of children and adolescents with insulin-dependent diabetes mellitus: A review by the Diabetes Care and Education Dietetic Practice Group. J Am Diet Assoc 1991; 91:1556–1564; with permission.

Table 7 Making Food Adjustments for Exercise: General Guidelines

TYPE OF EXERCISE AND EXAMPLES	IF BLOOD GLUCOSE IS:	INCREASE FOOD INTAKE BY:	SUGGESTIONS OF FOOD TO USE
Exercise of short duration and of low-to-moderate intensity (walking a half mile or leisurely bicycling for less than 30 min)	Less than 100 mg/dl	10–15 g of carbohydrate per hour	1 fruit or 1 starch/bread exchange
	100 mg/dl or above	Not necessary to increase food	
Exercise of moderate intensity (1 hour of tennis, swimming, jogging, leisurely bicycling, golfing, etc.)	Less than 100 mg/dl	25–50 g of carbohydrate before exercise, then 10–15 g per hour of exercise	½ meat sandwich with a milk or fruit exchange
	100–180 mg/dl	10–15 g of carbohydrate	1 fruit or 1 starch/bread exchange
	180–300 mg/dl	Not necessary to increase food	
	300 mg/dl or above	Do not begin exercise until blood glucose is under control	
Strenuous activity or exercise (about 1 to 2 hours of football, hockey, racquetball, or basketball games; strenuous bicycling or swimming; shoveling heavy snow)	Less than 100 mg/dl	50 g of carbohydrate; monitor blood glucose carefully	1 meat sandwich (2 slices of bread) with a milk and fruit exchange
	100–180 mg/dl	25–50 g of carbohydrate, depending on intensity and duration	½ meat sandwich with a milk or fruit exchange
	180–300 mg/dl	10–15 g of carbohydrate	1 fruit or 1 starch/bread exchange
	300 mg/dl or above	Do not begin exercise until blood glucose is under control	

From Franz MJ, Norstrom J. Diabetes actively staying healthy (DASH): Your game plan for diabetes and exercise, Minneapolis: International Diabetes Center 1990; with permission.

of adherence. Suggestions to help prevent or improve poor adherence include:

- Adjusting diabetes nutrition education to the child's lifestyle.
- Being realistic that the child will desire sweets. Teach how to include sweets occasionally, and encourage parents to limit sweets in the house.
- Encouraging parents to be positive role models.
- Guiding the parents and the child in the appropriate level of responsibility for the child.

■ PHYSICAL ACTIVITY

Physical activity, the third side of the triad of diabetes management, is frequently underestimated by health care professionals. Planning physical activity into the nutritional care plan is essential. In persons with IDDM, regular physical activity increases glucose utilization and increases insulin sensitivity. Other effects of physical activity include decreased insulin requirement, reduction of low-density lipoproteins, increase in high-density lipoproteins, decreased blood pressure, improved weight control and self-image.

Blood glucose monitoring is essential to safely regulate blood glucose levels during exercise. Ideally, a person would expend approximately the same amount of energy at the same time each day. For practical reasons, this is rarely possible. Education about exercise is necessary to avoid the risks of immediate and delayed hypoglycemia and worsening of hyperglycemia and ketosis. Persons with proliferative retinopathy and sensory neuropathy should be given special instruction regarding the appropriate type and amount of exercise.

Food intake may need to be increased before, during, or after exercise. In general, persons with IDDM tend to overeat before exercise. See Table 7 for suggested food adjustments for exercise. The best way to determine how much extra food is needed is to monitor blood glucose levels before, during, and after exercise, especially in the planning stages of developing the meal plan.

In addition to increasing food intake, it is imperative that exercisers consume an adequate amount of fluids before, during, and after exercise. For every 1 pound of weight loss during exercise, 2 cups of fluid are needed for replacement.

All persons with IDDM should carry adequate identification and a source of readily available carbohydrate (i.e., sugar, glucose tabs, gels). Candy is generally not recommended for this purpose.

Suggested Reading

American Diabetes Association. Medical management of insulin-dependent (type 1) patients, 2nd ed. Alexandria, Va: American Diabetes Association, 1994.

A comprehensive review of pathogenesis, management objectives and tools, special problems, and complications of insulin-dependent (type 1) patients.

American Diabetes Association. Nutrition recommendations and principles for people with diabetes mellitus [position statement]. Diabetes Care 1994; 17:517–522.

Position statement on goals of medical nutrition therapy and recommended treatment for type 1, type 2, and pregnancy.

Holler HI, Pastors JG, eds. Diabetes medical nutrition therapy:A professional guide for management and nutrition education resources. Chicago: American Diabetes Association Inc, The American Dietetic Association; 1997.

A guide for health care professionals on the processes of nutritional assessment, goal setting, intervention, and evaluation; how to use a variety of meal-planning approaches to effect positive medical outcomes.

Bertorelli AM, Czarnowski-Hill JV. Review of present and future use of non-nutritive sweeteners. Diabetes Educator 1990; 161:415–420.

A review of the history, properties, uses, advantages, and safety of sweeteners already approved and those awaiting approval by the FDA. The role of sweeteners in nutrition therapy for diabetes mellitus and guidelines for safe consumption.

Connell JE, Thomas-Doberson D. Nutritional management of children and adolescents with insulin-dependent diabetes mellitus: A review by the Diabetes Care and Education Dietetic Practice Group. J Am Diet Assoc 1991; 91:1556–1564.

A comprehensive review of management goals and the nutrition education process in children and adolescents with insulin-dependent diabetes, from infants to teenagers.

Diabetes Care Education Practice Group of American Dietetic Association. Meal planning approaches for diabetes management, 2nd ed. Chicago: American Dietetic Association, 1994.

A review of meal-planning approaches for use in basic and in-depth education phases, including case-study applications.

Franz MI, Horton ES, Bantle JP, et al. Nutrition principles for the management of diabetes and related complications [technical review]. Diabetes Care 1994; 17:490–518.

A review of over 200 published studies that support the 1994 Position Statement on Nutrition Recommendations and Principles for people with diabetes mellitus.

Position of the American Dietetic Association: Use of nutritive and non-nutritive sweeteners. J Am Diet Assoc 1993; 93:816–821.

A statement from the American Dietetic Association recognizing the appropriate use of nutritive and non-nutritive sweeteners when consumed in moderation and within the context of a diet consistent with U.S. Dietary Guidelines for Americans.

Powers MA. Handbook of diabetes medical nutrition therapy. Rockville, Md: Aspen Publishers, 1996.

A complete reference textbook on nutrition knowledge and skills for diabetes care and education.

THE DIABETES NURSE EDUCATOR

Julie S. Meyer, M.S.N., R.N., C.D.E.

In diabetes, more than any other chronic illness, excellent care can only be achieved through daily, lifelong attention by a motivated patient. Therefore, patient education is an essential component of the treatment plan, and the diabetes nurse educator is an essential component of the treatment team.

It is well accepted that the team approach is the best way to assist the patient in learning self-management skills, and it is important to acknowledge that the patient is the most important member of the diabetes care team. Although the physician, the nurse specialist or educator, and the nutritionist are integral to the team, they serve only in the capacity of consultant to the patient, because the patient has ultimate control over whether or not to follow the treatment regimen.

Additional members of a more comprehensive diabetes care team (Table 1) are the podiatrist, ophthalmologist, pharmacist, exercise physiologist or physical therapist, and social worker or counselor. Each of these specialists is involved in various aspects of diabetes education for the patient and family members.

The Standards of Medical Care for Patients with Diabetes Mellitus, as published by the American Diabetes Association, includes the requirement that each aspect of the management plan is understood by the patient and care provider and that the education plan is consistent with the National Standards for Diabetes Patient Education.

The nurse specialist or educator can play a key role in assisting the physician to meet the standards by assessing and providing for the educational needs of the patient and

Table 1 Members of the Diabetes Care Treatment Team

ESSENTIAL TEAM
Patient
Diabetes nurse educator
Physician
Nutritionist
COMPREHENSIVE TEAM
Patient
Diabetes nurse educator
Physician
Nutritionist
Podiatrist
Ophthalmologist
Pharmacist
Exercise physiologist or physical therapist
Social worker/counselor

Table 3 Topics for Inclusion in Patient/Family Educational Program

General facts
Psychological adjustment
Nutrition
Exercise
Medications
Monitoring
Acute complications
Chronic complications
Sick-day rules
Hygiene
Foot care
Community resources

Table 2 American Association of Diabetes Educators Standards

STANDARDS OF EDUCATION FOR DIABETES EDUCATORS
Assessment
Use of resources
Planning
Implementation
Documentation
Evaluation and outcome

by planning and coordinating the various services that the patient may need to manage his or her diabetes.

A "diabetes educator" is a health professional who is directly involved in teaching patients and/or professionals about diabetes.

A "certified diabetes educator" (CDE) is a health professional who has met the eligibility requirements and passed the National Certification Examination for Diabetes Educators earning the credential "Certified Diabetes Educator." This credential is instrumental in assuring the public that the CDE has attained a certain minimum standard of knowledge and expertise in all areas of diabetes education.

A "diabetes clinical nurse specialist" (CNS) is a registered nurse who has a minimum of a master's degree with a focus on clinical diabetes. A CNS is an advanced practitioner who has a broader range of knowledge and skills and can function more autonomously to assist the patient in clinical management. The CNS may also be a CDE.

The American Association of Diabetes Educators has developed and published national Standards of Practice for Diabetes Educators in order to assure quality in the professional practice of diabetes education (Table 2). The document includes Practice Guidelines for each specific standard. The role of the diabetes educator is reflected in the Standards of Education, which are as follows:

Standard I: Assessment
The diabetes educator should conduct a thorough, individualized needs assessment with the participation of the patient, family, or support systems, when appropriate, prior to the development of the education plan and intervention.

Standard II: Use of Resources
The diabetes educator should strive to create an educational setting conducive to learning, with adequate resources to facilitate the learning process.

Standard III: Planning
The written educational plan should be developed from information obtained from the needs assessment and based on the components of the educational process: assessment, planning, implementation, and evaluation. The plan is coordinated among diabetes health-team members, including the patient, family, and support system.

Standard IV: Implementation
The diabetes educator should provide individualized education based on a progression from basic survival skills to advanced information for daily self-management.

Standard V: Documentation
The diabetes educator should completely and accurately document the educational experience.

Standard VI: Evaluation and Outcome
The diabetes educator should participate in at least an annual review of the quality and outcome of the education process.

These standards provide the framework for carrying out an individualized education component. The topics that need to be included in the educational program for the patient and family are as described in the following paragraphs and summarized in Table 3:

1. General facts about diabetes including definition, classification signs and symptoms, and the importance of receiving on-going medical care.
2. Psychological adjustment. The chronicity of diabetes and the life-style changes that may be required can have a devastating emotional impact on the patient and the family. The family needs to be included in every aspect to provide support and encouragement for the patient. Referral to a social worker or psychologist may be appropriate.
3. Nutrition is the cornerstone of diabetes management. An individualized meal plan should be developed and instruction should be provided (by a dietitian if possible) on the effect of food intake on blood glucose levels and the relationship between nutrition, physical activity, and medication.

4. Exercise guidelines and special precautions that need to be taken to prevent hypoglycemia. Referral to an exercise physiologist or physical therapist may be appropriate.
5. Medications. Instruction on type, dose, and action of insulin or oral hypoglycemic agents. If insulin is required, the instruction will be more comprehensive to include injection technique, correct disposal of needles, storage and care of insulin, causes, symptoms, and treatment of insulin-related hypoglycemia. Discussion may include alternate insulin delivery systems such as needleless injectors and external or implantable insulin pumps.
6. Monitoring is essential in achieving and evaluating blood glucose control. Instruction includes self-monitoring of blood glucose and urine testing for ketones. The method that is most appropriate for each individual patient should be discussed and the appropriate methods, equipment, and supplies are selected. Additional methods of monitoring diabetes control, such as glycosylated hemoglobin and serum fructosamine levels, should be explained. A target range for glycemic control should be set.
7. Acute complications. The patient needs to know the causes, symptoms, treatment, and prevention of hypoglycemia, hyperglycemia, and diabetic ketoacidosis. Emphasis should be on prevention. Prompt treatment of hypoglycemia should be stressed.
8. Chronic complications. Explanation of the risk for chronic complications, the importance of prevention strategies, a schedule for monitoring and screening exams, and the frequency of medical management visits should be discussed.
9. Sick-day rules. Maintenance of adequate glycemic control during illness or surgery, guidelines for adjustments in frequency of self–blood-glucose monitoring, and possible insulin adjustments with related changes in food intake should be discussed.
10. Hygiene. Instruction includes the importance of general hygiene, skin care, and dental care.
11. Foot care. The risk for lower extremity amputation is high for persons with diabetes, therefore, thorough instruction on foot care, choice of shoes, how to recognize potential problems, and seeking prompt attention is important. Referral to a podiatrist for baseline evaluation is recommended and regular follow-up with the podiatrist should be part of the plan.
12. Community resources. The patient and family should be made aware of diabetes-related organizations and support groups available in the community, such as the American Diabetes Association and the Juvenile Diabetes Foundation. Information about financial assistance through third-party reimbursement, ways to access the health care system, and referral to an ADA-approved program may be needed.

It is clear that the diabetes educator must have a comprehensive knowledge base about current medical management and teaching-learning principles. Excellent communication and counseling skills are necessary to promote the behavioral changes necessary for optimal health outcomes, psychosocial adaptation, and quality of life. A quality patient-education program depends on the professional practice standards of the diabetes educator.

In addition to the six Standards of Education for Diabetes Educators, the American Association of Diabetes Educators has also published Standards of Professional Practice for Diabetes Educators (Table 4). They are as follows:

Table 4 Standards of Professional Practice for Diabetes Educators

Multidisciplinary collaboration
Professional development
Professional accountability
Ethics

Standard VII: Multidisciplinary Collaboration
The diabetes educator should collaborate with the multidisciplinary team of health care professionals and integrate their knowledge and skills to provide a comprehensive educational experience.
Standard VIII: Professional Development
The diabetes educator should assume responsibility for professional development and pursue continuing education to acquire current knowledge and skills.
Standard IX: Professional Accountability
The diabetes educator should accept responsibility for self-assessment of performance and peer review to ascertain the delivery of high-quality diabetes education.
Standard X: Ethics
The diabetes educator should respect and uphold the basic human rights of all persons.

With the increasing public awareness of the right to quality health care and the right to be informed, physicians are becoming ever more aware of the increasing time commitment required for patient education. Studies have shown that in outpatient physician offices it is the physician who provides the majority of patient education. This is time consuming, costly, and too often inadequate. The publication of standards of medical care for patients with diabetes includes an education, tracking, and monitoring component that may increase liability if these components are not carried out. The advantage of having a qualified diabetes nurse educator as a partner in the care of diabetic patients is that the nurse educator can:

1. Assess the patient and family needs and develop individualized educational plans.
2. Provide comprehensive and individualized patient instruction with on-going telephone contact for questions as they arise.
3. Assess appropriateness of various meters, supplies, and equipment for each patient.
4. Be available by phone to answer questions and help the patient in problem solving.
5. Track and schedule screening tests for complications as indicated by the National Standards.
6. Coordinate referrals to other specialists such as ophthalmologists and podiatrists.
7. Provide consistency and psychological support to the patient and family.
8. Assist the patient in adjusting insulin dosage according to established protocols.

The diabetes nurse educator plays a major role in improving the quality of patient care by allowing more frequent communication with the patient and thereby increasing patient satisfaction. In fact, by working in collaboration with and under protocols of the physician, the nurse educator can provide almost complete clinical management of the patient with diabetes.

Suggested Reading

American Association of Diabetes Educators. The scope of practice for diabetes educators and the standards of practice for diabetes educators. The Diabetes Educator 1992; 18:52–56.

Describes the standards of practice for diabetes educators including specific practice guidelines.

American Diabetes Association. Standards of medical care for patients with diabetes mellitus. Diabetes Care 1995; 18:8–15.

A position statement that describes the minimum standards of medical care for people with diabetes.

Cypress M, Wylie-Rosett J, Engle S, Stager T. The scope of practice of diabetes educators in a metropolitan area. The Diabetes Educator 1992; 18:111–114.

A study to determine the extent of the medical management role of the diabetes educator versus the educator role.

Farkas-Hirsch R, Hirsch I. Role of diabetes educator in patient management. In: Lebovitz H. (ed) Therapy for diabetes mellitus and related disorders. Alexandria, Va: American Diabetes Association, 1991:82.

Describes the diabetes team, lists examples of educational and support services provided by the diabetes educator, and describes reasons to refer patients to a diabetes educator.

Hiss R, Frey M, Davis W. Diabetes patient, education in the office setting. The Diabetes Educator 1986; 12:281–285.

A study to determine the current status of diabetes education in the office setting.

Ratner R, Ritter El-Gamassy, E. Legal aspects of team approach to diabetes treatment. The Diabetes Educator 1990; 16:113–116.

Discusses the possible increased risk for legal liability related to the establishment of national standards of practice and the existence of a certification process for diabetes educators.

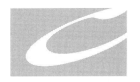

TYPE 2 DIABETES MELLITUS

DIET THERAPY OF TYPE 2 DIABETES MELLITUS

Robert R. Henry, M.D.
Kay Griver, R.D.

Non–insulin-dependent (or type 2) diabetes mellitus (NIDDM) is the most common form of diabetes and occurs in approximately 80 to 90 percent of the estimated 5 to 10 million Americans diagnosed with the disease. Although NIDDM affects both sexes about equally, it occurs more frequently in certain ethnic populations including Blacks, Hispanics, and Native Americans. The onset of NIDDM can occur at any age but in the majority of cases is diagnosed after the onset of the fourth decade. NIDDM includes a heterogenous group of patients who are further classified according to whether or not obesity is present. By this criteria, some 70 to 80 percent of patients are defined as obese NIDDM with the remainder having the nonobese or lean variety.

Reference is often made to nutritional management as the cornerstone of the diabetes treatment plan. Statements of this nature underscore the role that dietary modification can have in achieving widespread and often dramatic benefits on the metabolic abnormalities present in NIDDM. They also emphasize that poor nutrition may contribute to the development of severity of glucose tolerance in genetically susceptible individuals. In most cases, NIDDM tends to be a slowly progressive disease with the severity of glucose intolerance increasing over time. Diet therapy is beneficial in all stages of this progression but is most efficacious during the earlier stages of development. Diet manipulation can be so effective, at times, that initiation of pharmacologic therapy is no longer required. In other cases, with prudent nutritional management, the dose of medication required to achieve and maintain adequate glycemic control can often be significantly reduced or discontinued altogether. Finally, appropriate diet therapy not only improves widespread metabolic derangements in NIDDM but may impede the development of numerous end-organ complications of this disease.

In this chapter, we review the role of diet therapy in NIDDM with the understanding that it is a rapidly evolving field with few areas of consensus and many controversial issues. Although the focus is on the current nutritional recommendations for NIDDM in general, emphasis is placed on the different strategies used for lean and obese subtypes as well as coexisting medical conditions requiring special consideration and unique management such as renal impairment, hypertension, and hyperlipidemia.

■ PATHOPHYSIOLOGY

It is now well established that NIDDM is characterized by three basic pathophysiologic abnormalities including impaired pancreatic insulin secretion; peripheral insulin resistance, primarily at liver and muscle tissue; and excessive hepatic glucose production. These abnormalities combine, in varying degrees of severity in each individual, to result in a wide range of fasting and postprandial hyperglycemia. For the purposes of this review of diet therapy, it is helpful to recognize that although the obese and nonobese varieties of NIDDM have the same basic pathophysiologic abnormalities, their pattern of expression and contribution to the genesis of hyperglycemia differ. This, in turn, can affect the strategies used to achieve the goals of nutrition management.

For example, obese NIDDM patients tend to exhibit severe insulin resistance (in both muscle and liver) in association with hyperinsulinemia. Although it may seem a paradox to have impaired insulin secretion and hyperinsulinemia coexist, this situation occurs because the large quantity of insulin produced by the pancreas is insufficient to overcome the insulin resistance that is present. Much of the insulin resistance and hyperinsulinemia result from the concomitant obesity that has been clearly shown to aggravate these abnormalities. Obesity per se does not cause hyperglycemia but contributes to its development in those individuals with the genetic predisposition to develop NIDDM. Thus, a major thrust of diet therapy in obese NIDDM patients includes a plan directed at reducing body weight.

In contrast, lean or nonobese NIDDM patients tend to have less insulin resistance, often mild to moderate in severity, combined with hypoinsulinemia due to deficient pancreatic insulin secretion. In these individuals, the focus is directed at optimizing the composition, form, content, and timing of food intake without an emphasis on reduction of caloric intake.

■ THERAPEUTIC APPROACH

Overview

In most cases, the nutritional recommendations for NIDDM are similar to those for healthy individuals. There is no recognized need for special foods based on any specific or unique requirements particular to NIDDM. Recent interest in the nutritional management of NIDDM has been rekindled by emerging evidence about the metabolic impact of diet manipulation on a variety of metabolic parameters in this disorder. Additional developments and refinements in pharmacologic therapy and increased usage of self-monitoring of capillary blood glucose make it possible for diets to be modified in such a manner that greater individualization and flexibility in meal planning has resulted.

As outlined by the American Diabetes Association, there are two objectives in the management of NIDDM. The first goal is to strive for a normal metabolic state and the other is to prevent or delay development of the micro- and macrovascular complications that frequently occur. Nutritional management serves as the foundation on which other therapeutic modalities such as exercise, oral hypoglycemic agents, and insulin therapy are added as required. Attempts to achieve the therapeutic objectives listed above, without adherence to a consistent and individualized meal plan, are unlikely to be successful.

A number of aspects of dietary therapy in NIDDM need to be considered before an effective nutritional plan can be implemented. The most difficult aspect of providing a comprehensive nutritional treatment plan based on current knowledge involves the many unresolved issues about what constitutes the optimal diet for NIDDM. Controversy persists about the content and types of carbohydrates, protein, and fat that should be used; the role of dietary fiber; and the need for micronutrient supplementation, as well as unresolved issues concerning diet form, timing of food intake, and meal-planning methods. Careful planning is also necessary in devising diet therapy for NIDDM subjects in need of special consideration such as those from minority groups, the elderly, the disabled, and those with significant complications. The current status of these topics, including our approach to these management issues in NIDDM, is discussed in this chapter.

Nutrition Implementation

Effective nutrition management requires a coordinated team approach with active participation by the physician, registered dietitian, and diabetes nurse educator. Participation by family members, particularly the husband or wife of the diabetic person, should be actively sought. Continuous emphasis and encouragement by all team members improves the likelihood of both short- and long-term compliance. An integrated team approach is also more likely to result in a realistic meal plan that allows for individual flexibility. As shown in Table 1, several factors need to be considered during development of an appropriate diet including the age, sex, activity level, degree of obesity, presence of complications, medications, and current nutritional status of the patient. Particular cultural, ethnic, and socio-economic aspects also need to be considered in tailoring the individual's requirements.

The initial interaction with the patient provides a unique opportunity for the physician to stress the importance of

Table 1 Factors Influencing the Choice of Diet Therapy of NIDDM

Age	Cultural and ethnic aspects
Sex	Medical complications
Activity level	Medications
Degree of obesity	

consistent caloric intake and diet composition on glucose, lipids, blood pressure, and other important metabolic variables. Together with the expertise of a registered dietitian or nutrition counselor, the basic principles and goals of dietary therapy are reviewed and the overall meal plan devised. There are no benefits derived from the prescription of an ideal diet if the patient is unable or unwilling to adhere to it. Therefore, the specific dietary intervention chosen for each patient will not only vary according to the type of NIDDM (lean versus obese), the presence of concomitant complications, and treatment with medications (such as oral hypoglycemic agents or insulin) but upon a realistic appraisal about the likelihood of long-term compliance.

Exchange lists remain the most commonly used method to counsel and educate individuals with NIDDM about meal planning. The exchange list includes six groups of foods categorized by their content of carbohydrate, protein, fat, and calories. A meal plan is developed by using a given number of exchanges per meal and exchanging foods within each list. Healthy Food Choices are a simplified version of food grouping that categorize the six food groups by calories in a poster format along with guidelines to lower fat, salt, and sugar intake and to increase fiber intake. By using specific food choices, a simplified meal plan can be developed. We find that the concept of food exchange is difficult for many individuals and we prefer to use Healthy Food Choices as a simplified means to both count calories and lower fat intake.

The Food Guide Pyramid developed by the United States Department of Agriculture is another choice for individuals with diabetes to use in meal planning. The major concept is to choose a diet with more complex carbohydrate such as whole grains, vegetables, and fruits as well as less sugar and fat to improve healthy choices in meal planning. Carbohydrate counting may also be used in meal planning in patients with NIDDM, especially those using insulin.

The focus of nutrition education should be to enable an individual to make the appropriate changes to achieve improved metabolic control. Records of food intake and self-monitoring are additional tools used by the dietitian to follow-up and assess individual problem areas. We also provide group classes on a weekly basis to discuss food choices, healthy snacks, and dining-out guidelines. Even when an appropriate dietary meal plan is devised, we believe it is best to alter eating habits gradually after identifying the major culprits first. Although unhealthy eating patterns can be uncovered from either actual food records or dietary recall, we prefer to identify priority areas based on the former method. To use dietary recall we must rely on memory, which is frequently inaccurate. Many patients also forget or do not appreciate that calorie-dense foods (e.g., sodas and snacks) can be major contributors to the dietary intake of carbohydrates, fat, and calories. A skilled registered dietitian can usually identify these oversights and rectify the situation.

If the patient is being seen at the time of initial diagnosis, we find it best to initiate diet therapy alone unless glycemic control is very poor (fasting glucose >200 mg per deciliter). Below this level, diet manipulation by itself may obviate the need for drug therapy. Above this level (>200 mg per deciliter), patients tend to be symptomatic, and we usually initiate diet therapy along with pharmacologic agents. When patients have had marked hyperglycemia that is unrecognized for a prolonged period, some of the failure to respond to dietary therapy alone may be the result of glucose toxicity. Initial treatment with oral hypoglycemic agents or insulin to reduce hyperglycemia may reverse the glucose toxicity and allow diet therapy to be more efficacious.

Because the great majority of NIDDM patients are obese, nutritional efforts in this group should be directed primarily at weight-loss strategies. Striving for ideal body weight is unrealistic, rarely achieved, and not necessary to achieve metabolic benefits. Even modest weight loss of 5 to 10 percent of initial body weight can be beneficial to multiple metabolic derangements and enhance the therapeutic efficacy of drug therapy. Placing demands on patients to achieve large weight loss leads to frustration and guilt, and is counterproductive. In our patients, we aim for weight loss of 10 to 20 percent of initial body weight with the understanding that not everyone can achieve this goal. However, in the majority of patients we have found that this degree of weight loss can be both achieved and maintained.

In lean or nonobese NIDDM patients, calorie restriction and weight loss are not indicated. It should be pointed out, however, that many individuals, particularly men, may be minimally obese or nonobese by standard criteria but have increased intra-abdominal adipose accumulation. These individuals have upper body segment or android obesity, which is associated with a greater risk of cardiovascular and other metabolic complications. In addition to determining the weight and height of patients, we also routinely measure waist and hip circumference. Weight loss is indicated when the waist-hip ratio is greater than 0.9 in men and greater than 0.85 in women. Our approach to the management of weight loss will be discussed later in this chapter. In lean or nonobese NIDDM patients without an increased waist-hip ratio, diet therapy is directed at weight maintenance.

Caloric Distribution

The daily distribution of caloric intake may constitute an important component of glycemic control in NIDDM. By spreading calories as evenly as possible throughout the day, sufficient time elapses for a more optimal response with less insulin required to achieve and maintain glycemic control. The habit of missing meals and compensating with subsequent excessive consumption, particularly in the evening hours, may be a major contributor to poor glycemic control in NIDDM, which could result in both hypoglycemic and hyperglycemic episodes.

Nutrient Composition of Diet

Recent research into the dietary management of NIDDM has focused attention on the optimal content of the diabetic diet. Despite considerable progress in this area, great differ-

ences in opinion exist, which to some extent may reflect the heterogeneous nature of NIDDM. It seems quite likely that no particular diet composition will be found to have uniformly favorable metabolic effects in all patients with NIDDM. Fortunately, with the monitoring techniques currently available, recommendations can now be based on individual responses of glucose, lipids, and other metabolic parameters to diet manipulation.

Carbohydrates

Current recommendations emphasize reduction of total and saturated fat and replacement with complex carbohydrate. Unfortunately, high carbohydrate diets containing little or no fiber have been shown to cause a deterioration in blood glucose control and elevation of triglyceride levels. When individual preferences permit, we strive for a carbohydrate content of 50 to 55 percent, encouraging foods particularly high in water-soluble fiber such as fruits, vegetables, and legumes. Wherever possible, high fiber carbohydrate should be used to reduce the cholesterol and saturated fat intake. In patients who are both willing and able to follow a diet of this nature, periodic monitoring of glucose and lipid levels should be conducted to evaluate individual metabolic responses.

It is also important to emphasize that not all complex carbohydrates have favorable glycemic effects. The glycemic response to various starches varies widely and may depend not only on the food source per se but the form, texture, and presence of other nutrients in the meal plan. Whenever possible, we encourage patients to test their glycemic response to particular foods consumed in a variety of forms using self-glucose monitoring of capillary glucose.

With regards to sucrose content of the diet, what is important is the total amount of carbohydrate rather than the source. Each type of carbohydrate is counted in the same manner. A food item containing sucrose may be substituted within a meal rather than added to the meal. Fructose should also be used in moderation due to its potential to elevate lipid levels in NIDDM. Fructose is a nutritive sweetener that can be incorporated into most foods with little change in taste or texture. Although we do not advocate the absolute avoidance of sucrose, we make every effort to keep its consumption less than 5 percent of total calories and to encourage its use only as part of mixed meals spaced throughout the day. When sucrose is included in the diet in this manner, we have found adverse effects on glycemia to be uncommon.

Fats

As indicated in Table 2, all individuals with NIDDM should have saturated fat and cholesterol restricted in their diet because of their propensity for cardiovascular disease.

Reducing these components can have favorable influences on a number of lipid parameters. However, as alluded to above, it remains controversial exactly how saturated fats should be replaced. Because high carbohydrate diets may elevate triglyceride levels, possibly in select susceptible individuals, replacement of saturated fat with monounsaturates is now being expounded as a better alternative. In accordance with current recommendations, we attempt to keep total saturated fatty acids below 10 percent of total calories. A realistic approach to reduce saturated fat intake requires a marked decrease in red meats, organ meats, high fat dairy

Table 2 Diet Composition for Non–Insulin-Dependent Diabetes Mellitus

	OPTION 1	OPTION 2
CARBOHYDRATE	55–60%*	45–50%*
Complex	50–55%	40–45%
Sucrose	≤5%	≤5%
Fiber	25g/1,000 Kcal or 40g/day	
PROTEIN	10–20%	10–20%
FATS	<30%	35–40%
Saturated	<10%	<10%
Polyunsaturated	≤10%	<10%
Monounsaturated	10–15%	15–20%

*Expressed as % of total calories.

Table 3 Monounsaturated Fatty Acid (MUFA) Content of Common Oils

OIL*	MUFA (g)
Olive	10
Canola	8
Peanut	6
Corn	3
Soybean	3
Sunflower	3
Safflower	2

Adapted from Reeves, JB, Weihrauch JL. Composition of Foods, Agriculture Handbook No. 8–4. Washington, DC: USDA, 1979.
* Amount of oil = 1 tbsp (14g).

products, and tropical oils (e.g., palm, palm kernel, coconut oil). In addition to replacement of saturated fat by complex carbohydrates, lean meat, fish, and low-fat or skim milk products can be used. As stated previously, small increment goals may be used in NIDDM patients to achieve the desired extent of fat modification.

Although polyunsaturated fatty acids lower cholesterol and may have other potential benefits for NIDDM, concern exists that no population has ever consumed these compounds in large amounts and for prolonged periods. Furthermore, a number of potential adverse effects, especially when consumed in large quantities, have been reported with polyunsaturates. Based on this information, we partially replace saturated fatty acids with polyunsaturates but restrict the intake to 5 to 10 percent of total calories. Fish oil (ω-3 fatty acids) enrichment of the diabetic diet could benefit plasma triglycerides, platelet aggregation, and blood pressure. Unfortunately, fish oils have also been documented to have adverse effects on glycemic control in NIDDM and a tendency to elevate LDL cholesterol. At the current time, we do not encourage the use of fish oil supplements but believe that consumption of natural occurring ω-3 fatty acids in the form of fish and other marine sources is warranted to reduce saturated fat intake.

Perhaps the most significant recent advance in the dietary management of NIDDM is the evidence that monounsaturates (oleic acid) may be a satisfactory replacement for saturated fatty acids in the diet. These fatty acids have been consumed in large amounts by people of the Mediterranean basin and appear to be safe and to exert beneficial effects on cardiac risk factors. Not only does it appear that modest amounts of oleic acid have the beneficial effects of reducing LDL cholesterol and triglyceride levels and raising HDL levels, but increased intake may add palatability to the diet and expand the variety of food choices available to patients. The oleic acid content of various oils is shown in Table 3. By using monounsaturates to replace saturated fatty acids, we have been able to keep the intake of carbohydrate in the diet to 45 to 50 percent of total calories. By including 15 to 20 percent of calories from monounsaturates together with approximately 10 percent polyunsaturates and 5 to 10 percent as saturated fats we are able to provide a total fat intake of 35 to 40 percent. We believe that for many individuals with NIDDM, a diet of this composition is easier to prescribe and follow. In addition, such a diet may have favorable effects on glycemia as well as lipid levels.

Protein

In general, it is felt that the consumption of protein by Americans is greater than necessary for overall health. For people with NIDDM, excess dietary protein could lead to a number of potential deleterious effects. Although the principal function of dietary protein is to ensure adequate growth and tissue maintenance, it also contributes to the regulation of glucose metabolism and the workload of the kidney. Approximately 20 percent of individuals with NIDDM develop diabetic nephropathy within 15 years of diagnosis and excess dietary protein intake may contribute to its rate of progression. In addition, evidence has accumulated that early protein restriction may delay progression of diabetic nephropathy. The recommended dietary allowance (RDA) for protein intake is 0.8 g per kilogram body weight per day for adults. For people with diabetes, protein should constitute 10 to 20 percent of total calories. Although it has not yet been conclusively demonstrated that protein intake can influence diabetic nephropathy, we believe that current evidence warrants reduction in the current level of intake. Our approach to protein intake is to provide the RDA for protein to NIDDM patients with early or no evidence of renal disease (serum creatinine <2 mg per deciliter). In most people, adherence to 0.8 g per kilogram per day is a significant decrease in protein intake and a reasonable level of restriction. As renal impairment progresses, protein intake is usually reduced further. If frank nephrotic syndrome and hypoalbuminuria develop, however, protein intake is increased back to 0.8 to 1.0 g per kilogram per day as

Table 4 Selected High-Fiber Foods

SOURCE		PORTION SIZE	EXCHANGE	TOTAL DIETARY FIBER
BREADS, GRAINS				
Breads:	Pumpernickel	1 slice	1 starch	3.8
	Whole wheat	1 slice	1 starch	1.5
Cereals:	Bran flakes	½ Cup	1 starch	3.5
	Oat bran (cooked)	½ Cup	1 starch	2.1
LEGUMES				
Beans:	Kidney (cooked)	⅓ Cup	1 starch	3.8
	Baked beans	¼ Cup	2 starch	2.9
	Lentils (cooked)	⅓ Cup	1 starch	2.6
RAW VEGETABLES				
	Carrots	1 Cup	2 vegetable	3.6
	Cauliflower	1 Cup	1 vegetable	3.3
COOKED VEGETABLES				
	Corn	½ Cup	1 starch	3.9
	Brussels sprouts	½ Cup	1 vegetable	3.6
	Spinach	½ Cup	1 vegetable	2.0
	Broccoli	½ Cup	1 vegetable	2.0
RAW FRUIT				
	Blackberries	¾ Cup	1 fruit	6.7
	Strawberries	1¼ Cup	1 fruit	4.1
	Nectarine	1 medium 2½	1 fruit	3.3
	Pear	(w/skin) ½ large	1 fruit	2.5
	Apple	(w/skin) 1 small	1 fruit	2.1
	Orange	1 medium	1 fruit	2.0

Adapted from Nutrition Guide for Professionals. Diabetes Education and Meal Planning, American Diabetes Association, Inc., The American Dietetic Association, 1988.

required. When severe renal insufficiency develops (serum creatinine >10 mg per deciliter) and dialysis can not be initiated, an extremely low protein intake of 0.3 to 0.4 g per kilogram per day (20 to 30 g/day) may be instituted with essential amino acids and their alpha-ketoanalogues supplemented. In NIDDM patients on dialysis, protein intake can be liberalized at 1.0 to 1.2 g per kilogram per day. It remains unclear whether the source of dietary protein (e.g., animal versus vegetable sources) influences renal workload and subsequent progression of diabetic nephropathy. Whenever possible, we prefer to use lean animal and vegetable protein in the diabetic diet.

Dietary Fiber

Current recommendations suggest that fiber intake up to 40 g per day or 25 g per 1,000 calories ingested should be encouraged in the diabetic diet. Increased dietary fiber intake appears to have multiple metabolic benefits including improved glycemic control, lower levels of atherogenic lipids, blood pressure reduction, and possibly weight reduction through enhanced satiety. Table 4 lists the dietary fiber content of a number of commonly selected foods. We recommend that the fiber content of the diet only be increased through consumption of natural foods. Again, as with other components of the diabetic diet, the increase in dietary fiber content needs to be gradual over a period of weeks to months. Rapid escalation in fiber intake can result in diarrhea, abdominal cramping, and flatulence. In prescribing an increased fiber intake, we try to ensure that it comes from a variety of sources and is consistent in amount from day-to-day. Finally, high-fiber diets require additional fluid intake to assist in passage through the intestines. Patients with abdominal disorders and autonomic neuropathy should not undertake a high-fiber diet.

Alcohol

Alcohol influences glycemic control and lipid levels, and it contributes to caloric intake. The American Diabetes Association guidelines recommend moderate use of alcohol when diabetes is well controlled. One drink is equivalent to the amount of alcohol in a 1.5 ounce shot of distilled beverage, 5 ounces of wine, or 12 ounces of beer. In order to avoid potential hypoglycemia, alcohol should be consumed with a meal. In NIDDM patients with a history of hypertriglyceridemia, pancreatitis, gastritis, or other conditions affected by alcohol, its use should be actively discouraged.

Sodium

The principal issue regarding sodium intake in the diet of NIDDM is development of hypertension. People with NIDDM are more susceptible to the development of hypertension, and its presence can exacerbate the progression of cardiovascular complications and diabetic nephropathy. The consumption of sodium in the American diet is excessive, in large part from processed fast foods. The intake recommended by the American Heart Association, 1,000 mg sodium per 1,000 kcal ingested, not to exceed 3,000 mg per day, seems prudent and is the approach we follow. This goal is initiated by avoiding the addition of excess salt, limiting intake of high sodium foods, replacing salt with other flavors, and decreasing the amount of convenience and fast foods.

Alternative Sweeteners

Alternative sweeteners are generally categorized as caloric (or nutritive) versus noncaloric (or non-nutritive). Caloric sweeteners include fructose and the sugar alcohols (e.g., sorbitol, mannitol) whereas aspartame, saccharin, and acesulfame-K are the principal noncaloric ones. Alternative sweeteners are widely used by the general public and the food industry, and their use is considered acceptable in the management of diabetes. It is not clear, however, whether sweeteners have beneficial effects on the metabolic status of NIDDM. Furthermore, their use should be tempered by the lack of information regarding possible long-term adverse effects. We advise against excessive use, particularly of any one form. We have no preferred sweetener but incorporate these substances on an individual basis after consideration of the meal plan, life-style, and glycemic control desired.

Micronutrients

Considerable experimental evidence exists to suggest that diabetes may be associated with deficiencies in trace elements and vitamins under certain circumstances. Situations that may predispose to micronutrient deficiency include chronic inadequate dietary intake as may occur in the elderly, the disabled or those with gastrointestinal disease; use of very–high-fiber diets; very–low-calorie diet (VLCD) therapy; acidosis; and uncontrolled hyperglycemia with glycosuria. In the majority of diabetic individuals, however, clinically significant micronutrient deficiencies are not present. Our approach is to assess those diabetic patients at particularly high risk of developing specific micronutrient deficiency and to replete only if deficiency can be clearly documented.

■ TREATMENT OF NIDDM WITH OBESITY

Weight Reduction

Table 5 outlines the indexes commonly used by us to indicate whether treatment of obesity is required. A variety of approaches are available to achieve weight reduction, differing primarily in the extent of caloric restriction and dietary composition (Table 6). In general, caloric recommendations range from approximately 400 kcal per day found in the VLCD formulations to the more nutritionally complete conventional diet plans with modest caloric restriction of 1,800 kcal per day. Although total fasting can be used for short periods (7 to 10 days) to achieve rapid weight loss and glycemic control in obese NIDDM, we have found this procedure to be more problematic and of no greater efficacy than achieved using VLCD.

Two major difficulties are encountered during weight reduction therapy. The first problem involves difficulty initiating and achieving significant weight reduction. This limitation occurs frequently with conventional diet plans, which have small daily caloric deficits. The most difficult aspect of weight-loss therapy involves maintenance of the reduced weight. A successful weight-maintenance program requires the resources that only a multidisciplinary team approach can provide. Regardless of the method of caloric restriction used, long-term success is enhanced when exercise and behavioral modification are combined with a diet program.

Table 5 General Treatment Indicators of Obesity	
Weight	≥ 130% ideal body weight*
Body Mass Index (Wt[kg])/Ht([M²])	≥ 28
Waist-Hip Ratios†	≥ 0.90 for men
	≥ 0.85 for women
Presence of complications of obesity (e.g., hypertension, sleep apnea, hyperlipidemia, etc)	

*Based on medium frame, Metropolitan Life Tables, 1983.
†Abdominal circumference (cm) divided by hip circumference (cm). Varies according to ethnic group.

In each individual, a target goal weight is set and the schedule to achieve target weight is negotiated. The person's age, life-style, exercise habits, timing of meals, cultural preferences, medications, and any other medical problems must be considered. This is accomplished by taking a thorough medical and dietary history. Gradual step-by-step goals are developed with the patient and frequent follow-up is mandatory. Food records are completed by recording calorie and fat intake, exercise patterns, and blood glucose levels. When conventional diets are used, the meal plan must be individualized with a focus on controlling portion size, as well as distribution of calories.

Most VLCDs now used in the treatment of obesity provide 400 to 800 kcal per day and contain high-quality protein and micronutrient supplements. The most popular VLCDs are commercially available preparations that are usually provided as a powder that is reconstituted to liquid with water or skim milk. On average, VLCDs provide a daily intake of 40 to 100 g of high-quality protein from milk, eggs, or soybeans; 50 to 100 g of carbohydrate mainly as sucrose, fructose, or maltodextrins; and small quantities of fat (usually <5 g) to ensure adequate intake of essential fatty acids. Some products also include up to 15 g soluble fiber per day. Many products are aggressively supplemented with minerals, vitamins, and trace elements, whereas others require additional supplementation.

Although VLCD therapy is not recommended as primary diet therapy for NIDDM, these diets are now recognized as an effective alternative form of therapy, particularly when weight loss and metabolic control cannot be achieved with conventional diet therapy. We find VLCDs to be particularly useful to achieve rapid short-term weight loss and control of excessive fasting hyperglycemia to reduce symptoms. We frequently resort to this form of diet therapy to improve insulin sensitivity, which enables glycemic control to be re-established with oral hypoglycemic agents or insulin.

Conventional diets that provide 1,200 to 1,800 kcal per day result in caloric deficits of approximately 500 to 1000 kcal per day with a weight loss of 1 to 2 lb per week. With VLCDs the caloric deficit and the rate of weight loss are approximately 2 to 3 times that of conventional diets. All forms of diet therapy, particularly in NIDDM patients on oral hypoglycemic agents or insulin, require close medical supervision and constant interaction between members of the health care team.

Clearly, the most difficult period of weight-loss therapy occurs during the transition from a calorie-reduced to a

Table 6 Comparison of Weight Loss Plans for Obese NIDDM

DIET PLAN	KCAL/DAY	% OF TOTAL CALORIES			FIBER
		CHO	PRO	FAT	
Conventional	1,200–1,800	50–55	15–20	25–30	25 g/100 kcal
Very low calorie	400–800	30–50	35–50	5–15	≤15 g/1,000 kcal

Table 7 Weight Loss Therapy Re-feeding Schedule

Pre-diet weight maintenance 25–35 kcal/kg B W
Re-feeding program:
       Week 1=10 kcal/kg B W
       Week 2=15 kcal/kg B W
       Week 3=20–25 kcal/kg B W
Post-diet weight maintenance 25–35 kcal/kg B W

B W = body weight.

weight-maintenance diet. Frequently, patients overeat, which leads to guilt and a sense of helplessness. During this re-feed period, frequently scheduled visits, patient call-ins, and self-monitoring techniques are crucial to maintaining weight. The calorie content of the diet is gradually increased during the re-feed period until a weight-maintenance level is achieved. We find that a structured plan of re-feeding, combined with exercise and behavioral support, improves compliance and long-term success. Support groups that share their experience and discuss the difficulty of weight maintenance can also be beneficial. Table 7 outlines our approach to the re-feeding process following weight-loss therapy in obese NIDDM patients.

Exercise

All individuals with NIDDM should have exercise included as part of their overall treatment program unless contraindicated for medical reasons. Exercise not only reduces glucose intolerance, improves insulin sensitivity, and lowers cardiac risk factors but in addition increases energy expenditure, which complements dietary efforts to reduce and maintain body weight. Moreover, a well-designed exercise program can have psychological as well as physiologic benefits that promote dietary adherence by facilitating a change in life-style pattern.

Although exercise is an important adjunct to diet therapy in the management of NIDDM, it must be prudently planned and tailored to the physical capabilities of an individual. Exercise must also be approached cautiously because of its potential for adverse effects. In addition to physical injury of a musculoskeletal nature, attention must be given to the possibility of silent cardiac ischemia, which could be aggravated by an overly aggressive exercise program.

We find that one of the most effective methods to prevent or minimize exercise-induced hypoglycemia is to institute a regular routine of exercise activities. We encourage all patients to self-monitor capillary blood glucose measurements just before and after each exercise session. This assists in preventing hypoglycemia and in reinforcing the benefits of exercise on glycemic control. Although exercise can acutely lower blood sugar in NIDDM, a regular program is required to obtain the more chronic beneficial effects on glu-

cose and lipid metabolism. We initiate exercise by beginning at a low level of intensity and gradually progressing. Initiating exercise with walking, stationary cycling, and lap swimming three to four times per week for 20 to 30 minutes (100 to 200 kcal expended) are safe and effective forms of exercise advocated for patients with NIDDM. Progression of exercise intensity should be closely monitored with adjustment of diet and medications as required. Individuals who request or desire a more intensive exercise program should be referred to a physical therapy fitness program that specializes in the treatment of medical disorders. A close liaison must be maintained between exercise program personnel and the diabetes treatment team.

■ SPECIAL CONSIDERATIONS

Elderly Patients

Because elderly individuals with NIDDM may be likely to develop nutritional deficiencies, special attention often is required to account for individual food preferences, ethnic background, and the presence of associated medical conditions requiring dietary restriction. It may not be easy to convince elderly patients to alter dietary habits that have existed for 65 years or more. Furthermore, compliance with specific dietary advice may be influenced by physical limitations and functional disabilities. Clearly, elderly NIDDM patients require nutritional advice that is tailored to their specific and unique needs yet assures adequacy and a well-balanced intake.

Minority Patients

NIDDM is the predominant form of diabetes in minority populations and its incidence and prevalence are rising rapidly. Appropriate diet therapy for minority groups is often unsuccessful because of failure to recognize the unique aspects of each minority or to tailor recommendations with the individual's specific cultural framework. The diet prescription must relate to the cultural and economic status of the minority patient. The information must also be presented in a manner that is understandable, appropriate for the patient's level of literacy, and implementable.

Acknowledgment

This work was supported by funds from the Department of Veterans Affairs and Veterans Affairs Medical Center, San Diego, CA.

Suggested Reading

American Diabetes Association. Nutritional recommendations and principles for people with diabetes mellitus. Diabetes Care 1994; 17:519–522.

Outlines the nutritional recommendations advocated by the American Diabetes Association for individuals with diabetes mellitus.

Beebe CA, Pastors JG, Powers MA, Wylie-Rosett J. Nutrition management for individuals with non-insulin-dependent diabetes mellitus in the 1990's: A review by the Diabetes Care and Education Dietetic Practice Group. J Am Diet Assoc 1991, 91:196–207.

Provides a consensus opinion about the current state of nutrition therapy for individuals with NIDDM.

Franz MJ, Horton ES, Bantle JP, Beebe CA, Brunzell JD, Coulston AM, Henry RR, Hoogwerf BJ, Stacpoole PW. Nutrition principles for the management of diabetes and related complications. [technical review]. Diabetes Care 1994; 17:490–518.

Reviews research related to nutrition and complications of diabetes.

Grundy SM. Diet therapy in diabetes mellitus: Is there a single best diet? Diabetes Care 1991; 14:796–801.

Reviews the current controversial aspects about the macronutrient composition of the diet used in NIDDM.

Grundy SM, Denke MA. Dietary influences on serum lipids and lipoproteins. J Lipid Res 1990, 31:1149–1172.

Reviews the influences of a variety of dietary fats on serum lipid and lipoprotein levels.

Henry RR, Gumbiner B. Benefits and limitations of very low-calorie diet therapy in obese NIDDM. Diabetes Care 1991; 14:802–823.

The practical aspects of using very–low-calorie diets and the role they can play in the treatment of obese NIDDM are reviewed.

Lebovitz HE: The Physician's Guide to Non–Insulin-Dependent (Type 2) Diabetes: Diagnosis and treatment, 2nd ed. Alexandria, Va: American Diabetes Association, 1988.

This book provides a synopsis of current concepts about the pathogenesis, diagnosis, and therapeutic modalities commonly used in non–insulin-dependent diabetes mellitus.

Mooradian AD, Morley JE. Micronutrient status in diabetes mellitus. Am J Clin Nutr 1987; 45:877–895.

The current status of micronutrient deficiencies in diabetes mellitus is reviewed in this article.

Riccardi G, Rivellese AA. Effects of dietary fiber and carbohydrate on glucose and lipoprotein metabolism in diabetic patients. Diabetes Care 1991; 14:1115–1125.

This article reviews the current role of fiber and carbohydrate in the diet of NIDDM and the effects on glucose and lipid metabolism.

BEHAVIORAL WEIGHT CONTROL

Rena R. Wing, Ph.D.

Obesity is a major risk factor for the development of type 2 diabetes, but successful weight reduction can often help in the management of this disease. In this chapter, I will review some of the strategies that I have found effective in the behavioral treatment of obese patients with diabetes.

■ ROLE OF THE PHYSICIAN AND HEALTH CARE TEAM

Behavior modification is best done by experts in this field, who have training and prior experience with leading behavioral weight control groups. However, the physician and health care team can play a major role in this process. These individuals are in a unique position to accomplish the following:

- Identify those patients needing to lose weight. The physician is able to access information about the patient's current weight, body-fat distribution, risk-factor profile, family history of disease, and weight change over the past several years. Therefore, physicians are in the best position to determine who should be referred for weight loss. Individuals who have a body mass index (BMI; kg/m^2) greater than 27 or who are more than 20 percent above ideal body weight should be encouraged to lose weight. Particular emphasis should be placed on those individuals with upper body obesity, defined as a waist-to-hip ratio of >0.8 in women and >1.0 in men.
- Motivate patients to lose weight. Previous research in the area of smoking cessation has shown that physicians can be extremely powerful behavior-change agents. Therefore, it is important that physicians use the "power" inherent in their role to strongly advise their overweight patients to lose weight.
- Make referrals to appropriate resources in the community. The physician and health care team should provide information to patients about various approaches to weight reduction and encourage patients to enroll in programs that include nutrition education, exercise, and behavior modification.
- Support the patient's weight-loss efforts. Weight loss is difficult; it is a long-term process, often with few tangible rewards. Therefore, members of the health care team

should try to encourage patients in their weight loss efforts. This may include simply praising the patient when they enroll in a weight loss program, when they lose weight (even if it is a small amount), or when they report being more physically active. In addition, it may be possible to provide patients with opportunities to "weigh-in" for free or for minimal charge as a way of supporting their efforts.

■ FORMAT OF A BEHAVIORAL WEIGHT-LOSS PROGRAM

In the following sections, I describe my own program and provide the reader with an overview of some of the steps involved in conducting a behavioral weight-control program.

Identifying Appropriate Patients
Participants in my behavioral weight-control programs are 35 to 70 years of age, and 30 to 100 percent over ideal body weight based on the 1983 Metropolitan Life Insurance norms. In addition, all patients have type 2 diabetes and have their physician's permission to participate in a behavioral weight-control program. Patients are screened to ensure that they have no physical or psychological problems that would make participation in a group treatment difficult or inappropriate.

Starting a Treatment Group
Typically, the behavioral weight-control groups I run have 15 to 20 members. There is usually a 2:1 female-male ratio. The group members differ dramatically in age, weight, and severity of diabetes; the heterogeneity seems to help, not hinder, the group process.

The 20 patients begin and complete treatment together (except for dropouts). No new members are admitted to the group.

Treatment Format
Groups usually meet weekly for 20 weeks and then bi-weekly or monthly for the remainder of the year. For the patient's convenience, meetings are held in the evening and last about 1 to 1.5 hours. Each meeting begins with a private, individual weigh-in. The weight is entered in the patient's personal record, and eating and exercise diaries from the prior week are collected. The group meeting commences after all patients are weighed.

Therapists
A multidisciplinary team of therapists is used. The primary therapist is usually a Ph.D.-level clinical psychologist, with training in behavior modification and prior experience with leading behavioral weight-control groups. The therapy groups are led by nutritionists (registered dietitians), exercise physiologists, and other master's-level clinicians.

Lesson Content
Behavioral weight-loss programs have a structured format, with a new behavioral skill presented at each lesson. The lessons build on each other. At each lesson a written handout is provided that presents the main points to be discussed. The therapist presents the material in a seminar style and encourages patients to provide examples, raise questions, and discuss their own experiences. The leader keeps the discussion relevant to the week's lesson, but may tailor the topic to deal with seasonal events (holidays) or issues raised by the participants. Often role playing or modeling is used to help teach new behavioral skills.

Adjusting Medications
The program physician reduces oral hyperglycemic medication and adjusts the insulin dose. The magnitude of the reduction depends on the blood sugar of the patient and the severity of caloric restriction to be used in the program. Reductions are often made before the start of the diet, in anticipation of the decrease in blood sugar. In some cases, diuretics and hypertensive medications are also reduced or discontinued.

Patients are taught to self-monitor their blood glucose (SMBG) and to record fasting levels at least two times per week. SMBG readings before and 2 hours after dinner are also used as needed. The SMBG records are reviewed to make further adjustments in diabetes medication. Glycosylated hemoglobin and lipids are measured periodically and used in large part to provide feedback to patients on the health changes accompanying weight reduction.

■ PRINCIPLES OF BEHAVIORAL WEIGHT CONTROL

This section describes some of the major strategies used in a behavioral weight-control program.

Emphasize Behaviors
Behavioral treatments focus on changing behaviors. In the case of weight loss, the target behaviors are (1) decreasing total caloric intake, (2) decreasing fat consumption, and (3) increasing exercise. In my program, these three behaviors all receive equal emphasis.

Self-Monitoring
To effectively change behavior, it is important that the patient and therapist have some way of measuring the target behavior. Such measurement provides information about the starting point and the changes that occur over time.

In the area of weight control, it is usually necessary to rely on the subject's self-report of his or her own behavior. Patients are therefore asked to keep a diary and to write down all the foods and drinks that they consume and the number of calories (and/or grams of fat) in those foods. Patients also record all the physical activities that they perform and the calories in those activities. This information is reviewed weekly by the therapist and by the patient to evaluate the changes that have occurred. Efforts are made to identify appropriate food choices and exercise opportunities and to praise the patient for these behaviors. Problem-solving techniques are applied to episodes of inappropriate eating to help patients determine why the inappropriate eating occurred and to plan strategies to deal more effectively with such situations in the future.

Setting Appropriate Goals

Behavioral treatment programs set goals for both behavior change and for weight loss. Several behavioral principles are important in setting goals. First, it is important that short-term rather than long-term goals be used, and second, it is important that patients are able to achieve the goals that are set. Therefore, we set a weight-loss goal for our patients on a weekly basis—usually 1 to 2 lb per week. The program director never discusses "ideal body weight," because it is very discouraging for a 200-lb woman to be told her ideal body weight is 120 lb; rather, this woman is informed of current research showing that weight losses of just 10 lb can improve blood sugar and blood pressure.

Calorie Intake Goals

In terms of behavior change, patients are given a daily and a weekly calorie intake goal. Women are encouraged to eat about 1,200 to 1,500 kcal per day and men, about 1,500 to 1,800 kcal. To set a calorie goal, the patient's current intake is estimated by assuming that a sedentary individual uses approximately 12 kcal per pound to maintain his or her body weight. Hence a 200-lb person uses approximately 2,400 kcal per day. To lose 1 lb per week, it is necessary to lower intake by 500 kcal per day (or 3,500 per week) and to lose 2 lb per week, it is necessary to lower intake by 1,000 kcal per day (or 7,000 per week). Therefore, we would encourage the 200-lb individual to reduce intake from 2,400 to 1,400 kcal per day, to produce a weight loss of 2 lb per week (Fig. 1).

I use a calorie-counting approach in my behavioral weight-loss program (not an exchange system diet). I find that the calorie-counting format provides patients with greater flexibility in planning their diets, and helps them to understand that overeating at one meal can be compensated for by decreasing intake at the subsequent meal. Patients are taught a great deal about nutrition in the course of the treatment program. They learn the differences between protein,

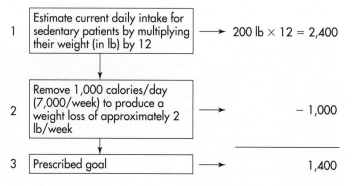

Figure 1
Setting a calorie goal

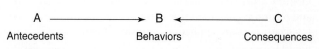

Figure 2
Simplified behavioral model

fat, and carbohydrates, and they are helped to develop an individually tailored eating plan that contains 20 to 30 percent of calories from fat.

Exercise Goals

We also set exercise goals for our patients. These goals are gradually increased over time, as the individual becomes more capable of exercising. Initially, patients in our program may be encouraged to walk one-fourth of a mile on 3 days per week; eventually, this goal is increased to 2 to 3 miles per day on 5 days per week. Walking is emphasized because we believe this is the most appropriate form of exercise for middle-aged, overweight individuals. However, individuals with orthopedic problems that make walking difficult are encouraged to swim or to use a stationary bicycle.

In setting goals for exercise, it is important to recognize that calorie expenditure depends primarily on distance covered, not speed. Therefore, we increase the distance patients walk rather than focusing on how fast they walk. We teach patients to use the formula: 1 mile = 100 calories as a way of estimating their calorie expenditure. (This estimate is accurate for people weighing 150 lb; heavier patients actually expend more calories per mile.) Gradually, exercise goals are increased until patients are asked to achieve 1,000 calories per week in extra exercise. This goal can be accomplished by walking 2 miles, 5 days each week.

Changing the Environment

Behavioral approaches are based on the assumption that behaviors are controlled by the environment; to change behavior, it is necessary to change the environment. Many of the lessons in a behavioral program focus on identifying the antecedents and consequences for inappropriate behavior and then modifying these environmental contingencies to produce more appropriate behaviors. This is shown diagrammatically in Figure 2.

Antecedents are cues in the environment that are believed to trigger behavior. For example, the sight and smell of food can trigger the desire to eat. Often these cues elicit eating even in the absence of hunger. For example, if you are in a movie theater, you may suddenly crave popcorn, or if you look at your watch and see it is 6:00 PM, you may want dinner, even if you had a late lunch. The goal of behavioral programs is to break these learned associations and help patients distinguish times when they are hungry from times when they are eating merely "out of habit."

Thoughts and moods can also be cues for eating. The thought "I've had a good day, I deserve a treat" can be a stimulus to eat inappropriately, as can boredom or depression.

Behavioral weight-control programs teach patients to recognize these types of hunger cues and to deal with them in more effective ways than by eating. Patients may be taught to associate the same cues with a new healthier behavior (6:00 PM is time to take a walk, rather than time to eat) or to remove the cue from their environment. Likewise, cues can be introduced into the environment to trigger new behaviors (e.g., an exercise chart on the wall may increase exercise behavior).

Consequences are events that come after the behavior and determine its recurrence. Events that are followed by positive consequences will increase in frequency, whereas those followed by negative consequences will decrease in frequency.

Again, it is important to realize that it is the short-term (not the long-term) consequences that are important in controlling the behavior. Therefore, foods that taste good are likely to be eaten with increased frequency, even if in the long term these foods increase the risk of heart disease.

In order to change behavior, behavioral weight-control programs are designed to develop positive consequences for the new behaviors that are desired. For example, patients are given new low-calorie foods to taste; the pleasant taste of these items should encourage their continued consumption. Praise is used as a positive reinforcer; any progress that patients make in changing their eating and exercise behavior and losing weight is praised. Feedback on the effect of behavior change on physiologic end points (including weight, glycemic control, and blood pressure) is provided. Finally, many behavioral weight-control programs include contingency contacting procedures. In my programs we often require small financial deposits ($50) from patients at the start of the program. This money is refunded to patients ($2.00 per week) if they attend the meeting and meet their calorie intake and expenditure goal, or if they achieve their weight-loss goal for the week.

Planning for the Long Term

The key to a behavioral weight-control program is helping the patient realize that the goal of the program is not adherence to a rigid diet for a 2- or 4-week period, but rather a permanent change in life-style. As part of this realization, the patient and therapist must accept that results of the behavior change program may not be apparent immediately, and that the path will not be a smooth or steady one. There will be times when the patient reverts back to old eating and exercise habits. Both the patient and the therapist must accept this and be prepared to deal with these periods.

One important component of planning for the long term is to develop a system of continued contacts. Many behavioral programs now include weekly meetings or weigh-ins for prolonged periods of time. When weight regain is observed, patients can be encouraged to re-enroll in a program, to reintroduce self-monitoring of intake, or to increase their activity levels.

■ COMBINING BEHAVIOR MODIFICATION WITH OTHER TREATMENT APPROACHES

The principles of behavioral weight control can be used in combination with other treatment approaches, such as very low calorie diets (VLCD) and pharmacologic treatments. Very–low-calorie diets are diets of less than 800 kcal per day, consisting primarily of high-quality protein. These diets have been shown to be quite safe when used with carefully selected patients and appropriate medical supervision, and for periods of only 3 to 4 months. Moreover, weight losses achieved on these diets are excellent. Several controlled studies have shown that utilizing VLCDs in combination with behavior modification produces far better long-term results than using VLCDs by themselves. However, an important question that remains unanswered is whether the combination of behavior modification plus a VLCD is more effective in the long term than behavior modification alone (i.e., behavioral modification and a balanced, moderate diet of 1,200 to 1,500 kcal).

Similarly, behavior modification techniques can be used in combination with pharmacologic agents for weight loss. Again, however, it is not clear whether this combination of behavioral techniques plus drugs results in better long-term weight loss than behavioral techniques alone.

Suggested Reading

Brownell KD. The LEARN program for weight control. Dallas: American Health Publishing Company, 1991.

This is a self-help manual that may be of assistance to individuals attempting to lose weight.

Perri MG, McAllister DA, Gange JJ, Jordan RC, McAdoo WG, Nezu AM. Effects of four maintenance programs on the long-term management of obesity. J Consult Clin Psychol 1988; 56:529–534.

This study shows that a long-term maintenance program, involving continued contact, aerobic exercise, and social support can help patients maintain their weight loss.

Wadden TA, Bell ST. Obesity. In: Bellack AS, Hersen M, Kazdin A, eds. International handbook of behavior modification and therapy. vol II. New York: Plenum Press, 1990: 449.

This chapter provides an excellent overview of recent research on obesity and the various treatment approaches that can be utilized for mild and moderate obesity.

Wadden TA, Foster GD, Letizia KA. One-year behavioral treatment of obesity: Comparison of moderate and severe caloric restriction and the effects of weight maintenance therapy. J Consult Clin Psychol 1994; 62:165–171.

Wing RR. Use of very-low-calorie diets in the treatment of obese persons with non-insulin-dependent diabetes mellitus. J Am Diet Assoc 1995; 95:569–572.

Wing RR, Koeske R, Epstein LH, Nowalk MP, Gooding W, Becker D. Long-term effects of modest weight loss in type 2 diabetic patients. Arch Intern Med 1987; 147:1749–1753.

This study shows that modest weight losses can improve glycemic control and CHD risk factors in type 2 diabetic patients.

EXERCISE IN THE MANAGEMENT OF TYPE 2 DIABETES MELLITUS

Stephen H. Schneider, M.D.
Antonio Morgado, M.D.

Exercise has been recommended in the treatment of diabetes mellitus for centuries. Data supporting the role of exercise in the treatment of type 2 non–insulin-dependent diabetes mellitus (NIDDM) has been strong enough to prompt the American Diabetes Association to formally recommend exercise in the overall treatment plan for this disease. In this chapter we describe the potential benefits of exercise for the patient with diabetes, address some of the problems and complications of exercise programs for this patient group, and discuss some specific recommendations for the practicing physician to use in developing programs for patients with NIDDM.

■ BENEFITS OF EXERCISE (Table 1)

Glucose Metabolism
The effects of regular exercise on glucose metabolism can be divided into two major categories; (1) those that are related to the bout of exercise itself; and (2) those that result from repeated bouts of exercise (e.g., training effect). Physical training results in changes in body composition and muscle oxidative capacity. Regular exercise results in a decrease of body fat, especially in the abdominal area. Decreased intra-abdominal fat is, in turn, associated with improved glucose tolerance and a reduction in associated cardiovascular risk factors. When exercise is intense it can result in muscle hypertrophy, thus enhancing the capacity for glucose disposal. Because glucose disposal per gram of skeletal muscle is not increased, this is probably due to the increase in muscle mass per se.

Table 1 Potential Benefits of Exercise in Non–Insulin-Dependent Diabetes Mellitus

Enhanced insulin sensitivity
  Decreased plasma insulin levels
  Improved glucose control
Prevention of diabetes mellitus
Reduced blood pressure
Decreased triglyceride and increased HDL cholesterol levels
Improved fibrinolysis
More efficient myocardial performance
Increased threshold for cardiac arrhythmias
Weight reduction
Enhanced self-image

Regular exercise improves insulin sensitivity independent of any measurable changes in weight or body composition. Following a single bout of moderately intense physical activity, there is an increase in insulin sensitivity that can last for 1 to 2 days or longer. Recent studies have demonstrated that exercise increases the number, translocation, and activity of glucose transport proteins. Changes in glucose transporters in muscle appear to be specific for the muscle group that has been exercised and are more pronounced in the red oxidative fibers that correlate best with muscle insulin sensitivity. Following exercise, glucose is primarily used to replete muscle glycogen. Glycogen synthase activity, the key enzyme in glycogen formation, is decreased in type 2 diabetes and is activated by exercise. Enhanced activity of glycogen synthase and glucose transport, combined with increased activity of the enzymes involved in glucose oxidation, may explain the exercise-induced increase in insulin sensitivity.

Because insulin resistance is a major pathophysiologic factor in the etiology of type 2 diabetes mellitus, exercise can be particularly useful in improving glycemic control in this group. Several well-controlled studies have shown a beneficial effect of regular exercise on glucose control in NIDDM patients, independent of measurable effects on body composition. In diabetic patients who exercise 3 to 4 times per week, for 30 to 40 minutes at 40 to 60 percent VO_2 max, a decrease in the glycohemoglobin of 1 to 2 percent generally is observed by 4 to 6 weeks with little additional improvement thereafter. Improved glucose levels occur with unchanged or even decreased levels of plasma insulin as a result of improved insulin sensitivity. Programs in which exercise is performed roughly every other day are required to observe a sustained improvement in insulin sensitivity. Unfortunately, following cessation of exercise programs that have lasted for as long as a year, inactivity of as little as 2 to 3 days can lead to a marked decline in insulin sensitivity to pre-exercise levels; changes in muscle enzyme patterns, mitochondrial number, and capillary density regress at a much slower rate.

Atherosclerotic Cardiovascular Disease
The major cause of premature morbidity and mortality in type 2 diabetes is accelerated atherosclerosis. Epidemiologic data strongly suggest that regular physical activity in the general population is associated with a decreased incidence of atherosclerotic cardiovascular disease. Patients with type 2 diabetes, as well as individuals with insulin resistance and milder forms of glucose intolerance, often have a clustering of cardiovascular risk factors including dyslipidemia, essential hypertension, and impaired fibrinolytic activity. Hyperinsulinemia and insulin resistance have been strongly linked to this group of risk factors. The ability of regular exercise to enhance insulin sensitivity and reduce hyperinsulinemia, in association with improvements in dyslipidemia, hypertension, and hypercoagulability, most likely explains the beneficial effect of regular exercise in the prevention or amelioration of atherosclerotic cardiovascular disease.

Dyslipidemia
The characteristic dyslipidemia associated with type 2 diabetes consists of elevated levels of plasma triglycerides, mild elevation of LDL cholesterol, and reduced levels of HDL cholesterol. Exercise has both direct (activation of lipoprotein lipase)

and indirect (through weight reduction and negative energy balance) effects to lower both VLDL and IDL and to increase HDL cholesterol. The acute effect of exercise on triglyceride levels follows a time course similar to plasma glucose. After a short delay, levels decrease and remain depressed for as long as 2 to 3 days. A decrease in plasma-LDL cholesterol during physical training is less consistently observed. The greater the intensity and duration of exercise, the more pronounced is the improvement in circulating lipid levels.

Coagulation System

A number of abnormalities of the coagulation system occur in patients with diabetes mellitus, including impaired fibrinolytic activity owing to increased activity of plasminogen activator inhibitor (PAI). Epidemiologic studies have demonstrated a negative correlation between VO_2 max and PAI levels, suggesting that a sedentary life-style is associated with impaired fibrinolysis. In general, most studies have shown that physical training improves fibrinolytic activity in patients with type 2 diabetes mellitus.

In summary, regular exercise is associated with improvements in the entire cardiovascular risk-factor cluster that is associated with type 2 diabetes. Several large epidemiologic studies, including the Nurses Health Survey and the Pennsylvania Alumni Follow-up Study, have shown a reduced incidence of ischemic heart disease and overall mortality in physically active patients. This observation has been confirmed in several smaller studies involving type 2 diabetic patients.

Prevention of Diabetes Mellitus

A sedentary life-style has been shown to predispose to the development of diabetes mellitus. Decreased physical activity also is a consistent feature of the aging population. Aging is associated with an increased incidence of glucose intolerance and overt type 2 diabetes, in large part owing to an age-related decrease in insulin sensitivity. Master athletes are virtually free of this age-related insulin resistance. Both prospective and cross-sectional studies support the notion that regular physical activity prevents the age-related decline in glucose tolerance and development of NIDDM.

Recent prospective studies have demonstrated that physical activity delays the clinical onset of type 2 diabetes in high-risk populations (Table 2). Subjects who report exercising just once a week had a 30 to 40 percent lower risk of developing diabetes than sedentary controls. The threshold for protection is unclear but may be as low as an additional caloric expenditure of 100 calories per week. Protection appears to be greater in obese individuals. Improved insulin sensitivity is the likely mechanism.

Weight Reduction and Body Composition

Obesity, and especially accumulation of fat in the intra-abdominal area ("android" pattern of obesity), is related to insulin resistance, hyperlipidemia, and hypertension in type 2 diabetes. Dietary programs for weight reduction have met with limited success. The addition of regular exercise to increase caloric expenditure can significantly enhance the value of a weight reduction program. However, the physician should be aware that the amount of energy that is expended in the modest exercise sessions patients with type 2 diabetes generally engage in, rarely exceeds 200 to 300 cal per day (Table 3). Although exercise increases energy expenditure for some time following a moderately intense exercise bout, the amount of calories consumed in this process has often been overstated. Resistance exercise as an adjunct to weight reduction in patients with type 2 diabetes might increase the percentage of weight lost as adipose tissue. Often the beneficial effects of exercise are underestimated because excess body fat is replaced, in part, by skeletal muscle. Exercise also results in a redistribution of body fat to the more gynecoid pattern that is associated with enhanced insulin sensitivity and a decreased cardiovascular risk profile.

Several factors may serve to mitigate the beneficial effect of regular exercise on weight reduction. At low-to-moderate exercise levels appetite is stimulated, resulting in increased food intake. Unfortunately exercise often is used as an excuse for dietary indiscretion. Recently there has been an increased use of very low-calorie diets in the treatment of obese patients with type 2 diabetes. However, these low-caloric diets decrease basal energy expenditure, limiting the rate of weight loss. Exercise has been advocated as a way of maintaining a higher metabolic rate. However, the addition of aerobic exercise to diets of less than 600 to 800 calories per day may result in a paradoxic decrease in energy expenditure that equals the calories expended during exercise. Exercise is most beneficial in promoting weight loss when used in combination with moderate caloric restriction.

Table 2 Individuals at Risk for Type 2 Diabetes Mellitus who Might Benefit from Increased Physical Activity

Family history of diabetes
Elderly patients with a sedentary life-style
History of gestational diabetes
Abdominal obesity
Essential hypertension
Impaired glucose intolerance
Ethnic background (Native Americans, Mexican Americans, African Americans)

Table 3 Duration of Exercise Required to Expend 200 Kcal Working at 60–70% VO_2 max

Approximate VO_2max (ml/kg/min)	Expended Energy (kcal/min)	Time to Expend 200 kcal (min)
62.5	15–17.5	12–14
50.0	12–14	15–17
37.5	9–10.5	19–23
25.0	6–7	29–34
18	4.5–5.5	38–45

Other important benefits of a chronic physical training program include reduction in blood pressure, improved myocardial vascularization and cardiac function, decreased threshold for arrhythmias, increased hematocrit, enhanced pulmonary function, and an improved sense of well being.

■ COMPLICATIONS OF EXERCISE
(Table 4)

The benefits of exercise need to be balanced against the risks. Although serious complications in a well-structured and monitored exercise program are rare, minor problems commonly arise and diligence on the part of both patient and physician is necessary to assure a good outcome.

Cardiovascular

In type 2 diabetic individuals the most feared complication of exercise is a cardiovascular or arrhythmic event. Non–insulin-dependent diabetes mellitus patients commonly have underlying atherosclerotic cardiovascular disease, which may be associated with a lowered threshold for ventricular fibrillation. In a large outpatient program run by the authors, 11 percent of patients referred without a history of coronary disease had exercise-related ischemia on formal evaluation. A relationship between silent ischemia and autonomic neuropathy, as defined by abnormal cardiac reflexes, has been found by some, but not all authors. In practice, the incidence of serious cardiac events in a well-monitored exercise program for patients with diabetes is very low, if a preceding stress test reveals no evidence of myocardial ischemia. In our experience with over 300 patients in a 10-year period, none of the subjects had a myocardial infarction or a life-threatening arrhythmia during a monitored exercise session.

Foot Injury

Injury to the feet is a major concern. Predisposing factors include peripheral vascular disease, decreased visual acuity, and especially diabetic neuropathy. Neuropathy results in the loss of normal pain and pressure sensation in the foot and places the patient at risk for trauma resulting from poorly fitting shoes and foreign objects. In addition, atrophy of the interosseous muscles of the feet causes changes in weight distribution that may lead to tissue breakdown. Finally the loss of proprioception may result in gait abnormalities that further place the foot at risk. Proprioceptive loss also predisposes patients to degenerative joint disease and traumatic joint injury.

Microvascular Complications

The possibility that exercise may worsen microvascular complications remains a controversial issue. Early surveys suggesting that physical activity may be a major cause of retinal hemorrhage in patients with diabetic retinopathy have not been confirmed in more recent studies. When hemorrhages occur, they do so most commonly in patients with proliferative retinopathy or advanced background retinopathy. However, heavy resistance training can result in increased retinal capillary pressure and hemorrhage even in patients with minimal disease. Increased retinal capillary pressure also may occur with situps and pushups. There also is concern about

Table 4 Potential Complications of Exercise in Type 2 Diabetic Patients
Cardiovascular
Myocardial ischemia or infarction
Cardiac dysrhythmias
Postural hypotension
Hypertensive response to exercise
Microvascular
Retinal hemorrhage
Proteinuria
Accelerated microvascular disease?
Metabolic
Hypoglycemia
Hyperglycemia
Ketosis
General
Muscle strains/sprains
Foot injury
Joint injury, degenerative arthritis
Poor dietary compliance

the effect of exercise on diabetic nephropathy. Exercise results in an increase in proteinuria, which appears to be proportional to the rise in systolic blood pressure. However, the proteinuria decreases rapidly after exercise. Whether the hemodynamic changes that occur during exercise accelerate the progression of renal disease remains an unanswered question. Treatment of hypertension in diabetic patients, especially those who wish to participate in an exercise program, is essential and generally results in decreased proteinuria. Because of their adverse metabolic effects on glucose tolerance and lipids and their propensity to cause hypoglycemia, beta-blockers should be avoided in NIDDM patients, especially those who exercise on a regular basis. Beta-blockers, as well as thiazide diuretics, often are associated with impaired exercise performance. Angiotensin-converting enzyme inhibitors and alpha-adrenergic–blocking agents do not impair exercise performance and effectively reduce the blood pressure response to exercise.

Metabolic Complications

Metabolic complications of exercise, especially hypoglycemia, are seen primarily in patients using insulin, although hypoglycemia during exercise has been noted in patients with type 2 diabetes taking oral agents. NIDDM patients who are poorly controlled may paradoxically increase levels of plasma glucose and ketones during exercise and the hypoglycemic effect of exercise is blunted. Very high-intensity exercises cause a brief increase in plasma glucose concentration even in well-controlled diabetic individuals. A more complete discussion of these complications can be found in the chapter *Exercise in the Management of Type 1 Diabetes Mellitus*.

■ EXERCISE RECOMMENDATIONS

Patient Evaluation

A thorough evaluation of the patient prior to the initiation of an exercise program is essential. The history should include a careful search for evidence of occult coronary artery disease,

Table 5 Medical Evaluation Prior to Formulating an Exercise Program

History and physical examination
Review of diet and medications
Cardiovascular risk-factor profile
Funduscopic examination
Podiatric evaluation
Neurologic evaluation
 Sensory/motor
 Autonomic
  Valsalva ratio
  R-R interval variation in deep respiration
Estimation of body composition
Assessment of glucose control and adequacy of insulinization
Formal exercise testing
 Pulse and blood pressure response
 ECG monitoring
 Post-exercise orthostatic blood pressure
 Post-exercise glucose concentration
 Post-exercise urine protein excretion

Table 6 Complications Encountered in 300 Patients Referred for an Exercise Program

Occult coronary disease	11%
Symptomatic peripheral vascular disease	14%
Sensory neuropathy	76%
Autonomic neuropathy	29%
Hypertension	42%
Resting proteinuria	8%
Post-exercise proteinuria	29%

Table 7 Life-style Questions to Ask When Evaluating Patients for an Exercise Program

Has the patient been involved in exercise in the past? If not, why not?
Does the patient exercise now? If not, why not?
What are the patient's expectations of exercise and are they realistic?
What are the patient's exercise preferences?
What kind of exercise skills does the patient have (i.e., can he/she swim)?
What time of the day is the patient able to set aside for exercise?
How does the time of exercise relate to meals and medication?
What are the social and economic limitations that might have an impact on the program?
Is the spouse interested in sharing in the planned activities?

autonomic dysfunction, hypoglycemia unawareness, foot problems, evidence of retinopathy, hypertension, and so on (Tables 5 and 6). In addition, life-style patterns need to be carefully considered (Table 7). On physical examination, complications that might interfere with exercise should be carefully sought. Cataracts or proliferative retinopathy need to be identified. The feet should be examined with special care to determine the presence of vascular compromise, neuropathy, and early skin lesions. The footwear should be examined and,

if necessary, special footwear or orthotics should be obtained. Evidence of autonomic neuropathy should be sought, as it may be associated with an increased risk of silent ischemia, sudden death, and post-exercise hypotension. Evaluation of cardiovascular reflexes by Valsalva and respiratory rate variation during deep respiration may be of value in assessing this risk and can readily be assessed in the office setting (see the chapter *Autonomic Neuropathy*).

Exercise Testing

Exercise testing is valuable for diabetic patients who wish to exercise at high intensities or who are at a high risk for complications. All sedentary patients over the age of 35 should have a formal exercise evaluation, as should patients of any age who have had diabetes for more than 10 years. Because of the high prevalence of coronary disease in this population, some form of graded exercise testing should be performed with electrocardiographic (ECG) monitoring. Clinical and ECG evidence of arrhythmias or ischemia and rise in blood pressure should be carefully sought. A near-linear response in pulse, oxygen consumption, and systolic blood pressure with increasing work to the point of maximal aerobic exercise capacity usually is seen. Diastolic blood pressure rarely rises more than a few millimeters of mercury even at relatively high work loads. A substantial elevation in diastolic pressure may be a sign of myocardial ischemia. A fall in blood pressure with increasing exercise may reflect left ventricular dysfunction, dehydration, or autonomic instability. Following the exercise test, subjects should be checked for the development of orthostatic hypotension. In some patients it may be useful to measure urinary protein excretion following exercise. Exercise testing should be done at a time when the patient is well hydrated, in the post-absorptive period, and when metabolic control is acceptable.

Exercise Prescription

The exercise prescription consists of four major components: type, intensity, frequency, and duration (Table 8).

Type

The type of exercise recommended represents a compromise between the patient's preferences and limitations, the latter of which are imposed by existing complications. In general, aerobic activities involving repetitive submaximal contractions of large muscle groups are recommended; these include swimming, cycling, walking, and running. In the past, resistance exercise has been avoided because of poor long-term compliance and the belief that this form of exercise did not improve the risk for cardiovascular events. However, recent data indicate that moderate resistance exercise is safe and has beneficial effects on hypertension, dyslipidemia, glucose tolerance, and insulin sensitivity. Resistance exercise can be combined with aerobic activities and may be particularly useful in patients with a low percentage of lean body mass, such as the elderly. Enhanced strength and muscle mass generate a feeling of well being, improve metabolic parameters, decrease the risk of falls or injury, increase bone mass, and sometimes help with weight control.

Presence of diabetic complications has a major impact on the exercise choice. Patients with severe peripheral neuropathy should be encouraged to choose swimming rather than

Table 8 The Exercise Prescription

TYPE

Must be adjusted to the patient's preference and existing medical conditions. Aerobic exercise is preferred; the addition of moderate resistance exercise should be considered.

INTENSITY

Start at 40–50% of the patient's VO$_2$ max and increase slowly to 60–65%, as tolerated. Keep systolic blood pressure <200 mm Hg.

DURATION

20–45 min per session.

FREQUENCY

3–4 sessions per week is required to observe beneficial metabolic effects. 4–5 sessions per week as needed for weight reduction.

PROGRAM

Stretching (5–10 min)

Warm up (5–10 min)

Exercise (20–45 min) (brief <2 min rest periods are permitted)

Warm down (10 min at 30% of full exercise intensity)

high impact exercises, such as jogging. Those with proliferative retinopathy should avoid sports that are likely to result in trauma to the eyes or cause fluctuations in intraocular pressure, such as deep sea diving and moderate-high intensity weight lifting. Use of properly fitted footwear and protective eye wear can make a major contribution to safety. Exercise, such as sky diving and scuba diving, should not be undertaken without consultation with a diabetes expert who is knowledgeable about exercise physiology.

Intensity

Exercise sessions should be preceded by stretching to avoid muscle sprains. Care should be taken to stretch properly, as breath holding during stretching can cause wide swings in blood pressure. The intensity of exercise is determined from the results of the initial exercise evaluation. Initiation of programs with a high exercise intensity is a common error. The aerobic exercise capacity (expressed per kilogram of body weight) of patients with type 2 diabetes is typically 10 to 15 percent less than sedentary age-matched populations. The cause of this extremely low aerobic capacity has not been defined. Therefore, the capacity for many untrained middle-age diabetic patients to engage in even light jogging may be limited.

The hemodynamic and metabolic improvements seen with physical activity have heterogeneous intensity thresholds. Large epidemiologic studies suggest that the major benefit to decrease cardiovascular events occurs with relatively low weekly energy expenditures (i.e., 500 to 1,000 cal over baseline). On the other hand, higher intensity thresholds exist for parameters such as increased HDL-cholesterol levels. The metabolic changes associated with exercise depend primarily on relative, not absolute, work loads and beneficial effects may be seen at very light absolute work intensities in the sedentary or older population for whom a brisk walk might represent 50 to 60 percent of maximal aerobic capacity. Exercise of sufficient intensity to cause some depletion of muscle glycogen appears necessary to generate enhanced insulin sensitivity. Exercise at less than 30 to 40 percent VO$_2$ max has minimal effects on glucose control. In general, a major

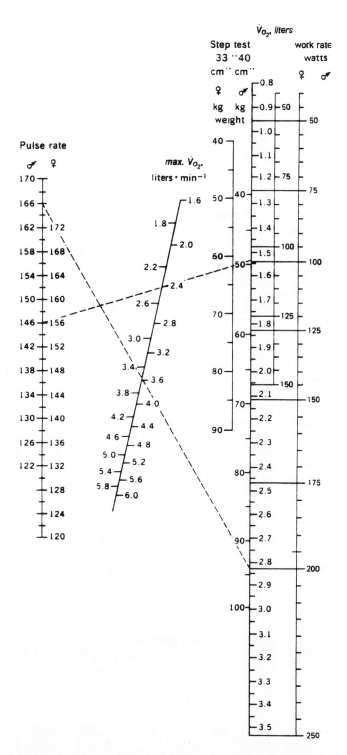

Figure 1

Adjusted nomogram for calculation of maximal oxygen uptake for submaximal pulse rate and O$_2$ uptake values (cycling, running, or walking). VO$_2$max can be estimated by drawing a line from the pulse rate to the VO$_2$ in liters measured during submaximal exercise on a bicycle or treadmill. When direct measurement of submaximal oxygen uptake is not available, it can be estimated by reading horizontally from the work-rate scale to the VO$_2$ in liters. *(From Åstrand P-O, Rodahl K. Textbook of work physiology: Physiological bases of exercise, 3rd ed. New York: McGraw-Hill, 1986:365; with permission.)*

improvement in glucose tolerance requires that individuals exercise at about 60 percent VO_2 max.

Most exercise programs start at an intensity of 40 to 50 percent of maximal aerobic capacity. Prescriptions generally are given in terms of a pulse rate. Pulse rates obtained during the initial exercise test generally can be extrapolated to the field. Determining the appropriate pulse rate is best done by using an exercise test that takes patients to their true maximal oxygen uptake. Patients who are using drugs that affect exercise capacity should take their medications when exercise testing is performed. Many patients are unable to exercise to maximal levels because of orthopedic injuries, ischemic heart disease, peripheral vascular disease, autonomic instability, or proliferative retinopathy. The linear relationship between pulse and oxygen uptake makes it possible to estimate maximal pulse rates from submaximal exercise tests (Fig. 1). In patients with long-standing type 2 diabetes and/or autonomic neuropathy, these nomograms may overestimate maximal exercise capacity. The patient's maximal pulse rate can be estimated by subtracting the patient's age from 220. Patients can be started at 40 to 50 percent of their maximal pulse rate (i.e., 40 to 50 percent of their aerobic work capacity) with gradual increments to 60 to 70 percent over 6 to 8 weeks. Once an adequate regimen has been established, the absolute work load can be increased gradually to maintain the target heart rate at a fairly constant level. Exercise at intensities that elevate the systolic pressure above 180 to 200 mm Hg should be avoided in patients with vascular complications. Resistance exercise in patients at risk for complications should be of modest intensity. Resistance that allows the patient to comfortably perform three to five sets of 12 to 15 repetitions is usually associated with acceptable hemodynamic changes. Anabolic steroids and protein supplements should be avoided, and hypertension should be controlled prior to initiating the exercise program. Exercise always should be followed by a warm-down period of at least 5 to 10 minutes. This speeds recovery from muscle fatigue, adds a pleasurable psychological effect to the exercise session, and may reduce the risk of post-exercise arrhythmias.

Duration

Limited information about the optimal duration of exercise suggests that improved glucose disposal is a function of the product of the intensity and duration, i.e., the total work performed. Therefore, longer sessions of modest intensity are as effective as higher intensity sessions of shorter duration. Exercise sessions of at least 15 to 20 minutes are necessary for a useful effect. Brief rest periods of less than 2 minutes duration at regular intervals during the training sessions do not decrease the training effect and may be helpful in obtaining better compliance.

Frequency

The frequency of exercise sessions is extremely important in maximizing its effect on glucose control. Much of the beneficial effect of exercise is related to the residual effect of each individual exercise bout. Therefore, exercise should be performed every other day to maximize its glucose lowering effect. Subjects who exercise at moderate intensity four times per week do better metabolically than those who exercise at higher intensity twice a week even when the total work performed is equivalent.

Timing

Morning exercise is often preferable. It is associated with less hypoglycemia and the effects will be most pronounced when the patient is eating. In some patients exercise may be more effective in controlling postprandial glucose levels if performed after a meal. However, many individuals feel uncomfortable if they exercise on a full stomach. In NIDDM patients who are taking insulin, an appropriate dosage adjustment must be made (see the chapter *Insulin Therapy in Type 2 Diabetes Mellitus*).

Feedback

Providing adequate feedback to the patient during an exercise program is an important part of any strategy aimed at improving compliance. Weight changes may be disappointing during physical training; an improvement in body composition and/or fat distribution may be helpful in demonstrating progress. Improvements in fitness can be demonstrated by reduced pulse rate, decreased blood pressure, and increased maximal oxygen uptake. Metabolic improvements from exercise may occur rapidly, and include decreased triglycerides and glucose levels. A reduction in HbA_{1c} is usually measurable by 6 weeks.

Compliance

Compliance remains the major problem with exercise programs, as with other strategies based on life-style modification. Inappropriate exercise recommendations and excessive costs associated with programs not currently eligible for third-party reimbursement are common problems. Involvement of the spouse, participation in group exercise programs, and provision of positive feedback are useful in improving patient compliance.

Suggested Reading

Bjorntorp P. Evolution of the understanding of the role of exercise in obesity and its complications [review]. Int J Obes Relat Metab Disord 19(suppl): 1995; 4:S1–S4.

Council for Exercise, American Diabetes Association, National Center. Guidelines for prescribing exercise for type II diabetes. Diabetes Care 1990; 13:785–789.

A technical review in which the specifics of the exercise program recommended by the American Diabetes Association are discussed.

Helmrich SP, Ragland DR, Paffenberger RS, Jr. Prevention of non–insulin-dependent diabetes mellitus with physical activity [review]. Med Sci Sports Exerc 1994; 26:824–830.

Horton ES. Role on management of exercise in diabetes mellitus. Diabetes Care 1988; 11:201–211.

An excellent review of practical and theoretical considerations when using exercise in the treatment of diabetes.

Manson JE, Rimm EB, Stampfer MJ, et al. Physical activity and incidence of non–insulin-dependent diabetes mellitus in women. Lancet 1991; 338:774–778.

A prospective study of 87,253 nurses. Physical activity was associated with a decreased incidence of type 2 diabetes over an 8-year follow-up.

Martin IK, Wahren J. Glucose metabolism during physical exercise in patients with non insulin-dependent (type II) diabetes. Adv Exp Med Biol 1993; 334:221–233.

McArdle WD, Katch FI, Katch VL. Exercise physiology, 4th ed. Baltimore: Williams & Wilkins, 1996.

A comprehensive text with many diagrams and nomograms useful for understanding exercise physiology and recommending exercise programs.

Ruderman NB, Schneider SH. Diabetes, exercise, and atherosclerosis [review]. Diabetes Care 1992; 15:1787–1793.

Schneider SH, Khachadurian AK, Amorosa LF, et al. Ten years experience with an exercise-based outpatient lifestyle modification program in the treatment of diabetes mellitus. Diabetes Care 1992; 15:1800–1810.

A 10-year experience with a physical training program consisting of 200 patients with type 2 and 55 patients with type 1 diabetes mellitus. Problems and typical metabolic and hemodynamic effects are reviewed.

Schwartz RS. Exercise training in the treatment of diabetes mellitus in elderly patients. Diabetes Care 1990; 13(suppl 2): 77–85.

The author reviews the literature and gives recommendations for physical training in older patients.

Spelsberg A, Manson JE. Physical activity in the treatment and prevention of diabetes. Compr Ther 1995; 21:559–562.

SULFONYLUREAS

Leif C. Groop, M.D.
Ralph A. DeFronzo, M.D.

Non–insulin-dependent diabetes mellitus (NIDDM) accounts for about 85 percent of all cases of diabetes mellitus. Patients with manifest NIDDM are characterized by both insulin resistance and impaired insulin secretion. The insulin resistance is manifested in the liver and in peripheral tissues. Hepatic insulin resistance results in overproduction of glucose in the basal state despite the presence of fasting hyperinsulinemia and is largely responsible for fasting hyperglycemia. Insulin resistance in peripheral tissues, predominantly muscle, results in impaired insulin-stimulated glucose uptake and accounts for postprandial hyperglycemia. Once hyperglycemia has developed, it will feed back to inhibit insulin secretion by the beta cells and down-regulate glucose transport and post-transport steps in muscle, i.e., "glucose toxicity." The optimal treatment for NIDDM should, therefore, not only improve beta-cell function and enhance peripheral glucose metabolism, but also break this vicious cycle of glucose toxicity. The results of a number of studies, including the U.S. Diabetes Control and Complications Trial, the Stockholm and Steno Intervention Studies, the Wisconsin Eye Study, the Japanese Intervention Study, and others have documented conclusively that microvascular—and to a lesser extent macrovascular—complications in both IDDM and NIDDM are related to the mean day-long blood glucose level, as measured by the HbA_{1c}. Therefore, it is critically important to reduce the plasma glucose concentration to normal or near-normal levels. Target goals (see the chapter *Goals of Diabetes Management*) have been established by the American Diabetes Association and the European NIDDM Policy Group with the purpose of preventing microangiopathic complications. Therefore, the fasting plasma glucose concentration should be reduced to less than 140 mg per deciliter and ideally to below 110 mg per deciliter. The two-hour postprandial glucose concentration should be less than 200 mg per deciliter and ideally less than 140 mg per deciliter. Diabetic retinopathy does not occur unless the fasting glucose is greater than 140 mg per deciliter and the postprandial glucose is above 200 mg per deciliter.

Presently available therapeutic agents, when used as monotherapy, will achieve these goals in only 20 to 30 percent of individuals. For more than 30 years, the sulfonylureas have been the mainstay of therapy for NIDDM patients throughout the world. Despite their widespread usage controversy still remains about the mechanisms by which the sulfonylureas lower blood-glucose levels in type 2 diabetic patients.

■ MODE OF ACTION

In vitro and in vivo studies conclusively have demonstrated that sulfonylureas stimulate the second phase of insulin secretion. The sulfonylureas bind to a specific sulfonylurea receptor on the pancreatic beta cell and exert their insulinotropic effects by closing adenosine triphosphate (ATP)-dependent potassium channels. This, in turn, causes depolarization of the beta cell, which promotes influx of calcium and stimulation of insulin secretion. The binding capacity of different sulfonylureas to their sulfonylurea receptor closely reflects their ability to stimulate insulin secretion.

When given acutely to nondiabetic and diabetic subjects, all sulfonylureas augment insulin secretion and potentiate the effect of glucose and amino acids to stimulate insulin secretion. In the postabsorptive state the resultant portal hyperinsulinemia suppresses hepatic glucose production and lowers the fasting glucose concentration, while the meal-potentiated insulin release decreases the postprandial glycemic excursion. With time the acute stimulatory effect of the sulfonylureas wanes and the plasma insulin levels, both fasting and postprandial, return to pretreatment values. Nonetheless, the improvement in plasma glucose levels persists. The same plasma insulin response in the face of a markedly lower plasma glucose level indicates a persistent stimulatory effect of the sulfonylureas on insulin secretion. The sulfonylureas also have been proposed to increase circulating plasma insulin levels by interfering with the hepatic degradation of insulin, although this mechanism has not conclusively been established.

Sulfonylureas also have been suggested to exert extrapancreatic effects on both the liver, peripheral and muscle tissues. However, it presently remains unclear whether these beneficial effects on glucose metabolism are primary or secondary to an improvement in glucose toxicity.

The most likely sequence of events is as follows: (1) the primary effect of the sulfonylureas is to stimulate insulin secretion by the pancreas (direct effect); (2) the resultant portal hyperinsulinemia suppresses hepatic glucose production, leading to a decline in fasting plasma glucose; (3) the improvement in glycemia ameliorates glucose toxicity, leading to enhanced insulin sensitivity in muscle (indirect effect). According to this scenario most of the extrapancreatic effects of the sulfonylureas are considered to be indirect. However, some in vitro studies have provided support for a direct action of sulfonylureas on insulin sensitivity. Although the relative importance of each of these actions to improve glycemia has yet to be precisely defined, it is likely that both pancreatic (direct) and extrapancreatic (both direct and indirect) effects contribute to the improvement in glucose tolerance. Since NIDDM patients are characterized by defects in both insulin secretion and insulin action, the sulfonylurea drugs, regardless of their mechanism of action, are effective in controlling hyperglycemia in type 2 diabetic patients.

■ PHARMACOKINETICS

Sulfonylureas are weak acids and display marked differences in absorption, metabolism, and elimination (Table 1). The first generation sulfonylureas (tolbutamide, chlorpropamide, tolazamide, acetohexamide) are much less potent on a milligram for milligram basis compared to the second generation sulfonylureas and are extensively protein bound. The second generation sulfonylureas (glipizide, glyburide, glimepiride) do not bind to circulating plasma proteins and, unlike the first generation sulfonylureas, are not associated with significant drug-drug interactions. When used in maximally effective doses all sulfonylureas, with the exception of tolbu-

tamide, are equally effective in lowering the blood-glucose level. The sulfonylureas differ significantly in their route of metabolism and excretion (see Table 1), and these differences may influence the choice of which sulfonylurea to use in a particular diabetic. In addition, a number of factors influence the absorption and bioavailability of sulfonylureas, including the type of formulation, the time of ingestion in relation to food, and the level of glycemia.

Timing of Drug Ingestion

Sulfonylureas should be taken 30 minutes prior to a meal. This consideration is particularly important when the sulfonylurea is initially started, because the acute release of insulin results in a lower postprandial plasma glucose excursion than when the drug is taken together with the meal. However, after several months of sulfonylurea therapy the acute insulin response wanes, and the need to take the drug prior to meals becomes less evident. During chronic treatment no difference in postprandial glucose concentrations have been noted when the drug is given before rather than with the meal. With the exception of chlorpropamide, the plasma half-life of the sulfonylureas is relatively short, in the range of 4 to 10 hours (see Table 1). However, most sulfonylureas maintain effective daylong glycemic control when given twice daily. This means that the tissue half-life of the sulfonylurea on the putative beta-cell receptor must be much longer.

Glipizide provides a good example. The elimination half-life varies from 2 to 4 hours, yet the plasma glucose lowering effect of 7.5 mg glipizide lasts about 12 to 14 hours. Some studies have demonstrated that even administration of glipizide once daily in the morning gives the same day-long hypoglycemic effect as giving the same dose three times daily. Nonetheless, we recommend that both glipizide and glyburide are given twice daily, with the morning and evening meals. A new long-acting glipizide has been developed and can be given once daily.

Most sulfonylureas are metabolized in the liver to active or inactive metabolites that are subsequently excreted in the urine. The exception is chlorpropamide, which is excreted unchanged in the urine. Both glyburide, and to a lesser extent glipizide, are excreted in significant amounts in the urine. These elimination characteristics can influence the choice of a given sulfonylurea in a particular diabetic patient.

DRUG	PLASMA HALF-LIFE (HR)	DURATION OF EFFECT (HR)	DAILY DOSE (MG)	DOSES/DAY (NO.)	ACTIVE METABOLITES
Acetohexamide	1–3	12–18	250–1500	2	+
Chlorpropamide	24–48	36–48	100–500	1	+
Tolbutamide	5–7	6–10	500–3000	3	-
Tolazamide	5–7	12–14	100–1000	1–2	-
Glipizide	2–4	12–14	2.5–40*	1–2	-
Glipizide-GITs	8–10†	24	5–20	1	-
Glyburide	10	12–24	2.5–20	1–2	-/+
Gliclazide	8–12	12–14	40–320	1–2	-
Glimepiride	9	16–24	1–8	1–2	+

Table 1 Pharmacokinetic Properties of Sulfonylurea Agents

*No further hypoglycemic effect at doses greater than 20 mg/day.
†Apparent half-life.

■ INSTITUTION OF THERAPY

All NIDDM patients with residual beta-cell function are potential candidates for sulfonylurea therapy. Known insulin-dependent (type 1) diabetic (IDDM) patients should not be treated with sulfonylureas; IDDM individuals require treatment with insulin. Approximately 10 percent of NIDDM individuals have slowly evolving IDDM and will have a poor response to sulfonylurea agents. Such patients can be recognized by the presence of circulating islet cell antibodies and glutamic acid decarboxylase (GAD) antibodies.

Clinical characteristics of diabetics who are most likely to respond to a sulfonylurea are shown in Table 2. Although it is commonly stated that diabetics with onset after age 30 respond better to sulfonylureas, numerous studies have shown that MODYs (maturity onset diabetes of youth) respond equally well. Shorter duration of diabetes (<5 years) predicts a better response, although many diabetics with a longer duration of diabetes also respond well to sulfonylureas. Diabetics who are very lean (less than 100 percent of ideal body weight) often are insulinopenic and respond poorly to sulfonylureas. Noncompliant patients who are unable to follow an appropriate diet also tend to do poorly when treated with sulfonylureas. Very–high-fasting glucose concentrations, greater than 300 mg per deciliter, also predict a poor response to sulfonylurea therapy.

In symptomatic patients with fasting glucose concentrations greater than 250 to 300 mg per deciliter, therapy should be initiated with insulin. Because of the deleterious effects of glucose toxicity on insulin secretion and/or intrinsic beta-cell failure, such individuals often respond poorly to sulfonylureas. After a short (6 to 8 weeks), intensified course of insulin plus dietary therapy to reduce the fasting glucose to below 140 mg per deciliter and elimination of glucose toxicity, sulfonylurea therapy can be substituted successfully for insulin treatment.

Successful sulfonylurea therapy means maintenance of the fasting glucose less than 140 mg per deciliter and ideally less than 110 mg per deciliter. Therapy should be initiated with a low dose, 2.5 to 5 mg of glipizide or glyburide, and increased every 4 to 7 days based on the decrease in fasting glucose concentration. Because of its long duration of action, it is best to wait 7 to 10 days before increasing the dose of chlorpropamide. After optimal glycemic control has been established, the dose of the sulfonylureas should be maintained constant as long as the fasting glucose concentration and HbA_{1c} remain within the normal range. In patients with good dietary compliance, especially those who lose weight, it may

Table 2 Diabetic Patients Most Likely to Respond to Sulfonylureas

Onset of diabetes after age 30 yr
Residual beta-cell function
Absence of GAD and islet cell antibodies
Duration of diabetes <5 yr
Normal weight or moderately obese
Demonstrated compliance with diet or exercise regimen
Fasting glucose <300 mg/dl

GAD = glutamic acid decarboxylase.

be possible to reduce or even discontinue the sulfonylureas. The development of hypoglycemia is an absolute indication to decrease the sulfonylurea dosage.

If the blood glucose concentration declines but does not reach target levels (<140 mg per deciliter), a second oral hypoglycemic agent should be added. The sulfonylurea should not be stopped or decreased in dosage. Metformin (see the following chapter) is particularly effective when added to a sulfonylurea. Because metformin (enhanced hepatic and peripheral tissue sensitivity to insulin) and the sulfonylureas (increased insulin secretion) have different mechanisms of action, the two drugs are completely additive. Approximately 20 to 30 percent of all NIDDM patients will be controlled with a sulfonylurea alone or metformin alone. With combined therapy, one can expect to achieve acceptable glycemic control (fasting glucose <140 mg per deciliter; HbA_{1c} <7 to 7.5 percent) in approximately 60 to 70 percent of newly diagnosed NIDDM patients. Acarbose (see the chapter *Alpha Glucosidase Inhibitors*) also can be added to sulfonylurea therapy. However, this oral hypoglycemic agent has its major effect on the postprandial plasma glucose concentration and only decreases the fasting glucose by 20 to 30 mg per deciliter. Therefore, if the fasting glucose remains very high on maximum-dose sulfonyl-urea therapy, it is best to start with the addition of metformin to the sulfonylurea. The institution of bedtime long-acting insulin to daytime sulfonylurea (BIDS therapy) also has been shown to be highly effective in restoring normoglycemia (see the chapter *Combination Therapy: Insulin-Sulfonylurea and Insulin-Metformin*).

Approximately 20 to 25 percent of diabetic patients fail to respond whatsoever to sulfonylureas. Such individuals represent primary failures. Because it is highly unlikely that they will respond to a second sulfonylurea drug, it is best to discontinue the sulfonylurea and start metformin (see the chapter *Metformin*) or insulin (see the chapter *Insulin Therapy in Type 2 Diabetes Mellitus*). In the 75 to 80 percent of individuals who have an initial good response to the sulfonylurea, the rate of secondary failure is high, 4 to 5 percent per year. The cause of this high secondary failure rate is unclear, but most likely is multifactorial and includes progressive beta-cell failure, tachyphylaxis to the sulfonylurea, and dietary noncompliance. Other causes of secondary failure are shown in Table 3. Because of the high rate of secondary failure, the physician must continue to monitor therapy closely and be prepared to change therapy as necessary to maintain good glycemic control. The results of the Diabetes Control and Complications Trial have demonstrated conclusively that tight glycemic control prevents microvascular complications in IDDM patients. Based on animal experiments, epidemiologic data, and human intervention studies, including the Wisconsin Eye Study and the Japanese Intervention Study, one can reasonably expect that tight glycemic control will be equally as effective in preventing diabetic microvascular complications in NIDDM patients.

There are a number of contraindications to the use of sulfonylureas (Table 4). In addition to IDDM these include pancreatic diabetes (insulin deficiency) and history of adverse reaction to a sulfonylurea or a sulfa-containing drug. Because their effect on the unborn fetus is unknown, sulfonylureas are contraindicated in pregnancy. Because major surgery, serious infection, stress, and trauma are associated with the release of counter-regulatory hormones, which cause severe insulin resistance and impair insulin secretion, such patients should be switched to insulin until the medical-surgical problem has resolved.

■ SPECIFIC SULFONYLUREA DRUGS

Each of the sulfonylureas have specific characteristics that may favor or present a relative contraindication to their use. The maximum dose and dose range (i.e., milligrams per day) is a function of the intrinsic potency. However, when used at maximally effective doses, all of the sulfonylureas with the exception of tolbutamide are equally effective clinically and lower the fasting plasma glucose concentration by approximately 60 to 70 mg per deciliter (Fig. 1).

Chlorpropamide has a very long half-life (approximately 36 hours) and is the drug with the longest duration of action. The drugs undergo extensive hepatic metabolism. The two major hepatic metabolites, along with chlorpropamide, all possess hypoglycemic activity and are excreted by way of the kidney. Chlorpropamide is contraindicated in patients with renal disease or in elderly diabetics (>60 to 65 years) because of the normal age-related decline in glomerular filtration rate.

Absorption of glyburide (glibenclamide) is highly dependent on the formulation used. The bioavailability of the micronized formulation is significantly better than the standard formulation. This has led to reduction in the tablet

size to 3 mg with a maximum dose of 12 mg per day, instead of 20 mg per day. Although it is recommended that glyburide be given twice daily, a single dose of 7.5 mg of glyburide lasts for about 24 hours and most patients do quite well when a single daily dose is given in the morning. The physician may wish to initiate therapy with a twice-daily schedule and, after maximum glycemic control is achieved, attempt to switch to once daily therapy.

Although glipizide has a very short half-life, it is effective when given twice daily. Although the maximal-approved dose is 40 mg per day, it is clear that the glipizide does not perform better when given in doses above 20 mg per day. In fact, recent studies suggest that the maximally effective dose of both glipizide and glyburide are closer to 10 mg per day. In nondiabetic subjects, glyburide enhances insulin secretion by the beta cell at plasma concentrations up to 100 to 200 nM, cor-

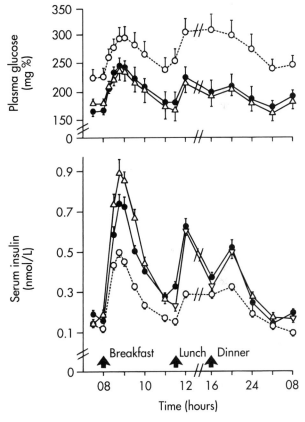

Figure 1

Plasma glucose and serum insulin concentrations (mean ± SEM) in 14 NIDDM patients after 6 months of glyburide (*solid line*) or glipizide (*dotted line*) treatment and after 1 month of placebo treatment (broken line). The areas under the plasma glucose curves were significantly smaller (p<0.01) and the areas under the plasma insulin curves were significantly greater (p<0.05) during glyburide and glipizide than during placebo therapy. There were no differences in any parameter between glyburide and glipizide. (*From Groop L, Groop P-H, Stenman S, et al. Comparison of pharmaco-kinetics, metabolic effects and mechanisms of action on glyburide and glipizide during long-term treatment. Diabetes Care 1987; 10:671–678; with permission.*)

Table 3 Causes of Secondary Sulfonylurea Failure
NATURAL HISTORY OF NIDDM
Progressive beta-cell failure: genetic
Progressive insulin resistance: genetic
PATIENT-RELATED FACTORS
Diet failure/weight gain
Poor compliance with medical regimen
Lack of exercise
Stress, intercurrent illness
THERAPY-RELATED FACTORS
Glucose toxicity
Tachyphylaxis to sulfonylurea following chronic exposure
Inadequate drug dose
Impaired sulfonylurea absorption by hyperglycemia
Simultaneous use of diabetogenic drugs (steroids, diuretics, beta-blockers)

Table 4 Contraindications to the Use of Sulfonylurea Drugs
Insulin dependent (type 1) diabetes mellitus
Pancreatic (insulin deficiency) diabetes
Adverse reaction/allergy to sulfonylureas or to sulfa drugs
Pregnancy
Major surgery or general anesthesia
Severe infection, stress, trauma
Predisposition to severe hypoglycemia, i.e., advanced liver or kidney disease

responding to an oral dose of 5 to 10 mg per day. At higher plasma levels, no further increase in insulin secretion was observed. In fact, several recent studies suggest that doses of glipizide and glyburide of 15 to 20 mg per day may even cause an increase, rather than a decrease in blood-glucose level. In escalating the dose of both glyburide and glipizide above 10 mg per day, the physician should closely monitor the plasma-glucose response. The above observations have important cost implications. Glipizide-GITs is a long-acting preparation that is administered once per day and is as effective as both glipizide and glyburide.

Several studies have shown that glyburide has more of an effect to inhibit hepatic glucose production than glipizide, which has more of an effect to enhance insulin secretion. This raises the possibility that these two agents would be beneficial when used in combination to treat NIDDM patients. There are few data available on this subject, but one small study comparing combined glyburide-glipizide with treatment with either agent alone did not demonstrate any improvement in glucose control in NIDDM patients.

◼ EFFECTS ON LIPID METABOLISM AND BODY WEIGHT

Patients with NIDDM are characterized by elevated plasma triglyceride and low plasma HDL-cholesterol concentrations. LDL concentrations are relatively normal, although their composition tends to be abnormal (small dense particles or subphenotype B). In general, the sulfonylureas have not been shown to have any consistent effect, either beneficial or deleterious, on plasma triglycerides or total LDL-HDL cholesterol. In most diabetic patients treated with sulfonylureas, body weight either does not change or it increases modestly.

◼ ADVERSE EFFECTS

Sulfonylureas usually are well tolerated and the frequency of adverse effects is low (Table 5). Skin reactions are nonspecific and rare. Hematologic complications, including thrombocytopenia, agranulocytosis, and hemolytic anemia have been described with tolbutamide and chlorpropamide but appear to be very rare with the second generation drugs. Gastrointestinal side effects, including dyspepsia and nausea, may occur, but they usually subside with time and almost never necessitate cessation of the drug. Abnormal liver-function tests and icterus occur uncommonly with all agents.

Chlorpropamide has a higher incidence of nonhypoglycemic side effects than the other sulfonylureas. In predisposed individuals, chlorpropamide causes an unpleasant flush in connection with alcohol intake. The flush is due to an accumulation of acetaldehyde because chlorpropamide inhibits the enzyme acetaldehyde dehydrogenase. Chlorpropamide also causes the release of antidiuretic hormone, and the resultant water retention can cause significant hyponatremia (SIADH), especially in elderly patients with underlying heart problems. Chlorpropamide also enhances the effect of the antidiuretic hormone in the distal tubule. In contrast to chlorpropamide, both glyburide and glipizide promote water excretion.

Table 5 Adverse Effects of Sulfonylureas
Hypoglycemia
Allergic reactions
Skin rash (rare)
Hematologic abnormalities
Hemolytic anemia
Thrombocytopenia
Agranulocytosis (rare)
Gastrointestinal
Nausea
Abdominal discomfort
Abnormal liver function tests
Facial flushing (chlorpropamide)
Antidiuresis, SIADH (first generation sulfonylureas)

SIADH = syndrome of inappropriate secretion of antidiuretic hormone.

◼ HYPOGLYCEMIA

Hypoglycemia represents the most common and serious side effect of sulfonylureas and, in elderly diabetic subjects, it can lead to permanent neurologic damage and even death. In elderly patients, hypoglycemia easily can be misdiagnosed as a cerebrovascular insult. About 20 percent of patients treated with sulfonylureas in Britain reported at least one episode of symptomatic hypoglycemia during a 6-month period. The true incidence of severe hypoglycemia (resulting in loss of consciousness) during sulfonylurea therapy is difficult to estimate, because most cases are never reported. Data from the Swedish Adverse Reaction Registry and from Switzerland report an incidence of 0.22 episodes per 1,000 patient years. This should be judged against 100 episodes per 1,000 patient years with insulin therapy. Most cases of severe and fatal hypoglycemia have been reported with the long-acting sulfonylureas, chlorpropamide and glyburide. The higher incidence of nocturnal hypoglycemia with glyburide versus glipizide has been related to its greater suppressive effect on hepatic glucose production.

It is important to emphasize that almost all severe cases of prolonged hypoglycemia have involved patients over the age of 70 years or patients with renal insufficiency. Other risk factors for the development of hypoglycemia include excessive alcohol intake, poor nutrition, intercurrent gastrointestinal disease, and drug interactions. A number of drugs can potentiate the hypoglycemic action of sulfonylureas by displacing them from their plasma-protein binding sites (e.g., salicylates, phenylbutazone, sulfonamides, clofibrate). Other drugs will interfere with the hepatic metabolism of sulfonylureas (e.g., phenylbutazone, dicumarol) or have intrinsic hypoglycemic activity (e.g., salicylates, alcohol). It is important to identify persons at risk for hypoglycemia and to avoid long-acting sulfonylureas in such individuals. Hypoglycemia can be minimized by following the preventive measures outlined in Table 6.

When hypoglycemia occurs, it should be treated promptly and aggressively. For mild reactions, ingestion of a readily absorbable carbohydrate is usually sufficient to reverse the symptoms. Intravenous glucose or glucagon may—along with hospitalization—be required for more severe reactions.

Table 6 Prevention of Sulfonylurea-Related Hypoglycemia

Identify high risk patients
    Elderly (>70 years of age)
    Renal or kidney disease
Start with lowest dose
Titrate slowly every 7–10 days
Avoid long-acting sulfonylureas, especially chlorpropamide
Use short-acting sulfonylureas, i.e., glipizide
Be cognizant of drug interactions (see Table 7)
Do not skip meals

In patients who develop hypoglycemia while taking chlor-propamide—especially those with renal insufficiency—the hypoglycemia may last for as long as 7 to 10 days. Such individuals require prolonged hospitalization and continuous IV glucose administration.

■ DRUG INTERACTIONS WITH SULFONYLUREAS

A variety of drugs are known to interact with the sulfonylureas, and cause either hyperglycemia or hypoglycemia (Table 7). Conversely, the sulfonylureas can alter the effectiveness of concomitantly administered medications. Certain drugs (e.g., aspirin) displace sulfonylureas from albumin-binding subjects. Conversely, sulfonylureas can displace other drugs from albumin-binding sites (e.g., coumadin) and result in prolonged bleeding times and hemorrhage.

Suggested Reading

Flatt PR, Shibier O, Sjecowskai, Berggun PO. New perspectives on the actions of sulfonylureas and hypoglycemic sulphonamides on the pancreatic beta cell. Diabetes Metab 1994; 20:257–162.

Review of the basic biochemical actions of the sulfonylurea drugs on the pancreatic beta cell.

Groop L. Sulfonylureas in NIDDM. Diabetes Care 1992; 15:737–754.

Excellent, comprehensive review of the use of sulfonylurea drugs in treatment of type 2 (non–insulin-dependent) diabetic patients.

Groop L, Groop P-H, Stenman S., et al. Comparison of pharmacokinetics, metabolic effects, and mechanisms of action on glyburide and glipizide during long-term treatment. Diabetes Care 1987; 10:671–678.

Well-designed, prospective, long-term, comparative study of glyburide and glipizide demonstrating that these two sulfonylurea agents have virtually identical effects on plasma glucose, insulin, and lipid levels in type 2 diabetic individuals.

Groop L, Wide E. Treatment strategies for secondary sulfonylurea failure. Should we start insulin or add metformin? Diabetes Metab 1991; 17:218–223.

Very practical overview of the treatment options available for type 2 diabetic patients who have failed to achieve satisfactory glycemic control on a sulfonylurea alone.

Table 7 Sulfonylureas and Drug Interactions

DETERIORATION OF GLYCEMIC CONTROL
Antagonists of insulin action: diuretics, beta-blockers, nicotinic acid, steroids, others
Inhibitors of insulin secretion: diuretics, beta-blockers, hypokalemia, phenytoin
Drugs that augment sulfonylurea metabolism: barbiturates, rifampin
DEVELOPMENT OF HYPOGLYCEMIA
Agents that displace sulfonylureas from albumin binding sites: aspirin, fibrates, trimethoprim
Inhibitors of renal excretion: probenecid, allopurinol
Insulin secretagogues: low dose aspirin, prostaglandin-like drugs
Inhibitors of gluconeogenesis: alcohol
Inhibitors of endogenous counter-regulatory hormones: beta-blockers
Competitive inhibitors of sulfonylurea metabolism: H2 blockers, alcohol
OTHER DRUG INTERACTIONS
Displacement of drugs from albumin binding sites: coumadin

Lebovitz HE. Stepwise and combination drug therapy for the treatment of NIDDM. Diabetes Care 1994; 17:1542–1544.

Succinct clinical review that examines the indications and efficacy of combination therapy with oral agents and insulin in the management of type 2 diabetic individuals.

Lebovitz HE, Melander A. Sulfonylureas: Basic aspects and clinical uses. In: Alberti KG, DeFronzo RA, Zimmet P, eds. International textbook of diabetes mellitus. Chichester, England: John Wiley, 1997:817.

Comprehensive, updated review of the mechanism of action, pharmacology, and clinical use of the sulfonylurea agents.

Melander A, Bitzen P-O, Faber O, Groop L. Sulfonylurea antidiabetic drugs: An update of their clinical pharmacology and rational therapeutic use. Drug 1989; 37:58–72.

A well-written, clinically relevant article that presents a rational approach for the use of sulfonylurea agents in the treatment of type 2 diabetic patients.

Shank M, Del Prato S, DeFronzo RA. Bedtime insulin—daytime glipizide: Effective therapy for sulfonylurea failures in NIDDM. Diabetes 1995; 44:162–172.

Well-designed, double-blind clinical study documenting the efficacy of adding bedtime insulin in type 2 diabetic patients who are poorly controlled with a sulfonylurea alone.

UK Prospective Diabetes Study Group. UK Prospective diabetes study: Overview of 6 years, of therapy of type II diabetes: a progressive disease. Diabetes 1995; 44:1249–1258.

Long-term prospective study comparing the effectiveness of sulfonylurea drugs, metformin, and insulin in the treatment of lean and obese type 2 diabetic patients.

Williams G. Management of non–insulin-dependent diabetes mellitus. Lancet 1994; 343:95–100.

Practical clinical overview of the management of type 2 diabetes mellitus.

METFORMIN

Agostino Consoli, M.D.

Metformin is a biguanide that is widely used in Europe and Canada to treat hyperglycemia in non–insulin-dependent diabetes mellitus (NIDDM) and recently has been approved for use in the United States. Two large prospective studies have demonstrated that metformin is equally effective when given as monotherapy or when given to NIDDM individuals who are poorly controlled on a sulfonylurea. The drug also had significant lipid-lowering effects, reducing plasma LDL cholesterol and triglyceride concentrations by 10 to 20 percent. Metformin does not cause weight gain and, in many diabetic patients, has been associated with weight loss. Metformin differs from the sulfonylureas in chemical structure, pharmacokinetics, and mechanism of action.

■ CHEMISTRY AND PHARMACOKINETICS

Metformin (N', N'-dimethylbiguanide) is a guanidine derivative in which two molecules of guanidine are linked together with the elimination of an ammonia group. It shares structural similarities with phenformin (beta-phenylbiguanide) and buformin (n-butylbiguanide), which are available in other countries in the world but are unlikely to gain acceptance in the United States because of a high incidence of adverse reactions. Approximately 60 percent of metformin is promptly absorbed by the gut following oral ingestion. The plasma half-life is 1.5 to 4 hours and the plasma concentration reaches a peak of 1 to 3 hours after oral ingestion. Metformin is not metabolized in the body, and does not bind to plasma proteins. Virtually 100 percent of the absorbed dose is excreted in the urine during the first 24 to 36 hours after oral administration. The half-life of metformin is directly correlated with creatinine clearance and it is prolonged in subjects with impaired renal function. In the United States, the use of metformin is contraindicated in individuals with a reduced glomerular filtration rate because of its potential to accumulate in plasma.

■ MECHANISM OF ACTION

Metformin is not truly a hypoglycemic agent, because it does not lower blood sugar in nondiabetic individuals. It should be considered an antihyperglycemic agent. It will lower the plasma glucose concentration from a high level to a normal level but not below normal. The mechanisms by which metformin lowers the blood glucose level in diabetic subjects are not yet completely understood. It is well documented that metformin does not stimulate insulin secretion and that its primary mechanism of action is related to (1) suppression of the elevated rate of basal hepatic glucose production and (2) increased peripheral muscle sensitivity to glucose. Although it has been suggested that impaired gastrointestinal absorption of glucose contributes to the hypoglycemic action of metformin, studies performed with isotopic techniques in humans have failed to support this. Some studies have shown that metformin increases insulin binding to its receptor, enhances insulin-receptor tyrosine kinase activity, and stimulates glucose transport in adipocytes and muscle cells. However, when muscle insulin resistance has been examined in NIDDM patients following metformin treatment, variable results have been reported. Some investigators have shown no significant improvement in insulin action, whereas others have reported a modest, 15 to 30 percent increase in insulin action. The reason for these variable results is unclear, but may be related to the reduction in body weight that commonly occurs in metformin-treated patients.

All studies that have examined the effect of metformin on basal hepatic production in NIDDM subjects uniformly have demonstrated a significant decline, which is closely correlated with the decrement in fasting plasma glucose concentration. The decline in basal hepatic glucose production results from an inhibition of both gluconeogenesis and glycogenolysis.

■ EFFICACY

Metformin treatment has proven effective, not only in improving blood glucose control, but also in inducing weight loss and in decreasing both the fasting and postprandial plasma lipid profile (Table 1). Some studies also have demonstrated a significant reduction in arterial blood pressure during metformin therapy, but this has not been a consistent effect.

Metformin does not lower the blood glucose level in nondiabetic subjects. In NIDDM patients a consistent hypoglycemic effect of metformin has been documented. The mean decline in fasting glucose and HbA_{1c} is approximately 70 mg per deciliter and 1.5 percent, respectively. The decrement in fasting glucose is directly related to the starting level. Thus, in diabetics with a fasting glucose of 300 mg per deciliter or more, the mean decrement is approximately 100 to 120 mg per deciliter. In diabetics with mild fasting hyperglycemia (i.e., 140 to 160 mg per deciliter), the mean decrement is approximately 20 to 30 mg per deciliter. The improvement in glycemia occurs with no change or a decrease in fasting and postprandial plasma insulin levels. On average, metformin treatment has produced a clinically significant decline in blood glucose levels and HbA_{1c} in approximately 80 percent of patients. However, the achievement of a fasting glucose concentration below 140 mg per deciliter is seen only in approximately 25 percent of individuals when metformin is used as monotherapy. In diabetic patients who have failed to achieve adequate control on sulfonylureas, addition of metformin while continuing the sulfonylurea, has been shown to be equally as effective in improving glycemic control as in diabetic patients treated with diet alone. The onset of action of metformin is not immediate. Within 2 to 3 days the blood glucose level begins to decline, reaching a nadir after approximately 2 weeks. This

Table 1 Beneficial Effects of Metformin in NIDDM

Decreases blood glucose
  Decreases fasting glucose by 60–70 mg/dl on average
  Decreases the increment in plasma glucose after meals
Does not increase (or even reduces) plasma insulin levels
Induces weight loss
Improves plasma lipid profile
  Decreases plasma LDL cholesterol
  Decreases plasma triglyceride
  Decreases postprandial hyperlipidemia

time course of metformin action is similar in diabetic patients treated with diet alone and in patients treated with a diet plus a sulfonylurea. Approximately 60 percent of NIDDM patients treated with combined metformin-sulfonylurea therapy achieve adequate glycemic control, i.e., fasting glucose about 140 mg per deciliter or less. Unlike the sulfonylureas, which are associated with a high rate of secondary failure, tachyphylaxis is unusual with metformin and the initial glucose-lowering effect is maintained for up to 5 years or longer.

In most patients who are treated with metformin the plasma insulin levels usually decline. Because metformin does not lower blood glucose levels in nondiabetic individuals and because it does not stimulate insulin secretion, hypoglycemia seldom, if ever, occurs during therapy with metformin alone.

Several clinical trials have shown a beneficial weight-reducing effect of metformin. The weight loss, which averages about 5 to 10 lbs, usually occurs during the first 6 months of the therapy and the body weight remains stable thereafter. A direct action of the drug on the satiety center has been proposed, but anorexia does not seem to be the only explanation for the weight loss. Decreased absorption of nutrients from the gastrointestinal tract can not explain the weight loss. A stimulatory effect of metformin on thermogenesis has been proposed, but not proven.

Metformin reduces the formation of atherosclerotic lesions in rabbit aorta and decreases the incorporation of labeled cholesterol into the aorta in vitro. Clinical trials consistently have demonstrated that treatment with metformin lowers both plasma VLDL triglyceride and LDL cholesterol levels. The beneficial effect on plasma lipids requires at least 2 weeks of treatment and is unrelated to the improvement in glycemic control or weight loss. A few studies also have demonstrated a small beneficial effect of metformin in increasing HDL cholesterol levels.

■ INDICATIONS FOR METFORMIN TREATMENT

In the absence of contraindications (see the following page), metformin can be used in any NIDDM patient who is poorly controlled on diet alone or with a diet plus a sulfonylurea. Because metformin effectively decreases blood sugar, induces weight loss, improves the plasma lipid profile, decreases plasma insulin levels, and works by improving insulin sensitivity in both muscle and liver, the drug should be considered as first line therapy in obese, dyslipidemic NIDDM patients.

Metformin also can be used in nonobese NIDDM, although these subjects often have a more severe defect in insulin secretion and might benefit more from sulfonylurea treatment.

Metformin also can be used in combination with a sulfonylurea in NIDDM patients who have failed to achieve the designed reduction in fasting glucose levels. In most studies, more than 50 percent of sulfonylurea failure subjects responded in a satisfactory manner to the addition of metformin. When initiating metformin therapy in diabetic patients who are taking a sulfonylurea, it is important that the sulfonylurea not be discontinued or reduced in dose.

It has been suggested that metformin might be effective in preventing the development of overt NIDDM in individuals with impaired glucose tolerance because of its ability to improve insulin sensitivity and decrease plasma insulin levels. For the same reason metformin has been advocated for use in individuals with the insulin-resistance syndrome or syndrome X (impaired glucose tolerance, dyslipidemia, essential hypertension, central obesity, hyperinsulinemia). However, proven clinical efficacy of metformin in these situations has not been established.

Metformin also has been recommended for use in insulin-requiring type 2 diabetic patients who are poorly controlled. Several studies have indicated that the addition of metformin can improve glycemic control and reduce plasma insulin concentrations. However, this use of metformin has not received formal approval by the FDA.

■ DOSAGE

Metformin comes in tablet sizes of 500 mg and 850 mg. Therapy should be initiated with lowest dose, either 500 mg or 850 mg, and given with the evening meal to minimize gastrointestinal side effects. It takes 1 to 2 weeks to see the maximal effect of any given dose. Therefore, dose escalation should not be carried out at intervals less than 1 to 2 weeks. The 500 mg tablets are preferred because the dose can be increased more gradually, therefore minimizing gastrointestinal side effects (see the following page). When increasing the dose of metformin, a second 500 mg tablet should be added with supper. After 1 to 2 weeks the blood glucose level should be checked and, if indicated, a third 500 mg tablet should be given with breakfast. If needed, a fourth 500 mg tablet can be taken with breakfast and a fifth 500 mg tablet added with the lunch meal. If the 850 mg tablets are used and additional dose escalation is indicated, the second tablet should be taken at breakfast and the third with lunch. The maximum dose of metformin is 2.5 to 2.55 g per day. However, most of metformin's effect will be seen with a daily dose of 1.5 to 2.0 g. It is important to emphasize that the dose should be increased slowly according to the blood-sugar response. Usually a dose of 1.5 to 2.0 g per day, which produces plasma metformin levels of approximately 5 μg per milliliter, achieves an acceptable clinical effect. Usually, no further improvement in blood glucose control is seen with doses greater than 2.5 g per day. Although 10 to 20 percent of the patients might not respond initially to metformin treatment, secondary failure with metformin is seldom observed and is much rarer than secondary failure with sulfonylureas.

■ SIDE EFFECTS

Side effects with metformin are almost entirely related to the gastrointestinal tract and occur in approximately 30 percent of individuals. These include metallic taste, anorexia, nausea, abdominal discomfort, and diarrhea. These side effects usually are mild, transient, and self-limiting, subsiding after the first 2 to 3 weeks of therapy. Small initial doses and administration with mealtime help to minimize these symptoms. If diarrhea or other gastrointestinal side effects persist, the dose of metformin should be titrated downward to the previous dose that was free of symptoms and held at that level until symptoms subside. After 2 to 3 weeks at the lower dose, upward titration should be attempted and usually is successful. Persistent diarrhea should raise suspicion about lactose intolerance. Skin rash and urticaria have been reported but are very rare. In less than 1 to 2 percent of the cases, side effects are severe enough to lead to withdrawal of the drug.

Lactic acidosis, a serious side effect of phenformin treatment, is very rare in diabetics treated with metformin. Because phenformin is very lipid soluble, it readily penetrates the mitochondrial membrane, and inhibits the electron transport chain, leading to an inhibition of glucose oxidation. This favors the conversion of pyruvate to lactate. Metformin, unlike phenformin, is highly lipid insoluble and does not affect the electron transport chain. Consistent with this, studies in NIDDM patients have shown that, at therapeutic doses, metformin does not inhibit glucose oxidation or lactate turnover. Not surprising, the incidence of lactic acidosis in NIDDM patients treated with metformin is extremely small, occurring with an incidence of three cases per 100,000 patient treatment years. This incidence is probably no higher than that in the general population. When lactic acidosis has been observed, it almost always has been reported in association with a major catastrophic illness, i.e., cardiogenic shock, septic shock, hypotension, severe liver disease, hypoxemia, and pulmonary insufficiency. All of these conditions are known to cause lactic acidosis. Lactic acidosis also has been reported in metformin treated patients who have chronic renal insufficiency or are on dialysis. Because metformin is excreted by way of the kidneys, it can accumulate in the plasma in individuals with impaired renal function. If blood levels reach those that are tenfold to twentyfold above the normal therapeutic dose, sufficient metformin can be pushed into cells and into the mitochondria by mass action to achieve levels that are high enough to interfere with lactate metabolism and cause clinically significant lactic acidosis.

When administered in therapeutic doses, a modest reduction in vitamin B_{12} levels uniformly occurs. However, the serum vitamin B_{12} levels almost always remain within the normal range, and the development of pernicious anemia is uncommon. If unexplained anemia should occur in a metformin treated patient, the vitamin B_{12} level should be checked.

■ CONTRAINDICATIONS

The major contraindications to metformin treatment are listed in Table 2. Because metformin is only eliminated by renal excretion, it is contraindicated in patients with impaired renal function in whom toxic levels of the drug might accu-

---

Table 2 Contraindications to Metformin Treatment

Renal insufficiency
Hepatic failure
Alcoholism
Severe cardiac disease
Severe pulmonary disease with hypoxemia
Severe trauma, systemic infection, or shock
Pregnancy
Vitamin B_{12} deficiency

---

mulate. In males with a serum creatinine concentration greater than 1.5 mg percent (1.4 mg percent in females), metformin is absolutely contraindicated. The drug should be used cautiously in elderly individuals over the age of 60 to 65 years, because the glomerular filtration rate can be significantly reduced even though the serum creatinine concentration is less than 1.4 to 1.5 percent. Due to the potential risk of lactic acidosis, metformin is also contraindicated in patients with severe cardiopulmonary disease or with acute systemic infection or trauma. In such individuals tissue anoxia markedly enhances the production of lactate. Chronic alcoholism and severe liver disease also represent contraindications to the use of metformin because altered hepatic lactate metabolism occurs in both of these conditions. Metformin should not be administered in pregnancy. In patients with vitamin B_{12} deficiency, metformin should be administered with caution due to the possible interference with absorption of the vitamin. Lastly, metformin should not be substituted for insulin therapy in type 2 insulin-dependent diabetic subjects. Insulin-dependent diabetic individuals have an obligate, life-long requirement for insulin.

■ CESSATION OF METFORMIN TREATMENT

Even in patients who are well controlled on metformin, there are certain instances when the drug should be stopped. Metformin should be stopped in any patient who develops a life-threatening medical problem associated with tissue hypoperfusion, i.e., shock of any etiology, hypotension, severe hypoxemia, liver failure, or renal insufficiency. Metformin also should be discontinued 48 hours prior to any radiocontrast procedure and not restarted until it is clear that there has been no injury to the kidney. This will avoid accumulation of the drug if the patient should experience dye-induced acute renal failure.

Suggested Reading

Bailey CJ, Turner RC. Metformin: A review. N Engl J Med 1996; 334:574–579.

A recent, comprehensive review of the basic and clinical aspects of metformin.

Clark B, Duncan L. Comparison of chlorpropamide and metformin treatment on weight and blood-glucose response of uncontrolled obese diabetics. Lancet 1968; 1:123–126.

The first relatively large randomized crossover study showing that metformin is not only as effective as chlor-

propamide in improving blood glucose control in obese NIDDM but it also induces weight loss.

DeFronzo RA, Barzilai N, Simonson C. Mechanism of metformin action in obese and lean non-insulin dependent diabetic subjects. J Clin Endocrinol Metab 1991; 73:1294–1301.

This is an original article demonstrating that 3 months of metformin treatment improves blood-glucose control by reducing hepatic glucose output.

DeFronzo RA, Goodman AM. Efficacy of metformin in patients with non-insulin dependent diabetes mellitus. N Engl J Med 1995; 333:541–549.

Two large, double-blind, randomized trials demonstrating the efficacy and safety of metformin when used as

monotherapy and in combination with a sulfonylurea in poorly controlled NIDDM patients.

Hermann L: Biguanides and sulfonylureas as combination therapy in NIDDM. Diabetes Care 1990; 13(suppl 3):37–41.

In this review article the advantages and the limitations of combined metformin-sulfonylurea therapy are discussed.

Hermann L, Melander A. Biguanides: Basic aspects and clinical uses. In: Alberti KG, Zimmet P, DeFronzo R, eds. International textbook of diabetes mellitus. Chichester, England: John Wiley and Sons, 1997:841.

An updated, comprehensive review about biguanide in general, and metformin in particular.

ALPHA-GLUCOSIDASE INHIBITORS

Janet Blodgett, M.D.

The alpha-glucosidase inhibitors are a new class of antihyperglycemic drugs that have a unique effect on the glycemic profile. Their major action is to lower postprandial plasma-glucose levels, while causing a modest reduction in the fasting plasma glucose concentration. Because these drugs inhibit the breakdown of complex carbohydrates within the intestine, their use results in delayed absorption of glucose within the small bowel and a consequent reduction in postprandial glucose levels. Acarbose (Precose) was approved by the Food and Drug Administration in September of 1995 and currently is available in the United States. Miglitol, another alpha-glucosidase inhibitor, currently is being investigated for possible clinical use.

■ POSTPRANDIAL GLUCOSE PROFILE

Non–insulin-dependent or type 2 diabetes mellitus (NIDDM) is characterized by fasting hyperglycemia in the basal state, and an excessive increase in plasma glucose concentration above baseline after ingestion of either glucose or mixed meals. Fasting hyperglycemia primarily results from overproduction of glucose by the liver, whereas postprandial hyperglycemia results from a combination of abnormalities, including reduced insulin-mediated glucose uptake by muscle, impaired suppression of hepatic glucose production, and "relative" or absolute insulin deficiency

owing to defective insulin secretion. Essentially all NIDDM individuals are insulin resistant, and this genetic defect is already well established in childhood. Early in the natural history of NIDDM the pancreas of diabetic individuals releases an excessive amount of insulin in response to a glucose load or mixed meal, although this release often is delayed. Glucose tolerance is known to deteriorate progressively with age. For each decade of advancing age, the fasting plasma glucose concentration increases little, approximately 1 mg per deciliter per decade of life. However, the 2-hour postprandial plasma-glucose level increases on average about 10 mg per deciliter per decade of life. Similar to the glucose intolerance of aging, people with impaired glucose tolerance have a normal or near-normal fasting plasma-glucose concentration with significant postprandial hyperglycemia. The transition to NIDDM is heralded by rises in the fasting glucose level, as well as by a worsening of the postprandial plasma-glucose profile.

■ MECHANISM OF ACTION

The brush border of the small bowel contains hydrolase enzymes known as alpha-glycosidases. These enzymes cleave oligo- and disaccharides into monosaccharides, which then are rapidly absorbed from the gastrointestinal tract. The alpha-glucosidase inhibitors competitively inhibit these enzymes. There are several intestinal alpha-glucosidases including glucoamylase, sucrase, maltase, isomaltase, and lactase. The inhibitory effects of acarbose on the various alpha-glucosidases are variable. For instance, acarbose inhibits 90 percent of the activity of glucoamylase but only 10 percent of the activity of lactase. Therefore, lactose intolerance is not a clinical problem in patients who take acarbose because the drug's inhibitory activity against lactose is minimal. This selective inhibition results in reduced carbohydrate digestion and a resultant delay in the absorption of simple sugars. The alpha-glucosidase inhibitors do not cause malabsorption. They simply delay absorption and shift it to the more distal portions of

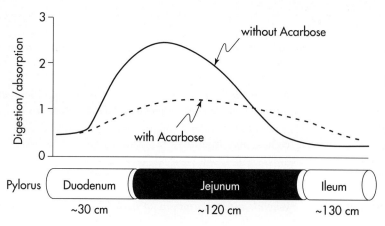

Figure 1
Delay in carbohydrate absorption with the use of acarbose. Absorption occurs along the entire length of the small bowel and not just in the upper portion in patients treated with acarbose. This results in an attenuation of the postprandial glucose rise. Absorption of monosaccharides is not significantly affected.

the small bowel. The result is that carbohydrate absorption occurs along the entire length of the small bowel rather than rapidly and primarily in the duodenum and upper jejunum (see Fig. 1). Some carbohydrates also may reach the large bowel. Among insulin-dependent diabetes mellitus (IDDM) and NIDDM patients who have been treated with the alpha-glucosidase inhibitors, their action results in a lower postprandial glucose rise that occurs over a longer period of time. On mean, the postprandial glucose rise is diminished by about 50 to 60 mg per deciliter by acarbose and other alpha-glucosidase inhibitors. With the reduction in the peak postprandial glucose levels, the amount of insulin released from the pancreas also is diminished. Acarbose and related agents exert only a modest effect on the fasting glucose level, decreasing it by approximately 20 to 30 mg per deciliter. A drop in glycosylated hemoglobin (HbA$_{1c}$) of 0.75 to 1 percent can be expected.

The alpha-glucosidase inhibitors not only delay carbohydrate absorption, but they also alter the gastrointestinal hormonal axis. These drugs decrease postprandial secretion of gastric-inhibitory polypeptide (GIP) and increase postprandial levels of glucagon-like peptide (GLP-1). GLP-1 is released in the distal portion of the gastrointestinal tract (ileum and colon) in response to nutrients and may play a role in the regulation of insulin secretion. This gut hormone also inhibits glucagon secretion. Gastric-inhibitory polypeptide is produced primarily in the upper gut (duodenum and jejunum) and its release is dependent on the absorption of nutrients. Gastric-inhibitory polypeptide potentiates insulin secretion, but only when plasma glucose levels are elevated. Because GIP exerts no effect on the alpha cell, glucagon levels are not affected by this gut hormone.

■ PHARMACOKINETICS

Only 1 to 2 percent of acarbose is absorbed as active drug. Because the drug acts locally in the small bowel, this low systemic bioavailability is desirable. Acarbose is metabolized in the gastrointestinal tract, principally by intestinal bacteria, but some also is degraded by digestive enzymes. A small fraction of these metabolites are absorbed and subsequently

Table 1 Clinical Features of Acarbose
No change in body weight
Reduction in postprandial plasma glucose and insulin levels
Modest decrease in postprandial triglyceride levels
When used as monotherapy, hypoglycemia is not a side effect.
If used with a sulfonylurea, the risk of hypoglycemia may be increased. Patients must be advised to reverse their reactions with dextrose or lactose (not complex carbohydrates).

excreted in the urine. The plasma half-life of acarbose is approximately two hours. Therefore, drug accumulation does not occur with the recommended three times a day dosing schedule, i.e., with each meal.

■ CLINICAL USE OF ACARBOSE (PRECOSE)

Acarbose (Precose) is available in 50- and 100-mg tablets. It is taken orally and must be chewed with the first bite of food at each of the three main meals. The recommended starting dosage is 25 mg three times a day. The tablets are scored on one side, making it easy to break the 50 mg tablets in half. The starting dosage should be increased to 50 mg orally three times a day after 4 to 8 weeks, based on the patient's one-hour postprandial glucose concentration and the patient's tolerability. The maximal recommended daily dosage is 100 mg orally three times a day. If there is no further reduction in blood-glucose level with this titration, it is recommended that the dosage be reduced to 50 mg orally three times a day. The maintenance dosage ranges from 50 to 100 mg orally three times a day. If patients forget to take the pill at the appropriate time, they should take the usual dose at the start of the next main meal. Because the drug works by inhibiting starch digestion, it is effective only if taken with meals. As a corollary, if the carbohydrate content of the meal is low, acarbose will have less of an effect on the postprandial plasma-glucose level. The total dosage of acarbose should not exceed 300 mg per day in an average sized (70 kg) person and 150

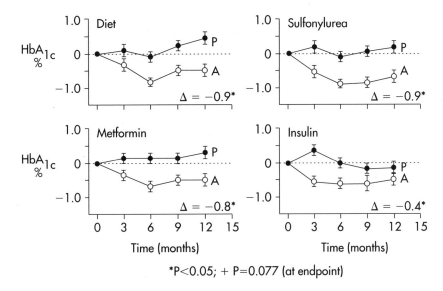

Figure 2

Mean change in HbA_{1c} from baseline in NIDDM patients treated with combination therapy using acarbose. NIDDM patients managed with diet alone *(upper left)*, metformin alone *(bottom left)*, a sulfonylurea alone *(upper right)*, and insulin alone *(bottom right)* were randomized to receive adjunctive therapy with acarbose for a period of 1 year. Compared to the placebo group *(P)*, acarbose *(A)* therapy resulted in an additional reduction of 0.8–0.9 percent in the HbA_{1c} level of the sulfonylurea, diet, and metformin groups. The reduction in HbA_{1c} in the insulin-treated group was not as great as in the other three groups. *(Adapted from Chiasson JL, Josse RG, Hunt JA, et al. The efficacy of acarbose in the treatment of patients with non–insulin-dependent diabetes mellitus. A multicenter controlled clinical trial. Ann Intern Med 1994; 121:928–935.)*

mg per day in people who weigh less than 132 lbs (60 kg). Patients weighing under 60 kg are at risk to develop an elevation in the serum transaminase levels. Liver enzyme (SGOT and SGPT) increases also have been reported in patients taking greater than the recommended maximal dosage of 100 mg three times a day. Table 1 summarizes some of the important clinical features of acarbose.

■ SIDE EFFECTS

The majority of reported side effects are gastrointestinal in nature, transient, and related to the mode of action of the drug. Carbohydrates that are not digested in the small bowel are metabolized by bacteria in the large bowel. This fermentation of undigested carbohydrates can cause bloating, abdominal discomfort, diarrhea, and flatulence. These side effects are dose-related, worsening with initiation of therapy and with dose increases. These side effects tend to diminish with continued use of the drug. No formal studies have been done to evaluate the benefit of antiflatulants (simethicone), antacids, or antidiarrheals to reduce the gastrointestinal tract side effects. As discussed previously, liver-function test abnormalities may occur in patients with low body weight (less than 60 kg) or in individuals taking greater than the maximal recommended daily dosage.

Hypoglycemia does not occur when acarbose is used alone because it has no effect on the pancreatic islet cells and does not stimulate insulin secretion. In patients who are on combination therapy with a sulfonylurea, hypoglycemia may occur. It is important to advise patients to treat their hypoglycemic symptoms with glucose (dextrose) or lactose and

not by ingestion of complex carbohydrates or sucrose. Digestion and subsequent absorption of these agents is delayed by the alpha-glucosidase inhibitors. The simplest remedy for hypoglycemia in a patient taking acarbose is the ingestion of glucose tablets.

Use of the alpha-glucosidase inhibitors is not associated with weight loss. Patients on these agents do not appear to be at risk for malabsorption of nutrients. When used in combination with a sulfonylurea, acarbose diminished the insulinotropic and weight-gaining effects of the sulfonylureas.

■ INDICATIONS

Currently, there are two approved indications for acarbose. As monotherapy, acarbose is beneficial as an adjunct to diet to reduce postprandial hyperglycemia. It also has been approved for use in combination with sulfonylureas in cases where either agent alone is inadequate to achieve optimal glycemic control. At the present time, acarbose is not FDA approved for use with either metformin or insulin, although there are a number of studies that clearly demonstrate that these combinations are effective treatment options. Figure 2 illustrates the findings of a multicenter Canadian study that compared the effects of acarbose added to dietary therapy, metformin, a sulfonylurea, and insulin. Their findings demonstrated that acarbose reduced HbA_{1c} levels by an additional 0.8 to 0.9 percent in subjects on dietary therapy, metformin, or a sulfonylurea. The additive effect of acarbose to insulin was significantly less than with a sulfonylurea or metformin. When added to insulin, acarbose decreased the HbA_{1c} by only 0.4 percent.

Table 2 Clinical Use of Acarbose

INDICATIONS
Monotherapy in patients with mild to moderate hyperglycemia
Adjunctive therapy in patients on a sulfonylurea but who have
    suboptimal glycemic control
CONTRAINDICATIONS
Patients with underlying disorders of the gastrointestinal tract
    including inflammatory bowel disease, colonic ulceration,
    partial bowel obstruction, and gastroparesis
Pregnancy and lactation
Serum creatinine > 2.0 mg/dl
History of diabetic ketoacidosis
Patients with cirrhosis

■ CONTRAINDICATIONS

There are a number of contraindications to the use of acarbose. Patients with underlying disorders of the bowel, including inflammatory bowel disease, colonic ulceration, partial bowel obstruction, or gastroparesis, should not be prescribed acarbose. Acarbose is contraindicated in pregnancy and among women who are breastfeeding. Patients with serum creatinine levels above 2.0 mg per deciliter should not receive the drug. Additional precautions are listed in Table 2.

There are relatively few drug interactions associated with the use of acarbose. In theory, the concomitant use of intestinal absorbents and digestive enzyme replacement therapy could decrease the effectiveness of acarbose. This interaction has not yet been examined formally. Cholestyramine may potentiate the decrease in postprandial insulin levels observed with acarbose. Neomycin may enhance the gastrointestinal side effects when used with acarbose.

Suggested Reading

Chiasson JL, Josse RG, Hunt JA, et al. The efficacy of acarbose in the treatment of patients with non–insulin-dependent diabetes mellitus. A multicentered controlled clinical trial. Ann Intern Med 1994; 121:928–935.

A review of the findings of a year-long multicenter trial on the efficacy of acarbose, an alpha-glucosidase inhibitor, on glycemic control in 354 patients with non–insulin-dependent diabetes. Glycemic control was improved in those patients on acarbose as demonstrated by reductions in postprandial blood-glucose concentrations and improved HbA$_{1c}$ levels. A significant change in serum C-peptide levels was not shown. Fasting lipid levels did not significantly change. No serious side effects were demonstrated among the study subjects.

Clissold SP, Edwards C. Acarbose: A preliminary review of its pharmacodynamic and pharmacokinetic properties, and therapeutic potential. Drugs 1988; 35:214–243.

A detailed review on the pharmacokinetics and clinical effects of acarbose, an alpha-glucosidase inhibitor. Use of this agent in type 1 diabetes, reactive hypoglycemia, and dumping syndrome is also discussed.

Lebovitz HE. A new oral therapy for diabetes management: alpha-glucosidase inhibition with acarbose. Clinical Diabetes 1995; 13:99–103.

A concise summary of the mechanism of action and clinical efficacy of acarbose is presented. Activity of acarbose on gut-enzyme activity is reviewed in detail.

INSULIN THERAPY IN TYPE 2 DIABETES MELLITUS

Jay S. Skyler, M.D.

Insulin therapy in the treatment of type 1 diabetes mellitus has been discussed in an earlier chapter, which also covered the pharmacology of insulin. Insulin therapy also may be used in patients with type 2 diabetes. In this chapter, treatment

The author is supported, in part, by NIH Grant HL-36588, U.S. Public Health Service. Portions of this chapter are based on the author's article, "Insulin Therapy in type II Diabetes," which appeared in Postgraduate Medicine 1997; 101:85–96.

strategies for insulin therapy of type 2 diabetes mellitus are discussed. It emphasizes three basic concepts that underlie the clinical rationale for insulin therapy: (1) glucose toxicity, (2) basal insulinemia, and (3) the variability of disease severity and progression. Also discussed is the rationale for insulin use in combination with other glucose-lowering agents.

Patients with type 2 diabetes have altered insulin secretory dynamics but retention of endogenous pancreatic insulin secretion; absence of ketosis (therefore, the disease has been called ketosis-resistant diabetes); and insulin resistance due to diminished target cell action of insulin. They are usually not dependent on insulin for prevention of ketosis or maintenance of life, but insulin may be used to control symptoms or to correct disordered metabolism. Temporary insulin therapy may be used to re-regulate patients who are decompensated in terms of glycemic control.

The two major pathogenetic mechanisms operative in type 2 diabetes are (1) impaired islet beta-cell function (impaired insulin secretion), and (2) impaired insulin action (insulin resistance or decreased insulin sensitivity). Both defects are present in most patients. However, type 2 diabetes is heterogeneous, such that different patients manifest varying degrees of these two impairments. In some patients

Table 1 Indices of Glycemic Control in Type 2 Diabetes

INDEX	NONDIABETIC	GOAL	ACTION SUGGESTED
Fasting/preprandial plasma glucose	<115 mg/dl (<6.4 mM)	80–120 mg/dl (<7.8 mM)	<80 or >140 mg/dl (<4.4 or >7.8 mM)
Bedtime plasma glucose	<120 mg/dl (5.6–7.8 mM)	100–140 mg/dl (5.6–8.9 mM)	<100 or >160 mg/dl (<5.6 or >8.9 mM)
HbA$_{1c}$ (%)*	<6.0%	<7.0%	>8.0%

*Referenced to a nondiabetic range of 4 to 6%.

insulin resistance is predominant, whereas in others there is greater impairment in beta-cell function. There probably are separate genetic defects responsible for these. In addition, environmental factors create further insulin resistance. There is progressive decrease in insulin sensitivity with age, and insulin resistance is induced by adiposity and by a sedentary life-style. Moreover, hyperglycemia can further impair both beta-cell function and insulin action, thereby creating a vicious cycle that aggravates hyperglycemia.

Replacement insulin therapy may substitute for impaired insulin secretion. With sufficient insulin therapy, it is possible to overcome insulin resistance. Yet, there are pharmacologic agents that are used to correct the metabolic defects in type 2 diabetes, e.g., insulin secretogogues (sulfonylureas), insulin sensitizers (thiozolidinediones), drugs that alter glucose metabolism (metformin), and drugs that alter glucose absorption (alpha-glucosidase inhibitors). Nevertheless, when these strategies fail to attain adequate glycemic control, insulin becomes the ultimate therapy used in type 2 diabetes.

■ TREATMENT OBJECTIVES

The beneficial effects and impact of effective glycemic control on chronic complications (retinopathy, nephropathy, and neuropathy) of type 1 diabetes have been firmly established. In patients with type 2 diabetes, the preponderance of the evidence suggests that similar relationships between glycemia and diabetic complications exist for both type 1 and type 2 diabetes. The results demonstrate that careful control of glycemia is important and should be sought in all patients with diabetes. Glycemic targets, as recommended by the American Diabetes Association, are shown in Table 1. The minimal treatment goals are to correct fasting and preprandial hyperglycemia to below the diagnostic threshold (140 mg per deciliter), while striving ideally for a normal fasting level (<115 mg per deciliter). Other goals are to minimize postprandial hyperglycemia and to obviate glycosuria. This is best reflected by normal or near-normal levels of glycated (glycosylated) hemoglobin (HbA$_{1c}$ or HbA$_1$). Various behavior (diet, exercise) and pharmacologic therapies are progressively used until the glycemic treatment goals are attained. Such "goal based-therapy" or "targeted glycemic control" is the basis for contemporary management of type 2 diabetes.

In addition to glycemic goals, attention must be paid to other variables, including lipids, blood pressure, smoking cessation, and attaining and maintaining weight as close as possible to ideal body weight. Normalizing weight in obese type 2 diabetes individuals is as crucial as controlling glycemia, because success with the former often leads to success with the latter.

Contemporary management of type 2 diabetes is based on the concept of targeted glycemic control. This involves therapy based on glycemic goals, using a step-wise approach of whatever therapy is necessary to achieve glycemic goals. A nutritional plan and the promotion of physical activity are the cornerstones in management. Pharmacologic therapy is required in most patients. This is based on severity of the disease and whether glycemic goals are met.

■ INDICATIONS FOR INSULIN IN TYPE 2 DIABETES

As noted, the primary pathophysiologic defects in type 2 diabetes are impairment in beta-cell function and impairment in insulin action (insulin resistance). Although it has been argued by some that insulin is not an effective therapy in type 2 diabetes because insulin deficiency per se is not the primary defect, it is possible with insulin therapy both to overcome insulin resistance and to provide insulin availability in the face of islet beta-cell dysfunction. Almost invariably, if enough insulin is used, glycemia can be regulated. However, most physicians and patients prefer other pharmacologic approaches first. Therefore, there are evolving indications for insulin therapy, which include:

- Hyperglycemia despite maximum doses of oral agents
- Decompensation due to intercurrent events, e.g., infection, acute injury, or other stress
- Development of severe hyperglycemia with ketonemia and/or ketonuria
- Uncontrolled weight loss
- Perioperative in patients undergoing surgery
- Pregnancy
- Renal or hepatic disease
- Allergy or other serious reaction to oral agents
- Latent autoimmune diabetes in adults (LADA, see p.112)

Insulin therapy also may be preferred by some patients or their physicians.

■ GLUCOSE TOXICITY AND TEMPORARY INSULIN THERAPY

Glucose Toxicity

Glucose toxicity is a well-established concept that has been shown to contribute to development of insulin resistance and impaired insulin secretion in animal models of diabetes. The data suggests that hyperglycemia per se is responsible for some of the impairment in beta-function and some of the resistance to insulin action. In humans with type 2 diabetes, a considerable body of evidence has accumulated indicating that a chronic physiologic increment in plasma glucose concentration leads to progressive impairment in insulin secretion and aggravation of insulin resistance, in part due to downregulation of the glucose-transport system. Therefore, impairments in insulin secretory response and insulin action are not static, but dynamic. Chronic hyperglycemia, of itself, aggravates the defects. Moreover, and most important, it has been shown that in poorly controlled diabetic patients, the attainment of improved glycemic control results in improvement in insulin secretion and amelioration of some of the insulin resistance. Therefore, insulin therapy can be effectively used to overcome glucose toxicity and restore the potential effectiveness of other therapeutic modalities, making maintenance of the improved metabolic state easier. Such a "feed-forward" system would explain the clinical aphorism that it is much easier to maintain glucose control than it is to attain glucose control.

Understanding of the concept of glucose toxicity provides a rationale both for (1) temporary use of insulin in type 2 diabetes both to initially attain glycemic control and to re-regulate decompensated patients, and (2) discontinuation of insulin therapy in some patients with type 2 diabetes.

Temporary Insulin Therapy

An important use of insulin is as temporary therapy to:

- Initially attain glycemic control in patients with severe type 2 diabetes
- Overcome glucose toxicity
- Re-regulate decompensated patients

Indeed, type 2 diabetes may be considered a disease of periodic decompensation with the need for re-regulation, usually with insulin. For this reason, all patients with type 2 diabetes should learn insulin administration techniques and be prepared to initiate insulin therapy in the face of expected periodic decompensation, which occurs both spontaneously and, particularly, with intercurrent illness or stress. Unfortunately, however, the temporary use of insulin is one of the more neglected principles of management of type 2 diabetes.

The hypothesis that short-term insulin therapy may induce long-lasting metabolic improvements in patients with type 2 diabetes has been tested. The degree of success varies depending on the stage of the disease. This approach works extraordinarily well early in the disease to initially attain glycemic control and to re-regulate decompensated patients with intercurrent illness or stress.

When used by long-standing patients in whom other therapy has failed to achieve adequate glycemic control, results with temporary insulin therapy are quite variable. These patients probably have progressive pancreatic beta-cell failure that is unrelated to glucose toxicity. After insulin withdrawal, some of these patients continue to sustain improvements in glycemic control, whereas in others blood-glucose levels increase but generally remain below preinsulin treatment values. With 4 weeks of insulin therapy, there is a decrease in ambient blood glucose levels and basal glucose-

production rate, and improvement both in insulin secretory response and in insulin action. The enhanced insulin secretory response and improved insulin action persist after cessation of insulin therapy. Unfortunately, patients may not sustain desired glycemic targets after stopping insulin therapy. In such circumstances, long-term insulin therapy is required.

When using insulin to initially attain glycemic control, vigorous insulin therapy is needed to overcome insulin resistance and glucose toxicity. The plan here is a program of "sequential therapy" in which insulin is used initially to attain glycemic control, with subsequent control maintained by oral agents, diet and exercise, or basal insulin therapy.

When using insulin to re-regulate decompensated patients with intercurrent illness, it is often possible to merely add the insulin to existing oral therapy. As such, insulin may be used for a few days to a few weeks. Dosage may either be as supplemental insulin based on prevailing level of preprandial glycemia (e.g., 1 to 2 U of short-acting insulin for every 50 mg per deciliter above the preprandial glucose target) or as relatively small total dose (e.g., 0.2 to 0.3 U per kilogram per day) added to the existing therapy, either as intermediate-acting insulin or a combination of short-acting insulin and intermediate-acting insulin.

Discontinuation of Insulin Therapy

Insulin therapy in type 2 diabetes need not be permanent. With correction of glucose toxicity, there is improvement in both endogenous insulin secretion and in insulin sensitivity. As a consequence, it may be possible to discontinue exogenous insulin therapy. Patients with type 2 diabetes who are candidates for discontinuing insulin are those who are clinically stable, including stable body weight, and in whom glycemic targets are being met. My guidelines for insulin discontinuation are to reduce insulin dose progressively by steps of 10 to 15 percent of the total daily dose, while carefully monitoring blood glucose to be sure that there is no deterioration in glycemia. Should blood glucose rise, the insulin dose is restored. If blood glucose does not rise, insulin dose reduction is continued by about 10 to 15 percent every 1 to 2 weeks. When the insulin dose has been decreased to less than 0.3 to 0.4 U per kilogram per day, consideration can be given to stopping insulin and replacing it with either a sulfonylurea alone, the combination of a sulfonylurea plus metformin, or the combination of a sulfonylurea plus troglitazone. I favor glipizide-GITS (or glimiperide) as the sulfonylurea. If the patient has near-normal levels of glycemia and a lower dose of insulin (approximately 0.25 to 0.3 U per kilogram per day) at the time of switching, it is often possible to use a sulfonylurea alone, albeit at a fairly high dose. The sulfonylurea has immediate effect, so that insulin may be discontinued after the first sulfonylurea dose. If the patient has glycemia that is not quite normal or if the insulin dose is a little higher (approximately 0.3 to 0.4 U per kilogram per day) at the time of switching, it is usually desirable to use the combination of a sulfonylurea plus either metformin or troglitazone. In this case, it should be appreciated that metformin requires 3 to 6 weeks for its full effect, while troglitazone requires 10 to 12 weeks for its full effect. Therefore, some insulin should be sustained for this period (generally about half of the dose).

■ BASAL INSULINEMIA

Basal Insulin Therapy

The level of fasting (basal) glycemia is crucial in type 2 diabetes, as it determines the level above which glycemia oscillates. Fasting hyperglycemia is due to increased hepatic-glucose production. Adequate overnight insulinemia is important in regulation of fasting hyperglycemia. "Basal insulin therapy" is that designed to correct fasting hyperglycemia. The concept dates back to the earliest use of sustained-action insulin and had a rationale strengthened by recent physiologic insights. A series of insulin regimens based on basal insulin therapy have been proposed in the management of type 2 diabetes. Basal insulin therapy may be provided as bedtime intermediate-acting insulin (e.g., NPH or Lente), long-acting Ultralente insulin to supplement basal insulin secretion, or continuous insulin infusion. Basal insulin therapy reduces overnight basal hepatic-glucose production by inhibiting gluconeogenesis; suppresses nocturnal increases of free fatty acids; and obviates the overnight waning of insulinemia responsible for the dawn phenomenon.

Adequate basal insulinemia is essential in glucose homeostasis. Thus, basal insulin therapy is an important component of therapy for type 2 diabetes. Yet, in the United States, more than 60 percent of insulin is prescribed as a single daily dose of intermediate-acting insulin in the morning. Such treatment fails to provide adequate basal insulinemia and may lead to excess risk of daytime hypoglycemia. Morning insulin is prescribed for convenience and because of fear of nocturnal hypoglycemia. However, it has been shown in a number of studies that bedtime intermediate-acting insulin is superior to morning intermediate-acting insulin in patients with type 2 diabetes.

The superiority of basal insulin therapy is a consequence of better glycemic control, with less weight gain and lower ambient levels of circulating insulin. In studies comparing morning versus bedtime intermediate-acting insulin, there has been better overall glycemic control with bedtime insulin, less frequent hypoglycemic events, lower daily insulin dose, less hyperinsulinemia, and less weight gain.

It is possible to use "basal insulin therapy" alone to correct fasting hyperglycemia, with endogenous insulin secretion being adequate to control meal-related, postprandial glucose excursions. The theme of bedtime insulin use has also been applied to studies with combinations of insulin and sulfonylureas, as discussed further in a later section.

■ ONGOING INSULIN THERAPY

Subclassification Based on Severity of Diabetes

For clinical purposes, the severity of type 2 diabetes can be related to the degree of hyperglycemia on a stable diet and activity program. This clinical subclassification has four categories: mild, moderate, severe, and very severe (Table 2). Because basal (fasting) glycemia is relatively constant from day to day on a stable diet and activity program, the fasting plasma glucose is the principal determinant. Also used is the postprandial glucose response to a meal. Although type 2

Table 2 Subclassification of Type 2 Diabetes

CATEGORY	FASTING (BASAL) PLASMA GLUCOSE*	POSTPRANDIAL GLUCOSE RESPONSE TO MEALS**
Mild	<140 mg/dl (<7.8 mM)	Restored to basal
Moderate	140–250 mg/dl (7.8–13.9 mM)	Restored to basal
Severe	>250 mg/dl (>13.9 mM)	Restored to basal
Very severe	(>250–300 mg/dl) (>13.9–16.7 mM)	Not restored to basal

*On a stable diet and activity program.
**Within 4 to 5 hours, within 20 to 25 mg/dl.

diabetes is characterized by a prolonged period of postprandial hyperglycemia (glucose intolerance), typically, patients have intact endogenous insulin response to meals such that postprandial glycemia is restored to basal levels (± 20 to 25 mg per deciliter) within 4 to 5 hours of meal consumption. When this does not occur, they are defined as "very severe" type 2 diabetes. Otherwise, they are subclassified on the basis of fasting plasma glucose.

"Mild" Type 2 Diabetes

"Mild" describes patients with fasting plasma glucose (FPG) less than 140 mg per deciliter, the threshold for diagnosis on the basis of fasting hyperglycemia alone. These individuals sometimes can be treated with a diet and activity program without pharmacologic intervention. When this proves inadequate, these patients may benefit from the addition of a sulfonylurea or metformin.

"Moderate" Type 2 Diabetes

"Moderate" type 2 diabetes describes patients with FPG in the range of 140 to 250 mg per deciliter. In addition to a diet and activity program, they almost invariably require pharmacologic intervention.

"Severe" Type 2 Diabetes

"Severe" type 2 diabetes describes patients with FPG more than 250 mg per deciliter, and with restoration of glycemia to basal levels within 4 to 5 hours of meal consumption.

Glycemic control can be most readily attained with insulin therapy providing around-the-clock insulinization. Long-term glycemic control then can be maintained either with a sulfonylurea and/or metformin, or with insulin.

"Very Severe" Type 2 Diabetes

"Very severe" type 2 diabetes describes patients with nonintact endogenous insulin response to meals, such that postprandial glycemia is not restored to basal levels within 5 hours of meal consumption. Fasting plasma glucose is usually quite elevated as well (above the 250 to 300 mg per deciliter range), but may not be. There is such profound insulin deficiency that these patients initially may be difficult to distinguish from patients with type 1 diabetes, although generally they do not manifest ketosis. Initially they are best treated like type 1 patients.

In all four subcategories of type 2 diabetes, it should be recognized that with adequate treatment there may be improvement both in islet beta-cell function and in peripheral insulin action at target cells. As a consequence, there may be sufficient improvement in glucose homeostasis that a patient can be reclassified to a less severe subcategory, with glycemic control maintained by a treatment program typical for that category.

A subtype of type 2 diabetes has been termed latent autoimmune diabetes in adults (LADA). It appears to be a slowly evolving variant of type 1 diabetes. These patients, if identified, should always be treated with insulin, because insulin may slow the progressive nature of the autoimmune process, and because actively secreting beta cells are more prone to autoimmune attack. Indeed, sulfonylurea therapy may hasten beta-cell failure in these patients. Latent autoimmune diabetes in adults can be suspected in patients with type 2 diabetes who are younger (onset in the third and fourth decade of life) and thinner, but may occur at any age and not only in thin individuals. The presence of a family history of type 1 diabetes or autoimmune endocrine disease favors the diagnosis. Antibodies directed against islet-cell antigens establish the diagnosis. Insulin therapy should be given as in type 1 diabetes.

Insulin Therapy Based on Severity of Diabetes

The approach to insulin therapy in type 2 diabetes is based on the severity of disease as determined by the clinical subclassification shown in Table 2. Table 3 lists the approaches to insulin therapy used in each category. These are discussed below.

"Moderate" Type 2 Diabetes

For patients with "moderate" type 2 diabetes (fasting plasma glucose 140 to 250 mg per deciliter), if insulin therapy is used, it is often sufficient to use "basal insulin therapy" to correct fasting hyperglycemia, with endogenous insulin secretion being adequate to control meal-related, postprandial glucose excursions. Basal insulin therapy may be provided as a bedtime dose of intermediate-acting insulin (e.g., NPH or Lente), as long-acting Ultralente insulin to supplement basal insulin secretion, or as a continuous insulin infusion. These insulin programs are schematically depicted in Figures 1 and 2. Doses required generally are in the range of 0.3 to 0.6 U per kilogram per day. When intermediate-acting insulin is administered at bedtime, its peak effect 8 to 10 hours later coincides with the prebreakfast period, thus controlling basal (fasting) glycemia.

"Severe" Type 2 Diabetes

For patients with "severe" type 2 diabetes (fasting plasma glucose >250 mg per deciliter), clinical experience has shown that around-the-clock insulinization is necessary. Therefore, in contrast to patients with "moderate" type 2 diabetes, bedtime intermediate-acting insulin cannot be used (although twice-daily intermediate-acting insulin may be used). Most patients with "severe" type 2 diabetes will require a more intensive insulin program (with addition of short-acting insulin—Regular or lispro) to attain glucose control. (Schemes for such

insulin programs are depicted in the chapter *Insulin Therapy in Type 1 Diabetes Mellitus*). Doses required are generally in the range of 0.5 to 1.2 U per kilogram per day. However, large doses, even in excess of 1.5 U per kilogram per day, may be required, at least initially, to overcome prevailing insulin resistance. Such high-dose therapy may be necessary only to attain control, with subsequent control maintained on lower doses, on a basal insulin program, or with oral hypoglycemic agents. Often, insulin therapy is continued as dosages in the range of 0.3 to 1.0 U per kilogram per day. The use of premixed insulin preparations (e.g., 70/30, which contains 70 percent NPH and 30 percent Regular insulin) may facilitate implementation of such programs. Such intensive insulin therapy may be necessary only to attain control, with subsequent control maintained on a basal insulin program or with sulfonylurea therapy. Another option is to attain glycemic control by the use of continuous insulin infusion, with subsequent maintenance of control as outlined above.

"Very Severe" Type 2 Diabetes

Patients with "very severe" type 2 diabetes are severely insulin deficient and need to be managed akin to patients with type 1 diabetes.

In all categories of patients with type 2 diabetes, there will be improvement of the pathophysiologic defects as glycemic control is attained and maintained. This facilitates ease of control and may permit patients initially treated with insulin to be maintained on oral hypoglycemic agents therapy or even a diet and activity program alone, as discussed above.

Effectiveness of Insulin Therapy in Type 2 Diabetes

Most patients with type 2 diabetes can be controlled with insulin, if adequate doses are given, and if the patient follows an appropriate dietary and exercise program. The latter facilitate insulin action. Failure to follow a diet may countermand the effects of insulin and lead to a vicious cycle of progressively increasing insulin doses, yet failure to control glycemia.

When intensive insulin therapy is used in type 2 diabetes, glycemic control is markedly improved with surprisingly lit-

---

Table 3 Approaches to Insulin Therapy in Type 2 Diabetes Based on Severity of Disease

MILD TYPE 2 DIABETES
Insulin virtually never needed

MODERATE TYPE 2 DIABETES
"Basal insulin therapy" usually sufficient
   Bedtime intermediate-acting insulin (NPH or Lente)
   Ultralente insulin
Endogenous insulin controls meal glucose excursions

SEVERE TYPE 2 DIABETES
Around-the-clock insulinization is necessary
   Twice daily intermediate-acting insulin (NPH or Lente)
   Ultralente insulin
   Continuous insulin infusion
Some patients require more intensive insulin
   Addition of short-acting insulin (Regular or lispro)

VERY SEVERE TYPE 2 DIABETES
Severely insulin deficient
Managed akin to patients with type 1 diabetes

tle hypoglycemia. Concomitantly, there is improvement in the lipid profile, but there often is weight gain. Several studies have demonstrated the superiority of insulin over oral medications in achieving satisfactory glycemic control.

Progressive Insulin Therapy

Type 2 diabetes is a progressive disease. Therefore, with time, in spite of maximum doses of various therapeutic agents, glycemic control may deteriorate. Therefore, in patients with type 2 diabetes in whom standard pharmacologic therapy with oral agents has failed to achieve adequate glycemic control, it is necessary to use insulin therapy. Initially, insulin ther-

apy may be commenced as "basal insulin therapy." However, if this also fails to achieve adequate glycemic control, insulin therapy can be intensified using a stepwise approach: combination therapy by addition of daytime sulfonylurea, twice daily insulin, and ultimately insulin three to four times daily. With this strategy, it is often feasible to achieve excellent glycemic control.

However, excellent glycemic control may not be sustained indefinitely. This has been demonstrated in the United Kingdom Prospective Diabetes Study (UKPDS), a randomized, multicenter, controlled trial on the effect of improved metabolic control on complications in type 2 diabetes,

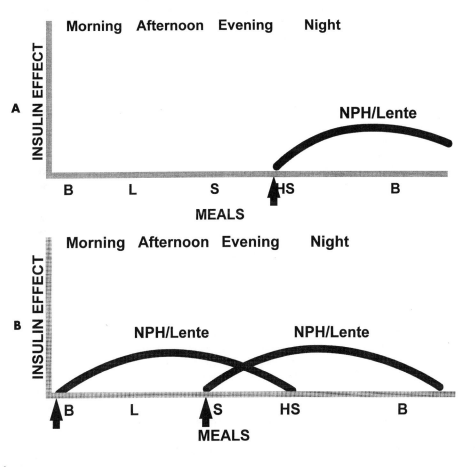

Figure 1
A, Schematic representation of idealized insulin effect provided by insulin regimen consisting of a bedtime injection of intermediate-acting insulin (NPH or Lente). **B**, Schematic representation of idealized insulin effect provided by insulin regimen consisting of two daily injections of intermediate-acting insulin.
Symbols: *B* = breakfast; *L* = lunch; *S* = supper; *HS* = bedtime snack. Arrows indicate time of insulin injection, 30 minutes before meals.

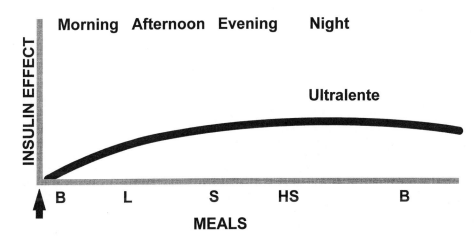

Figure 2
Schematic representation of idealized insulin effect provided by basal long-acting Ultralente insulin.
Symbols: *B* = breakfast; *L*=lunch; *S* = supper; *HS* = bedtime snack. Arrows indicate time of insulin injection, 30 minutes before meals.

involving over 4,000 patients enrolled from the time of diagnosis. Over 9 years of follow-up, regardless of the assigned therapy, the fasting plasma glucose and HbA$_{1c}$ levels increased and maintaining near-normal glycemia was, in general, not feasible. This is a consequence of progressive beta-cell failure. In this circumstance, even insulin therapy did not achieve the therapeutic goal of near-normal glycemia because of the difficulty in treating marked hyperglycemia and the risk of hypoglycemic episodes. With time, then, progressive beta-cell failure results in inability to optimally control glycemia in type 2 diabetes.

Insulin Programs for Elderly Patients with Type 2 Diabetes

Insulin therapy is often used in the elderly as a last resort, after failure of dietary management and maximum doses of oral hypoglycemic agents. The aim of therapy in the elderly is to relieve symptoms and prevent both hypoglycemia and acute complications of uncontrolled diabetes, e.g., hyperosmolar states. Schedules for the injection of insulin should be kept as simple as possible, because self-administration may be difficult and dosage errors are not uncommon. Premixed insulins may be particularly desirable due to their simplicity of use.

■ INSULIN THERAPY IN COMBINATION WITH ORAL AGENTS

Combination Therapy of Insulin with Sulfonylureas

Sulfonylureas work by enhancing endogenous insulin secretion. Therefore, it does not seem obvious that combining insulin and sulfonylureas would offer much benefit. At one time, however, it was thought that a primary action of sulfonylureas was to improve insulin action. That, however, has proven to be a secondary effect consequent to lowering ambient glycemia and overcoming glucose toxicity. Nevertheless, the idea of combining insulin and sulfonylureas has long been considered as a therapeutic option for type 2 diabetes. Most early studies failed to show a consistent therapeutic benefit. However, as demonstrated by three recent meta-analyses of randomized trials, combination therapy does result in a statistically significant improvement in glycemic control. Yet, although the addition of a sulfonylurea to insulin seemed to reduce hyperglycemia, insulin dose, or both, long-term benefits from such combination therapy were not demonstrated conclusively. Therefore, the authors of the first two meta-analyses concluded that the benefit was quantitatively marginal and that this approach warranted but lukewarm recommendation. The authors of the third meta-analysis more strongly endorsed combination therapy, concluding that this approach leads to improved metabolic control as reflected by a significant lowering of both fasting plasma-glucose values and glycated hemoglobin levels, and that this was achieved with a significantly smaller daily insulin dose without a significant change in body weight, and with enhanced endogenous insulin secretion. Therefore, these three analyses have provided inconsistent conclusions and have failed to resolve the controversy. Part of the problem is that different subject groups were studied, using different treatment programs.

Nevertheless, over the past decade there has been rekindled interest in combination therapy of insulin and sulfonylureas. Partly, this is because recent studies of combination therapy have most often used bedtime administration of intermediate-acting insulin, with daytime administration of a sulfonylurea. This is termed "BIDS" therapy, i.e., bedtime insulin, daytime sulfonylurea. This strategy combines bedtime intermediate-acting insulin, to decrease hepatic-glucose production and thus control fasting hyperglycemia, with preprandial sulfonylurea to stimulate pancreatic insulin secretory response to meals. BIDS may be considered either (1) in patients already on maximum dose of sulfonylurea, but in whom there is rising fasting plasma glucose, or (2) in patients who have already been treated with bedtime intermediate-acting insulin with adequate control of fasting plasma glucose but escape of glycemic control postprandially and throughout the day.

Combination Therapy of Insulin with Biguanides

Biguanides work by decreasing hepatic glucose production and thus reduce fasting glycemia. They are also associated with an improvement in insulin action, but this appears to be a secondary effect consequent to lowering ambient glycemia and overcoming glucose toxicity. The idea of combining insulin with biguanides, e.g., metformin, also has long been considered as a therapeutic option for type 2 diabetes. This strategy has been considered because metformin can act in the presence of insulin and thus might facilitate its effects. As a consequence, there have been a number of studies in both type 1 and type 2 diabetes in which the possible synergistic effect of metformin added to insulin therapy has been examined. Although some studies have shown that insulin requirements were decreased during the administration of metformin, these have not been rigorously controlled and are generally unimpressive. What little effect is seen seems to be maximal shortly after commencing the addition of metformin. Some authors have also claimed that metformin smoothes glycemic profiles, but this is denied by others. Because the only alleged benefit is to decrease insulin requirements, and most studies are inadequate, there can not currently be much enthusiasm for this combination. More studies are needed.

Combination Therapy of Insulin with Thiozolidinediones

The primary mechanism of action of thiozolidinediones (glitazones) is as insulin sensitizers to correct insulin resistance and improve target cell insulin action. Because they improve insulin action, the idea of combining insulin with thiozolidinediones, e.g., troglitazone, is a logical therapeutic option for type 2 diabetes. In fact, the initial basis for approval of troglitazone by the FDA was for "insulin rescue," i.e., its use in reducing insulin dose and allowing insulin discontinuation in approximately 15 percent of patients studied.

Combination Therapy of Insulin with Alpha-Glucosidase Inhibitors

Yet another possible strategy is to combine insulin with alpha-glucosidase inhibitors, e.g., acarbose. This strategy has been considered because acarbose acts to decrease postprandial glycemia by inhibiting digestion of complex carbohydrates and disaccharides, therefore retarding gastrointestinal glucose absorption. Because excess postprandial glycemia remains a problem in both type 1 and type 2 diabetes, even in insulin treated patients, this is a logical approach. Indeed, there are reports of better postprandial glycemic control when acarbose is added to insulin therapy. Unfortunately, the data are inadequate to draw firm conclusions, and are drawn mostly from relatively short-term studies. Nevertheless, the logic of the approach is sound and it must therefore be given some consideration. More studies are required.

■ ADDITIONAL POINTS

Concerns About Insulin Therapy in Type 2 Diabetes

The "insulin resistance syndrome" is a cluster of metabolic disorders, including type 2 diabetes mellitus, central obesity, hypertension, dyslipidemia, and atherosclerotic cardiovascular disease. The resistance to insulin action engenders compensatory hyperinsulinemia. In epidemiologic studies, therefore, hyperinsulinemia has been associated with hypertension, dyslipidemia, and with cardiovascular disease. This has led some authors to be critical of insulin therapy in type 2 diabetes on the grounds that insulin may have atherogenic effects and that relative hyperinsulinemia is already present in this insulin-resistant state. Yet, the state of cellular resistance to insulin action subtends the observed hyperinsulinemia. In fact, patients with moderate to severe degrees of hyperglycemia have reduced endogenous insulin secretion, thereby providing a logical basis for insulin administration. Moreover, sufficient insulin doses can overcome any insulin resistance that is present. In addition, there is substantial evidence that it is the insulin resistance per se, rather than hyperinsulinemia, that accounts both for blood pressure elevation and dyslipidemia in the insulin resistance syndrome. For example, one of the effects of insulin is vasodilation. Therefore, impaired insulin-mediated vasodilation could contribute to the elevation of blood pressure observed in the insulin resistance syndrome. Likewise, another of the effects of insulin is inhibition of lipolysis. Therefore, impaired insulin inhibition of lipolysis could lead to elevated plasma-free fatty acid (FFA) concentrations, which provides increased substrate, thus enhancing very–low-density lipoprotein (VLDL) synthesis, and leading to hypertriglyceridemia and the dyslipidemia observed in the insulin resistance syndrome. Indeed, effective insulin therapy results in correction of hypertriglyceridemia, rather than aggravation of it.

Insulin Pumps in Type 2 Diabetes

Continuous subcutaneous insulin infusion (CSII) has been compared to conventional insulin therapy in type 2 diabetes. CSII patients are more likely to achieve the established glucose treatment targets and may have greater improvement in serum triglycerides. Continuous subcutaneous insulin infusion is a viable modality for insulin delivery in patients with type 2 diabetes, either as basal delivery alone or combined with preprandial boluses.

Intensive insulin therapy with implantable insulin pumps (IIP) has been studied in patients with type 2 dia-

betes. Compared to multiple daily insulin (MDI) injections, IIP had significant advantages in reducing glycemic variability, clinical hypoglycemia, and weight gain, while improving aspects of quality of life. The use of IIP may be extreme for routine practice, but may prove quite useful in special circumstances or in research studies.

Insulin Preparations

In type 2 diabetes, because insulin therapy may be interrupted, it is best to use the least immunogenic insulin available. Therefore, highly purified preparations should be used. Animal insulins should be avoided and only human insulins used.

Short-acting insulin may be given as human Regular insulin or as the insulin analog lispro. The latter has a more rapid onset of action and shorter duration of action than Regular insulin. This may offer an advantage because there is often prolonged hyperglycemia in type 2 diabetes causing greater glycemic exposure. This may be minimized with insulin lispro.

■ CONCLUSIONS

Insulin therapy can control glycemia in patients with type 2 diabetes. Because of insulin resistance, high doses may be required to attain satisfactory glycemic control. However, also because of insulin resistance, hypoglycemia is much less common than in insulin-treated patients with type 1 diabetes. Insulin therapy need not be permanent, as glucose toxicity can cause temporary worsening of severity of disease. On the other hand, with long duration of diabetes, there is progressive beta-cell failure, which may mandate the use of permanent insulin therapy if satisfactory glycemic control is to be achieved.

SUGGESTED READING

American Diabetes Association. Consensus statement: The pharmacological treatment of hyperglycemia in NIDDM. Diabetes Care 1995; 18:1510–1518.

An ADA consensus statement.

American Diabetes Association. Clinical practice recommendations: 1997. Diabetes Care 1997; 20(suppl 1):S1–S70.

ADA's annually updated clinical practice recommendations.

DeFronzo RA. Lilly lecture 1987. The triumvirate: Beta-cell, muscle, liver. A collusion responsible for NIDDM. Diabetes 1988; 37:667–687.

Discusses pathophysiologic issues related to insulin therapy in type 2 diabetes.

Genuth S. Insulin use in NIDDM. Diabetes Care 1990; 13:1240–1264.

Outlines insulin treatment approaches in type 2 diabetes.

Hanning I, Alberti KG, Tunbridge WMG. Intermediate-acting insulin given at bedtime: Effect on blood glucose concentrations before and after breakfast. BMJ 1983; 286:1173–1176.

Deals with bedtime-insulin strategy.

Henry RR, Gumbiner B, Ditzler T, Wallace P, Lyon R, Glauber HS. Intensive conventional insulin therapy for type II diabetes. Metabolic effects during a six-month out-patient trial. Diabetes Care 1993; 16:21–31.

Discusses pathophysiologic issues related to insulin therapy in type 2 diabetes.

Holman RR, Turner RC. Insulin therapy in type II diabetes. Diabetes Research and Clinical Practice 1995; 28 (suppl):S179–S184.

Outlines insulin treatment approaches in type 2 diabetes.

Johnson JL, Wolf SL, Kabadi UM. Efficacy of insulin and sulfonylurea combination therapy in type II diabetes. A meta-analysis of the randomized placebo-controlled trials. Arch Intern Med 1996; 156:259–264.

Discusses combination therapy.

Lebovitz H (ed). Therapy for diabetes mellitus and related disorders, 2nd ed. Alexandria, Va: American Diabetes Association, 1994.

An American Diabetes Association monograph.

Ohkubo Y, Kishikawa H, Araki E, et al. The Kumomoto Study: Intensive insulin therapy prevents the progression of diabetic microvascular complications in Japanese patients with non–insulin-dependent diabetes mellitus: A randomized prospective 6-year study. Diabetes Res Clin Prac 1995; 28:103–117.

Discusses pathophysiologic issues related to insulin therapy in type 2 diabetes.

Peters AL, Davidson MB. Insulin plus a sulfonylurea agent for treating type 2 diabetes. Ann Intern Med 1991; 115:45–53

Discusses combination therapy.

Pugh JA, Ramirez G, Wagner ML, Tuley M, Sawyer J, Friedberg SJ. Is combination sulfonylurea and insulin therapy useful in NIDDM patients? Diabetes Care 1992; 15:953–959.

Discusses combination therapy.

Raskin P (ed). Medical management of non–insulin-dependent (type II) diabetes mellitus, 3rd ed. Alexandria, Va: American Diabetes Association, 1994.

An American Diabetes Association monograph.

Riddle MC. Evening insulin strategy. Diabetes Care 1990; 13:676–686.

Discusses bedtime-insulin strategy.

Riddle MJ. Combine therapy with insulin plus a sulfonylurea: The next step after failure of a sulfonylurea? The Endocrinologist 1993; 3:103–107.

Discusses combination therapy.

Seigler DE, Olsson GM, Skyler JS. Morning versus bedtime isophane insulin in type 2 (non–insulin-dependent) diabetes mellitus. Diabetic Medicine 1992; 9:826–833.

Discusses bedtime-insulin strategy.

Skyler JS. On the pathogenesis and treatment of non-insulin-dependent diabetes mellitus. In: Skyler JS, ed. Insulin Update 1982: Princeton, NJ: Excerpta Medica, 1982:247.

Skyler JS. Non–insulin dependent diabetes mellitus: A clinical strategy. Diabetes Care 1984; 7(suppl 1):118–129.

Skyler JS. Insulin treatment. In: Lebovitz HE, ed. Therapy for diabetes mellitus and related disorders, 2nd ed. Alexandria Va: American Diabetes Association, 1994:131.

Skyler JS: Insulin therapy in type II diabetes. Postgraduate Medicine 1997; 101(2):85–90, 92–94, 96.

Skyler JS: Targeted glycemic control in type 2 diabetes. Ann Intern Med 1997; in press.

The preceding five references provide successive iterations of the author's approach to insulin therapy in type 2 diabetes.

Tattersall RB, Gale E. Patient self-monitoring of blood glucose and refinements of conventional insulin treatment. Am J Med 1981; 70:177–182.

Discusses bedtime-insulin strategy.

Turner R, Cull C, Holman R. United Kingdom Prospective Diabetes Study 17: A 9-year update of a randomized, controlled trial on the effect of improved metabolic control on complications in non–insulin-dependent diabetes mellitus. Ann Intern Med 1996; 125(1 Pt 2):136–145.

Discusses pathophysiologic issues related to insulin therapy in type 2 diabetes.

Yki-Järvinen H, Esko N, Eero H, Marja-Riitta T. Clinical benefits and mechanisms of a sustained response to intermittent insulin therapy in type 2 diabetic patients with secondary drug failure. Am J Med 1988; 84:185–192.

Discusses pathophysiologic issues relating to insulin therapy in type 2 diabetes.

Yki-Järvinen H, Kauppila M, Kujansuu E, et al. Comparison of insulin regimens in patients with non–insulin-dependent diabetes mellitus. N Engl J Med 1992; 327:1426–1433.

Deals with bedtime-insulin strategy.

COMBINATION THERAPY: INSULIN-SULFONYLUREA AND INSULIN-METFORMIN

Matthew C. Riddle, M.D.

Ralph A. DeFronzo, M.D.

■ RATIONALE FOR COMBINATION THERAPY

The achievement of normoglycemia in non–insulin-dependent diabetes mellitus (NIDDM, or type 2 diabetes) patients has been difficult to accomplish because no single agent currently available can normalize the day-long plasma-glucose profile in the majority of patients. The rationale for combination therapy is as follows: combinations of drugs can be used to achieve greater therapeutic power, greater convenience, and greater safety. Greater therapeutic power is needed when individual agents (such as sulfonylureas, metformin, and acarbose) are not completely effective. Consequently, two agents with different mechanisms of action must be combined effectively to achieve the desired result when either agent alone is unsuccessful. Convenience also can be improved when the use of a second agent simplifies the regimen, with either fewer daily doses or a reduction in the number of injections of insulin. Greater safety from side effects may result from using lower doses of two or more agents rather than maximal doses of one alone.

The use of insulin and sulfonylureas in combination fulfills these criteria and has proven effective in the treatment of diabetic patients who are poorly controlled on a sulfonylurea alone. Insulin is an excellent and powerful agent that is capable of lowering the plasma-glucose concentration in everyone if given at sufficient dosage and as a mixed-split (Regular and long-acting) regimen. Its difficulties are inconvenience and potential risks. Despite improvement of the formulations of insulin and the devices for administering them, taking multiple daily injections remains a complex, uncomfortable, and wearisome task for many patients. When used as a single agent for obese patients with typical NIDDM accompanied by moderate or severe insulin resistance, large doses of insulin, often 100 to 150 U daily, are required to achieve normal glucose levels, and these large doses are usually associated with weight gain. Moreover, hypoglycemia can be a serious problem, especially for elderly patients. Conversely, sulfonylureas alone are often ineffective in normalizing the glucose profile. Approximately one of four persons started on a sulfonylurea fail to respond (i.e., experience primary failure), and among those who have a good initial response there is a high rate of secondary failure, 5 to 10 percent per year. Combining insulin with a sulfonylurea has proven useful in achieving good glycemic control while minimizing the incidence of hypoglycemia and avoiding excessive weight gain. Combination therapy with bedtime insulin-daytime sulfonylurea (BIDS) also should improve compliance by allowing a simpler regimen.

■ ADDITION OF SULFONYLUREA TO INSULIN THERAPY

A large number of studies with varying experimental design have examined combined insulin-sulfonylurea therapy, most of them focusing on patients who are unsuccessful with insulin alone. This experience has been reviewed by Peters and Davidson (Table 1). When the results from over 20 studies were analyzed collectively, the authors found that combination therapy reduced fasting plasma glucose an average of 31 mg per deciliter (1.7 mM) and the glycated hemoglobin by about 1 percent. Insulin dosage was also reduced by, on average, about 25 percent. The Diabetes Control and Complications Trial showed that a 1 percent decline of HbA_{1c} is associated with significant reductions of diabetic retinopathy, nephropathy, and neuropathy.

In these studies, a large variation in the response of individual subjects to combination therapy was observed, suggesting that the effectiveness of this method depends on the susceptibility of the patients selected. In general, after 15 years of known diabetes, which corresponds to about 10 years of insulin use, combination therapy using a sulfonylurea rarely gives better results than the use of insulin alone. This decline of response correlates with the loss of endogenous insulin and C-peptide reserve. Thus, the shorter the duration of diabetes, the more likely that this form of combination therapy will be helpful.

When initiating sulfonylurea therapy in patients in NIDDM who are taking insulin, the same guidelines should be followed as when starting sulfonylurea treatment in a newly diagnosed patient (see the chapter *Sulfonylureas*). The patient should start with a low dose that can be titrated gradually upward every week or two. No change should be made in the insulin dose until the fasting glucose has decreased to

Table 1 Summary of Studies Using Combination Insulin/Sulfonylurea Versus Insulin Therapy Alone		
	PARALLEL TRIALS	**CROSSOVER TRIALS**
Fasting plasma glucose	−23 mg% (8)	−36 mg% (14)
Glycosylated hemoglobin (%)	−1.1% (8)	−0.8% (14)
Insulin dose (%)	−33% (7)	−15% (8)

140 mg per deciliter, the minimally acceptable goal of therapy. When the fasting plasma glucose falls below 140 mg per deciliter, the insulin dose should be reduced progressively while increasing the dose of sulfonylurea is continued. Using this approach, good control will be maintained while the daily insulin dose will be reduced to the minimum necessary for the individual patient.

■ ADDITION OF METFORMIN TO INSULIN THERAPY

Although there is less experience with the addition of metformin to insulin-requiring patients with NIDDM, recent clinical studies suggest that this combination may also be an effective strategy. Unlike the sulfonylureas, which primarily work by augmenting insulin secretion, the major mechanism of metformin action involves improved insulin sensitivity in liver and muscle (Table 2). Patients with NIDDM typically have moderate to severe insulin resistance. In these patients, metformin would be expected to enhance the effects of both endogenously secreted and exogenously injected insulin. Early experience with combined metformin-insulin therapy has been encouraging and indicates that the majority of insulin-requiring NIDDM patients will have a significant reduction of their insulin requirement while experiencing an improvement of glycemic control (Table 3). Added benefits of metformin treatment are a reduction of plasma triglyceride and cholesterol levels and lack of the weight gain that is frequently associated with insulin treatment. A significant minority of such patients, perhaps 10 to 20 percent, may be able to stop taking insulin entirely. Shorter duration of diabetes and a lower daily insulin dose appear to be the best predictors of insulin withdrawal.

When added to insulin, metformin should be started in the same way as described for newly diagnosed patients (see the chapter *Metformin*). A 500 mg tablet should be taken twice daily, with breakfast and with the evening meal. Because the maximum hypoglycemic effect of metformin may not be reached until 2 to 4 weeks, the dose should be titrated upward by 500 mg daily no more frequently than every 2 weeks, while the glucose response is closely monitored. The insulin dose should not be altered until the fasting plasma glucose declines to 140 mg per deciliter. At this level, the insulin may be gradually reduced while the metformin dose is further increased if desired.

■ ADDITION OF INSULIN TO SULFONYLUREA THERAPY

Although many patients already taking insulin may benefit from adding a sulfonylurea or metformin, even more are likely to benefit from adding insulin to oral treatments. Until recently, the sulfonylureas were the only oral hypoglycemic agents available for treating NIDDM. However,

---

Table 2 Mechanism of Action of Antidiabetic Agents

	INSULIN SECRETION	HEPATIC GLUCOSE PRODUCTION	PERIPHERAL GLUCOSE UPTAKE
Sulfonylurea	↑	↓*	±↑
Metformin	0	↓	↑
Acarbose	0	0	0
Insulin	↓	↓	↑
SU-INSULIN	↑ (Daytime)	↓ (Bedtime)	±↑
MF-INSULIN	↓	↓↓	↑

*Indirect effect secondary to portal hyperinsulinemia.
SU = sulfonylurea; *MF* = metformin.

Table 3 Effect of Antidiabetic Therapy on Glycemic Control

	DECREASE IN FASTING GLUCOSE	DECREASE IN HBA$_{1C}$
Sulfonylurea	by 60–70 mg/dl	1–1.5%
Metformin	by 60–70 mg/dl	1–1.5%
Acarbose	by 20–30 mg/dl	0.5–1.0%
Bedtime insulin daytime SU	to < 140 mg%	≥ 1.5%
Bedtime insulin daytime MF	to < 140 mg%	≥ 1.5%
Bedtime insulin daytime SU and MF	to < 140 mg%	≥ 1.5%

SU = sulfonylurea; *MF* = metformin.

most patients eventually fail to maintain acceptable glycemic control (fasting plasma glucose < 140 mg per deciliter or 7.8 mM; HbA₁c 7.0 to 7.5 percent) on a sulfonylurea. At this time in the natural history of NIDDM, continuing the sulfonylurea while adding an injection of insulin at bedtime has proved very effective, restoring control more reliably than a single injection of insulin alone and more simply than multiple injections of insulin.

The rationale behind BIDS therapy is as follows. Because of its ability to augment daytime insulin secretion, the sulfonylurea should be continued to take advantage of its glucose-lowering effect, albeit incomplete, during the day. The persistent fasting hyperglycemia that is characteristic at the time of failure of sulfonylurea monotherapy is largely due to excessive hepatic glucose production during the sleeping hours. This elevated rate of nocturnal hepatic glucose production occurs in the presence of significant fasting hyperinsulinemia, indicating the presence of insulin resistance. Because the liver is 3 to 4 times more sensitive to insulin than is muscle, administration of sufficient amounts of long-acting insulin, usually NPH or Lente, at bedtime can overcome hepatic insulin resistance without causing a major stimulation of peripheral (muscle) glucose uptake and thus risking hypoglycemia. This regimen is highly successful in reducing the fasting plasma concentration and achieving day-long glycemic control. The results of a typical double-masked, placebo-controlled study of bedtime NPH insulin and daytime glipizide are shown in Figure 1.

The following method of implementing this regimen has proved safe and reliable. Patients with poor glycemic control despite maximal doses of a sulfonylurea (e.g., 20 mg glyburide or glipizide daily or the equivalent; see the chapter *Sulfonylureas*) should begin taking 5 to 10 units of NPH insulin subcutaneously in the evening at approximately 10:00 PM, while continuing their oral medication. NPH insulin begins to work after 2 hours, peaks at 6 to 10 hours, and is largely gone after 12 to 14 hours. Injecting NPH insulin at 10:00 PM ensures significant nocturnal hyperinsulinemia and sustained inhibition of hepatic glucose output with a peak suppressive action between 4:00 and 8:00 AM. Because Lente insulin has a similar time-course of action, it can be used in place of NPH insulin. Some patients with slower absorption of insulin may find it necessary to take evening insulin somewhat earlier, such as between 6:00 and 8:00 PM, to suppress hepatic glucose production and reduce fasting glucose most effectively.

All patients who take evening insulin must be proficient in doing home glucose monitoring and should measure fasting blood glucose every morning. Based on this measurement, the evening NPH dose can at first be increased by 5 U every 4 to 7 days. After fasting glucose by capillary blood measurement reaches 160 to 180 mg per deciliter, smaller increments of 2 to 4 U every 4 to 7 days are recommended. When the fasting glucose reaches 140 mg per deciliter, the insulin dose should be increased by 1 to 2 U every 4 to 7 days. It should be remembered that a capillary blood-glucose con-

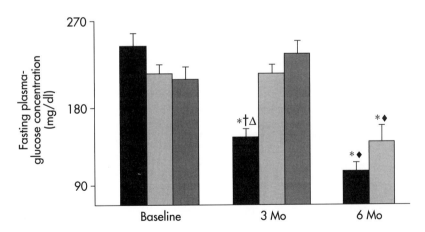

Figure 1
Fasting plasma-glucose concentration before the start of therapy (Baseline), after 3 months of therapy (3 mo), and after 6 months of therapy (6 mo) in type 2 patients treated with bedtime insulin–daytime sulfonylurea (solid bars), bedtime insulin–no daytime sulfonylurea (cross hatched bars), and daytime sulfonylurea–no bedtime insulin (stippled bars). During the first 3 months of therapy insulin was administered at a fixed dose, 20 U/1.73 m² subcutaneously at bedtime (10 to 11 PM). During the subsequent 3 months the bedtime insulin dose (mean = 40 ±5/day) was gradually titrated upward until the fasting plasma-glucose concentration was less than 120 mg per deciliter or until hypoglycemic symptoms were encountered. Glipizide was given at a dose of 20 mg BID.

* p < 0.05–0.0005 versus baseline for the same group.
† p < 0.001 versus bedtime insulin alone for the same phase.
Δ p < 0.05–0.001 versus glipizide for the same phase.
◆ p < 0.05–0.01 versus 3 mo for the same group.

centration of 120 mg per deciliter (6.7 mM) corresponds to a plasma glucose concentration (measured by the laboratory) of 140 mg per deciliter (7.8 mM). The approach described above uses capillary blood-glucose measurements done by the patient at home to guide day-to-day insulin adjustment.

Long-term glycemic control is best judged by measurement of the HbA$_{1c}$ every 3 months. A majority (70 to 80 percent) of NIDDM patients who are inadequately controlled on a sulfonylurea alone can restore acceptable glycemic control (fasting plasma glucose < 140 mg per deciliter; HbA$_{1c}$ < 7.0 to 7.5 percent) with BIDS therapy. The dose of NPH insulin required is usually in the range of 30 to 60 U. A simple method for some patients is to administer the dose of NPH with an insulin pen that is kept on a bedside table for use just before sleep.

Modifications of the above regimen have also been used successfully. One that is often helpful is use of premixed 70/30 (70 percent NPH/30 percent Regular) insulin just before the evening meal (6:00 to 7:00 PM), instead of NPH insulin later in the evening. This approach is best suited to obese, inactive persons with slow absorption of insulin and, often, a large proportion of daily calories taken at that meal. The Regular insulin included in this dose helps to dispose of the carbohydrate contained in the meal, whereas the NPH has an appropriate absorption pattern for nocturnal effect for such patients. Another regimen that has been used effectively is the administration of human Ultralente insulin with the evening meal. This insulin has a broad peak at 12 to 16 hours and maintains its effect for up to 24 hours.

■ COMBINED THERAPY WITH INSULIN PLUS METFORMIN-SULFONYLUREA

The introduction of metformin into the United States market has changed the approach to the management of NIDDM. Because of its lipid-lowering and weight-loss promoting effects, metformin has become the preferred drug for initial treatment for the poorly controlled, obese, hyperlipidemic NIDDM patient. Metformin alone often fails to achieve the desired level of glycemic control, and a sulfonylurea may be added while continuing metformin. In the same way, when patients who have started treatment with a sulfonylurea alone no longer maintain good enough control, it has become accepted practice to add metformin while continuing the sulfonylurea. By switching from oral monotherapy to combined therapy with sulfonylurea plus metformin, perhaps 60 to 70 percent of patients can restore acceptable glycemic control.

The remaining 30 to 40 percent who have some response to combined metformin-sulfonylurea therapy but are still not adequately controlled may benefit from adding bedtime NPH insulin while continuing both oral agents. Although this regimen has not been extensively used in clinical practice, preliminary experience suggests that good glycemic control can be restored in most patients with an NPH dose in the same range as is effective with standard BIDS therapy, 30 to 60 U daily.

■ QUADRUPLE THERAPY: INSULIN-ACARBOSE-METFORMIN-SULFONYLUREA

Acarbose, an alpha-glucosidase inhibitor that slows intestinal absorption of carbohydrates, has been used successfully with diet alone, metformin alone, a sulfonylurea alone, or insulin alone (see the chapter *Alpha-Glucosidase Inhibitors*). Although there is little clinical experience, it is reasonable to consider adding acarbose to the regimen for patients who are inadequately controlled on combined metformin-sulfonylurea therapy and need a further 20 to 30 mg per deciliter reduction in fasting glucose and/or an improvement in postprandial hyperglycemia. If combined acarbose-metformin-sulfonylurea therapy does not produce an acceptable level of control, a number of options are available: (1) add bedtime insulin to triple oral agent therapy; (2) discontinue acarbose and add bedtime insulin; (3) discontinue all oral agents and start a mixed-split insulin regimen. No data are yet available to define how to choose between these options for an individual patient.

All patients with NIDDM, especially those who are not controlled on a treatment with oral agents and required addition of bedtime insulin, need continued and intensified efforts to improve diet and exercise patterns. When successful, these nonpharmacologic interventions can be more effective than any pharmacotherapy and remain important even after establishing pharmacotherapy.

Suggested Reading

Bailey TS, Mezitis NHE. Combination therapy with insulin and sulfonylureas for type II diabetes. Diabetes Care 1990; 13:687–695.

Overview of combination therapy for the treatment of type 2 diabetes mellitus.

Bailey CJ, Turner RC. Metformin. N Engl J Med 1996; 334:574–579.

Excellent, up-to-date review article on the pharmacology, clinical indications, efficacy, and side effects of metformin.

Chiasson J-L, Josse RG, Hunt JA, et al. The efficacy of acarbose in the treatment of patients with non–insulin-dependent diabetes mellitus. Ann Intern Med 1994; 121:928–935.

Summary of the Canadian experience with acarbose in the treatment of type 2 diabetic patients.

Lebovitz HE. Stepwise and combination drug therapy for the treatment of NIDDM. Diabetes Care 1994; 17:1542–1544.

Succinct clinical review that examines the indications and efficacy of combination therapy with oral agents and insulin in the management of type 2 diabetic patients.

Lebovitz HE, Pasmantier R. Combination insulin-sulfonylurea therapy. Diabetes Care 1990; 13:667–675.

Old, but still useful review examining the benefits of combined insulin-sulfonylurea agents.

Peters LA, Davidson MB. Insulin plus a sulfonylurea agent for treating type 2 diabetes. Ann Intern Med 1991; 115: 43–53.

Review of studies examining the efficacy of combined insulin/sulfonylurea treatment in type 2 diabetes mellitus.

Riddle MC. Evening insulin strategy. Diabetes Care 1990; 13:676–686.

Very practical overview of the usefulness of bedtime insulin regimen in the treatment of type 2 diabetic patients.

Riddle M, Hart J, Bingham P, et al. Combination therapy for obese type 2 diabetes: suppertime mixed insulin with daytime sulfonylurea. Am J Med Sci 1992; 303:151–156.

A clinical study demonstrating that Regular/NPH insulin given with supper can effectively control nocturnal hyperglycemia and produce near-normal fasting-glucose levels in type 2 diabetic patients.

Riddle MC, Hart JS, Bouma DG, et al. Efficacy of bedtime NPH insulin with daytime sulfonylurea for a subpopulation of type II diabetic subjects. Diabetes Care 1989; 12:623–629.

One of the earliest clinical studies demonstrating the efficacy of bedtime insulin in achieving normoglycemia in poorly controlled type 2 diabetic subjects who are inadequately controlled on a sulfonylurea alone.

Rosenthal TC. Combining insulin and oral agents in diabetes: indications and controversies. Am Fam Phys 1992; 46:1721–1727.

Well-written review of combination insulin-oral agent therapy for the practicing physician.

Scheen AJ, Lefebvre PJ. Antihyperglycemic agents. Drug interactions of clinical importance. Drug Safety 1995; 12:32–45.

Well-written clinical article that details the most frequently encountered adverse interactions between the oral hypoglycemic agents and a variety of commonly prescribed therapeutic medications.

Shank M, DeFronzo RA. Bedtime insulin/daytime glipizide: effective therapy for sulfonylurea failures in NIDDM. Diabetes 1995; 44:165–172.

Well-designed double-blind clinical study documenting the superiority of bedtime insulin-daytime sulfonylurea over insulin alone or sulfonylureas alone.

Yki-Jarvinen H, Kauppila M, Kujansuu E, et al. Comparison of insulin regimens in patients with non–insulin-dependent diabetes mellitus. N Engl J Med 1992; 327:1426–1433.

Well-designed clinical trial examining the most common insulin regimens used in the treatment of type 2 diabetic patients.

TROGLITAZONE (REZULIN)

Ralph A. DeFronzo, M.D.

Troglitazone (Rezulin) recently has been approved by the U.S. Food and Drug Administration (FDA) for the treatment of non–insulin-dependent diabetes mellitus (NIDDM). Troglitazone belongs to a class of drugs called the thiazoladinediones and at least two other thiazoladinediones, pioglitazone and BRL 49653, currently are in clinical trials in the United States. In animal models of type 2 diabetes mellitus, troglitazone has been shown to be a potent hypoglycemic agent that works by enhancing tissue sensitivity in muscle. Troglitazone has no effect on plasma-glucose levels in insulin-deficient (type 1) diabetic animal models or in normal animals, although it does enhance insulin sensitivity in the latter. Muscle has been implicated as the primary site of enhanced insulin action, although a suppressive effect on hepatic-glucose production also has been demonstrated. Troiglitazone has no stimulatory effect on insulin secretion.

The cellular mechanism of action of troglitazone appears to be mediated through a novel nuclear receptor known as the peroxisome proliferator activated receptor (pPAR). The precise biochemical mechanisms through which pPAR enhances insulin sensitivity have yet to be defined.

■ METABOLIC EFFECTS IN TYPE 2 DIABETES MELLITUS

Initial studies in a small number of obese type 2 diabetic subjects demonstrated that troglitazone, when used as monotherapy, decreased the fasting plasma glucose concentration and improved oral glucose tolerance by decreasing basal hepatic-glucose production and enhancing insulin sensitivity in muscle, respectively. A similar improvement in oral glucose-tolerance tests and insulin sensitivity was observed in obese subjects with impaired glucose tolerance. In both of these studies, there was a moderate reduction in plasma triglyceride concentration and a slight rise in HDL cholesterol level. Three large, placebo-controlled, prospective, randomized, multicenter trials carried out in Japan, Europe, and the United States have examined the effect of long-term (3 months) treatment of NIDDM subjects with troglitazone monotherapy. All three of these studies are very consistent and demonstrate a decline in fasting glucose concentration of 25 to 40 mg per deciliter and HbA$_{1c}$ of 0.75 to 1 percent.

Fasting plasma insulin declined by 2 to 4 uU per milliliter. Plasma triglyceride concentration declined by 20 to 30 percent in all three studies, and in two of the three studies HDL cholesterol increased by 5 to 10 percent. Blood pressure did not change significantly and a small, but significant, weight gain (1 to 2 lbs over 3 months) was observed. In one study, addition of troglitazone to poorly controlled NIDDM subjects taking sulfonylureas showed a decline in fasting glucose (29 mg per deciliter) that was similar to that observed in diet-treated diabetic individuals receiving troglitazone. No data are available regarding combination therapy of troglitazone with metformin. In the United States, troglitazone has not been approved for use as a monotherapy or as combination therapy with sulfonylureas or metformin.

■ TROGLITAZONE AND INSULIN-TREATED TYPE 2 DIABETES MELLITUS

The use of troglitazone as adjunctive therapy in NIDDM patients who are being treated with insulin recently has been approved by the FDA. Two large, long-term (6 months), double-blind, placebo-controlled studies demonstrated that the addition of troglitazone (200 to 600 mg per day) to insulin-treated (mean dose, 75 U per day) NIDDM subjects decreased the daily insulin dose by 40 to 50 percent, and 15 percent of individuals were able to discontinue insulin completely. Forty-one percent of diabetics experienced a decrease in injection frequency from 3 to 1 shots per day and another 19 percent from 3 to 2 shots per day. Despite the reduction in daily insulin dose, HbA_{1c} declined on mean by 0.8 percent (troglitazone dose, 200 mg per day) and 1.4 percent (troglitazone dose, 600 mg per day).

On the basis of these results, troglitazone has been approved for use in NIDDM patients whose plasma-glucose levels are inadequately controlled ($HbA_{1c} > 8.5$ percent) despite a daily insulin dose in excess of 70 U per day given as multiple injections. The starting dose of troglitazone is 200 mg per day. If after 2 weeks adequate glycemic control (fasting plasma glucose < 140 mg percent) is not achieved, the dosage should be increased to 400 mg per day. The maximum recommended dosage is 600 mg per day. The tablets come in sizes of 200 mg and 400 mg.

It should be emphasized that the primary goal of therapy with troglitazone is to normalize the fasting-glucose and HbA_{1c} levels, not to reduce the insulin dose. Therefore, in very poorly controlled NIDDM patients, the dose of insulin (FPG > 180 to 200 mg per deciliter) should not be reduced until the fasting glucose has declined to 140 mg per deciliter. In diabetic subjects with an FPG less than 180 mg per deciliter, our experience indicates that a 15 to 20 percent reduction in insulin dose is advisable at the time that troglitazone is started in order to avoid hypoglycemia. It should be remembered that the bedtime dose of long-acting (NPH or Lente) insulin is the primary determinant of the fasting glucose concentration (by suppressing the excessive rate of hepatic glucose production that occurs during the sleeping hours). Therefore, it is essential to decrease the evening dose of NPH or Lente insulin when the fasting glucose declines to 140 mg per deciliter. Relative to the evening dose of long-acting insulin, the morning or lunch insulin doses contribute only modestly to the day-long glycemic control. Consequently, we have found that it is easy to decrease (or discontinue) the morning and/or lunchtime insulin dose as long as the evening insulin dose is maintained. However, when the fasting glucose concentration declines to less than 140 mg per deciliter, it is essential to decrease the evening dose of NPH or Lente as well. All patients receiving insulin therapy should perform home blood-glucose monitoring. It is essential that all insulin-treated diabetic individuals who are started on troglitazone measure their blood-glucose concentration at least four times per day and that they receive appropriate instruction about the warning symptoms of hypoglycemia (tachycardia, palpitation, sweating, tremor, anxiety, altered mental status) and how to treat it (rapidly absorbable simple sugar).

Safety

Troglitazone is well tolerated and no major side effects have been observed in the three large multicenter trials carried out in the United States, Europe, and Japan. A small decline (2 to 3 percent) in hematocrit and hemoglobin is commonly observed. This has been attributed to fluid redistribution and dilution. Neither edema nor cardiac symptoms have been observed. Repeated echocardiograms performed over a 2-year period have demonstrated no deleterious effects on cardiac function. Increased liver-function tests may occur, and troglitazone had to be withdrawn in 20 out of 2,510 (0.8 percent) patients during clinical trials in North America. Although troglitazone is not contraindicated in diabetic patients with liver disease, it should be used cautiously in this group. Because very little troglitazone and its metabolites (< 5 percent) are excreted in the urine, no dosage adjustment is required in diabetic patients with renal failure. When the drug is approved for use as monotherapy, patients with impaired renal function (in whom metformin is contraindicated) would be ideal candidates for treatment with troglitazone.

Absorption

Troglitazone is absorbed rapidly following oral administration, reaching a maximum plasma concentration within 2 to 3 hours. Because food enhances absorption by 30 to 85 percent, troglitazone should be given with meals. Cholestyramine markedly decreases the absorption of troglitazone and coadministration of the two drugs should be avoided, or separated by a period of 3 hours.

Suggested Reading

Iwamoto Y, Kosaka K, Kuzuya T, et al. Effects of troglitazone. A new hypoglycemic agent in patients with NIDDM poorly controlled by diet therapy. Diabetes Care 1996; 19:151–156.

Japanese multicenter trial documenting the efficacy of troglitazone in reducing HbA_{1c} and plasma triglycerides in NIDDM patients.

Kumar S, Boulton AJM, Beck-Nielsen H, et al, for the Troglitazone Study Group. Troglitazone, an insulin action enhancer, improves metabolic control in NIDDM patients. Diabetologia 1996; 39:701–709.

Large European multicenter study demonstrating the efficacy of troglitazone in poorly controlled NIDDM patients.

Nolan JJ, Ludvik B, Beerdsen P, et al. Improvement in glucose tolerance and insulin resistance in obese subjects treated with troglitazone. N Engl J Med 1994; 331:1188–1193.

Clinical study in obese subjects with impaired glucose demonstrating that troglitazone improves insulin sensitivity and glucose tolerance.

Saltiel AR, Olefsky JM. Perspectives in diabetes. Thiazolidinediones in the treatment of insulin resistance and type II diabetes. Diabetes 1996; 45:1661–1669.

Excellent review of the mechanism of action and clinical efficacy of troglitazone in the treatment of NIDDM.

Suter SL, Nolan JJ, Wallace P, et al. Metabolic effects of new oral hypoglycemia agent CS-045 in NIDDM subjects. Diabetes Care 1992; 15:193–203.

Initial clinical study demonstrating the mechanism of action (improved muscle sensitivity to insulin and enhanced suppression of basal hepatic glucose production) in poorly controlled NIDDM patients.

Valiquett T, Balagtas C, Whitcomb R. Troglitazone dose-response study in patients with NIDDM. Diabetes 1995; 44(suppl 1):109A.

Large U.S. multicenter trial demonstrating that doses of troglitazone ranging from 200 to 800 mg per day cause a dose-related reduction in fasting plasma glucose and HbA_{1c} levels

DYSLIPIDEMIA

Barry S. Horowitz, M.D.

Henry N. Ginsberg, M.D.

Epidemiologic studies have indicated that diabetes mellitus is associated with threefold to fourfold increases in risk for coronary artery disease. The increase in risk is particularly evident in younger age groups and in women. Females with diabetes mellitus lose the protection that characterizes nondiabetic females. Individuals with diabetes have a 50 percent greater in-hospital mortality, and a twofold increased rate of death within 2 years of surviving a myocardial infarction. Overall, coronary artery disease is the leading cause of death in individuals with diabetes mellitus who are over the age of 35 years.

Much of this increased risk can be accounted for by the presence of well-characterized risk factors for coronary artery disease in diabetics. A significant proportion of the increased risk, however, remains unexplained. Diabetics, particularly those with non–insulin-dependent diabetes mellitus (NIDDM), commonly have abnormalities of plasma lipids and lipoprotein concentrations, and dyslipidemia outweighs all of the other major cardiovascular risk factors (i.e., hypertension, glucose intolerance, obesity) in this patient population. Individuals with poorly controlled insulin-dependent diabetes mellitus (IDDM) also frequently present with a dyslipidemia, but the pattern differs from that in NIDDM. In the next section we briefly review normal lipid and lipoprotein physiology to provide a basis for treatment of the common dyslipidemias that are associated with diabetes mellitus, both NIDDM and IDDM.

■ LIPOPROTEIN COMPOSITION

Lipoproteins are macromolecular complexes that carry various lipids and proteins in plasma. The major classes of lipoproteins are defined by their physical-chemical characteristics (Table 1). The lipids form the core of the lipoprotein molecule and are represented by esterified cholesterol and triglycerides. Because the hydrophobic triglyceride and cholesteryl ester molecules are not soluble in water, the lipid core must be surrounded by more hydrophilic phospholipids, free cholesterol, and proteins. The proteins that comprise the lipoproteins are called apoproteins or apolipoproteins. They help to solubilize the core lipids and play a critical role in the regulation of plasma-lipid and lipoprotein transport.

Apolipoprotein (apo) B100 is required for the secretion of hepatic-derived very–low-density lipoproteins (VLDL), and is the major protein of intermediate density lipoproteins (IDL) and low-density lipoproteins (LDL). Apo B48 is a truncated form of apo B100 that is required for secretion of chylomicrons from the small intestine. Apo A-I is the major structural protein in high-density lipoprotein (HDL). Apo A-I also is an important activator of the plasma enzyme, lecithin cholesteryl-acyl transferase (LCAT), that plays a key role in reverse cholesterol transport (i.e., transport of cholesterol from tissues to the liver). Apo C-II, apo C-III, and apo E are important constituents of chylomicrons VLDL and HDL.

■ LIPOPROTEIN METABOLISM

Chylomicron Metabolism

Dietary fats (triglycerides and cholesterol) are absorbed into the cells of the small intestine and are incorporated into the core of nascent chylomicrons (Fig. 1) After secretion from mucosal cells, chylomicrons acquire apo C-II, apo C-III, and apo E. After they enter the circulation, chylomicron triglycerides are removed from the plasma by the enzyme lipopro-

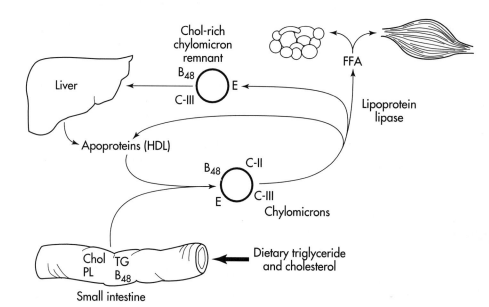

Figure 1
A schematic representation of the transport of exogenously derived lipids from the intestine to peripheral tissues and liver by means of the chylomicron system. The cyclic movement of several apoproteins between HDL and chylomicrons also is represented. *(From Ginsberg HN. Lipoprotein physiology and its relationship to atherogenesis. Endocrinol Metab Clin North Am 1990; 19:211.)*

Table 1 Characteristics of the Major Lipoproteins

LIPOPROTEIN	DENSITY (G/DL)	LIPID (%)	
		TG	CHOL
Chylomicrons	0.95	80–95	2–7
VLDL	0.95–1.006	55–80	5–15
IDL	1.006–0.019	20–50	20–40
LDL	1.019–1.063	5–15	40–50
HDL	1.063–1.21	5–10	15–25

Lipids (%): percent composition of lipids; apolipoproteins and phospholipids make up the rest.
TG = triglycerides; *CHOL* = cholesterol; *VLDL* = very–low-density lipoprotein; *IDL* = intermediate density lipoprotein; *LDL* = low-density lipoprotein; *HDL* = high-density lipoprotein.

tein lipase (LPL), which is present on the luminal surface of vascular endothelial cells. Lipoprotein lipase is activated by apo C-II. Upon activation by apo C-II, LPL hydrolyzes the triglycerides in the chylomicrons to glycerol and fatty acids, which subsequently are oxidized to generate energy or stored as synthesized triglyceride. The remaining chylomicron remnants are taken up by the hepatocytes and removed from the circulation. Apo E is required for the hepatocyte to recognize and clear the chylomicron remnant.

Transport of Chylomicrons in Diabetes Mellitus

Chylomicron and chylomicron-remnant metabolism frequently is altered in patients with diabetes. In poorly controlled IDDM, lipoprotein lipase activity is reduced, and postprandial chylomicron and, therefore, triglyceride levels are increased. Insulin therapy in IDDM activates lipoprotein lipase and rapidly clears the plasma of chylomicron triglycerides.

Defective removal of chylomicrons and chylomicron remnants is a characteristic finding in patients with NIDDM. Both fasting and postprandial hypertriglyceridemia, as well as reduced plasma concentrations of HDL cholesterol, are common in NIDDM. Lipoprotein lipase activity, however, is nor-

mal or only slightly reduced in untreated NIDDM. It has been difficult to identify a direct effect of NIDDM on chylomicron metabolism. Apo E plays a critical role in the hepatic uptake of chylomicron remnants, and recent studies have suggested that impaired chylomicron remnant removal contributes to the hyperlipidemia in NIDDM. There is some suggestion that the activity of hepatic triglyceride lipase, which plays an important role in remnant removal, is increased in NIDDM and may contribute to low HDL cholesterol levels. Dietary lipid (i.e., chylomicron) metabolism in NIDDM is complicated by coexistent obesity and familial hyperlipidemia, which commonly accompany NIDDM.

Metabolism of VLDL, IDL, and LDL (Apo B100–Containing Lipoproteins)

Very–low-density lipoproteins, the major source of endogenous triglyceride, are synthesized and secreted by the liver (Fig. 2). VLDL triglycerides derive from the combination of glycerol with free fatty acids that have either been taken up from plasma or newly synthesized in the liver. Cholesterol in VLDL is either synthesized de novo from acetate or delivered to the liver by chylomicron remnants or other lipoproteins. Together, these lipids are incorporated into the core of a nascent VLDL particle, while apo B and phospholipids form

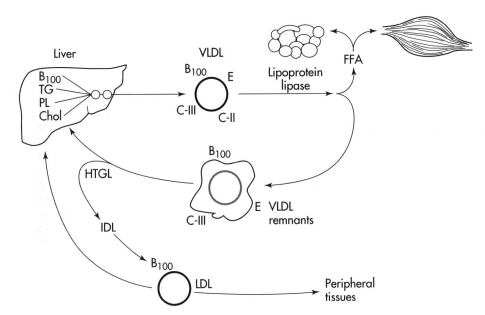

Figure 2
Transport of endogenous hepatic lipids by means of VLDL, IDL, and LDL. Note the changes in apoproteins, other than apo B100, as VLDL is converted to IDL and LDL. The sites of action of the two lipases, lipoprotein lipase (LPL) and hepatic triglyceride lipase (HTGL), are denoted as well, although the role of HTGL has not been completely defined. *(From Ginsberg HN. Lipoprotein physiology and its relationship to atherogenesis. Endocrinol Metab Clin North Am 1990; 19:211.)*

its surface. Regulation of VLDL synthesis and secretion by the liver has not been completely defined. However, substrate delivery is a major regulator of hepatic VLDL triglyceride synthesis. High glucose, by mass action, enters the beta cell and provides the carbon skeleton for glycerol synthesis, while high plasma-free fatty acid concentrations provide the source of lipid for VLDL triglyceride synthesis. Therefore, in poorly controlled NIDDM the accelerated flux of glucose and free fatty acids into the hepatocyte provides the driving force for increased VLDL synthesis.

Once in the plasma, VLDL loses triglyceride after interacting with LPL, which is activated by apo CII. Hydrolysis of VLDL triglyceride generates smaller and more dense VLDL, eventually leading to the formation IDL. Intermediate density lipoproteins are similar to chylomicron remnants, but unlike chylomicron remnants, not all IDL are removed by the liver. Some of the IDL particles undergo further catabolism to become LDL. Some lipoprotein lipase activity is necessary for normal functioning of the metabolic cascade leading from VLDL to IDL to LDL. Apo E, hepatic triglyceride lipase, and LDL receptors also play important roles in this process. Apo B is essentially the sole protein on the surface of LDL and the lifetime of LDL in plasma is primarily determined by the availability of LDL receptors. Approximately 60 to 70 percent of LDL catabolism from plasma occurs by way of the LDL receptor pathway, whereas the remaining tissue catabolism is non-receptor mediated. One of the non-receptor pathways recognizes glycosylated and/or oxidatively modified lipoproteins.

Transport of Apo B100–Containing Lipoproteins in Diabetes Mellitus: Relationship to Diabetes Control

Plasma levels of VLDL triglyceride are commonly increased in diabetic patients. In IDDM, elevated triglyceride levels correlate closely with the levels of glycemic control, and marked hyperlipemia can be found in ketotic diabetic patients. The basis for increased VLDL levels in poorly controlled, but not ketotic, IDDM subjects usually is hepatic overproduction of these lipoproteins. However, reduced clearance can play a significant role in more severe cases. In the latter situation, LPL activity is reduced and returns to normal with insulinization. With intensive insulin treatment in IDDM, plasma triglyceride levels often are in the "low-normal" range and lower than average production rates of VLDL have been demonstrated in such instances. Even in such circumstances, however, several qualitative abnormalities in VLDL composition may persist. These include enrichment in free and esterified cholesterol and an increased free cholesterol:lecithin ratio. The latter may be an indication of increased risk for coronary artery disease.

In hyperglycemic NIDDM patients overproduction of VLDL, together with increased secretion of both triglyceride and apo B, are primarily responsible for the increased plasma VLDL levels. In well-controlled NIDDM individuals LPL levels are normal or slightly reduced. In severely hyperglycemic patients decreased LPL-mediated hydrolysis of VLDL triglycerides may contribute significantly to the hypertriglyceridemia. The presence of obesity, insulin resistance, and concomitant familial forms of hyperlipidemia in NIDDM makes study of the pathophysiology difficult. The interaction of these overlapping traits makes therapy less effective. Therefore, in contrast to the situation in IDDM, where intensive therapy normalizes VLDL levels and metabolism, therapy of NIDDM with either insulin or oral agents only partly corrects VLDL abnormalities in the majority of patients.

In NIDDM, LDL metabolism, like that of its precursor VLDL, is complex. The presence of hypertriglyceridemia leads to the formation of small, dense triglyceride-rich LDL particles (so-called "pattern B profile"), which may be more atherogenic than normal LDL. Overproduction of LDL apo B is seen in patients with NIDDM, even in diabetics with mild degrees of hyperglycemia. This is particularly common if there is concomitant elevation of VLDL. Fractional removal of LDL, mainly by way of LDL receptor pathways, may be increased, normal, or reduced in NIDDM. Increased fractional catabolism of LDL usually is seen in diabetics with significant hypertriglyceridemia. As noted above, insulin is required for normal LDL receptor function, and reduced LDL fractional removal from plasma has been observed in more severe NIDDM. Glycosylation of LDL also contributes to the decreased fractional catabolism of LDL in NIDDM patients.

Diabetic LDL may be more atherogenic than LDL from normal subjects. Glycosylated LDL are taken up by macrophage scavenger receptors and contribute to foam-cell formation. Glycosylated LDL also are more susceptible to oxidative modification and catabolism by means of macrophage-scavenger receptors. Finally, the smaller, more dense triglyceride-enriched LDL may be more atherogenic, possibly because of a greater propensity to oxidation.

Metabolism of HDL (Apo A–Containing Lipoproteins)

HDL comprises an extremely complex lipoprotein class. Although HDL can be assembled and secreted by the small intestine, the majority of HDL are formed in the plasma by the coalescence of individual phospholipid-apolipoprotein complexes containing apo A-I, apo A-II, and apo A-VI. Two other plasma proteins, LCAT and cholesteryl ester transfer protein (CETP), can also join these complexes. The HDL_3 that is formed serves as the acceptor of cell-membrane–free cholesterol. This is the initial step in the reverse cholesterol transport process (Fig. 3), whereby cholesterol in tissues (blood vessels, muscle, fat, etc.) is removed and transported to the liver. The cholesterol in peripheral cells exists in the form of free cholesterol that is transferred to HDL_3 from the cell membrane. The free cholesterol in HDL_3 is then esterified by LCAT, allowing the HDL_3 to accept more free cholesterol from the tissues. With increasing generation of cholesteryl ester, HDL_3 becomes HDL_2. HDL_2 can deliver its cholesteryl ester to the liver by means of a process called selective uptake (the cholesteryl ester enters the cells without uptake of the entire particle) or can transfer the cholesterol esters to triglyceride-rich lipoproteins (chylomicrons and VLDL in the fed and fasted states, respectively). In humans the latter route appears to be the major pathway for movement of cholesteryl ester out of HDL_2. This process is mediated by cholesterol ester transfer protein (CETP). The CETP-transferred cholesteryl esters can be taken up by the liver as chylomicron remnants, VLDL rem-

nants, or IDL, or the LDL is taken up by tissues through the LDL receptor. In patients with diabetes, hypertriglyceridemia usually is accompanied by a reduction in HDL cholesterol. Recent evidence indicates that poorly controlled NIDDM and IDDM individuals with combined hypertriglyceridemia and reduced HDL cholesterol have increased transfer of cholesteryl ester from HDL to triglyceride-rich lipoproteins. In NIDDM, low HDL levels also can be present in the absence of fasting hypertriglyceridemia. The low plasma HDL cholesterol levels in NIDDM do not appear to be related to glycemic control or to the mode of treatment. A consistent finding has been the inverse relationship between the plasma insulin concentration and HDL cholesterol level. The degree of insulin resistance also is related inversely to the HDL concentration. Fractional catabolism of apo A-I, the major lipoprotein in HDL, is increased in NIDDM patients with low HDL, and apo A-I levels are reduced consistently in NIDDM. These abnormalities in HDL metabolism often are not reversed by correction of hypertriglyceridemia. The metabolism of HDL in NIDDM is complicated by the coexistence of obesity and familial dyslipidemias in this group.

■ RATIONALE OF TREATMENT

Over the last decade a number of lipid-lowering trials have provided conclusive evidence that an improvement in the plasma lipid profile (decrease in total/LDL cholesterol and triglyceride concentrations; increase in HDL cholesterol) will reduce the incidence of fatal and nonfatal myocardial infarctions by slowing the rate of progression, stabilizing, or even causing a regression of atherosclerotic plaques. Although most of these studies were carried out in nondiabetic subjects, recent lipid-lowering trials have reproduced these findings in diabetic individuals. These trials have demonstrated that a 1 percent decrease in total serum cholesterol will decrease coronary heart disease mortality by 2 percent, while a 1 percent increase in HDL cholesterol is associated with a 2 to 3 percent decrease in coronary heart disease mortality. Although the role of triglycerides in coronary artery disease is more controversial, there is growing evidence from a number of studies, including the Framingham Study, that hypertriglyceridemia represents an independent risk factor for atherosclerotic cardiovascular disease. This is especially true

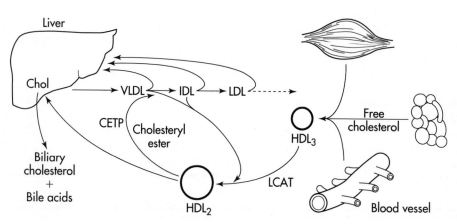

Figure 3
Simplified representation of HDL metabolism and the role of HDL in reverse cholesterol transport. Free cholesterol is accepted from peripheral tissues by HDL_3, and after esterification, may be transferred to apo B100 lipoproteins. Cholesteryl ester also may be delivered directly to the liver by HDL itself. (*From Ginsberg HN. Lipoprotein physiology and its relationship to atherogenesis. Endocrinol Metab Clin North Am 1990; 19:211.*)

in diabetic patients in whom hypertriglyceridemia is the most common dyslipidemia and correlates well with coronary artery disease. Hypertriglyceridemia also is associated with a decrease in HDL cholesterol, the presence of small dense LDL (pattern B), and other known cardiovascular risk factors including central obesity, insulin resistance, hyperinsulinemia, increased plasminogen inhibitor activator-1, and hypertension (i.e., the Insulin Resistance Syndrome or Syndrome X). In the Helsinki Heart Study a decrease in plasma triglyceride concentration of 30 to 35 percent together with a rise in HDL cholesterol of 10 to 20 percent was associated with a 34 percent decrease in cardiovascular mortality.

In summary, lipid abnormalities are much less common in IDDM compared to NIDDM individuals. However, IDDM may be associated with elevated VLDL triglyceride and LDL cholesterol if diabetic control is very poor or if the patient is ketotic. In contrast, NIDDM commonly is associated with lipid abnormalities. The most common lipid disturbance in NIDDM is one of high triglycerides and reduced HDL cholesterol levels: the diabetic dyslipidemia. If the hypertriglyceridemia is severe, acute pancreatitis, eruptive xanthomas, hepatosplenomegaly, lipemia retinalis, and milky plasma may occur.

LDL elevations are not more commonly present in people with NIDDM than they are in nondiabetics; however, compositional changes in the LDL particles of diabetics may increase the propensity for atherogenesis.

Table 2 National Cholesterol Education Program (NCEP) Guidelines Modified for the Initiation of Treatment of Dyslipidemia in Diabetic Patients

LDL cholesterol >160 mg/dl (<2 cardiovascular risk factors)
LDL cholesterol >130 mg/dl (≥2 cardiovascular risk factors)*†
LDL cholesterol >100 mg/dl (clinical cardiovascular disease)
Triglycerides >200 mg/dl‡
HDL cholesterol <35 mg/dl in males and <40 mg/dl in females‡

*We recommend institution of therapy when the LDL cholesterol is above 110 mg/dl in diabetic patients with two or more cardiovascular risk factors
†Cardiovascular risk factors include: diabetes, obesity, male sex, hypertension, decreased HDL cholesterol, family history of premature heart disease, coronary/cerebrovascular/peripheral vascular heart disease.
‡Specific treatment values for triglycerides and HDL cholesterol are not provided in the NCEP guidelines.

Table 3 General Approach to the Treatment of Diabetic Dyslipidemia

Optimize diet (see Table 5)
Encourage weight loss
Exclude other endocrine or medical diseases that cause dyslipidemia (see Table 4)
Discontinue drugs that cause dyslipidemia if possible
Recommend cessation of smoking
Suggest increasing physical activity
Prescribe oral hypoglycemic agents that improve the dyslipidemia, i.e., metformin, troglitazone

---

Because dyslipidemia represents the major risk factor for coronary artery disease in diabetic patients and, because patients with diabetes invariably have other associated cardiovascular risk factors, aggressive treatment of all lipid abnormalities is essential in both NIDDM and IDDM individuals.

■ GOALS OF THERAPY

The goals of therapy were discussed in the chapter *Goals of Diabetes Management*. Every diabetic patient should have a lipid profile that includes the measurement of plasma total/LDL/HDL cholesterol and triglycerides following an overnight (12 hours) fast. Chylomicronemia is suspected by the presence of milky plasma and is detected by the presence of a yellow creamy layer on the top of the plasma or serum after it has been stored in the refrigerator (4 °C) overnight. For primary prevention, the National Cholesterol Education Program (NCEP) recommends treatment when the LDL cholesterol is greater than 160 mg per deciliter in the absence of other cardiovascular risk factors or if the LDL cholesterol is greater than 130 mg per deciliter and two major risk factors are present (Table 2). For secondary prevention, treatment is recommended if LDL cholesterol is greater than 100 mg per deciliter. Because diabetes mellitus and male sex are major risk factors, this means that all male diabetics without clinical cardiovascular disease with a LDL cholesterol above 130 mg per deciliter require treatment. Moreover, because it is unusual to find female (as well as male) diabetic patients who do not have at least one other major cardiovascular risk factor (obesity, hypertension, decreased HDL cholesterol, family history of premature coronary heart disease, smoking), essentially all diabetics with an LDL cholesterol greater than 130 mg per deciliter will require treatment. Because dyslipidemia represents the major cardiovascular risk factor in diabetic patients, we believe that a more aggressive approach is indicated and we strongly recommend treatment for anyone with an LDL cholesterol greater than 130 mg per deciliter. Indeed, it is not unreasonable to assume that all patients with NIDDM have cardiovascular disease and initiate therapy in any diabetic patient with an LDL cholesterol above 100 mg per deciliter. No strict guidelines exist for other lipid disturbances in diabetic patients. However, we routinely treat individuals with plasma triglyceride concentrations above 200 mg per deciliter and HDL cholesterol concentrations less than 35 mg per deciliter, especially if other cardiovascular risk factors are present.

■ GENERAL APPROACH (Table 3)

Obesity per se is associated with an increase in triglycerides and decrease in HDL cholesterol. Because 70 to 80 percent of NIDDM patients are overweight, a major effort should be made to encourage diabetics to lose weight. Even small reductions in body weight can lead to significant improvement in the plasma lipid profile. A careful search should be made for other endocrine disorders, i.e., hypothyroidism, or medical diseases, i.e., renal or hepatic disease, that can cause hypertriglyceridemia or hypercholesterolemia (Table 4). Because both smoking and sedentary life-style are associated with dyslipidemia, a major effort should be made to encourage all diabetics to stop smoking and increase their physical activity. Both of these are associated with reduced HDL cholesterol and represent independent risk factors for coronary artery diseases. Excessive alcohol causes hypertriglyceridemia and alcohol intake should be limited to one drink per day. Certain drugs, including the thiazides, beta adrenergic blockers, and corticosteroids, can cause both hypercholesterolemia and hypertriglyceridemia (Table 4). Others cause either hypercholesterolemia (progestins, cyclosporine), hypertriglyceridemia (estrogens), or reduced HDL cholesterol (androgens, progestins). A careful review of all medications should be made to exclude drug-induced dyslipidemia.

Medications used to treat the diabetes may improve the diabetic dyslipidemia. Sulfonylureas either have no effect on the plasma lipid profile or cause a small reduction in the fasting plasma triglyceride concentration. Metformin, independent of its effect on the plasma-glucose concentration, causes a modest reduction in both the plasma VLDL triglyceride and LDL cholesterol concentrations. The newly approved drug, troglitazone, may lower triglycerides and increase HDL cholesterol. Acarbose has no major effect on the plasma-lipid profile, but some studies have shown a small reduction in the plasma triglyceride level. Insulin therapy usually reduces the plasma VLDL triglyceride concentration and causes a small increase in the HDL cholesterol. Even if the plasma-glucose profile is normalized by sulfonylurea, metformin, or insulin therapy, it is unusual to see a complete correction of the dyslipidemia.

■ DIET THERAPY

Diet therapy is the foundation for the treatment of diabetes, irrespective of the presence of dyslipidemia. The presence of abnormalities in plasma lipids, however, increases the importance of intensive diet intervention. Unlike diabetic glycemic control, decreases in the plasma triglyceride and cholesterol levels in response to dietary intervention can be observed even in the absence of weight loss. Therefore, reductions in dietary fat and saturated fat intake, along with reduced cholesterol consumption, can be associated with lower plasma triglyceride and LDL cholesterol even if caloric intake is unchanged.

High-Carbohydrate Versus High-Fat Diet

The recommendations of the American Diabetes Association (ADA) for the nutritional management (Table 5) of individuals with diabetes mellitus are in agreement with those of the American Heart Association (AHA) and NCEP. The Step 1 AHA diet calls for up to 50 percent to 60 percent of total daily energy to be in the form of carbohydrates (primarily complex carbohydrates). Fat calories should not exceed 30 percent of the total energy consumption and of this no more than 10 percent should be saturated fat. Both cholesterol and polyunsaturated fats decrease LDL receptor activity, leading to impaired LDL clearance from the blood. Therefore, saturated fats should be reduced with the remainder of the energy from fat derived from monounsaturated and polyunsaturated fats. Less than 300 mg of cholesterol should be taken per day, while protein consumption should account for 10 percent to 15 percent of calories. If after 2 to 3 months the desirable hypolipidemic effect is not observed, a more rigorous Step 2 AHA diet, limiting saturated fat to 7 percent of total calories and cholesterol to under 200 mg per day, should be instituted.

Some controversy has arisen that high-carbohydrate diets may have a deleterious effect on both diabetic control and the common lipid abnormalities seen in type 2 diabetic patients. Several studies have shown that fat-restricted, high-carbohydrate diets raise the plasma triglyceride levels in nondiabetic individuals with hypertriglyceridemia, as well as in those with normal plasma triglyceride levels. In NIDDM high-carbohydrate diets cause higher postprandial glucose levels and ele-

Table 4 Secondary Causes of Dyslipidemia in Diabetes Mellitus

	HYPERCHOLESTEROLEMIA	HYPERTRIGLYCERIDEMIA	LOW HDL CHOLESTEROL
Obesity	+	+	+
Associated medical disorders			
Hypothyroidism	+	+	
Nephrosis	+	+	
Liver disease	+	+	
Smoking			+
Physical inactivity		+	+
Alcohol		+	
Medications			
Thiazides	+	+	
Beta-blockers	+	+	+
Corticosteroids	+	+	
Progestins	+		+
Estrogens		+	
Androgens			
Cyclosporine	+		+

+ = use associated with lipid change.

vated fasting triglyceride levels. The etiology of hypertriglyceridemia with high-carbohydrate diets has been linked to increased VLDL production without a concomitant increase in apolipoprotein B production. This results in larger, triglyceride-enriched VLDL particles that have an increased triglyceride to apo B ratio. Because high-carbohydrate diets lower HDL cholesterol in normal individuals, an additional concern also has been raised about the use of such diets in diabetic patients. The potential deleterious effects of a high-carbohydrate diet on glycemic control and diabetic dyslipidemia have been confirmed in a multicenter study by Garg, Grundy, and colleagues. Consequently, the AHA offers diabetic patients an alternative diet in which the carbohydrate content is reduced to 40 to 45 percent of total calories, while the amount of polyunsaturated and monounsaturated fat is increased proportionately. This lower carbohydrate, higher-fat diet has no deleterious effect on the plasma-glucose profile or HbA_{1c}.

In contrast to NIDDM individuals, there is a no evidence that a high-carbohydrate diet causes deterioration of diabetic control or worsening of dyslipidemia in IDDM patients as long as the carbohydrates are of the complex variety and the insulin dose is adjusted to maintain normoglycemia. In general, simple sugars should be avoided in diabetic patients, both IDDM as well as NIDDM.

Specific Types of Dietary Fat

Replacement of saturated fat by fats enriched in the ω6 fatty acid series of polyunsaturated fatty acids (PUFAs) has been demonstrated consistently to reduce plasma total and LDL cholesterol in both nondiabetic and diabetic individuals. A polyunsaturated/saturated fat ratio (P:S) of >0.8 has been shown to both decrease LDL synthesis and to enhance LDL catabolism. However, if the dietary P:S ratio is too high (greater than 2.0), HDL levels generally have been shown to decline. No decrease in HDL cholesterol has been noted if a more modest P:S ratio (1.0 to 2.0) is used. Diets high in monounsaturated fatty acids (MUFAs) have the same total and LDL cholesterol-lowering effects as high-PUFA diet, without the HDL-lowering effect. We do not recommend the use of diets high in total fat. If, however, such a diet were to be used, monounsaturated fat should make up the majority of the additional fatty acids. The basis for this choice derives

---

Table 5 Dietary Recommendations for Treatment of Dyslipidemic Diabetic Patients

Modest caloric restriction if overweight

Carbohydrate = 50–60% of daily energy intake, primarily complex carbohydrates*

High fiber content (approximately 20 g/1,000 cal)

Fat = 30 percent of daily energy intake with less than 10 percent as saturated fat

Cholesterol <300 mg/day

ω3 fatty acids should not be supplemented beyond that present in the normal diet

Protein = 10–15% of daily energy intake

---

*If glycemic control or dyslipidemia worsens, the dietary carbohydrate content should be reduced to 40 to 45% of total daily energy intake and monounsaturated and polyunsaturated fat should replace saturated fat in this diet.

from the natural occurrence of a high monounsaturated fat diet in several Mediterranean populations, who have been shown to have a decreased incidence of atherosclerotic complications, and the lack of any human experience with diets containing more than 10 percent polyunsaturated fat.

A unique type of PUFA that has aroused much interest is the ω3 fatty acids series. These fatty acids, found primarily in fish oil, are comprised mainly of eicosapentaenoic acid and docosahexenoic acid. α-linolenic acid, present in vegetables, such as linseed, also is an ω3 fatty acid. This series of fatty acids has the ability to reduce platelet aggregability and, when consumed in large quantities, can cause a profound decrease in plasma VLDL triglyceride concentration in both diabetic and nondiabetic subjects with severe hypertriglyceridemia. In patients with mild hypertriglyceridemia, reductions in VLDL are often associated with increases in plasma LDL cholesterol and apo B levels. When administered to diabetic patients, ω3 fatty acids consistently have caused a worsening of diabetic control. Although ingestion of fish in the diet should not be restricted, use of ω3 fatty acid supplements in diabetics is not advised at this time.

Dietary Fiber

The benefits of a diet high in fiber (30 to 40 g) in both IDDM and NIDDM patients have been well documented. It is the nondigestible polysaccharide fractions of cell wall components that provide most of the therapeutic effects. Both soluble and insoluble fiber decrease gastrointestinal tract transit time, and thus reduce glucose absorption, leading to improved glycemic control. There is lowering of serum cholesterol and triglycerides as well. The soluble fraction of fiber appears to be responsible for lowering plasma total and LDL cholesterol levels. Diets that are high in fiber also have been shown to increase satiety in nondiabetic individuals and to promote weight loss, although few studies have been done with diabetics. It is recommended that diabetics take approximately 20 g of fiber per 1,000 kcal. It is preferable that this be in the form of dietary intake rather than supplements. However, this recommendation is five to six times the present fiber intake in the United States, and is unlikely to be attainable without exogenous supplementation. The only side effects with such high-fiber diets are related to the gastrointestinal tract; bloating, and abdominal discomfort. Diabetics with significant gastroparesis are unlikely to be able to tolerate a diet high in fiber.

Weight Loss

The multiple benefits of weight reduction in diabetic individuals are well established (see the chapter *Behavioral Weight Control*). Overweight diabetic individuals have increased VLDL production with hypertriglyceridemia, as well as increased LDL synthesis, that may or may not be accompanied by an increase in plasma LDL concentration. The increases in VLDL and LDL production are reversed with weight loss. Although HDL levels can initially fall with weight reduction, they usually return to baseline or increase above this if weight loss is maintained. The decrease in plasma triglyceride concentration often is dramatic in diabetic patients who lose a large amount of weight. However, a significant decrease in plasma triglyceride levels may be seen even in individuals in whom the weight loss is modest. In addition to the beneficial effects on lipids, weight loss has been shown to improve glycemic control and reduce insulin resistance.

It also should be noted that much of the work with diet and diabetes has been done with NIDDM patients, and although relevant literature with IDDM patients has been cited, systematic studies are needed with these patients before recommendations can be extrapolated from them.

At the present time, it seems reasonable to recommend the diet approved by both the ADA and the AHA as a first approach to all diabetics, irrespective of their plasma lipid concentrations (Table 5). If there is an adverse response to the recommended diet, such as worsening diabetic control or hypertriglyceridemia, a diet lower in carbohydrate and higher in monounsaturated fat can then be substituted. As a cautionary note, it must be emphasized that fat has more than twice the caloric density than carbohydrate (9 kcal per gram versus 4 kcal per gram), and the use of high-fat diets may predispose to weight gain.

The AHA and ADA recommend that evaluation of the impact of dietary therapy on the plasma-lipid profile be performed after 3 months. Our experience is that this is much too long. With respect to reduction in body weight, if significant weight loss has not occurred within the first month, diet therapy is unlikely to be successful in achieving weight reduction. At this point it is best to reemphasize the importance of dietary therapy and have the patient return in 4 weeks to be re-evaluated. It may take longer to see the effect of dietary treatment on plasma lipids than on weight loss (see subsequent discussion). If after 8 weeks of diet therapy weight loss has not occurred and the plasma lipid level has not changed, consideration should be given to the institution of pharmacologic therapy.

■ EXERCISE

Exercise is recommended in NIDDM patients to enhance weight loss and to improve glycemic control. Exercise also can significantly improve the lipid abnormalities present in diabetic patients. Exercise increases glucose uptake by muscle ten- to twentyfold depending on its intensity and duration. As exercise continues, fat rather than carbohydrate becomes the predominant fuel that is burned. In both lean and obese diabetic subjects exercise training causes significant reductions in the VLDL triglyceride concentration and, to a lesser extent, in LDL cholesterol. HDL cholesterol also has been shown to increase. These beneficial effects on lipids are observed in both NIDDM and IDDM individuals. Exercise in combination with weight loss is particularly effective in improving lipid levels in NIDDM individuals. In order to see significant effects on plasma lipids, the exercise should be performed 3 to 4 times per week, 30 to 40 minutes per bout of exercise, at 30 to 40 percent of the subject's VO_2max, and should be aerobic in nature.

Table 6 Pharmacologic Agents for the Treatment of Dyslipidemia

DRUGS	LIPOPROTEINS AFFECTED	DOSE	SIDE EFFECTS
Bile Acid Resins	↓↓ LDL		GI effects
Cholestyramine	± ↑ TG	8–24 g/d	Drug/vitamin
Colestipol*	± ↑ HDL	10–30 g/d	malabsorption
Nicotinic Acid	↓ LDL	1–6 g/d	Worsened glycemic
	↓ TG		control
	↑ HDL		Flush
			Hepatitis
			GI side effects
HMG-CoA Reductase	↓↓ LDL		↑ LFTs
Inhibitors	↓ TG		Myositis
	↑ HDL	20–40 mg/dl	GI effects
		10–40 mg/dl	Insomnia
Lovastatin		5–40 mg/dl	
Pravastatin		20–40 mg/dl	
Simvastatin		10–80 mg/dl	
Fluvastatin			
Atorvastatin			
Fibric Acid	± ↓ LDL		↑ LFTs
Derivatives	↓ TG	600 mg bid	GI side effects
	↑ HDL	1000 mg bid	Drug interactions
Gemfibrozil			
Clofibrate			

*Colestipol also is available in one-gram tablets.
GI = gastrointestinal; *HDL* = high density lipoprotein cholesterol; *LDL* = low density lipoprotein cholesterol; *LFTs* = liver function tests; *TG* = triglyceride.

■ DRUG THERAPY

If an adequate trial of diabetic control, diet, weight loss, and exercise are unsuccessful in correcting the dyslipidemia, pharmacologic intervention should be considered. The length of time needed for the patient to make these life-style changes should depend on the initial presentation of the patient, the severity of the dyslipidemia, and the presence of other risk factors for coronary heart disease or the presence of coronary heart disease itself. If the patient has poorly controlled glycemia, eats a diet that is very high in saturated fat and cholesterol, leads a sedentary life, and is obese, more effort and time may be devoted to life-style changes prior to initiation of specific hypolipidemic drug treatment. Lipid-lowering agents will be less efficacious, or often ineffective, if these related factors are not optimally controlled. On the other hand, if the dyslipidemia is severe and/or the patient is at very high risk for coronary heart disease, earlier institution of pharmacotherapy is prudent. If the patient already has clinically significant coronary heart disease or other vascular disease, drug treatment is indicated concomitantly with other interventions. Another impetus for earlier specific hypolipidemic drug treatment is the association between the severity of the lipid abnormalities and the presence of a separately inherited lipid disorder. Plasma triglyceride or LDL cholesterol levels above the 90th percentile or HDL cholesterol below the 10 to 20th percentile are indications of a separate (but interactive) lipid problem. In any event, physicians should not wait forever to control the plasma-glucose concentration or to achieve weight loss before advancing to specific lipid-altering treatment. Before discussing each lipid-altering agent it should be remembered that although the combination of hypertriglyceridemia plus low HDL cholesterol profile is much more common in diabetics than in nondiabetics, pure hypercholesterolemia is not uncommon and should be treated accordingly (Table 6).

Bile Acid Resins

Cholestyramine and colestipol are used primarily to lower LDL cholesterol. They bind bile acids in the intestine, thereby interrupting the enterohepatic recirculation of these molecules. This intestinal activity triggers the following sequence of responses: the liver increases conversion of cholesterol to bile acids, which results in a diminution of a regulatory pool of hepatic cholesterol. This causes upregulation of hepatic LDL receptors, which leads to a decrease in plasma LDL concentrations (15 to 25 percent). Usual doses of the bile acid resins are between two and six scoops or packets of resin daily or 8 to 24 g per day for cholestyramine and 10 to 30 g per day for colestipol. Cholestyramine is mixed with sucrose, but there is a "light" form that is made with Nutrasweet. Bile acid binding resins are not absorbed and, therefore, have no systemic toxicities. A drawback to the use of bile acid binding resins is the increase in hepatic VLDL triglyceride production and plasma triglyceride levels commonly associated with their use. This is particularly relevant in diabetics, in whom the most common lipid abnormality is hypertriglyceridemia with low HDL cholesterol. The major side effect of these agents is bloating and constipation, which may pose a significant problem in the diabetic patient with gastroparesis. Bile acid resins should, therefore, only be used alone in diabetics with pure elevations of total and LDL cholesterol. They are recommended as first line agents for hypercholesterolemia, although the availability of the HMG-CoA reductase inhibitors (see further discussion) provides an excellent alternative.

Nicotinic Acid (Niacin)

Niacin would seem to be an ideal agent for the diabetic with hyperlipidemia because it lowers triglycerides (by 20 to 40 percent), raises HDL cholesterol (by 10 to 25 percent), and lowers LDL cholesterol (by 15 to 20 percent). Therapeutic doses are between 1 and 6 g per day given in three divided doses. The mechanism of action of nicotinic acid generally is thought to be through lowering hepatic VLDL apo B production. Unfortunately, niacin has a number of serious side effects that limit its utility in both diabetics and nondiabetics. In diabetics, niacin consistently worsens glycemic control by inducing insulin resistance. Nonetheless, niacin has been shown to effectively lower triglycerides, reduce total and LDL cholesterol, and increase HDL cholesterol. In some type 2 diabetics who already are on insulin, niacin may be considered, as any worsening of glycemic control could be countered by modifying the insulin dose. Niacin should not be considered a first-line drug in diabetic patients, particularly if they are diet-controlled or are on oral agents. A prostaglandin-mediated flush, which is transient, is very common. Gastric irritation, exacerbation of peptic ulcer disease, dry skin, hyperuricemia with precipitation of gouty attacks, and elevation of hepatic transaminases occur in about 3 to 5 percent of patients. Niacin causes clinically significant hepatitis in about 1 out of every 200 patients. In one study of male NIDDM patients, niacin was highly effective in lowering triglycerides and total and LDL cholesterol, and in raising HDL cholesterol. This was at the expense, however, of a deterioration in glycemic control, with an increase in glycosylated hemoglobin level.

HMG-CoA Reductase Inhibitors

Lovastatin, pravastatin, simvastatin, fluvastatin, and atorvastatin are the only drugs in this category available for use in the United States. They work to competitively inhibit HMG-CoA reductase, the rate limiting enzyme in cholesterol synthesis. This results in both decreased hepatic production of apo B–containing lipoproteins and upregulation of LDL receptors. The overall effect is a dramatic lowering of plasma levels of LDL cholesterol. VLDL triglyceride concentrations also are reduced in many subjects with moderate hypertriglyceridemia. HMG-CoA reductase inhibitors usually are not efficacious in severe hypertriglyceridemia. These agents can lower LDL cholesterol by up to 50 percent and decrease triglycerides by up to 30 percent. Reductase inhibitors can raise HDL cholesterol by up to 10 percent, but should not be considered as first line agents for increasing HDL cholesterol. Atorvastatin is the most potent HMG-CoA reductase inhibitor.

Starting doses are 20 mg per day for lovastatin, pravastatin, fluvastatin, 5 mg per day for simvastatin and 10 mg per day of atorvastatin. The main side effects are myositis and nonclinically significant hepatitis, which occur in fewer than 1 percent of patients. Transaminitis occurs in 1 to 3 percent of individuals taking these agents. These agents do not have any deleterious effect on diabetic control. In NIDDM patients with elevated plasma LDL cholesterol concentrations, with or without moderate hypertriglyceridemia (in the 250 to 500 mg per deciliter range), these agents cause significant decrease in plasma total/LDL/VLDL cholesterol and triglyceride levels. HDL cholesterol is not increased. The HMG-CoA reductase inhibitors are, therefore, excellent first-line drugs for the treatment of diabetic patients with isolated high levels of LDL cholesterol, hypercholesterolemia with moderate hypertriglyceridemia (<500 mg per deciliter), or hypercholesterolemia with combined hyperlipidemia. As discussed further, they also can be used in conjunction with other hypolipidemic agents under some circumstances.

Fibric Acid Derivatives

Gemfibrozil and clofibrate are the agents that currently are available in the United States. Several others are available in Europe and Canada. As a class, the fibric acid derivatives have potent lipid-altering effects that are quite useful in diabetics. In a literature review of studies with gemfibrozil in diabetics, triglycerides were lowered by 17 to 57 percent and HDL cholesterol rose by 6 to 19 percent while decreases in LDL levels were more variable. Although their mechanism of action is unclear, these agents appear to work by both decreasing hepatic VLDL production and increasing the activity of lipoprotein lipase. The usual dose is 600 mg twice daily of gemfibrozil, and 1.0 g twice daily of clofibrate. The latter is not used much at present. These agents are lithogenic and are contraindicated in patients with gallstones. Because they are tightly bound to plasma proteins, levels of other drugs (e.g., Coumadin) should be monitored carefully. LDL cholesterol levels can increase when fibrates are used in patients with hypertriglyceridemia, and this should be looked for closely. Most studies have indicated either no change or a slight improvement in glycemic control following therapy with fibric acid derivatives.

Because diabetic dyslipidemia is characterized by elevated triglyceride and reduced HDL cholesterol levels, fibrates play an important role in this patient group. Of concern is the rise in LDL cholesterol concentration that can accompany reduced triglyceride levels during fibrate therapy. Two points should be considered in that regard: first, in the Helsinki Heart Study, following gemfibrozil therapy, hypertriglyceridemic patients with and without concomitant elevations in LDL cholesterol achieved the same reduction in coronary heart disease; thus, the lack of reduction in LDL cholesterol during fibrate therapy may not be an indication of reduced efficacy; and second, if LDL cholesterol levels increase, this can be reversed by adding either bile acid resins or reductase inhibitors.

In a randomized blinded trial, gemfibrozil was compared to lovastatin in hypercholesterolemic NIDDM patients with minimally elevated plasma triglyceride levels (approximately 200 mg per deciliter). Gemfibrozil caused a greater reduction in triglycerides, while lovastatin resulted in a greater decline in LDL and total cholesterol. Both agents were effective in increasing HDL cholesterol, although gemfibrozil was about twice as potent. In NIDDM patients with moderate hypertriglyceridemia (250 to 500 mg per deciliter) gemfibrozil also significantly decreased the plasma triglyceride levels without change in HDL cholesterol, but LDL cholesterol increased significantly. In NIDDM patients with severe hypertriglyceridemia (>500 mg per deciliter) a greater reduction in plasma triglycerides was observed, but LDL also increased more. These observations underscore the need to measure the LDL cholesterol concentration in diabetic patients after the

start of gemfibrozil (or other fibrates). If an increase in the LDL cholesterol is observed, an HMG-CoA reductase inhibitor should be started. One can expect combined therapy to further reduce the plasma triglyceride concentration and to effectively lower both total and LDL cholesterol, compared to gemfibrozil alone. No deleterious effects on glycemic control have been reported with combined HMG-CoA reductase inhibitor/gemfibrozil therapy. There is a small increased incidence, 3 to 5 percent, of myositis with the use of combination therapy. It is not clear if the risk of hepatitis or transaminitis is increased as well.

Other Agents

Probucol is an agent that inconsistently lowers LDL cholesterol modestly (10 to 20 percent). The mechanism whereby LDL cholesterol is lowered is poorly defined, although increased nonreceptor clearance of LDL has been proposed. Probucol also is an antioxidant, and may be useful in preventing the oxidative modification of LDL, which appears necessary for uptake into macrophages. However, a recent report indicated that probucol did not reduce atherosclerosis in men at high risk for coronary artery disease. In addition to its lack of proven efficacy, probucol also lowers HDL cholesterol, although the significance of the effect on HDL is unclear. In light of the fact that low levels of HDL cholesterol are an almost universal problem in diabetics with NIDDM, the use of this agent should be reserved until further study into its mechanisms of action are completed.

■ SUMMARY OF PHARMACOLOGIC INTERVENTION

For the diabetic with isolated hypertriglyceridemia and low HDL cholesterol, fibric acid derivatives should be the first choice in most patients. In many cases, this will be all that is necessary. If the LDL cholesterol concentration also is elevated, or increases during treatment with fibric acid drugs, the physician has several choices. First, a bile acid binding resin can add to the fibrate. This will lower LDL cholesterol without (in the presence of the fibrate) significantly affecting triglyceride levels. Long-term compliance with bile acid resins is a problem. The second alternative would be either to switch to an HMG-CoA reductase inhibitor (this would be the logical choice if the triglyceride elevation before or during fibrate treatment was only moderate, less than 300 mg per deciliter), or to add an HMG-CoA reductase inhibitor to the fibrate. The latter combination is very effective in correcting severe combined hyperlipidemia, but carries a slightly increased risk of myositis. We believe that this combination can be used successfully, particularly if the patient knows clearly that they must stop the medications, drink large quantities of liquids, and call their physician if diffuse, severe muscle pain occurs. Liver function tests should be obtained regularly with use of fibrates or reductase inhibitors when used alone or in combination. The use of nicotinic acid should be reserved for patients with severe, combined hyperlipidemia in whom other lipid-lowering drugs have failed, because this agent consistently causes a deterioration in glucose tolerance.

In those patients who present with a combined elevation of both LDL cholesterol and plasma triglycerides, an HMG-

CoA reductase inhibitor is probably the most effective single agent. Again, niacin could also be used as a sole drug, with caution taken as described above. A fibric acid derivative can be added if triglycerides are not sufficiently reduced by either of those drugs alone, and fibrates could be used initially with bile acid binding resins. The use of fibric acid derivative alone is quite effective in those patients found to have type III hyperlipidemia.

Therapy for the diabetic patient with an isolated reduction in HDL cholesterol is not clearly defined. Fibrates have not been demonstrated to be very effective in raising HDL cholesterol levels in nondiabetics with isolated reductions in HDL, although no similar studies have been carried out in diabetics. Niacin may be more effective in elevating HDL cholesterol concentrations when they are the low in the absence of hypertriglyceridemia, but all of the caveats of niacin use in diabetes mellitus would apply here as well. If the HDL cholesterol concentration can not be increased in these subjects, lowering of the LDL cholesterol concentration should be pursued aggressively, with the goal of reducing it to approximately 100 mg per deciliter. It must be clear, however, that there are no end-point trials supporting any approach to the treatment of an isolated reduction in HDL cholesterol either in nondiabetics or diabetics.

Finally, in those diabetics with isolated high levels of LDL cholesterol, either a bile acid resin or an HMG-CoA reductase inhibitor may be used as primary treatment. The combination of these two agents has been shown to be very effective in those individuals who have extremely high levels of LDL cholesterol, resistant to monotherapy. Triglyceride levels need to be observed closely in patients who are placed on resins.

SUGGESTED READING

Albu J, Konnarides C, Pi Sunyer X. Weight control. Metabolic and cardiovascular effects. Diabetes Metab Rev 1995; 3:335–347.

A review of the effects of weight loss on carbohydrate and lipid metabolism.

American Diabetes Association: Nutritional recommendations and principles for people with diabetes mellitus. Diabetes Care 1994; 17:519–522.

The most recent review of studies providing the basis for the ADA dietary recommendations.

Anderson JW, Gustafson NJ, Bryant CA, Tietyen-Clark CA. Dietary fiber and diabetes: A comprehensive review and practical application. J Am Diet Assoc 1987; 87:1189–1197.

A review of the literature regarding the effects of dietary fiber on plasma lipid and glucose levels in patients with diabetes mellitus.

Consensus Report: Role of cardiovascular risk factors in prevention and treatment of macrovascular disease in diabetes. Diabetes Care 1989; 12:573–579.

A report focused on the diagnostic criteria and treatment modalities to be used to prevent cardiovascular disease in patients with diabetes mellitus.

Expert Panel on Detection, Evaluation, and Treatment of High Blood Cholesterol in Adults. Summary of the second report of the National Cholesterol Education Program (NCEP) expert panel. JAMA 1993; 269:3015–3023.

This is the most recent report from the panel convened to promote the screening, diagnosis, and treatment of hypercholesterolemia in people at risk for cardiovascular disease.

Garg A. Management of dyslipidemia in IDDM patients. Diabetes Care 1994; 17:224–234.

A review of treatment approaches to control hyperlipidemia in patients with IDDM.

Garg A, Bantle JP, Henry RR, et al. Effects of varying carbohydrate content of diet in patients with non–insulin-dependent diabetes mellitus. JAMA 1994; 271:1421–1428.

The results of a multicenter trial comparing diets higher in carbohydrate with diets higher in monounsaturated fats in patients with NIDDM.

Garg A, Grundy SM. Treatment of dyslipidemia in patients with NIDDM. Diabetes Rev 1995; 3:433–445.

A review of the effects of lipid-lowering drugs on plasma lipid, lipoprotein, and glucose levels in patients with NIDDM.

Ginsberg HN. Lipoprotein physiology in nondiabetic and diabetic states: relationship to atherogenesis. Diabetes Care 1991; 14:839–855.

This is a detailed review of plasma lipid and lipoprotein metabolism in normal individuals and in patients with type 1 and type 2 diabetes mellitus. The effects of treatment of diabetes on plasma lipids are also discussed.

Grundy SM. Dietary therapy in diabetes mellitus. Diabetes Care 1991; 14:796–801.

A review of the literature and recommendations regarding the optimal approaches to dietary therapy in diabetes mellitus.

Howard B. Pathogenesis of diabetic dyslipidemia. Diabetes Rev 1995; 3:423–432.

A review of the pathophysiology of lipoprotein disorders in patients with NIDDM.

Laakso M. Epidemiology of diabetic dyslipidemia. Diabetes Rev 1995; 3:408–422.

A review of the incidence, prevalence, and natural history of lipid disorders in patients with diabetes mellitus.

Lampman RM, Schteingart DE. Effects of exercise training on glucose control, lipid metabolism, and insulin sensitivity in hypertriglyceridemia and non–insulin-dependent diabetes mellitus. Med Sci Sports Exercise 1991; 23:703–712.

A study demonstrating the effects of exercise on glucose, insulin, and lipid metabolism in patients with NIDDM.

Wallidius G, Erickson U, Olsson AG, et al. The effect of probucol on femoral atherosclerosis: The Probucol Quantitative Regression Swedish Trial (PQRST). Am J Cardiol 1994; 74(R):875–883.

The results of the PQRST study of probucol and peripheral vascular disease.

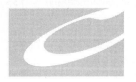

DIABETIC COMPLICATIONS

DIABETIC NEPHROPATHY: DIAGNOSTIC AND THERAPEUTIC APPROACH

Ralph A. DeFronzo, M.D.

Diabetic nephropathy is the most common cause of end-stage renal failure in the United States and is responsible for approximately 30 percent of all new patients entering end-stage renal failure programs. Although dialysis and transplantation prevent death from uremia (see the chapter *Diabetic Nephropathy: End Stage*), the five-year survival in such patients is much worse than in nondiabetic patients and approaches 20 percent. Therefore, it is important to recognize the earliest stages of diabetic nephropathy and to institute appropriate therapy. Once proteinuria has been established, relentless progression to end-stage renal failure is inevitable.

Diabetic nephropathy develops in 40 to 50 percent of patients with type 1 or insulin-dependent diabetes mellitus (IDDM) who have had diabetes for 20 years or more. Clinically significant renal disease is less common in type 2 or non–insulin-dependent diabetes mellitus (NIDDM), occurring in 5 to 10 percent. However, in certain populations with an increased prevalence of NIDDM, such as Native Americans, Mexican Americans, and African Americans, the prevalence of renal disease is much greater and approaches that in IDDM.

■ PATHOGENESIS

A rational approach to the therapy of diabetic renal disease depends on a thorough understanding of its pathogenesis. Therefore, those factors that have been implicated in the development of diabetic nephropathy will briefly be reviewed (Table 1).

Essentially all diabetic patients, both type 1 and type 2, who develop renal insufficiency demonstrate evidence of poor glycemic control, as documented by persistently elevated fasting plasma glucose levels (>160 to 180 mg per deciliter) and glycosylated hemoglobin levels (HbA$_{1c}$ >8.0 percent). The results of the Diabetes Control and Complications Trial (type 1 diabetics) and the Japanese Intervention Study (type 2 diabetics) conclusively have demonstrated that tight glycemic control serves as primary prevention for all microvascular complications; including nephropathy, retinopathy, and neuro-pathy. These observations are consistent with a meta-analysis of seven smaller studies. Genetic factors also are important and diabetic nephropathy tends to aggregate in families of diabetics with IDDM, as well as NIDDM. Although these genetic factors can not be reversed, a strong family history of renal involvement should alert the physician to pay close attention to the monitory signs of renal involvement. Hemodynamic abnormalities also have been implicated in the pathogenesis of diabetic nephropathy. Poor glycemic control is associated with a rise in renal blood flow and increased intraglomerular pressure, which combine to augment the glomerular filtration rate (GFR). The increase in intraglomerular pressure has been shown to contribute to the demise in renal function by directly injuring the glomerulus. These hemodynamic changes are exacerbated by excessive protein intake. Systemic hypertension per se directly causes

---

Table 1 Etiologic Factors in the Development of Diabetic Renal Disease

Poor glycemic control (fasting plasma glucose levels >140–160 mg/dl; HbA$_{1c}$ >7.5–8%)
Genetic factors
Hemodynamic abnormalities (increased renal blood flow, glomerular filtration rate, and intraglomerular pressure)
Altered vascular permeability
Systemic hypertension
Excessive protein intake
Metabolic disturbances (abnormal polyol metabolism, formation of advanced glycation end products, increased cytokine production, activation of protein kinase C)
Release of growth factors
Abnormalities in carbohydrate/lipid/protein metabolism
Structural abnormalities (glomerular hypertrophy, mesangial expansion, glomerular basement membrane thickening)
Disturbances in ion pumps (increased Na$^+$-; H$^+$ ion pump and decreased Ca^{++} ATPase pump)
Hyperlipidemia (hypercholesterolemia and hypertriglyceridemia)

---

renal damage and will exacerbate local renal hemodynamic changes. Metabolic disturbances, including abnormal polyol metabolism and formation of advanced glycosylation end products, which develop secondary to poor glycemic control, also have been implicated in the pathogenesis of diabetic nephropathy. Release of growth factors and various cytokines, as well as abnormalities in carbohydrate-lipid-protein metabolism, contribute to the development of structural abnormalities (glomerular hypertrophy, mesangial expansion, glomerular basement membrane thickening) that characterize diabetic nephropathy. Recently, an increase in the Na^+, H^+ pump activity has been demonstrated in diabetic patients with renal disease and this may prove to be an important genetic marker. Overactivity of the Na^+, H^+ pump has been shown to be associated with systemic hypertension, cardiomegaly, and possibly accelerated atherosclerosis.

■ NATURAL HISTORY OF DIABETIC NEPHROPATHY

The natural history of renal disease has been well characterized in those patients with IDDM and NIDDM who are destined to develop renal insufficiency. At the time of initial diagnosis there are no renal histologic abnormalities, but renal blood flow (RBF) and GFR are elevated (Fig. 1). Within 3 years, histologic changes (increased mesangial matrix material and glomerular basement membrane thickening) of diabetic nephropathy are evident but GFR and RBF remain elevated.

Over the subsequent 10 to 15 years there is progressive histologic damage but renal hyperfiltration persists, and there are no laboratory clues to suggest the presence of renal involvement. Approximately 15 years after the diagnosis of diabetes, albuminuria (>300 mg per day) is detected, and the elevated rates of RBF and GFR have returned to normal (Fig. 1). This is an ominous sign and heralds the onset of progressive renal insufficiency. At this stage no intervention has been shown to prevent the eventual progression to end-stage renal failure, although pharmacologic therapy may slow the rate of decline of GFR. Within 5 years after the onset of albuminuria approximately half of individuals will have experienced a 50 percent reduction in the GFR and a doubling of their serum creatinine. Within a mean of 3 to 4 years, half of these patients will have progressed to end-stage renal failure. At or just before the time of onset of overt albuminuria, most patients will develop hypertension, and the increase in blood pressure markedly accelerates the progression of renal disease. Effective treatment of the hypertension has been documented to slow, although not prevent, the progression to end-stage renal failure. Once clinically significant albuminuria (>300 mg per day) has developed, tight glycemic control can not prevent or slow the development of renal insufficiency.

Recent studies have demonstrated that there is a "preclinical" stage of diabetic nephropathy characterized by microalbuminuria (Table 2). Normal individuals do not excrete more than 10 to 20 mg per day of albumin. However, routine laboratory tests do not detect these small amounts of albuminuria unless it is in excess of 300 mg per day. Therefore, there is

Table 2 Definition of Microalbuminuria

	URINARY AER (MG/24 H)	URINARY AER (µG/MIN)	URINE ALBUMIN:CREATININE RATIO (MG/MG)
Normoalbuminuria	<30	<20	<0.02
Microalbuminuria	30–300	20–200	0.02–0.20
Macroalbuminuria	>300	>200	>0.20

The mean value for urinary albumin excretion rate (AER) in normal individuals is 10±3 mg/day or 7±2 µg/min.

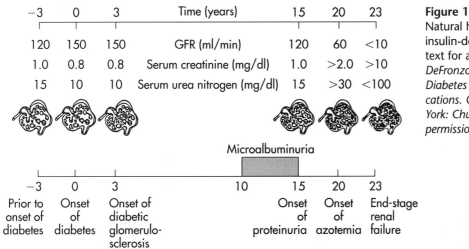

Figure 1
Natural history of diabetic nephropathy in insulin-dependent diabetes mellitus. See text for a detailed discussion. *(Adapted from DeFronzo RA. Diabetes and the kidney. In Diabetes mellitus: management and complications. Olefsky JM, Sherwin RS, eds. New York: Churchill Livingstone, 1985:169; with permission.)*

a range of albumin excretion, 30 to 300 mg per day, that is distinctly abnormal, yet can not be detected by routine means. This range (30 to 300 mg per day or 20 to 200 µg per min) has been referred to as microalbuminuria and is the first laboratory evidence of diabetic renal disease. Fortunately, microalbuminuria can be detected using more sophisticated techniques (radioimmunoassay, enzyme-linked immunosorbent assay), and a highly accurate screening urine test for microalbuminuria now exists (Micral, Boehringer Mannheim). It is advisable to determine microalbuminuria using a timed collection (i.e., 24 hours) because this allows one to simultaneously measure the creatinine clearance. However, the urine albumin to creatinine ratio (microalbuminuric range = 0.02 to 0.20 mg per) on a spot urine is nearly as good as a timed urine collection. Most important, tight glycemic control with insulin during the microalbuminuric stage has been shown to prevent the development of overt diabetic nephropathy in IDDM subjects. Once the urine albumin excretion exceeds 300 mg per day no study has demonstrated that tight glycemic control can slow the progression to end-stage renal failure. Therefore, it is essential that all IDDM diabetic patients be screened yearly for microalbuminuria starting 5 years after the onset of diabetes. Annual screening is recommended for NIDDM patients from the time that the diabetes is initially diagnosed.

The natural history of diabetic nephropathy in NIDDM closely follows that in IDDM with several exceptions. Clinically detectable albuminuria is common at the time of diagnosis, but only a minority (5 to 10 percent) of Caucasian patients with NIDDM progress to end-stage renal failure. The incidence of progression of microalbuminuria to renal insufficiency is much higher (15 to 20 percent) in African Americans, Mexican Americans, and Asians, and exceeds 50 percent in certain Native American tribes. In all NIDDM individuals, irrespective of ethnic background, microalbuminuria is a strong predictor of death from stroke and myocardial infarction. Approximately 80 percent of individuals die from atherosclerotic cardiovascular complications within 10 years after the onset of microalbuminuria.

■ EVALUATION OF LOSS OF RENAL FUNCTION

Every patient with diabetes who develops proteinuria or a rise in the serum creatinine concentration should have a thorough evaluation to define the cause of the renal failure. It is unwise to assume that all diabetic subjects who experience a deterioration in renal function have diabetic nephropathy. A comprehensive evaluation should be undertaken to exclude other causes of renal disease (Table 3). In general, they can be divided into prerenal, postrenal, and intrarenal (glomerulonephritis, tubulointerstitial disease, and vasculitis).

History and Physical Examination

The history and physical exam should focus on drugs taken (non–steroidal anti-inflammatory drugs and analgesics), toxin exposure, administration of radiographic contrast media, hereditary diseases, prior history of renal disease, allergic manifestations, skin rash, arthritis, fever, and involvement of other organ systems. Intravascular volume and cardiac status should be assessed to ensure that renal perfusion is adequate. Symptoms indicative of urinary tract obstruction, especially in the male, or neurogenic bladder should be elicited. History of oliguria suggests another cause of the renal failure.

In IDDM clinical evidence of renal disease within the first 5 years after the diagnosis of diabetes does not occur and is unusual (<5 to 10 percent) within the first 10 years. This is not true in NIDDM because the true onset of diabetes is difficult to document with certainty. Importantly, diabetic nephropathy does not occur in the absence of retinopathy. If examination of the dilated pupil by an eye specialist fails to document any evidence of diabetic retinopathy, another cause of the renal failure is likely. Proteinuria is the hallmark of diabetic nephropathy and in its absence the diagnosis cannot be made.

Laboratory Assessment
Urinalysis
The urinalysis in diabetic nephropathy is usually benign. Occasional red blood cells may be seen. Abundant red blood cells or red blood cell casts indicate glomerulonephritis. Numerous white blood cells and bacteria imply urinary tract infection, and a urine culture should be obtained. If renal tubular epithelial cells accompany white blood cells, one of the tubulointerstitial causes of renal disease should be suspected. Heavy proteinuria is consistent with diabetic renal disease or glomerulonephritis. The absence of proteinuria virtually excludes the diagnosis of diabetic nephropathy. Numerous uric acid or calcium crystals should suggest renal calculous disease.

Serum Chemistries and Blood Tests
The serum urea nitrogen and creatinine concentrations are helpful in excluding prerenal and postrenal causes of renal failure. In intrinsic renal disease they rise in parallel in a ratio of 10 to 15 to 1, whereas a disproportionate rise in the serum urea nitrogen is observed in patients with intravascular volume depletion, congestive heart failure, and urinary tract obstruction. Hyperkalemia and hyperchloremic metabolic acidosis, in the absence of a significant increase in the serum creatinine concentration (3 to 4 mg per deciliter), suggest the presence of interstitial nephritis or hypoaldosteronism. The latter is quite common in diabetic nephropathy. Serum calcium and uric acid concentrations should be measured to rule out hypercalcemic and uric acid nephropathy, respectively.

Table 3 Causes of Renal Failure

Prerenal
    Volume depletion
    Hypotension
    Congestive heart failure

Postrenal
    Bladder outlet obstruction
    Ureteral obstruction

Intrarenal
    Glomerulonephritis
    Tubulointerstitial disease
    Vasculitis

Peripheral eosinophilia suggests an allergic interstitial nephritis. In patients with suspected glomerulonephritis total serum complement and C3, antinuclear antibody, ASLO titer, antiglomerular basement membrane antibody titer, and cryoglobulins should be obtained. A very high erythrocyte sedimentation rate suggests one of the vasculitides. Microangiopathic hemolytic anemia and thrombocytopenia are observed in hemolytic uremic syndrome and thrombotic thrombocytopenic purpura.

Other Diagnostic Maneuvers

Renal ultrasound is a simple, noninvasive method to exclude urinary tract obstruction. It also allows one to quantify renal size. Small kidneys imply chronic, advanced renal disease. Patients with early diabetic nephropathy have normal or more often increased kidney size. Radionuclide imaging with radiolabeled technetium allows assessment of renal blood flow. If, after a thorough evaluation, the cause of the renal failure remains undefined, a renal biopsy should be considered. Because diabetic nephropathy is generalized and involves all parts of all glomeruli, the diagnosis cannot be missed. It is characterized by an increase in mesangial matrix material, glomerular basement membrane thickening, and hyalinosis of the afferent and efferent arterioles. The renal histology also will allow one to differentiate between vasculitis, glomerulonephritis, or interstitial nephritis and will provide information concerning the specific etiology of glomerulonephritis or tubulointerstitial nephritis.

■ TREATMENT OF MICROALBUMINURIA (30 TO 300 MG PER DAY)

Microalbuminuria represents the earliest stage of diabetic nephropathy that can be detected. IDDM patients have a fifteen- to twentyfold increase in the incidence of developing clinically overt albuminuria (>300 mg per day) after 10 years; the incidence of clinically overt albuminuria after 10 years in NIDDM individuals is increased five- to tenfold. In NIDDM subjects microalbuminuria is a strong predictor of cardiovascular mortality, and 80 percent of microalbuminuric type 2 diabetics are dead within 10 years. At the time of initial onset of microalbuminuria the majority of IDDM patients are not

hypertensive; the incidence of hypertension at the time of onset of microalbuminuria is higher than in NIDDM patients and more closely approximates that seen in older individuals with hypertension and obesity. As the microalbuminuria worsens there is a progressive increase in the incidence of hypertension in both IDDM and NIDDM patients.

Because there is significant day to day variation (approximately 40 to 50 percent) in urinary microalbumin excretion, it is recommended that at least two baseline determinations be performed to solidify the diagnosis. This also will provide a more accurate baseline against which to judge subsequent therapeutic interventions. It should be noted that a number of factors, including stress, systemic or urinary tract infection, acute metabolic decompensation, fever, exercise, hypertension, and cardiac failure, can increase the urinary albumin excretion rate.

Glycemic Control

Strict glycemic control is the most critical factor in treating diabetic patients, both type 1 and type 2, during the microalbuminuric stage. IDDM patients in the highest quartile for hyperglycemia have a four- to fivefold increased risk of developing overt proteinuria and eventual renal insufficiency compared to those in the lowest quartile. Hyperglycemia also predicts clinical proteinuria in NIDDM. In every animal model of diabetes, tight glycemic control has been shown to prevent the development of renal disease. In IDDM patients with overt clinical albuminuria (>300 mg per day) or renal insufficiency, no study has demonstrated that normalization of the plasma glucose profile can alter the progression to end-stage renal failure. However, a number of prospective studies (most notably, the Diabetes Control and Complications Trial) have shown that in IDDM patients with microalbuminuria (30 to 300 mg per day) tight glycemic control with insulin, which maintains the glycosylated hemoglobin level below 7.0 to 7.5 percent, prevents the development of clinical albuminuria (Fig. 2). Moreover, in type 1 diabetic patients without microalbuminuria, tight glycemic control prevents the progression to microalbuminuria, i.e., primary prevention. Although some concern has been raised about extrapolation of these results to NIDDM patients, both the Japanese Intervention Study and the Wisconsin Eye Study have demonstrated the importance of normoglycemia or

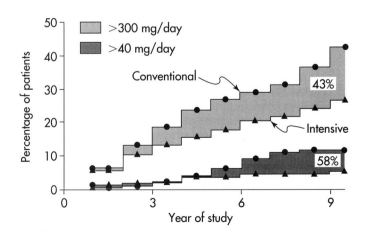

Figure 2
Effect of conventional versus intensive glycemic control on urinary albumin excretion rate in IDDM patients with normoalbuminuria and microalbuminuria. Tight glycemic control significantly reduced the development of microalbuminuria in normoalbuminuric patients (primary prevention) and slowed the progression from microalbuminuria to overt proteinuria (secondary prevention). (*Adapted from The Diabetes Control and Complications Trial Research Group, N Engl J Med 1993; 329:977–896, with permission.*)

near-normoglycemia in the prevention of microvascular complications (renal and retinal) in type 2 diabetic subjects.

The implication of these studies is that strict glycemic control, if implemented sufficiently early, can prevent completely the progression to clinical overt proteinuria and end-stage renal failure. Based on these observations, IDDM patients with a normal urinary albumin excretion rate and, especially those with microalbuminuria, should be aggressively treated with insulin to maintain as near-normal glycemic profile as possible and to achieve a glycosylated hemoglobin value less than 7.0 percent (Table 4). Such intensive therapy requires a highly motivated patient, multiple insulin injections, and home glucose monitoring, because the risk of hypoglycemia is significant. In NIDDM patients, similar glycemic control should be achieved with diet, exercise, hypoglycemic agents (sulfonylureas, metformin, acarbose) and, if necessary, insulin. Immediate benefits of tight glycemic control on urinary albumin excretion may not be obvious, and 1 to 2 months may be necessary to see a reduction in microalbuminuria.

Dietary Protein

In both diabetic and nondiabetic models of renal disease, a high-protein diet exacerbates, whereas a low-protein diet ameliorates the progression of chronic renal disease. In humans, many studies have documented that a low-protein diet slows the rate of decline of GFR in patients with all types of chronic renal disease, including diabetic nephropathy. When dietary protein is restricted to 0.6 to 0.8 g per kilogram body weight per day in patients with diabetic nephropathy, the rate of decline in GFR is blunted and urinary protein excretion is diminished. In microalbuminuric diabetic patients with normal renal function, institution of a low-protein diet causes a reduction in urinary albumin excretion without any change in GFR. Based on these observations moderate protein restriction, 0.8 to 1.0 g per kilogram per day, is advocated in diabetic patients with microalbuminuria (urinary albumin excretion = 30 to 300 mg per day) (Table 4). Replacement of animal protein with vegetable protein is recommended, because this has the same effect as a low-protein diet to slow the rate of decline of GFR in diabetic patients. Patients with normal renal function and no microalbuminuria should avoid a high-protein intake and substitute vegetable protein for animal protein.

Antihypertensive Therapy

Hypertension is a characteristic feature of diabetic nephropathy and is the single most important factor known to accelerate the progression of renal disease. In IDDM the onset of hypertension characteristically occurs at the time of onset of microalbuminuria or shortly thereafter. In NIDDM hypertension may occur at any time and more closely parallels the patient's age and obesity index. However, once microalbuminuria develops in NIDDM patients the incidence of hypertension increases significantly. Multiple factors, including increased total body sodium content and enhanced responsiveness to angiotensin II and norepinephrine, have been implicated in the development of hypertension. Recent studies have implicated insulin resistance and hyperinsulinemia in the pathogenesis of the hypertension. Treatment of hypertension at the microalbuminuric stage (30 to 300 mg per day of albumin) can completely arrest progression of the renal disease in both IDDM and NIDDM patients, whereas treatment at the stage of clinical albuminuria (>300 mg per day) can only slow the rate of deterioration.

Antihypertensive therapy should begin at the earliest indication of a rise in blood pressure and should be aggressive. The most prudent goal is to lower the patient's blood pressure to the level present prior to the onset of proteinuria and/or renal insufficiency. For many patients, especially if they are young, this will be less than the standard value of 120 to 130/80 to 85 mm Hg. If the patient's normal blood pressure is not known, the recommended goal should be 120 to 130/80 to 85 mm Hg (Table 4). This corresponds to a mean arterial blood pressure of 90 to 95 mm Hg. Special caution is advised in treating elderly hypertensive patients who may have underlying cerebrovascular and cardiovascular disease.

Nonpharmacologic Treatment

Nonpharmacologic intervention should be stressed. Weight loss, especially in the obese NIDDM patient, regular physical activity (walking 2 to 3 miles per day at 20 minutes per mile, 4 to 5 times per week), and salt restriction (4 to 5 g per day or 68 to 85 mEq per day) can be very effective in lowering the blood pressure. In addition, weight loss and exercise increase insulin sensitivity, enhance glycemic control, and improve the dyslipidemia. If these nonpharmacologic measures do not normalize the blood pressure pharmacologic intervention is indicated.

The ideal antihypertensive agent should not only lower the blood pressure but reverse the specific pathophysiologic derangements responsible for the hypertension. It should slow or halt the progression of renal disease and be metabolically neutral, i.e., not aggravate the insulin resistance, hyper-

Table 4 Treatment of Diabetic Patients with and without Microalbuminuria and with Overt Diabetic Nephropathy

	MICROALBUMINURIA ABSENT	MICROALBUMINURIA PRESENT	CLINICAL PROTEINURIA/ RENAL INSUFFICIENCY
Glycemic control	HbA_{1c}<6.0-7.0%	HbA_{1c}<6.0–7.0%	HbA_{1c}<8.0%
Blood pressure (mm Hg)*			
Range	120–130/80–85	120–130/80–85	120–130/80–85
Mean arterial pressure	90–95	90–95	90–95
Dietary protein intake (g/kg/day)	≤1.0–1.2	≤0.8–1.0	0.6–0.8†

*If the patient's normal blood pressure before the onset of hypertension is known, this should be established as the therapeutic end point.
†If the patient is on an ACE inhibitor, dietary protein intake can be higher, 0.8 to 1.0 g per kilogram per day.

insulinemia, and dyslipidemia, all of which have been implicated in the accelerated atherosclerosis that characterizes both NIDDM and IDDM. Patients should monitor their blood pressure daily at home, and the physician should adjust the blood pressure medication weekly.

Pharmacologic Therapy

Angiotensin Converting Enzyme Inhibitors. This class of drugs most closely approximates the ideal anti-hypertensive agent. They decrease peripheral vascular resistance by inhibiting the production of angiotensin II, decrease intraglomerular pressure, prevent glomerular hypertrophy, reduce proteinuria and microalbuminuria, and slow the rate of decline in GFR. Numerous studies have shown that the ACE inhibitors halt the progression or cause a reduction in the rate of microalbuminuria in both IDDM and NIDDM patients. The most abundant data have been collected with captopril and enalapril. Similar, although less extensive, data have been accumulated with the other ACE inhibitors. There are two primary mechanisms by which the ACE inhibitors decrease microalbuminuria and preserve renal function: (1) they decrease the vasoconstrictor effect of angiotensin II on the efferent arteriole, leading to a reduction in intraglomerular pressure; and (2) they decrease the systemic blood pressure.

The ACE inhibitors also improve insulin sensitivity, ameliorate hyperinsulinemia, and promote a more favorable serum lipid profile by reducing LDL cholesterol and triglyceride levels and increasing HDL cholesterol. The beneficial effects of ACE inhibitors on insulin sensitivity and serum lipids have been best demonstrated with captopril.

ACE inhibitors may cause hyperkalemia, especially in patients with type IV renal tubular acidosis, i.e., the syndrome of hypoaldosteronism. In some patients (i.e., those with renal artery stenosis, severe congestive heart failure, or advanced renal insufficiency) the GFR may be highly dependent upon angiotensin II-mediated efferent arteriolar tone, and ACE inhibition may cause a precipitous decline in GFR. In patients who are prone to develop hyperkalemia or deterioration in renal function, the decline in glomerular filtration rate is observed shortly after starting the drug. Therefore, patients who are treated with an ACE inhibitor should have their serum potassium and creatinine concentrations checked approximately one week after initiation of therapy.

Currently available ACE inhibitors and specific doses are listed in Table 5.

Calcium Channel Antagonists. In diabetics with hypertension the intracellular calcium concentration is increased and is thought to be related to decreased activity of $Ca^{++}ATPase$. An increase in intracellular calcium concentration enhances the pressor responsiveness to vasoactive hormones such as angiotensin II and norepinephrine. This pathophysiologic derangement provides the rationale for the use of calcium channel antagonists. These agents are quite effective in reducing blood pressure in hypertensive diabetics. Like the ACE inhibitors, calcium channel blockers have been shown to have a specific effect to decrease proteinuria and improve renal function in diabetics with microalbuminuria or overt albuminuria. This class of drugs does not adversely affect the plasma lipid profile or impair glucose tolerance, although several studies carried out in small numbers of diabetic patients suggest that nifedipine may aggravate the insulin resistance. Peripheral edema may occur during therapy.

The calcium channel antagonists, along with the ACE inhibitors, are the preferred drugs of choice in the treatment of hypertensive diabetic patients with microalbuminuria (or overt albuminuria or renal insufficiency).

Specific doses of currently available calcium channel blockers are listed in Table 5.

Diuretics. Diabetic patients with hypertension have an increase in total body sodium content. This is aggravated when proteinuria and renal insufficiency develop. Increased intracellular sodium content enhances the vascular responsiveness to angiotensin II and norepinephrine. Based on the central role of sodium retention in diabetic hypertension, diuretic therapy presents a rational therapeutic option. However, diuretics cause a deterioration in glucose tolerance, a worsening of pre-existing insulin resistance, an increase in LDL-cholesterol and triglyceride levels, and a decrease in HDL-cholesterol. Several recent studies have indicated that treatment of the hypertensive diabetic with or without albuminuria may significantly increase the mortality from coronary heart disease. Therefore, the use of diuretics as "first line" agents in the treatment of hypertensive diabetic patients without edema and/or renal insufficiency has been questioned by many authorities. At our institution diuretics are used for the treatment of peripheral edema or renal failure. In such situations diuretic therapy almost always becomes a necessary component of the therapeutic regimen. Blood-glucose and lipid levels should be monitored closely after the start of diuretic therapy. Concomitant use of captopril has been shown to offset the deleterious effect of diuretics on glucose tolerance and serum lipids. Diuretics also have the undesirable side effect of hypokalemia. This can increase peripheral vascular resistance and lead to arrhythmias. Frequent determination of serum electrolyte concentrations and appropriate KCl supplementation can effectively correct this side effect.

The choice of diuretic agents and their recommended dose range are shown in Table 5. When the serum creatinine concentration is greater than 1.8 to 2.0 mg per deciliter, thiazides become ineffective and the more powerful loop diuretics, furosemide and ethacrynic acid, are required to promote a diuresis. Potassium-sparing diuretics (spironolactone, triamterene, amiloride) are not advocated in the diabetic who may have underlying hypoaldosteronism.

Beta-Adrenergic Blockers. Beta-blockers have been shown to effectively reduce blood pressure and improve diabetic nephropathy in a number of clinical trials. However, these agents predispose to hypoglycemia, impair recovery from hypoglycemia, exacerbate hypoglycemic unawareness (especially in patients with autonomic neuropathy), inhibit insulin secretion in NIDDM patients, cause hyperkalemia by impairing extrarenal potassium uptake, exacerbate insulin resistance and hyperinsulinemia, worsen glucose tolerance, and induce adverse changes in the plasma lipid profile. Consequently, beta-adrenergic antagonists are not good "first-line" or even "second-line" drugs for diabetic hyper-tension. Beta-blockers may be warranted in combination with other agents in the diabetic patient with progressive renal insufficiency and severe hypertension that is unresponsive to multiple drug therapy. The hypertensive diabetic with angina also may be treated with beta-blocking agents, but the plasma-glucose and lipid profile should be monitored closely after the institution of such therapy. In the post myocardial infarction

period beta-blockers should be used because they are the only class of drugs that have been shown to decrease mortality from sudden death.

When beta-adrenergic antagonists must be used, selective beta 1 blockers (rather than nonselective beta-1, beta-2

Table 5 Recommended Antihypertensive Agents for Hypertensive Diabetic Patients

DRUG	USUAL DOSAGE RANGE (MG)	SIGNIFICANT SIDE EFFECTS	OTHER CONSIDERATIONS
Angiotensin-converting enzyme inhibitors			
Captopril	25–50 2–3x/day	Rash	Can improve insulin sensitivity, glucose tolerance, and plasma lipid levels. If total daily dose of enalapril and benazepril is ≥20 mg, split into 2 daily doses.
Enalapril	5–40/day	Neutropenia	
Benazepril	20–80/day	Proteinuria	
		Hyperkalemia	
		Fall in GFR	
Ca^{++}-channel antagonists			
Verapamil	40–120 3x/day	Increases serum digoxin level	Long-lasting formulations of these drugs are available. No significant adverse effects on glucose or lipid metabolism are known.
		Negative inotropic effect	
		May cause A-V block	
Diltiazem	30–90 3x/day	Constipation	
		May cause A-V block	
Nicardipine	20–40 3x/day	Peripheral edema	
Nifedipine	10–30 3x/day	Peripheral edema	
Diuretics			
Hydrochlorothiazide	12.5–50/day		Thiazides are not effective when GFR decreases to <40–50 ml/min. Higher doses of furosemide may be required when nephrotic syndrome and/or renal insufficiency are present.
Chlorthiazide	500–200/day	Hyponatremia	
Chlorthalidone	12.5–50/day	Hypokalemia	
Metolazone	2.5–10/day	Glucose intolerance	
Furosemide	20–80/day up to 40–160 2x/day	Increased low-density lipoprotein cholesterol and triglycerides	
Ethacrynic acid	25–100/day up to 50–200 2x/day	Decreased high-density lipoprotein cholesterol	
Bumetanide	0.5–2/day up to 1–4 2x/day	Insulin resistance	
β_1-selective antagonists			
Metoprolol	50–100 2x/day	May cause A-V block	At higher doses, β_1-selectivity is lost; bronchospasm may be precipitated, hypoglycemia may occur, symptoms of hypoglycemia are masked
Atenolol	50–100/day	May exacerbate congestive heart failure	
Central adrenergic antagonists			
Clonidine	0.1–0.6 2x/day	Drowsiness	Rebound hypertension may occur if these drugs are abruptly stopped.
Guanabenz	4–16 2x/day	Dry mouth	
Methyldopa	250–500 3x/day		
Peripheral α_1-antagonists			
Prazosin	1–5 2–3x/day	Orthostatic hypotension	These can improve insulin sensitivity and plasma lipid profile
Terazosin	1–5/day at bedtime	First-dose phenomenon of syncope	
Doxazosin	2–8/day at bedtime		
Vasodilators			
Apresoline	10–50 3–4x/day	Headache	
		Reflex tachycardia	
Minoxidil	5–30 2x/day	Excess hair growth	Minoxidil is very effective in patients with refractory hypertension and renal insufficiency

antagonists such as propranolol, nadolol, timolol, pindolol) are recommended because they have quantitatively less prominent metabolic side effects. The recommended dosages of atenolol and metoprolol are shown in Table 5. At higher doses both of these agents start to lose their beta selectivity.

Vasodilators. If an adequate response to combined therapy with ACE inhibitors, calcium channel blockers, and diuretics is not achieved, a peripheral vasodilator can be added (see Table 5). In diabetic patients with renal failure and severe, refractory hypertension, minoxidil is particularly effective. The major side effect of minoxidil is hair growth.

Adrenergic Antagonists. A number of central adrenergic antagonists (aldomet, clonidine, guanabenz) and peripheral alpha-1 antagonists (prazosin, terazosin, doxazosin) are available for the treatment of hypertension in the diabetic patient (see Table 5 for dosages). The alpha-antagonists have been shown to enhance insulin sensitivity, leading to an improvement in glucose tolerance, and to lower plasma-lipid levels. In several small studies, they also have been shown to reduce microalbuminuria.

Diabetics with clinically overt nephropathy (urine albumin excretion >300 mg per day or serum creatinine >1.8 mg per deciliter) also should strive for good glycemic control (see Table 4). However, there is little evidence that strict glycemic control slows the progression of renal disease at this stage. Intensive insulin therapy in IDDM patients at the macroalbuminemic stage has not been shown to decrease the rate of decline of GFR. Moreover, the risk of hypoglycemia is increased because of decreased insulin clearance, impaired glucose counter-regulation, and hypoglycemic unawareness related to autonomic neuropathy. Diabetic patients with macroalbuminuria and especially those with an elevated serum creatinine concentration often have underlying cardiovascular disease. Therefore, the physician should strive for moderate glycemic control and a glycosylated hemoglobin level less than 8.0 percent. However, such patients frequently have associated diabetic retinopathy that usually progresses as the renal disease advances. Consequently reasonable glycemic control still remains a cornerstone of therapy.

■ TREATMENT OF MICROALBUMINURIA WITHOUT HYPERTENSION

Tight glycemic control and modest protein restriction should be instituted as described in the previous section on the treatment of microalbuminuria (see Table 4). Which antihypertensive agent to use and how the dosage should be adjusted needs amplification.

In IDDM and NIDDM individuals with microalbuminuria (30 to 300 mg per day) and a normal blood pressure, the natural history of progression to overt albuminuria and eventual impairment of renal function is no different than that in microalbuminuric patients with hypertension. Therefore, aggressive treatment with a drug that has a specific renal protective effect is indicated. Only two classes of antihypertensive drugs, the ACE inhibitors and the calcium channel blockers, have been shown to specifically reverse the hemodynamic alterations (i.e., increased intraglomerular

pressure) that characterize diabetic nephropathy in both IDDM and NIDDM. Because the greatest amount of data has been accumulated with the ACE inhibitors and because this class of drugs improves insulin sensitivity, glucose tolerance, and dyslipidemia, the ACE inhibitors are the preferred drugs of choice. If cough, hyperkalemia, or deterioration in renal function are a problem, a calcium channel blocker can be substituted.

Captopril and enalapril have been most extensively studied in the treatment of microalbuminuria and their use will be described to illustrate the general approach. Once microalbuminuria has been documented, the patient should be started on a low dose of captopril (12.5 mg three times a day) or enalapril (5 mg per day). The patient should return in 4 to 8 weeks for a repeat determination of microalbuminuria. If no microalbuminuria is present, the dose of the ACE inhibitor should be held constant and the patient should be asked to return in 6 months and yearly thereafter if no microalbuminuria is detected.

If microalbuminuria is present in unchanged or decreased amount on the return visit, the dose of captopril (25 mg three times a day) or enalapril (10 mg every day) should be doubled and a repeat determination of microalbuminuria should be performed in 4 to 8 weeks. This procedure should be repeated every 4 to 8 weeks and the dose of captopril or enalapril increased by 12.5 mg three times a day or 5 mg every until the microalbuminuria disappears completely or decreases, but remains stable in three consecutive urine determinations, or until side effects of the medication are encountered.

■ TREATMENT OF DIABETICS WITH OVERT ALBUMINURIA OR RENAL INSUFFICIENCY

Glycemic Control

In diabetic patients with clinical proteinuria (AER >300 mg per day), and especially in those with established renal insufficiency, tight glycemic control has not been shown to slow the progression of renal disease. Moreover, patients with renal insufficiency are extremely difficult to control and hypoglycemic episodes are not infrequent. Therefore, less stringent glycemic control is recommended. However, it must be remembered that such patients remain at high risk to develop diabetic retinopathy. Therefore, good control is still advocated in diabetic patients with renal insufficiency, but the physician must be especially cognizant of the increased risk of hypoglycemia. Some caution should be interjected about diabetic patients with only modest levels of clinically overt albuminuria (300 to 500 mg per day), because it is unknown precisely at what level of albuminuria tight glycemic control ceases to be effective in preventing and/or slowing the progression of diabetic nephropathy. Because some of these patients with low levels of clinical albuminuria (300 to 500 mg per day) may well benefit from normalization or near normalization of the blood-glucose level, tight glycemic control probably should be pursued in this group as well. A reasonable goal in diabetic patients with urinary albumin excretion rate above 500 mg per day with or without renal insufficiency is to maintain the HbA_{1c} below 80 percent and the fasting glucose at approximately 140 mg per deciliter.

Antihypertensive Therapy

The general approach, goals of therapy, and choice of antihypertensive agents are essentially the same as described earlier in diabetic patients without renal insufficiency and overt albuminuria (Table 5). In many patients the blood pressure will be normalized, yet significant albuminuria will persist. In such individuals the ACE inhibitor or calcium channel blocker should be progressively increased until the albuminuria has disappeared or has declined significantly but has remained stable despite escalation of the dose of antihypertensive medication, or until hypotension or other side effects limit additional dose increases.

Protein Restriction

The therapeutic approach and benefits of dietary protein restriction in slowing the decline in renal function in patients with overt albuminuria and renal insufficiency are similar to those described earlier. However, a large multicenter trial sponsored by the National Institutes of Health failed to demonstrate any benefit of a low-protein diet (0.58 g per kilogram) to slow the decline in renal function over a 36-month follow-up period in patients with renal failure secondary to diabetes (3 percent of the total group) or to nondiabetic causes (97 percent of the total group). The failure of this study to demonstrate any benefit of a low-protein diet on preservation of renal function stands in contrast to previously published studies with much smaller numbers of patients. It is likely that any beneficial effect of the low-protein diet in this large prospective study was obscured by the concomitant use of antihypertensive medications, which were taken by 80 percent of the participants. In particular, 44 percent of the study patients were taking an ACE inhibitor, and this class of drugs has been shown to have a specific renal protective effect in diabetic patients (see previous discussion). Based on these results, it seems prudent to recommend only modest protein restriction (0.9 to 1.0 g per kilogram per day) in diabetic subjects who are taking an ACE inhibitor, while reserving more severe protein restriction (0.6 g per kilogram per day) to patients who are not receiving any antihypertensive medications.

Lastly, all diabetic patients with hypertension and overt albuminuria (>300 mg per day) and/or renal insufficiency (serum creatinine >1.6 to 1.8 mg per deciliter) should be referred to a nephrologist or a diabetes specialist who has expertise in treating diabetic nephropathy. If the patient's blood pressure fails to normalize using the above approach or if evidence of hypertensive organ system damage (i.e., retinopathy, congestive heart failure, nephropathy) is present,

referral to a nephrologist or diabetes specialist is indicated. Accelerated or malignant hypertension is cause for immediate referral and hospitalization for parenteral antihypertensive treatment.

■ MONITORING RENAL FUNCTION

In IDDM patients without microalbuminuria or overt albuminuria and normal renal function at the time of initial diagnosis, a repeat determination for microalbuminuria and creatinine clearance should be performed yearly starting 5 years after the diagnosis, because microalbuminuria and renal dysfunction are rare within the first 5 years of diabetes (Table 6). In NIDDM patients without microalbuminuria, a repeat determination for microalbuminuria and creatinine clearance should be performed yearly, because most of these individuals will have had their disease for many years prior to initial diagnosis.

In diabetic patients with microalbuminuria, overt albuminuria, or renal insufficiency, serum creatinine, urea nitrogen, and electrolyte concentrations and 24-hour urine creatinine and protein-albumin excretion rates should be obtained every 6 months or more frequently if indicated.

■ URINARY TRACT INFECTION

Infection of the urinary tract is common in diabetic patients, especially women, and unusual gram negative organisms and Candida are not uncommon. The urine should be examined on every visit to the physician's office and, if white blood cells are noted, a culture should be obtained. Prompt and appropriate antibiotic therapy should be instituted based on known sensitivities of the organism. Hyperglycemia interferes with a variety of white blood cell functions possibly making irradiation of the infection difficult. Therefore, tightened glycemic control is indicated.

■ NEUROGENIC BLADDER

Neurogenic involvement of the bladder can cause urinary tract obstruction and a rapid, irreversible decline in renal function if it is not recognized and treated. The suspicion of neurogenic bladder should be heightened in patients with peripheral neuropathy and especially in those with other man-

Table 6 Monitoring Renal Function in Postpubertal Patients		
TEST	**INITIAL EVALUATION**	**FOLLOW-UP***
Urinary microalbuminuria (timed collection)		
Creatinine clearance	After initial glycemic control and within 3 months of diagnosis	Type 1 diabetes: yearly after 5 yr / Type 2 diabetes: yearly from time of diagnosis
Serum creatinine		

*More frequent evaluation is indicated in diabetic patients with a creatinine clearance <70 to 80 ml/min or serum creatinine 1.5 to 1.6 mg/dl.

ifestations of autonomic dysfunction. Clinical symptoms include a weak urinary stream, frequent voiding of small amounts of urine, loss of sensation of bladder fullness, and recurrent urinary tract infections. The diagnosis can be made by the finding of a large post void residual (>150 ml) following bladder catheterization and confirmed by a cystometrogram that reveals a large, atonic bladder with decreased force of contraction following distension with sterile water. Patients with neurogenic bladder should be instructed in the manual Crede voiding maneuver and should empty their bladder every 8 hours. If this conservative measure proves ineffective, urecholine (10 to 15 mg orally, three times a day) or phenoxybenzamine (10 to 40 mg orally, three times a day) can be tried.

■ PAPILLARY NECROSIS

Impaired blood flow to the medullary tissues can lead to anoxic damage and eventually necrosis of the papilla. If the papilla sloughs, it can obstruct the renal pelvis and the patient will present with flank pain and a clinical picture similar to that observed with a renal calculus. Hematuria will be pres-ent. The diagnosis can be established with a renal ultrasound study or intravenous pyelography if necessary. If the patient is afebrile and does not appear toxic, symptomatic treatment with analgesics and hydration usually is sufficient for the papilla to be passed. If, however, the obstruction persists, and, especially if there is accompanying infection, antibiotic therapy and surgical intervention may be necessary.

■ HYPERKALEMIA

Hyperkalemia is common in diabetic patients with nephropathy and can result from disturbances in both extrarenal and renal potassium metabolism. Insulin, aldosterone, and epinephrine all enhance potassium uptake by extrarenal tissues and these hormones often are deficient. In addition, the hypertonicity that occurs secondary to hyperglycemia will cause a shift of potassium from intracellular to extracellular environment. Concomitant metabolic acidosis, either secondary to aldosterone deficiency or chronic renal failure, will exacerbate the hyperkalemia as hydrogen ions move into cells to be buffered in exchange for potassium. Diabetic patients with nephropathy often have the syndrome of hypoaldosteronism, which impairs renal potassium excretion. The deficiency in aldosterone will be magnified if concomitant renal failure is present and tubular mass is reduced sufficiently to impair potassium secretion. Metabolic acidosis also impairs renal tubular potassium secretion.

Treatment of hyperkalemia involves redistribution of potassium into cells and augmentation of urinary potassium excretion. The insulin regimen should be optimized to restore normoglycemia. This will redistribute potassium back into cells and in some patients may improve the defect in aldosterone secretion. Metabolic acidosis should be corrected with sodium bicarbonate, 1.8 to 4.8 g per day (or 24 to 64 mEq per day). The maintenance dose can be adjusted empirically depending on the change in plasma bicarbonate concentration. Correction of acidosis will redistribute

potassium into cells and relieve the inhibition of renal potassium secretion. In patients with hypoaldosteronism renal tubular potassium secretion becomes critically dependent on sodium and fluid delivery to the distal nephron segments. Therefore, an adequate intake of salt and water should be administered to maintain renal perfusion and GFR. Dietary potassium intake should be reduced to less than 60 mEq of potassium per day. In most patients these conservative measures will be sufficient to restore normokalemia. If significant hyperkalemia ($\geq$ 6.0 mEq per liter) persists and especially if there are electrocardiographic or neuromuscular signs of hyperkalemia, institution of Florinef, 0.1 to 0.2 mg per day, should be considered. In many patients with hyperkalemia secondary to hypoaldosteronism the renal tubular cell is refractory to Florinef and higher doses may be required. Sodium retention and congestive heart failure are a problem with these higher doses and the risks may outweigh the benefit of therapy. In such cases the Florinef should be discontinued and more severe dietary potassium restriction instituted. In some patients it may be necessary to continue the Florinef and start diuretic therapy to prevent sodium retention. Drugs that predispose to the development of hypoaldosteronism (nonsteroidal anti-inflammatory agents, ACE inhibitors, beta-adrenergic blockers, heparin) or inhibit renal tubular potassium secretion (spironolactone, triamterene, amiloride) should be avoided in the hyperkalemic patient.

SUGGESTED READING

Bressler R, DeFronzo RA. Drugs and Diabetes. Diabetes Rev 1994; 2:53–84.

Exhaustive review of the adverse effects of drugs on carbohydrate and lipid metabolism in diabetic individuals

Castellino P, Shohat J, DeFronzo RA. Hyperfiltration and diabetic nephropathy: Is it the beginning? Or is it the end? Sem Nephrol 1990; 10:228–253.

Critical examination of the contribution of increased intraglomerular pressure and glomerular hyperfiltration in the pathogenesis of diabetic nephropathy.

DeFronzo RA. Diabetic nephropathy: etiologic and therapeutic considerations. Diabetes Rev 1995; 3:510–565.

Exhaustive review of the etiology, clinical manifestations, and therapy of renal disease in type 1 and type 2 diabetic patients.

Feldt-Rasmussen B, Borch-Johnsen K, Decker T, et al. Microalbuminuria: an important diagnostic tool. J Diabetic Comp 1994; 8:137–145.

Excellent review of usefulness of microalbuminuria in the early identification and treatment of diabetic patients at risk to develop renal disease.

Klahr S, Levey AS, Beck GJ, et al. The effects of dietary protein restriction and blood-pressure control on the progression of chronic renal disease. N Engl J Med 1994; 330:877–884.

Large, NIH-sponsored trial demonstrating the failure of a low-protein diet to slow the progression of diabetic nephropathy. The lack of efficacy of a low-protein diet in this widely quoted publication most likely results from the inclusion of patients who already were being treated with an angiotensin-converting enzyme inhibitor or a calcium channel blocker.

Klein R. Hyperglycemia and microvascular and macrovascular disease in diabetes. Diabetes Care 1995; 18:258–268.

Comprehensive review of the central role of hyperglycemia in the development of microvascular (kidney and eye) and macrovascular complications in patients with long-standing diabetes mellitus.

Lewis EJ, Hunsicker LG, Bain RP, Rohde RD. The effect of angiotensin-converting-enzyme inhibition on diabetic nephropathy. N Engl J Med 1993; 329:1456–1462.

Well-designed, large, double-blind, prospective study documenting the efficacy of angiotensin-converting enzyme inhibitors in slowing the progression of diabetic nephropathy.

Mogensen CE, Poulsen PL. Epidemiology of microalbuminuria in diabetes and in the background population. Curr Opin Nephrol Hypertens 1994; 3:248–256.

Summary of epidemiologic studies examining the prevalence of microalbuminuria in the patients with diabetes mellitus and in the general population. The importance of microalbuminuria as a predictor of both macrovascular and microvascular complications is emphasized.

Ohkubo Y, Kishikawa H, Araki E, et al. Intensive insulin therapy prevents the progression of diabetic microvascular complications in Japanese patients with non–insulin-dependent diabetes mellitus: A randomized prospective 6-year study. Diab Res Clin Pract 1995; 28:103–117.

Companion study to the DCCT, demonstrating that tight glycemic control with insulin prevents microvascular complications in type 2 non–insulin-dependent diabetic patients.

Ravid M, Savin H, Jutrin I, et al. Long-term stabilizing effect of angiotensin-converting enzyme inhibition on plasma creatinine and on proteinuria in normotensive type II diabetic patients. Ann Intern Med 1993; 118:577–581.

Five-year prospective, double-blind, randomized trial establishing the efficacy of angiotensin-converting enzyme inhibitors in preventing diabetic nephropathy in type 2 diabetic patients.

Wang PH, Lau J, Chalmers TC. Meta-analysis of effects of intensive blood-glucose control on late complications of type I diabetes. Lancet 1993; 341:1306–1309.

Meta-analysis of all published studies that have examined the benefit of improved glycemic control in the prevention of diabetic microvascular complications. This combined analysis provides overwhelming support for the important role of glycemic control in decreasing the incidence of diabetic microvascular complications.

DIABETIC NEPHROPATHY: END-STAGE

Mariana S. Markell, M.D.
Eli A. Friedman, M.D.

Diabetic nephropathy is the leading cause of end-stage renal failure in the United States, and the number of patients with diagnosed diabetic nephropathy will continue to rise until appropriate preventive interventions are instituted on a regular basis. End-stage renal disease (ESRD) is the last stage of renal malfunction in diabetes and follows sequential glomerular hyperfiltration, progression to microalbuminuria, and then macroproteinuria, and eventually a relentless decline in the glomerular filtration rate. The sequence of signs and progression of renal disease is similar in patients with type 1 insulin-dependent diabetes mellitus (IDDM) and type 2 non–insulin-dependent diabetes mellitus (NIDDM), although, in the latter case, patients typically are older and may have pre-existent hypertension or systemic atherosclerosis that contributes to kidney damage and accelerates the course of the disease.

In the 30 to 40 percent of IDDM patients who eventually develop proteinuria—duration of diabetes correlates with development of ESRD—with an average latency of 15 to 20 years. In NIDDM patients, the duration also correlates with the development of renal failure. However, the prevalence of ESRD is more variable in NIDDM, ranging from a low of approximately 5 percent in Caucasians to over 50 percent in certain American Indian tribes.

Many factors have been implicated in the progression of diabetic nephropathy. Persistent hyperglycemia, protein glycosylation, systemic hypertension, and intraglomerular hypertension caused by increased sensitivity of the efferent arteriole to angiotensin II, all have been shown to contribute to the progressive glomerular injury.

■ PREPARATION FOR UREMIA THERAPY

Time of Discussion with Patient

The issue of renal replacement therapy should be addressed at the initial detection of macroalbuminuria (> 300 to 500 mg of albumin per day), despite the fact that patients may not require dialysis or transplantation for many years. This gives the patient time to learn about his or her options and come to terms with the reality that at some time in the future he or she will have to make a decision regarding choice of therapy.

Therapeutic Options

Options for renal replacement therapy include hemodialysis (in-center or at-home), continuous ambulatory peritoneal dialysis (CAPD), kidney or kidney-plus-pancreas transplantation, or the decision to forego renal replacement therapy altogether. The pros and cons for each of these therapeutic options are outlined in Table 1. We use a nurse-educator, familiar with each of these choices, to ensure that patients are well educated prior to making a decision. In addition, booklets that discuss options for the treatment of ESRD are available from the National Kidney Foundation and are very useful in patient education.

Institution of Dialysis

Once a patient has decided which option he or she wishes to pursue, appropriate preparatory steps are taken (Table 2). The decision to initiate dialytic therapy in a patient with diabetes may be difficult to time because the complications of diabetes may mimic symptoms that usually are used to gauge the degree of uremia. Gastroparesis can cause nausea and vomiting, poor glucose control may contribute to fatigue, and heart failure may promote the appearance of volume overload. Most ESRD patients with diabetes require dialysis with a higher level of residual renal function than patients with other forms of renal disease. Because diabetic patients generally become sicker with multiple organ-system involvement at a lower serum creatinine value than nondiabetic individuals, we usually initiate dialysis when the creatinine clearance falls to approximately 20 ml per minute or the serum creatinine reaches 5 to 6 mg per deciliter, depending on the patient's muscle mass. It is important to intervene with dialysis before the onset of weight loss from anorexia and hypercatabolism, before the development of fluid overload and

refractory hypertension, and before a general loss of energy occurs. Once such complications begin, there is a rapid deterioration in organ system function that may be difficult to reverse. It is especially important to initiate dialysis before the onset of significant retinopathy or neuropathy, because complications are markedly worsened by the uremic state.

Surgical Referral for Vascular Access

If the patient has chosen hemodialysis, we refer him or her to a vascular surgeon for placement of an arteriovenous fistula or prosthetic graft in the nondominant arm. A native arteriovenous fistula is preferred, because of the lower incidence of infection or thrombosis. Patients with longstanding diabetes, however, often have calcification or atherosclerosis of the arterial tree, and a fistula can not be created, or does not induce sufficient venous dilation to allow adequate dialysis. This necessitates the placement of a Teflon vascular graft. Occasionally patients with subclinical peripheral vascular disease develop a "steal" syndrome following the placement of hemodialysis access in the forearm because arterial blood is shunted from the hand. This syndrome presents with pain, coolness, and muscle weakness of the affected extremity, and if severe enough, may lead to digital gangrene requiring amputation of fingers and occasionally the hand. In many patients this complication can be corrected by tying off the artery distal to the fistula, whereas in some patients closure of the fistula or removal of the graft is required.

Initiation of Dialysis

Following creation of an arteriovenous fistula, it is preferable to wait at least 5 to 6 weeks before its first use. With a prosthetic graft, the access can be used as early as 2 weeks postplacement. However, it is best to wait at least 4 weeks

---

Table 1 Comparison of End-Stage Renal Disease Therapy Options for Patients with Diabetes

	RENAL TRANSPLANT	CAPD	HEMODIALYSIS
ADVANTAGES	1. Greater independence from treatment facility 2. Best rehabilitation 3. Patient survival often > 10 yr	1. Major surgery not required 2. Minimizes "volume" shifts (good control of hypo- and hypertension) 3. Intraperitoneal insulin administration may improve metabolic control 4. Technique can be taught rapidly 5. No requirement for vascular access	1. Major surgery not required 2. Patients with type 2 diabetes have survived > 10 yr 3. Rehabilitation improved since introduction of erythropoietin
DISADVANTAGES	1. Steroids complicate metabolic control 2. Cyclosporine exacerbates hypertension and hyperlipidemia 3. Infection risk 4. Does not prevent recurrent diabetic nephropathy or "cure" other diabetic complications 5. Risk of diabetes in HLA-identical sibling donor 6. Cannot be performed in patients with severe cardiovascular disease or chronic infection	1. High technique failure rate and mortality 2. High peritonitis rate 3. Risk of patient "burn out" because of repetitive nature or technique 4. Diabetic complications progress	1. Requires a committed partner (home hemodialysis) 2. About 30% of patients experience gradual unexplained deterioration 3. Other complications of diabetes progress 4. Requires vascular access

CAPD = continuous ambulatory peritoneal dialysis.

because wound healing often is delayed in the uremic diabetic. Premature use of either type of access can lead to hematoma complicated by graft thrombosis and/or infection. If emergency hemodialysis is required, a subclavian or internal jugular catheter should be placed using a semipermanent type of double-lumen catheter to minimize blood-vessel injury and subsequent subclavian stenosis. If a flexible catheter cannot be placed, femoral vein cannulation can be performed. However, we prefer to avoid this approach, because inadvertent arterial puncture or groin infection at the puncture site are potentially disastrous in a patient with longstanding diabetes and peripheral vascular disease.

For patients who elect CAPD, a peritoneal catheter is placed transcutaneously into the peritoneal cavity by surgeons in the operating room. We allow at least 2 weeks to elapse prior to initiation of training for CAPD and utilization of the catheter, in order for ingrowth of fibroblasts into the cuff to occur. This lessens the chance of leakage of peritoneal fluid once treatment is initiated.

Renal Transplantation

If the patient elects kidney transplantation, we encourage him or her to approach family members for donation, because of the severe organ shortage, which may result in very long waiting times for cadaveric renal transplantation and also because the best results in diabetic patients, both for graft and patient survival, have been reported following living related donation. The pretransplant work-up should be begun at approximately the same time the patient is referred for vascular access surgery. However, if a donor is identified, the transplant should be performed prior to the development of uremic symptoms.

Cardiovascular Evaluation

In addition to our standard requirements for pretransplant screening (Table 3), we also require all patients with diabetes who are older than 30 years of age to undergo evaluation by a cardiologist because of the very high incidence of coronary artery disease in this group. The work-up should include stress testing with follow-up angiography if indicated. We have found it prudent to intervene either with angioplasty or with revascularization procedures, both coronary and peripheral bypass surgeries, prior to the stress of transplantation.

Kidney versus Kidney-Pancreas Transplantation

In type 1 diabetic patients, it is important for the physician to consider whether the person is a candidate for combined kidney-pancreas transplant. Most transplant centers do not perform isolated pancreas transplantation. The advantages afforded by pancreatic-kidney transplantation include freedom from or markedly decreased insulin requirement, better glucose control, especially for patients whose blood sugar have been labile due to gastroparesis, unpredictable gastric emptying, and slight relaxation of dietary restriction. The disadvantages include increased technical difficulty of the surgery, a higher surgical complication rate, and the theoretical risk of hyperinsulinemia, because the insulin is secreted directly into the systemic circulation if the pancreas is positioned to empty into the bladder.

Table 2 Preparation for Uremia Therapy

PATIENT EDUCATION
  Nurse educator
  Literature
  Tour of hemodialysis, CAPD, and transplant units
  Discussions with patients
CHOICE OF THERAPY
  Dialysis
    Initiation of phosphate-lowering therapy
    Referral for vascular-access surgery or peritoneal catheter
      placement
    Follow-up teaching
      Access care
      Nutritional counseling
      Blood-glucose monitoring
    Initiation of erythropoietin therapy if Hct < 30%
    Alteration of insulin or oral hypoglycemic doses
  Transplantation (see Table 3)
    Living related donor
    Tissue typing of prospective donors
    Anti-islet cell antibodies and glucose tolerance test in HLA
      identical type 1 siblings
    Cadaveric: kidney alone and pancreas-kidney
    Preparation with dialysis while awaiting organ

■ INITIATION OF DIALYTIC THERAPY

Protein, Phosphorus, and Calcium Metabolism

Prior to initiation of dialysis, dietary protein usually is restricted to 0.6 to 0.8 g per kilogram per day. After dialysis has been started, dietary protein intake can be increased to 1 to 1.5 g per kilogram per day, with increased amounts allowed for patients on CAPD because of protein loss into the dialysate. If the patient remains nephrotic or has a serum albumin less than 3.2 mg per deciliter, protein should not be restricted. All patients are placed on a 2 g sodium, 2 g potassium diet, with restriction of phosphorus. Calcium carbonate, at least 500 mg, or calcium acetate (667 mg), two or three tablets with or after each meal, for phosphate binding is indicated if the serum phosphate is about 5 mg or more per deciliter. If the serum phosphate concentration remains high, or if the calcium-phosphate product is greater than 70, we use aluminum-containing antacids. However, prolonged use of these agents is associated with aluminum deposition in bone that can exacerbate dialysis-related bone diseases.

We attempt to maintain a corrected serum calcium concentration of 9.5 to 10.5 mg per deciliter, because this level is associated with lowered risk of hyperparathyroidism and osteitis fibrosa cystica. Vitamin D preparations, initially oral dihydrocholecalciferol (0.25 to 1.0 mg per day), are given if the serum calcium level cannot be maintained by oral calcium supplementation alone. Once a patient begins hemodialysis, he or she can be placed on the intravenous form of vitamin D.

Anemia

All predialysis patients should be screened for iron deficiency and, if detected, they should receive appropriate replacement. Our preference is to use Niferex Forte 1 capsule twice

Table 3 Pretransplant Work-up; Specific Considerations for Diabetic Patients are Highlighted

ALL PATIENTS	SPECIAL CONSIDERATIONS
Medical summary (including family history) and physical exam	History of cancer: cancer-free for 5 years or more
Social work summary: citizenship status, support systems, financial status, psychosocial evaluation, patient's expectations of transplant, if blind or handicapped: who will assist with medications	History of stroke or transient ischemic attack: neurologic evaluation including Doppler studies of carotid arteries
Recent chest radiograph (within 6 months) and PPD status	History of cardiac disease, diabetes (age > 30 yr) or all patients over age 60 years: cardiologic evaluation including echocardiogram if indicated by heart murmur, stress test (thallium or persantine), cardiac catheterization if indicated.
Current laboratory values and hepatitis serologies	Anuria, male patient with obstructive symptoms or history of diabetes: voiding cystourethrogram and urologic evaluation
HIV and cytomegalovirus testing	History of peripheral vascular disease or claudication: Doppler flow studies of lower extremities
Recent electrocardiogram (within 6 months)	
Recent Pap smear and mammography, if performed	
Recent dental exam	

PPD = Purified protein derivative.

a day, which is a polysaccharide iron complex supplemented with folate and vitamin B_{12}. If the hematocrit remains below 30 volume percent, patients should be given human recombinant erythropoietin by means of subcutaneous injection. The starting dose is 4,000 U twice or thrice weekly, and the dose should be tapered as the hematocrit rises above 33 volume percent. Hematocrit levels above 38 volume percent should be avoided because of increased viscosity, seizures, and accelerated hypertension. Once the patient is started on hemodialysis, the erythropoietin and iron dextran can be administered intravenously if necessary. For patients on CAPD, the subcutaneous route is continued.

Nurse Educator

The nurse educator is an integral part of of the ESRD management team. It is essential that the uremia specialist, who educates the patients about the choice of ESRD therapy, continues to offer support to the patient who is approaching dialysis. Instruction about the care of the hemodialysis access and what to expect of the dialytic process should be provided, and tours of the dialysis unit or the CAPD training area, as well as interaction with patients who are undergoing treatment, should be included.

We also use another nurse educator, who is a diabetes specialist, to aid in adjustment of insulin or oral hypoglycemic medications as renal failure progresses. Degradation of insulin is in part dependent upon the kidney and in part upon the liver. Decreased renal mass directly impairs insulin degradation, while uremia impairs hepatic catabolism of insulin. As renal function worsens, insulin degradation becomes progressively impaired and hypoglycemia is not uncommon. In CAPD patients who are receiving glucose through their peritoneal dialysis fluid, insulin doses must be adjusted accordingly.

Monitoring Other Diabetic Complications

It is important to closely monitor diabetic complications that affect other organ systems while preparing a patient for renal replacement therapy. Complications arising from peripheral neuropathy, retinopathy, or foot infection may delay later rehabilitation or curtail the choice of renal replacement therapy. Therefore, regular podiatric and ophthalmologic care is extremely important.

■ HEMODIALYSIS

Efficacy

During hemodialysis, diabetes creates difficulties that are not encountered in nondiabetic patients and the dialysis prescription and follow-up of the patient with diabetes must be altered to avoid these problems (Table 4). Autonomic neuropathy complicates performance of standard hemodialysis because of recurrent hypotension. Early hypotension within the first hour of dialysis treatment usually reflects autonomic neuropathy, not intravascular volume depletion. Absence of reflex tachycardia or venoconstriction further complicate the dialysis procedure in the neuropathic patient. This problem is exacerbated in patients treated with beta-blockers or calcium channel blockers, which affect the sino-atrial node, and such agents should be avoided in diabetic hemodialysis patients, if possible. Late hypotension following vigorous ultrafiltration usually reflects intravascular volume depletion, but this may also be accentuated by abnormal counterregulatory reflexes.

Because acetate dialysate buffer has been associated with myocardial depression, peripheral vasodilatation, and worsening of hypotension, bicarbonate dialysate buffer is preferred for patients with diabetes. Some patients require dialysis against a "high conductivity" bath (with a sodium concentration between 140 and 144 mEq per deciliter) to help reduce the number and severity of hypotensive episodes, especially in the early dialytic period. Patients treated in this fashion, however, often become thirsty during the interdialytic interval and may develop volume overload prior to their next treatment. Newer dialysis machines allow for "sodium modeling," which allows initiation of dialysis at a high conductivity (150 mEq per deciliter) and slow decrease to "normal" conductivity during the last half hour of treatment

Hypotensive episodes may lead to shortened dialysis time and necessitate frequent volume replacement resulting in a chronically underdialyzed, hypertensive, volume-overloaded

Table 4 Special Considerations for Hemodialysis Treatment of Patients with Diabetes

DIALYSIS PRESCRIPTION
Bicarbonate dialysate (avoidance of acetate)
Minimal heparinization
Increased conductivity or "sodium modeling" for recurrent hypotension
Maintenance of hematocrit > 30 vol% if possible
Scrupulous access care
Close attention to indicators of dialysis efficiency
Avoidance of drugs which interfere with reflex response to hypotension (beta-blockers, verapamil)
ROUTINE FOLLOW-UP
Ophthalmologic evaluation at 6-month intervals
Podiatric evaluation monthly
Lipid profile with nutritional counseling twice yearly
Evaluation of glycosylated hemoglobin monthly

patient. The problems associated with establishing vascular access for hemodialysis and the tendency of patients with autonomic neuropathy to develop repetitive bouts of intradialytic hypotension decrease dialysis efficiency and increase the diabetic patient's risk for insidiously progressive underdialysis. This may eventuate in wasting syndromes and "failure to thrive." Dialytic efficiency should be monitored by measuring pre- to post-dialysis differences in BUN (urea reduction ratio, which ideally should be greater than 65 to 70 percent) and creatinine concentrations or KT/V (in which K is the dialyzer clearance, T is the duration of dialysis, and V is the urea space) on a monthly basis.

Atherosclerosis and Lipids

Atherosclerotic disease accounts for the majority of deaths in diabetic hemodialysis patients. Pre-existent hypercholesterolemia may remit following initiation of dialytic therapy. However, hypertriglyceridemia often worsens and becomes refractory to treatment. The recommended diet for patients with hypertriglyceridemia is calorie-fat restriction, but for the diabetic patient with renal disease who already must restrict protein, simple sugars, potassium, sodium, and phosphorus, these added restriction leave very little to eat. Lipid-lowering agents, such as gemfibrozil, are effective in treating hypertriglyceridemia in dialysis patients. In patients with hypercholesterolemia one of the HMG CoA reductase inhibitors is indicated. Long-term compliance with bile acid resins usually is poor. Glycosylated hemoglobin concentration (HbA$_{1c}$) should be determined every 2 to 3 months. If the HbA$_{1c}$ is grossly elevated, the patient's insulin or oral hypoglycemia regimen should be re-evaluated.

Infection

Infectious complications commonly are encountered in diabetic hemodialysis patients. Sepsis may result from either an infected indwelling subclavian-internal jugular catheter or prosthetic vascular graft or from any of the other usual sites of infection seen in nondiabetic individuals. Sepsis from an infected arteriovenous fistula is unusual. When infection occurs, the outcome is often poor, because hyperglycemia coupled with uremia impairs wound healing and the immune response.

Retinopathy

Retinopathy in uremic diabetic patients often progresses rapidly, regardless of the type of renal replacement. The exception is combined kidney-pancreas transplant where the pancreatic graft functions well and establishes normal-or near-normal glycemia. Repeated heparinization is considered to be an exacerbating factor for retinopathy in hemodialysis patients, especially those with pre-existent vitreous hemorrhage. Over-heparinization can be avoided by closely following activated clotting times and using highly biocompatible dialysis membranes. Poor blood glucose and blood-pressure control contribute to retinopathy as well. Ophthalmologic follow-up should be obtained at least every 6 months.

Rehabilitation

Rehabilitation of hemodialysis patients with diabetes remains poor. Most patients are able to perform only the most routine of self-care tasks. Physical therapy may help some patients, but often the course is progressively downhill after a patient with diabetes starts on hemodialysis. The introduction of recombinant human erythropoietin has significantly improved the quality of life for diabetic ESRD patients.

■ CAPD

CAPD involves the instillation and later removal of osmotically active dialysate into the peritoneal cavity 3 to 5 times each day. The advantages and disadvantages of the technique are outlined in Table 1. We refer patients for CAPD who are motivated, have a history of compliance with medical therapy, understand the technique, and comply with strict aseptic techniques. In addition, there is a subset of patients who cannot tolerate hemodialysis because of medical conditions, including patients in whom hemodialysis vascular access cannot be created, patients with intractable hypotension, and individuals with severe cardiac disease. Patients who are not candidates for CAPD include those with recurrent peritonitis and those with severe visual impairment or physical disability that limits dexterity. The latter problems present insurmountable obstacles if there is no person at home to serve as a helper.

For CAPD patients with diabetes, we recommend the addition of insulin directly into the peritoneal dialysate solution. Intraperitoneal insulin delivery allows for a continuous basal rate of absorption of insulin into the portal circulation and often improves diabetic control. Intraperitoneal Regular insulin dosage is determined by calculating the total insulin dose (Regular plus NPH), which the patient takes subcutaneously and dividing by the number of exchanges that the patient will make each day. Thus, if a patient takes a total of 40 U of insulin and will make four exchanges each day, his intraperitoneal insulin dose will be 10 U per exchange. The osmotically active solute in peritoneal dialysis solution is 1.5 percent glucose. Patients who must remove excess fluid may require dialysate glucose concentrations as high as 4.25 percent. This will result in hyperglycemia if the insulin dose is not approximately adjusted. Patients should measure their blood-glucose concentration at the mid point of each dialysis period (fluid in abdomen) and adjust the amount of intraperitoneal insulin accordingly. If their blood glucose is greater than 200 mg per deciliter, they will require subcutaneous insulin as well. We also follow glycosylated hemoglobin levels every 2 to 3 months in CAPD patients as a guide for prescribing more or less insulin.

Although CAPD affords several advantages to the patient with diabetes, the technique is associated with a high rate of recurrent infectious complications, including peritonitis or "tunnel" (catheter) infection, which poses a risk of systemic sepsis. If turbid dialysis outflow fluid and/or abdominal pain occur, patients should save the bag of dialysate for culture and perform the next exchange with a new bag of dialysate into which 1 g of vancomycin has been instilled. The patient is then evaluated at the CAPD unit as soon as possible. Often no other therapy is required, as staphylococcal and streptococcal species are the most common causative agents.

Other problems encountered in the diabetic CAPD patient (Table 4) include progressive reduction in dialytic efficiency due to decreased peritoneal surface exchange area after repeated peritoneal infection and patient "burn-out" following years of 3 to 5 daily exchanges of peritoneal solution. These problems require transfer to hemodialysis or renal transplantation. Because of the high-glucose load, hyperlipidemia, primarily hypertriglyceridemia, is common in the CAPD patients with diabetes, and should be treated with gemfibrozil.

Rehabilitation of CAPD patients is similar to that of patients on hemodialysis, and includes physical therapy if indicated.

■ TRANSPLANTATION

Living-related transplantation is the therapy of choice for the diabetic patient with ESRD, unless the patient has serious chronic infection or intractable cardiac disease. All HLA-identical sibling donors should be screened for anti-islet cell antibodies and undergo intravenous glucose tolerance testing prior to kidney donation. If results of either test are abnormal, kidney donation is not advisable.

The initial immunosuppression regimen for cadaveric transplantation may include standard triple therapy with methylprednisolone/prednisone, azathioprine, and anti-lymphocyte globulin, followed by introduction of cyclosporin A when renal function is stablized, or substitution of the newer antimetabolite mycophenolate mofetil for azathioprine. Cyclosporine is tapered over the ensuing 6 months to achieve a blood level of 100 to 200 mg per milliliter or a total dose of 4 to 6 mg per kilogram. The "Neoral" preparation, which is a liposomal preparation, may be preferable in diabetics, as absorption is enhanced. If azathioprine is used, it is tapered to achieve a final dose of 0.5 to 1.0 mg per kilogram, unless the patient develops evidence of hepatotoxicity or bone-marrow suppression. Prednisone is tapered to achieve a final dose of 5 to 10 mg per day by 6 months post-transplant. In some patients with diabetes who have had no rejection episodes in the first 6 months after transplant, we attempt to discontinue steroids altogether, especially if they are receiving mycophenolate mofetil or have a living-donor transplant.

The drug tacrolimus is not yet approved for primary kidney transplant and is associated with a high rate of post-transplant diabetes; however, it allows better tapering of steroids than cyclosporin A.

Table 5 Complications Associated with Renal Replacement Therapies in Patients with Diabetes

HEMODIALYSIS
Poor vascular access development
"Steal" syndrome
Progressive retinopathy
Interdialytic hypotension
Hyperlipidemia and cardiovascular disease
Infected or thrombosed vascular access
Poor rehabilitation (in-center)
CAPD
Infections
   Peritonitis
   "Tunnel" infection
Difficulty in controlling blood glucose
Worsening of peripheral vascular and cardiovascular disease
Lower back pain
KIDNEY TRANSPLANTATION
Infections
   Common: urinary tract, skin, osteomyelitis
   Less common: opportunistic (pneumocystis, CMV, tuberculosis, fungal) wound
Cardiovascular: myocardial infarction, angina, stroke, peripheral vascular disease
Cancer: skin, solid organ, and lymphoma
Gout
Cataracts
Hypertension and hyperlipidemia
Rejection: acute and chronic
Recurrent diabetic nephropathy

In kidney transplantation recipients with diabetes, graft loss occurs because of chronic or acute rejection, or recurrent diabetic nephropathy. It is not uncommon for patients to lose grafts to recurrent diabetic nephropathy within 6 years of transplantation. Because the natural history of diabetic nephropathy may be accelerated after renal transplantation, tight glycemic control is essential.

Complications that occur most commonly in transplanted diabetic patients (Table 5) include infectious and cardiovascular diseases. We maintain all renal transplant recipients on trimethoprim-sulfamethoxazole prophylaxis for 6 months after transplantation for protection against *Pneumocystis carinii* as well as most bacterial urinary pathogens. We do not routinely use immune globulin for cytomegalovirus (CMV) or ganciclovir as prophylactic therapy at our center.

Other common complications of kidney transplantation include worsening of glycemic control, hyperlipidemia, and post-transplant hypertension. Blood-glucose concentrations must be monitored closely and the insulin or oral hyperglycemic therapy adjusted accordingly. This is especially crucial during the rapid taper of prednisone and cyclosporine that occurs in the first 6 months following transplantation. Both of these immunosuppressive agents cause insulin resistance. Hyperlipidemia in diabetics who receive a kidney transplant usually presents as combined hypertriglyceridemia and hypercholesterolemia. Such dyslipidemia requires aggressive therapy with diet, gemfibrozil, and/or an HMG CoA reductase inhibitor (see the chapter *Dyslipidemia*). Hypertension is a common finding, occurring in up to 80 percent of all cyclosporine-treated recipients and is treated in a fashion similar to nontransplanted patients with diabetes (see the chapter *Hypertension in Patients with Diabetes*).

Suggested Reading

Friedman EA. Management choices in diabetic end-stage renal disease. Nephrology, Dialysis and Transplantation 1995; 10(suppl 7): 61–69.

Manske CL, Wang Y, Thomas W. Mortality of cadaveric kidney transplantation versus combined kidney-pancreas transplantation in diabetic patients. Lancet 1995; 346:1658–1662.

Markell MS. Diabetes and dialysis. In: Nissenson AR, Fine RN, Gentile DE, eds. Clinical dialysis, Norwalk, Ct: Appleton and Lange, 1995; 3:795.

Markell MS, Friedman EA. Management of the diabetic patient with ESRD. Seminars in Nephrology 1990; 10:274–286.

Remuzzi G, Reggenenti P, Mauer SM. Pancreas and kidney/pancreas transplants. Experimental medicine or real improvement? Lancet 1994; 535:27–31.

CATARACT IN THE DIABETIC PATIENT

Kristin Story Held, M.D.

It is estimated that cataract, an opacity in the lens of the eye, causes half of all blindness in the world, and 40 million people will be blind due to cataract by the year 2025. The development of cataract is age related. Cross-sectional studies show that 10 percent of all Americans have cataracts. This percentage increases to 50 percent in people between the ages of 65 and 74 years and to 70 percent of persons older than 75. Fifteen percent of people ages 52 to 85 years have cataracts that decrease their visual acuity to 20/30 or less, and 96 percent of patients over age 60 years show some evidence of lens opacification on slit-lamp examination. Patients who refuse surgery for operable cataracts constitute the second largest group of blind individuals in the United States. Fortunately, cataract surgery is curative and is probably the single–most-effective operation performed in medicine today (Fig. 1).

Diabetes is a major cause of blindness in the United States. Diabetic persons are 25 to 30 times more likely to progress to blindness than nondiabetics of similar age and sex. In addition to diabetic retinopathy, diabetics are at increased risk for both cataract and glaucoma. In older onset diabetic patients, cataract is the most frequent cause of severe visual loss.

The lens is involved in diabetes in two major ways. First, diabetes produces a dynamic fluctuation in the refractive state of the eye with a tendency toward myopia (nearsightedness) with increased blood-glucose levels and a tendency toward hyperopia (farsightedness) with decreased blood-glucose levels. Secondly, the risk of cataract is two to four times greater in diabetics than nondiabetics, and, in fact, the risk may be 15 to 20 times greater in diabetics less than 40

years old. Senile cataracts are considered physiologic changes of aging. The type of cataract most commonly seen in diabetes is clinically indistinguishable from those found with advancing age except that they are seen with greater frequency at an earlier age and progress to maturity more rapidly. Increasing age, increasing duration of the diabetes, the presence of diabetic retinopathy, and female gender are all associated with the increased risk of developing a cataract in diabetics. Poor control of diabetes is a predisposing factor as well. In young diabetic patients, the duration of diabetes is the most important determinant of the presence of cataract. In older diabetic patients, the age at examination is the most important determining factor of the presence of cataract followed by the severity of diabetic retinopathy.

The "true diabetic" or "snowflake" cataract occurs in younger patients, usually in the second decade of life, and occasionally in infants. There is an acute course with progression from fine punctate anterior and posterior superficial cortical opacities to a mature lens in a few days. This is usually preceded by a sudden progressive myopia. This type of cataract resembles the "sugar cataract" produced in experimental animals.

■ ETIOLOGY

Despite the scope of the problem and considerable research, the etiology of cataract is still unclear. Human cataract formation is a multifactorial progressive process in which independent events accumulate over time to result in loss of transparency of the lens. A better understanding of the causes of cataract will lead to the development of preventive measures. Risk factors implicated in cataract development are listed in Table 1.

Physiologically, two basic processes are involved in cataract formation. First, an imbalance of electrolytes in the cortex leads to overhydration of the lens and eventually liquefaction of the lens fibers. Secondly, modification of lens proteins results in aggregation and formation of large light-scattering particles in the nucleus. Regional increases in water content and formation of protein aggregates seem to

Table 1 Factors Related to Cataract Development

RISK FACTORS

Age
Female gender
Geographic location (particularly tropical areas in developing
    countries)
UV radiation
Ionizing radiation
Nutrition
Diabetes
Drugs and/or alcohol
Smoking
Ocular trauma
Topical or oral steroid use
Intraocular inflammation
Syphilis
Myopia
Low education
Nonwhite race
Nonprofessional occupation
Gout medications
Family history of cataract
Hypertension
Occupational exposure to sunlight

PROTECTIVE FACTORS

Multivitamin supplementation (particularly dietary intake of
    riboflavin, vitamins C, E, and carotene, which have antiox-
    idant potential, as well as niacin, thiamine, and iron)
Rigorous control of the blood sugar
Effective management of the diabetes
Weight control

be the principal factors leading to the loss of transparency of the lens. Biochemically, a diabetic senile cataract shows a significant increase in sorbitol, glucose, and fructose in the lens compared to nondiabetic senile cataract.

Lens epithelial cells have a high concentration of aldose reductase, an enzyme that converts sugars to their alcohols when sugars are present in high concentrations. Sucrose is converted to sorbitol, which can not easily diffuse out of cells, leading to an increased intracellular concentration. Water then diffuses into the cell secondary to osmotic forces, resulting in electrolyte imbalance and resultant damage to the lens. That aldose reductase inhibitors inhibit cataract formation is strong support for this theory.

■ MANAGEMENT

Decreased vision that results from cataract has a profound impact on the patient and his or her daily activities. Early

Table 2 Chief Symptoms Associated with Cataract

Decreased vision not associated with ocular pain or irritation
Double vision in one eye (monocular diplopia)
Colored halos surrounding light
Increased visual acuity when pupillary dilation occurs in dim light
Glare and decreased acuity when pupillary constriction occurs
    in bright light
Increased refractive power in the lens, which may allow reading
    without spectacle correction

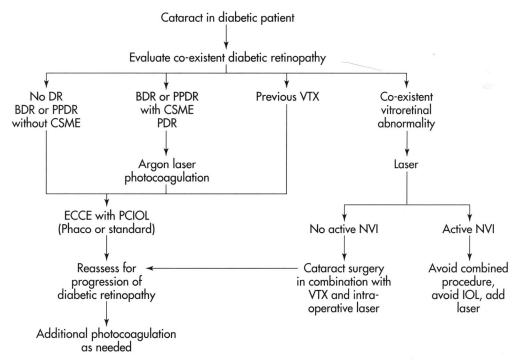

Figure 1
Cataract in diabetic patient. *DR* = Diabetic retinopathy; *BDR* = Background diabetic retinopathy; *PPDR* = Preproliferative diabetic retinopathy; *CSME* = Clinically significant macular edema; *ECCE with PCIOL* = Extracapsular cataract extraction with posterior-chamber intraocular lens implantation; *NVI* = Neovascularization of the iris; *PHACO* = Phacoemulsification; *VTX* = vitrectomy; *IOL* = intraocular lens.

medical management includes frequent refraction and treatment with spectacles or contact lenses. Strong bifocals may help as will increased illumination. Dilation of the pupil with a weak 2.5 percent solution of neosynephrine may improve vision of patients with small central opacities by allowing light to pass through the peripheral portion of the lens. Patient education and reassurance regarding prognosis is important at this point. Currently, there is no medical therapy available to prevent the formation or progression of cataract, although active research is ongoing and anticataract agents currently being advocated are catalin, phacolysin, bendazak, phakan, aspirin, and antioxidants such as vitamin E.

■ SURGERY

Approximately 1.25 million cataracts are surgically treated in the United States each year and cataract extraction is the leading surgical procedure for Americans over the age of 65 with ninety percent of cases performed on an outpatient basis. Blood-glucose level is determined preoperatively, intraoperatively, and postoperatively, and patients who are difficult to control may be best served by local anesthesia. Particularly brittle diabetics may require admission to the hospital for control of their diabetes through the perioperative period.

There are four major indications for cataract surgery as shown in Table 3. When it is determined that cataract surgery is indicated in the diabetic patient, one must carefully evaluate the status of any concurrent diabetic retinopathy. Diabetic patients without retinopathy achieve visual results comparable to those of nondiabetic patients. The visual prognosis is worse in diabetics with retinopathy. The visual outcome depends on the state of the retinopathy, particularly the maculopathy. The pre-existence of diabetic retinopathy preoperatively is a risk factor for its progression postoperatively.

Patients with maculopathy or severe retinopathy may have valuable visual improvement after surgery and a clear optical axis may allow adequate laser treatment to stabilize vision. In the diabetic patient with background or preprolif-erative diabetic retinopathy with clinically significant macular edema, focal laser therapy should be given preoperatively. The patient with proliferative diabetic retinopathy (PDR) with high-risk characteristics should be treated preoperatively with panretinal photocoagulation. If rubeosis is present, panretinal photocoagulation should be administered, and the patient should be observed for regression of the neovascularization. One may then proceed safely with extracapsular cataract extraction and posterior-chamber intraocular lens implantation. If the cataract is so dense that it precludes adequate laser photocoagulation, as much laser treatment is given as possible, and then one proceeds with surgery. For mature cataracts, ultrasonography is useful to determine the nature of vitreoretinal abnormalities in the posterior half of the eye. Additional laser therapy is given immediately postoperatively, and the patients are followed closely and retreated for any progressive retinopathy promptly. A posterior-chamber intraocular lens is considered safe and can still allow adequate evaluation and treatment of the retina. Many vitreoretinal specialists prefer a plano posterior one-piece all-PMMA lens with a large 7 mm optic and no positioning holes. This lens type facilitates visualization during future vitreoretinal surgery, particularly if gas-fluid exchange is performed. If capsular opacification occurs, a large capsulotomy may be performed with the Nd:YAG laser. Postoperatively, the patient will use topical steroid drops for several weeks and should avoid heavy lifting, bending, or straining in the immediate postoperative period. Most patients may resume full activities at 4 to 6 weeks following surgery.

Coexisting cataract and vitreoretinal complications from proliferative diabetic retinopathy are a common management problem. In patients with nonclearing vitreous hemorrhage, tractional retinal detachment, or preretinal membrane, cataract surgery may be combined with pars plana vitrectomy, intraocular lens implantation, and intraocular laser therapy with good result. Cataract extraction may be performed before vitrectomy or combined with vitrectomy to allow adequate view for vitreoretinal surgery and faster resolution of vitreous hemorrhage; however, removal of the lens has been associated with an increased risk of neovascular glaucoma and rubeosis iridis. The presence of active iris neovascularization is a contraindication to this type of combined surgery. Additionally, retinal detachment that extends to the ora serrata or peripheral traction may be best managed without the placement of an intraocular lens.

The combined cataract-vitrectomy procedure has traditionally been performed by pars plana lensectomy, which requires excision of the lens capsule precluding placement of a posterior-chamber intraocular lens. This increases the risk of postvitrectomy neovascular glaucoma in high-risk eyes. Further, visual rehabilitation in these patients is complicated as many of the patients are unable to wear an aphakic contact lens. Patients with unilateral aphakia and reduced visual potential, as from diabetic maculopathy, may not be motivated to wear a contact lens postoperatively. Additionally, patients with peripheral neuropathy secondary to longstanding diabetes may be unable to handle contact lenses and may be at increased risk of contact-lens induced corneal abrasion. Aphakic spectacles cause constriction in the visual field and optical distortion that is poorly tolerated in patients with diabetic macular disease. Preferably, pars plana vitrectomy can

---

Table 3 Cataract Surgery

CATARACT SURGERY: INDICATIONS
1. Patient desire for improved vision—most common
   Vision is decreased by a cataract
   The eye has potential vision
2. Lens threatens to cause secondary glaucoma or uveitis
3. Dense cataract obscures view of retina precluding assessment of retinopathy or glaucoma
4. Dense cataract precludes adequate treatment; i.e., photocoagulation, vitrectomy, or other retinal surgery

CATARACT SURGERY: CONTRAINDICATIONS
1. Patient refuses surgery
2. Spectacles or contact lenses provide satisfactory function that does not compromise patient's function and retina can be adequately assessed and treated through the cataract
3. Surgery will not improve visual function; e.g., a no-light perception phthisical eye
4. Patient medically unfit for surgery

be combined with pars plana lensectomy in which the anterior capsule is preserved for sulcus fixation of a posterior-chamber intraocular lens or combined with phacoemulsification and placement of a posterior chamber intraocular lens. The benefit of phacoemulsification combined with pars plana vitrectomy is preservation of the posterior capsule and visual rehabilitation from a posterior-chamber intraocular lens.

Brunescent lenses are frequently seen in patients with diabetes. The color of the nucleus changes from yellow to amber and reddish-brown and finally dark. These lenses are hard and not easily tumbled (during lens extraction) or phacoemulsified. They may be best removed by a sliding extracapsular technique. Careful patient selection is important when performing phacoemulsification in the diabetic patient specifically when combined with pars plana vitrectomy. Hard brunescent lenses, which are more commonly seen in diabetics, may require extensive ultrasonic energy, lens manipulation, and prolonged irrigation that contributes to corneal edema and predisposes the patient to a risk of lens dislocation, capsular tears, and zonular dehiscence. Furthermore, many diabetics have miotic pupils, which make anterior capsulotomy and cataract surgery more difficult. Posterior-chamber intraocular lenses are preferable to anterior-chamber lenses in diabetics, particularly in patients with predisposition to glaucoma or past history of proliferative disease. Active iris neovascularization is probably a contraindication to placement of an intraocular lens, and particularly an anterior chamber intraocular lens. Intracapsular cataract surgery should be avoided in diabetic patients as most vitreous surgeons agree that extracapsular procedures are less likely to result in progressive neovascular glaucoma. Most patients who have had a vitrectomy will develop cataract. Great care should be taken to avoid rupturing the posterior capsule in patients who have had a previous vitrectomy as the vitreous cavity is liquid filled, and there is little capsular support.

Diabetics have an increased incidence of postoperative complications than do nondiabetics. The major complications are related to the continuing neovascularization. Early, extensive preoperative laser and early postoperative laser therapy help prevent this. The intraocular lens does not interfere with laser therapy as long as there is a large capsulotomy in the setting of posterior capsule opacification. Early postoperative assessment and treatment of any maculopathy is essential. An intact capsule may help prevent the risk of progressive neovascularization, but early PRP is important regardless. The incidence of postoperative anterior segment complications is significantly higher in the diabetic than in the nondiabetic, particularly pigment dispersion, fibrin formation, development of posterior synechiae, and pupillary block. Corneal epithelial abnormalities are seen with greater frequency and the incidence of short-term postoperative corneal edema is increased.

Diabetics may be more sensitive to postoperative medications and develop punctate epithelial erosion more easily requiring meticulous postoperative care. Shallow anterior chamber may occur secondary to problems with poor wound healing. Pupillary block may occur secondary to increased inflammation, and it is probably beneficial to place peripheral iridectomies prophylactically in diabetic patients undergoing cataract surgery. Posterior capsular opacification may occur in one-third to one-half of patients after extracapsular surgery. Diabetic patients may safely undergo Nd:YAG capsulotomy; however, the maintenance of a two-chamber eye may be beneficial, and polishing of the posterior capsule may be favorable in selected patients. Posterior-chamber intraocular lenses have largely resolved the problems with visual rehabilitation. Diabetics also have an increased incidence of postoperative endophthalmitis. Concurrent systemic infection should be treated preoperatively and appropriate cultures should be obtained. One should consider utilizing preoperative, intraoperative, and postoperative antibiotics. Diabetes mellitus is said to be one of the contributing factors to expulsive hemorrhage, one of the most catastrophic surgical complications of cataract surgery. Finally, epithelial downgrowth occurs more commonly in patients with diabetes because of their tendency for poor wound healing. It is important to recognize these complications early and treat promptly, and final results will be satisfactory. Frequent follow-up after cataract surgery is essential.

In summary, there is an increased incidence of cataract in diabetic patients. Cataracts occur at an earlier age and progress more rapidly than in nondiabetics. These cataracts not only affect the quality of the patients' lives by decreasing their ability to perform activities of daily living, but also impair the ophthalmologist's ability to assess and treat diabetic retinopathy, which is the leading cause of blindness in our country in the 25- to 74-year-old age group. Fortunately, when combined with appropriate adjunctive laser photocoagulation or vitrectomy with endolaser in selected cases, cataract extraction with posterior-chamber lens implantation can produce excellent results in the diabetic patient. This can usually be performed on an outpatient basis under local anesthesia with minimal disruption to the patient's daily dietary, physical, and medical routine.

SUGGESTED READING

Cunliffe IA, Flanagan DW, George NDL, et al. Extracapsular cataract extraction with lens complications in diabetes with and without proliferative retinopathy. Brit J Ophthalmol 1991; 75:9–12.

In this article a favorable outcome after cataract surgery in diabetics and good results with intraocular lens implantation are reported.

Klein BE, Klein R, Moss SE. Prevalence of cataracts in a population-based study of persons with diabetes mellitus. Ophthalmol 1985; 92:1191–1196.

In this article an increased risk of cataract in diabetes, risk factors for cataracts, and possible preventive measures are discussed.

Klein R, Moss SE, Klein BEK, DeMets DL. Relation of ocular and systemic factors to survival in diabetes. Arch Intern Med 1989; 149:266–272.

In this article the association of ocular complications of diabetes with decreased survival in diabetics is defined and the importance of frequent examinations to detect the complications is emphasized.

Koening SB, Mieler WF, Han DP, Adams GW. Combined phacoemulsification, pars plana vitrectomy, and posterior chamber intraocular lens implantation. Arch Ophthalmol 1992; 110:1101–1104.

Favorable results and advantages associated with combined phacoemulsification, pars plana vitrectomy, and PCIOL insertion are reported.

Leske MC, Chylack LT, Wu SY. The lens opacities case-control study: Risk factors for cataract. Arch Ophthalmol 1991; 109:244–251.

Risk factors and protective factors associated with cataract are identified in this study.

Pollack A, Doton S, Oliver M. Course of diabetic retinopathy following cataract surgery. Brit J Ophthalmol 1991; 75:2–8.

This article is a report of five patients with progression of diabetic retinopathy following surgery. Appropriate follow-up and management are recommended.

Sprafka JM, Fritsche TL, Bakr R, Kurth D, Whipple D. Prevalence of undiagnosed eye disease in high-risk diabetic individuals. Arch Intern Med 1990; 150:887–891.

The high prevalence of ocular morbidity among diabetics who have no ophthalmic care is discussed and steps toward solving this problem are suggested.

Tasman W, Joeger EA, eds. Duane's clinical ophthalmology. [revised edition], Philadelphia: JB Lippincott Company 1991.

This is an excellent general ophthalmology reference.

DIABETIC RETINOPATHY

W.A.J. van Heuven, M.D.
Ralph A. DeFronzo, M.D.

Diabetic retinopathy is the leading cause of blindness in the United States, accounting for approximately 8,000 new cases of blindness each year. Over 700,000 Americans have proliferative diabetic retinopathy (PDR) and another 500,000 have diabetic macular edema (DME). Diabetic patients with PDR and DME are at markedly increased risk to develop progressive visual loss and blindness.

In its early stages diabetic retinopathy is usually asymptomatic. It is at this early stage that PDR and DME are most treatable with laser surgery. Unfortunately, less than half of all diabetic patients in the United States receive appropriate ophthalmologic care. It is essential that all type 2 diabetic patients at the time of diagnosis and all type 1 diabetic patients with a duration of diabetes more than 5 years have an ophthalmologic examination by a specialist trained in the diagnosis and treatment of diabetic retinopathy on a yearly basis. The most important function of the primary care physician is to ensure that all diabetic patients receive an annual eye examination. Early laser photocoagulation can reduce the risk of severe visual loss in patients with high-risk PDR by over 50 percent.

■ NATURAL HISTORY OF DIABETIC RETINOPATHY

The natural history of diabetic retinopathy is well defined by the Wisconsin Epidemiologic Study of Diabetic Retinopathy (WESDR) (Fig. 1, *top*). At the onset of type 1 diabetes,

retinopathy is not present and rarely occurs before 5 years of duration. After 10 years some retinopathy is present in approximately 60 percent of type 1 patients and by 20 years the incidence approaches 100 percent. Approximately 20 percent of type 2 diabetic patients have some form of retinopathy at the time of diagnosis. This is attributed to the fact that many type 2 patients are asymptomatic and have had diabetes for many years before they are diagnosed. After 20 years the incidence of any retinopathy in type 2 diabetic subjects increases to 60 to 80 percent (Fig. 1, *top*).

Proliferative retinopathy is uncommon within the first 10 years in type 1 diabetic patients but rises to 50 to 60 percent at 20 years. It is less common in type 2 diabetes, occurring in 10 to 20 percent of patients at 20 years (Fig. 1, *bottom*). It is notable that in type 2 diabetic individuals on insulin, the incidence of retinopathy is significantly greater than in subjects not taking insulin. This most likely reflects poorer glycemic control in the insulin-treated group, requiring the institution of insulin therapy, and a longer duration of diabetes. Macular edema is equally common in type 1 and type 2 diabetes mellitus and affects 10 to 20 percent of all diabetics by 20-years duration of disease.

■ RISK FACTORS FOR PROLIFERATIVE RETINOPATHY

The risk factors for PDR are listed in Table 1. Poor glycemic control is the most important risk factor (Fig. 2). With the currently available oral agents used alone or in combination with each other (see the chapters *Sulfonylureas, Metformin, Alpha-Glucosidase Inhibitors,* and *Troglitazone [Rezulin]*) or in combination with insulin (see the chapter *Combination Therapy: Insulin-Sulfonylurea and Insulin-Metformin*), adequate glycemic control (FPG <140 mg per deciliter; HbA_{1c} <7.0 to 7.5 percent) is achievable in essentially all diabetic individuals. The important role of good glycemic control in the prevention of diabetic retinopathy has been conclusively demonstrated in the Diabetic Control and Complications

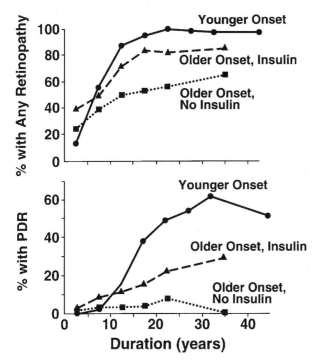

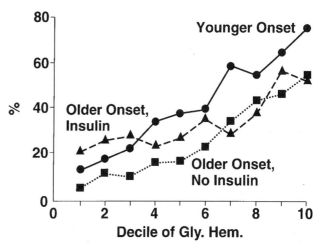

Figure 2

Prevalence of diabetic retinopathy based upon the decline of glycosylated hemoglobin at baseline. Subjects with the poorest glycemic control (highest decile) at baseline had the highest prevalence of diabetic retinopathy after 10 years. *(From Klein R, et al. Arch Ophthalmol 1989; 107:244–249, with permission.)*

Figure 1

Percentage of diabetic individuals with any retinopathy (*top*) and proliferative diabetic retinopathy (PDR) (*bottom*) as reported in the Wisconsin Epidemiologic Study of Diabetic Retinopathy. Younger onset refers to insulin-dependent patients under the age of 30 with a typical presentation for type 1 diabetes mellitus (islet cell or glutamic acid decarboxylase antibodies were not obtained to more definitively establish the diagnosis of IDDM). Older onset refers to diabetic individuals with an onset of diabetes over the age of 30, who were initially controlled with oral agents and who had a typical presentation of type 2 diabetes mellitus. *(From Klein R, et al. Arch Ophthalmol 1989; 107:244–249, with permission.)*

Table 1 Risk Factors for Proliferative Retinopathy

RISK FACTOR	CORRELATION
Age	Younger onset (type 1)
Ethnicity	Hispanics, Native Americans
Duration	>10 years
Hyperglycemia	Very positive and linear
Blood pressure	Positive, modest
Smoking	Weak
Proteinuria	Very positive

Data from the Wisconsin Epidemiologic Study of Diabetic Retinopathy.

Trial (see the chapter *Goals of Diabetes Management*). Proteinuria is the second most important risk factor for proliferative diabetic retinopathy. Renal disease and retinopathy occur so frequently that they have been referred to as the renal-retinal syndrome. Patients with proteinuria should be treated with an angiotensin-converting enzyme inhibitor or

a calcium channel blocker even if hypertension is not present (see the chapter *Diabetic Nephropathy: Diagnosis and Therapeutic Approach*). Hypertension should be treated aggressively because it also accelerates the progression of diabetic eye disease (see the chapter *Hypertension in Patients with Diabetes*).

■ CLASSIFICATION OF DIABETIC RETINOPATHY

For simplicity diabetic retinopathy can be divided into four categories (Table 2). Nonproliferative (background) diabetic retinopathy represents the earliest stage of eye involvement and is subdivided into three categories: mild, moderate, and severe. *Microaneurysms*, which represent focal dilatations of capillary walls, are the hallmark feature of mild nonproliferative diabetic retinopathy. Microaneurysm formation correlates closely with the loss of pericytes, which represent the supporting structure for retinal capillaries. Compromise of capillary-wall integrity by ischemia also contributes to aneurysmal formation. Microaneurysms often occur in association with dot and blot (smaller and larger) hemorrhages and, during a routine ophthalmologic examination, it often is impossible to distinguish between microaneurysms and small-dot hemorrhages. This distinction requires fluorescein angiography, which is not indicated at this stage of diabetic retinopathy, unless macular edema (see further discussion) presents a threat to central vision. Hard exudates may be observed during any stage of nonproliferative or proliferative diabetic retinopathy, and result from leakage of plasma through ischemic and permeable capillary walls. As water is reabsorbed from the extravasated plasma, proteins and lipids are left behind, leading to the appearance of yellow, deep, intraretinal deposits adjacent to areas of leakage.

The development of moderate nonproliferative diabetic retinopathy is characterized by more advanced intravascular and perivascular changes (i.e., microaneurysms, dot and blot hemorrhages, exudates) and the presence of retinal alterations that are related to hypoxia and capillary changes. The retinal veins become dilated and tortuous (beading) and intraretinal microvascular abnormalities (IRMA), which appear as clusters of microaneurysms and tortuous hypercellular vessels, develop. Clinically, it is not possible to tell whether IRMA represent dilated pre-existing vessels or intraretinal new vessels. The term is used to encompass both of these abnormalities.

"Cotton-wool spots", which are whitish, fuzzy-edged, superficial retinal lesions, appear at this stage and represent hypoxic necrosis of retinal nerve fibers caused by capillary closure.

When venous beading, cotton-wool spots, IRMAs, and retinal hemorrhages become more prominent, the stage of severe nonproliferative diabetic retinopathy has been reached and widespread retinal ischemia is present. Although the growth of new vessels on the retina is not present, such individuals are at high risk to develop vision-threatening proliferative retinopathy. *Referral to an ophthalmologist for consideration for early laser surgery is essential in diabetic patients with severe nonproliferative retinopathy.* The 4-year rate of progression from nonproliferative to proliferative diabetic retinopathy is shown in Table 3. It can be appreciated that even diabetic patients with mild nonproliferative diabetic retinopathy are at significant risk for progression to proliferative retinopathy within a relatively short period of time and, therefore, should be followed by a trained retinal specialist at regular intervals (see further discussion).

The appearance of new vessels (neovascularization) on the retina or optic disc and/or preretinal fibrous tissue proliferation indicates that diabetic retinopathy has entered the proliferative stage. The new vessels extend over the surface of the retina between the retina and the vitreous gel. Because neovascular vessels have abnormally leaking walls, they affect the surface of the gel, causing it to shrink and pull away from the retina. This type of vitreous detachment may pull on the fragile new capillaries, causing them to rupture, with resultant preretinal and vitreous hemorrhage. Proliferation of fibrous tissue and its subsequent contraction lead to traction on the retina, which can result in retinal hole formation and detachment. Hemorrhage, fibrous tissue proliferation, and retinal detachment, even if they only are modest in extent, present a major threat to vision if they occur in the region of the macula. Proliferative diabetic retinopathy usually progresses

through an active phase followed by remission. Any evidence of PDR mandates immediate referral to an ophthalmologist, specialized in the treatment of diabetic retinopathy. High-risk characteristics for diabetic patients with PDR retinopathy are shown in Table 4. Any of these findings indicates that the patient is at extremely high risk for visual loss and dictates immediate referral to a retinal specialist.

"Diabetic maculopathy" refers to the collection of intraretinal fluid in the macular area (macular edema) and can occur with or without lipid exudates, nonperfusion of parafoveal capillaries, fibrous tissue proliferation, and intraretinal or preretinal hemorrhages. Macular edema can be seen at any stage of diabetic retinopathy, is equally common in type 1 and type 2 diabetic patients, and represents a major cause of visual loss. Because the direct ophthalmoscope does not allow a three-dimensional view of the retina, and because the indirect ophthalmoscope does not produce enough magnification, macular edema is easily missed, even by diabetologists. However, it can be diagnosed readily by a trained ophthalmologist who examines the eye through a dilated pupil using a slit-lamp and precorneal lenses. The presence of hard exudates in the area of the macula, especially if extensive, provides a clue to the diagnosis of macular edema. The suspicion of macular edema is an indication for prompt referral to an ophthalmologist.

■ OPHTHALMOLOGIC REFERRAL SCHEDULE

A schedule of routine ophthalmologic evaluation for primary care physicians is presented in Table 5. A follow-up eye examination, based on the retinal status, is provided in Table 6. Patients with more advanced nonproliferative diabetic retinopathy and those with proliferative retinopathy require more frequent follow-up visits. Fundus photography is performed routinely in patients with mild/moderate nonprolif-

---

Table 2 Classification of Diabetic Retinopathy

Nonproliferative (background) retinopathy
Proliferative retinopathy
Advanced diabetic eye disease
Maculopathy*

*May occur in individuals with nonproliferative or proliferative diabetic retinopathy.

Table 3 Four-Year Progression Rates from Nonproliferative to Proliferative Diabetic Retinopathy

BASELINE RETINOPATHY	YOUNGER ONSET-INSULIN	OLDER ONSET-INSULIN	OLDER ONSET-NO INSULIN
None	<1%	0	1%
NPDR-very mild	5%	0	0
NPDR-mild	20%	2%	11%
NPDR-moderate	42%	20%	25%
NPDR-severe	50%	48%	36%

Based on data from the Wisconsin Epidemiologic Study of Diabetic Retinopathy.
NPDR = nonproliferative diabetic retinopathy; younger onset primarily reflects type 1 diabetic individuals, whereas older onset primarily includes type 2 diabetic patients.

erative retinopathy and serves as the "gold standard" to follow the progression of diabetic retinopathy. Fluorescein angiography is an important tool to document the location and extent of vascular involvement, differentiate IRMA from neovascularization, determine the presence of macular edema, and assist the ophthalmologist in planning laser treatment.

■ TREATMENT OF DIABETIC RETINOPATHY

Laser photocoagulation represents the mainstay of therapy in patients with diabetic retinopathy. Panretinal or scatter laser therapy is the most frequently employed form of treatment, although focal laser therapy is commonly used to treat macular edema. With panretinal laser therapy, hundreds of small burns (200 to 500 μm in diameter) are scattered throughout the retina, leaving one-half to one burn widths between burns. The beneficial effect of panretinal laser photocoagulation is related to (1) direct obliteration of new vessels, (2) destruction of ischemic retinal cells, which produce new-vessel stimulating factors, (3) improved retinal oxygenation secondary to destruction of highly metabolically active photoreceptor cells, and (4) increased production of new-vessel inhibiting factors by retinal epithelial cells.

The Diabetic Retinopathy Study (DRS) was the first large-scale trial to demonstrate that panretinal laser photocoagulation in eyes with PDR could reduce the rate of severe visual loss by over 50 percent (Fig. 3). The Early Treatment Diabetic Retinopathy Study (ETDRS) demonstrated that eyes with severe nonproliferative retinopathy and mild proliferative retinopathy also benefited from panretinal laser treatment. The ETDRS did not find laser therapy to be of benefit in diabetic patients with mild-to-moderate nonproliferative retinopathy. In fact, some decrease in visual acuity and visual field was observed in this latter group. The ETDRS also demonstrated the beneficial effects of both focal and grid-laser therapy in preserving visual acuity in eyes with macular edema. Eyes with capillary leakage sites in the center of the maculae were at highest risk to lose visual acuity and benefited most from laser treatment. Lastly, the Diabetic Retinopathy Vitrectomy Study (DRVS) demonstrated the

Table 4 High-Risk Characteristics for Visual Loss in Diabetic Patients with Proliferative Retinopathy
Neovascularization on optic disc or within 1 disk diameter (≥¼ disk area)
Neovascularization >1 disc diameter with fresh hemorrhage
Neovascularization on disc (<¼ disc area) with fresh hemorrhage

Table 5 Eye Examination Schedule

TYPE OF DIABETES	INITIAL EYE EXAM	FOLLOW-UP EYE EXAMS
IDDM*	5 years post diagnosis	Yearly†
NIDDM	At time of diagnosis	Yearly†

*All type 1 diabetic patients (IDDM) with mild-moderate proliferative retinopathy or suspicion of macular edema should receive an immediate referral to a retinal specialist regardless of the time of diagnosis
†Annual follow-up exam is indicated if no retinal abnormalities or minimal nonproliferative diabetic retinopathy are present.

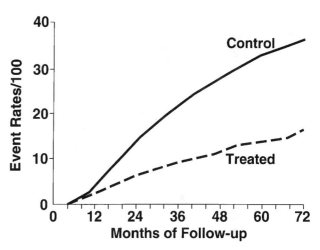

Figure 3
Effect of laser photocoagulation on the cumulative rate of severe visual loss. The treated eye showed a greater than 60% decrease in the rate of progression to severe visual loss. (From Klein R, et al. Arch Ophthalmol 1989; 107:237–243, with permission.)

Table 6 Recommended Frequency of Follow-Up Visits for Patients with Diabetic Retinopathy Based on the Retinal Status

RETINAL STATUS	FOLLOW-UP (MONTHS)	FUNDUS PHOTOGRAPHY	FLUORESCEIN ANGIOGRAPHY	LASER
Normal/min NPDR	12	No	No	No
Mild-mod NPDR without ME	6–12	Rarely	No	No
Mild-mod NPDR with ME	3–4	Yes	Yes	Yes
Severe NPDR	3–4	Yes	Yes	Yes
Non–high-risk PDR	3–4	Yes	Yes	Selected patients
High-risk PDR	2–4	Yes	Yes	Yes

NPDR = nonproliferative diabetic retinopathy; PDR = proliferative diabetic retinopathy; ME = macular edema.

efficacy and timing of vitrectomy in patients who experience a vitreous hemorrhage. Neither aspirin nor platelet inhibitors have been shown to be of benefit in the treatment of diabetic retinopathy. It should be emphasized, however, that one baby aspirin (81 mg) per day has been shown to decrease the incidence of macrovascular (stroke and myocardial infarction) complications in type 2 diabetic patients.

■ COMMON VISUAL SYMPTOMS REQUIRING OPHTHALMOLOGIC REFERRAL

Blurred vision and floaters are common complaints in diabetic patients (Table 7). Although these symptoms frequently are dismissed in nondiabetic individuals, they require prompt evaluation in patients with diabetes mellitus. Although blurred vision most commonly results from poor glycemic control and osmotic fluid shifts, which alter the refractive index of the lens, it also may signify the presence of more serious underlying conditions including macular edema, cataracts, or glaucoma. Floaters may indicate vitreous hemorrhage or retinal tears, which mandate immediate ophthalmologic referral and appropriate laser/surgical intervention.

■ NONRETINAL OCULAR COMPLICATIONS

Involvement of the eye in diabetes mellitus is not limited to the retina. All structures of the eye manifest increased susceptibility to the metabolic and circulatory alterations that occur in diabetic patients (Table 8).

Mononeuropathies
Mononeuropathies of cranial nerves III, IV, and VI are relatively uncommon (0.4 percent of all diabetic subjects), but dramatic in their presentation. The presenting feature is diplopia with or without eye pain or headache. Third-nerve palsy is the most common and the eye is directed down and out. There is ptosis of the eyelid, but the pupillary reflex is spared, distinguishing it from more serious intracranial lesions. Sixth-nerve palsy (eye turned inward toward the nose) is the next most frequent, with fourth-nerve palsy being relatively rare. Mononeuropathies result from microinfarcts of nerves that innervate the ocular muscles. Complete recovery can be expected within 1 to 9 months, and cranial nerve palsies that do not resolve in 6 to 9 months are probably not of diabetic origin. Treatment of ophthalmoplegia is directed toward relief of diplopia by patching the affected eye and a mild analgesic for the eye pain or headache, if needed.

Susceptibility to Corneal Ulceration
Diabetic subjects also have an increased susceptibility to corneal abrasion. This is related to two factors: decreased corneal sensitivity and impaired regeneration of the corneal epithelium and its basement membrane. Therefore, safety glasses and goggles are recommended in hazardous work environments and for sporting activities. Also, physicians should have a high index of suspicion when a diabetic patient complains of eye tearing, even without pain, because a significant corneal abrasion may be present, which, given the increased susceptibility of diabetics to infection, may become a painless corneal ulcer leading to an ocular perforation.

Presbyopia
Early presbyopia (inability to focus at near) and fluctuating vision are common occurrences in diabetic patients. The latter is most frequently associated with rapid swings in the blood-glucose concentration or chronically poor glycemic control. Chronic hyperglycemia leads to the accumulation of polyols and fructose within the lens, leading to osmotic fluid shifts that alter the refractive index of the lens. It is wise to wait at least 3 to 4 weeks after the achievement of good glycemic control before referring the patient to the optometrist for refraction for new glasses.

Cataracts
Cataracts occur twice as frequently in diabetic patients. Their diagnosis and management is discussed in the chapter *Cataract in the Diabetic Patient.*

Glaucoma
Glaucoma is significantly increased in individuals with diabetes, largely because chronic open angle glaucoma (which represents over 90 percent of all glaucomas) is 2 to 4 times more common in diabetic than in nondiabetic individuals. In addition, one of the secondary forms of glaucomas, neovascular glaucoma, is significantly increased in diabetics. Most other secondary glaucomas, such as those related to uveitis, cataract formation, or trauma, have the same incidence in the diabetic and nondiabetic population.

Chronic open-angle glaucoma, which can be asymp-

Table 7 Visual Symptoms in Diabetic Patients

SYMPTOM	ETIOLOGY	TREATMENT
Blurred vision	Poor glycemic control	Oral agents, insulin
	Cataracts, glaucoma	Ophthalmologic referral
	Macular edema	Prompt referral
Floaters	Vitreous hemorrhage	Urgent ophthalmologic referral
	Retinal detachment	Laser/surgical intervention
	Retinal hole	
Ocular pain	Corneal abrasion	Urgent referral
	Glaucoma	Medical/surgical intervention

Table 8 Nonretinal Ocular Complications

Mononeuropathies: cranial nerves III, IV, VI
Susceptibility to corneal ulceration
Early presbyopia
Fluctuating vision
Glaucoma
Cataracts

tomatic for many years, is best diagnosed by an ophthalmologist who combines the findings of increased intraocular pressure, cupping of the optic nerve, and visual-field defects in order to establish the diagnosis. Because of its increased incidence, it is important that all diabetics have regular eye exams to check for glaucoma. Treatment for chronic open-angle glaucoma in diabetics is the same as in nondiabetics and includes topical and systemic carbonic anhydrase inhibitors (Trusopt or Diamox), miotics (pilocarpine), beta-adrenergic blockers (Timoptic), and, if maximal medical therapy does not work, filtering surgery to provide an alternate outflow channel for aqueous humor.

Acute glaucoma, on the other hand, is symptomatic and associated with severe ocular and periocular pain, a fixed mid-dilated pupil, a cloudy cornea, a red eye, and blurred vision. Immediate referral to an ophthalmologist is necessary, because this represents one of the few surgical emergencies in ophthalmology. The diagnosis can be made by finger palpation and is confirmed by determining a markedly increased intraocular pressure, usually at or above 60 or 70 mm Hg. If a nonophthalmologist makes this diagnosis, while the patient is being transferred to an ophthalmalogist on the same day, oral Diamox (500 mg) should be given to decrease aqueous production in an attempt to reduce ocular pressure. The ophthalmologist will then determine the cause of the glaucoma to see whether or not it is simple angle-closure glaucoma, neovascular glaucoma, or one of the other secondary glaucomas. In angle-closure glaucoma the treatment is laser peripheral iridectomy. In most other secondary glaucomas, treatment is directed at controlling the inciting cause, such as inflammation. In neovascular glaucoma, therapy involves eradication of the neovascularization that is narrowing the anterior chamber filtration angle and is blocking aqueous outflow on the surface of the iris. In addition to panretinal photocoagulation and/or goniophotocoagulation, the treatment of neovascular glaucoma consists of the same topical and systemic medications normally used in chronic glaucoma. If none of these interventions control the intraocular pressure adequately, filtration surgery or ciliary body ablation surgery may be necessary; however, the results are not as good as in surgery for uncontrolled open-angle glaucoma.

Suggested Reading

Davis MD, Kern TS, Rand LI. Diabetic retinopathy. In Alberti KG, DeFronzo RA, Zimmet P. eds. International textbook of diabetes mellitus, John Wiley and Sons, 1997.

Excellent in-depth review of the pathogenesis, clinical manifestations, and treatment of diabetic retinopathy.

The Diabetes Control and Complications Trial Research Group. The effects of intensive treatment of diabetes on the development and progression of long-term complications in insulin-dependent diabetes. N Engl J Med 1993; 329:977–986.

Large (>1,400 patients) multicenter trial that conclusively demonstrates that tight glycemic control in type 1 diabetic individuals markedly reduces the incidence of retinopathy, nephropathy, and neuropathy. Similar results have been shown by other investigators in type 2 diabetic patients.

The Diabetic Retinopathy Study Research Group. Report no. 8: Photocoagulation treatment of proliferative diabetic retinopathy: Clinical applications of diabetic retinopathy study (DRS) findings. Ophthalmology 1981; 88:583–600.

Large multicenter trial documenting the efficacy of laser treatment in diabetic patients with diabetic retinopathy.

Early Treatment Diabetic Retinopathy Study Research Group: Photocoagulation for diabetic macular edema: ETDRS Report no. 1. Arch Ophthalmol 1985;103:1796–1806.

Large multicenter trial documenting the efficacy of laser treatment in diabetic patients with severe nonproliferative diabetic retinopathy, mild proliferative retinopathy, and macular edema.

Early Treatment Diabetic Retinopathy Study Research Group: Early photocoagulation for diabetic retinopathy: ETDRS Report no. 9. Ophthalmology 1991; 98:766–785.

See preceding reference.

Early Treatment Diabetic Retinopathy Study Research Group: Fundus photographic risk factors for progression of diabetic retinopathy: ETDRS Report no 12. Ophthalmology 1991; 98:823–833.

Large multicenter trial that identifies the high risk characteristics for progression to severe visual loss in diabetic patients.

Early Vitrectomy for Severe Vitreous Hemorrhage in Diabetic Retinopathy. Two-year results of a randomized trial. Diabetic Retinopathy Vitrectomy Study (DRVS Report no. 2): Diabetic Retinopathy Research Group. Arch Ophthalmol 1985; 103:1644–1652.

Large multicenter trials that define the clinical usefulness of vitrectomy in the management of diabetic patients.

Early Vitrectomy for Severe Proliferative Diabetic Retinopathy in Eyes With Useful Vision: Results of a randomized trial: Diabetic Retinopathy Vitrectomy Study (DRVS Report no. 3): Diabetic Retinopathy Research Group. Ophthalmology 1988; 95:1307–1320.

See preceding reference.

Klein R. Hyperglycemia and microvascular and macrovascular disease in diabetes. Diabetes Care 1995; 18:258–268.

Well-written summary of the Wisconsin Epidemiologic Study of Diabetic Retinopathy. This study delineates the natural history of retinopathy in type 1 and type 2 diabetic patients and identifies the major risk factors for the progression of diabetic retinopathy.

Klein R, Klein BEK, Moss SE, Cruickshanks KH. Relationship of hyperglycemia to the long-term incidence and progression of diabetic retinopathy. Arch Intern Med 1994; 154:2169–2178.

See preceding reference.

DIABETIC PERIPHERAL NEUROPATHY

Martin J. Stevens, M.D.
Eva L. Feldman, M.D.
Douglas A. Greene, M.D.

Diabetic neuropathy encompasses a group of clinical and subclinical syndromes, each of which is characterized by diffuse or focal damage to peripheral somatic or autonomic nerve fibers resulting from diabetes mellitus (Table 1). Clinical neuropathic syndromes in general represent the culmination of one or more chronic underlying pathogenic processes whose reversibility is somewhat limited once signs and symptoms are prominent. None of these syndromes are pathognomonic for diabetes, since indistinguishable neuropathic syndromes occur idiopathically or in association with other disorders in nondiabetic individuals. Therefore, their diagnoses are often ones of exclusion of other neuropathic disorders. The cumulative prevalence of clinical diabetic neuropathy parallels the degree of duration of antecedent hyperglycemia, and the Diabetes Control Complications Trial (DCCT) has definitively established the important role of improved metabolic control in the primary prevention and/or amelioration (secondary prevention) of symptomatic neuropathy. The roles of newer therapies, such as aldose reductase inhibitors, remain unclear at the present time.

■ ETIOLOGY AND PATHOGENESIS

The pathogenesis of diabetic neuropathy is almost certainly multifactorial and remains a subject of considerable controversy. Diabetic neuropathy occurs with similar frequency in insulin-dependent and non–insulin-dependent diabetes, has been described in secondary forms of diabetes, correlates closely with the degree and duration of antecedent hyperglycemia, and is thus generally ascribed to the diabetic state per se rather than to the underlying diabetogenic processes themselves. The results of the DCCT have established the importance of poor metabolic control in the development of diabetic neuropathy. However, factors other than glycemic control also appear to play a role in the pathogenesis of diabetic neuropathy. Therefore, clinical neuropathy can emerge without an unambiguous preceding period of especially poor metabolic control, and, paradoxically, improved metabolic control is sometimes associated with the development or worsening of painful neuropathic symptoms.

Still, taken collectively, available studies provide strong evidence implicating the abnormal metabolic milieu of the diabetic state in the pathogenesis of diabetic neuropathy. The

specific metabolic abnormalities (e.g., hyperglycemia or insulin deficiency per se, abnormal lipid or amino acid metabolism, or secondary effects of other growth factors and hormones) remain to be established. Similarly, it is unclear whether these metabolic abnormalities exert their effects on peripheral nerve neurons or Schwann cells or act through secondary abnormalities on the vascular, perineurial, or extracellular matrix components of peripheral nerve. These questions require detailed metabolic, cellular, morphologic, and molecular answers that are difficult to obtain from studies in patients with diabetes. In animal models of diabetes, a wide range of metabolic abnormalities has been linked with disturbances in nerve conduction velocity, resistance of nerve impulse conduction to ischemia, impaired axonal transport, and altered nerve structure. Most authorities believe that hyperglycemia, by altering flux through the polyol pathway and decreasing myo-inositol levels within the cell, plays an important role in the development of peripheral neuropathy. Glycation of neuroproteins and ischemia also contribute to the degenerative neuropathic changes.

■ DEFINITION, CLASSIFICATION, AND STAGING

By far the most common neuropathic syndrome associated with diabetes mellitus is distal, symmetric, primarily sensory polyneuropathy. This is often accompanied by autonomic neuropathy (see the following chapter). Diabetic neuropathy also encompasses a series of rare acute focal neuropathies involving the spinal roots, plexes, and individual (occasionally multiple) peripheral and cranial nerves. The association of these mononeuropathies with diabetes most likely reflects enhanced susceptibility of the diabetic peripheral nervous system to mechanical and/or ischemic insults. A demyelinating motor neuropathy, infrequently reported in diabetic subjects, is now generally attributed to the coincidental occurrence of chronic inflammatory demyelinating polyradiculoneuropathy (CIDP). In diabetic

---

Table 1 Classification of Diabetic Neuropathies

Mononeuropathy or mononeuritis multiplex
  Isolated cranial or peripheral nerve involvement (e.g., cranial nerves, ulnar, median, femoral, or peroneal)
  If confluent, may resemble polyneuropathy
Radiculopathy or polyradiculopathy
  Thoracic
  Lumbosacral
Clinical syndrome of diabetic amyotrophy
  Femoral mononeuropathy
  Lumbosacral plexopathy and/or radiculopathy
  Anterior horn cell neuronopathy
Polyneuropathy
Autonomic neuropathy
  Diffuse sensorimotor
  Painful sensory

From Greene DA, Sima AAF, Albers JW, Pfeifer MA. Neuropathy. In: Rifkin H, Porte D, eds. Ellenberg and Rifkin's diabetes mellitus, 4th ed. Connecticut: Appleton & Lange, 1990:710–755; with permission.

(or nondiabetic) subjects, dismissal of these focal and motor neuropathies as diabetes related (idiopathic) requires the exclusion of vasculitis, coagulation disorders, paraneoplastic syndromes, and other acknowledged causes of focal neuropathy with appropriate laboratory testing.

The management of focal neuropathies is directed at the exclusion of treatable metabolic, vascular, or mechanical factors. It is especially important to exclude nerve entrapment syndromes (e.g., median nerve entrapment at the wrist, or carpal tunnel syndrome), which occur with increased frequency in diabetic subjects. Diabetic mononeuropathies are managed conservatively, accompanied by prudent improvement in metabolic control.

The commonest forms of diabetic neuropathy are distal symmetric polyneuropathy and autonomic neuropathy. Their management constitutes a fundamental element of the overall therapeutic approach to diabetes mellitus.

Distal Symmetric Polyneuropathy

Diabetic distal, symmetric, primarily sensory, peripheral polyneuropathy can be defined as a disease of progressive nerve fiber injury, atrophy, and loss that manifests itself through deteriorating neural function and worsening sensory-motor deficit, with or without accompanying dysesthetic or paresthetic symptoms. Nerve fiber damage may be sufficiently mild that it is unapparent by careful clinical history and physical examination but evident by sensitive testing of nerve function or with nerve biopsy, in which case the disease is staged as subclinical. The appearance of clinical symptoms or neurologic deficits, affecting the most distal anatomic sites first, defines clinical neuropathy. Clinical neuropathy corresponds to a definable level of nerve fiber damage on sural nerve biopsy.

The extent of neuropathologic damage in clinically apparent diabetic neuropathy suggests that it represents a late stage in a chronic underlying degenerative process and that the neuropathologic threshold for clinically detectable neurologic deficits is high. The disease ultimately culminates in tertiary complications of peripheral distal sensory and motor denervation, including loss of sensation, anesthesia, limb deformity, ulceration, neuroarthropathy, and amputation. While sensory loss corresponds closely with the degree of underlying nerve fiber damage, neuropathic pain appears to represent an independent process that correlates better with nerve fiber regeneration. Therefore, scored neurologic examinations, quantitative sensory testing, and electrophysiologic studies provide reliable indicators of nerve fiber damage in diabetic neuropathy, whereas symptom assessment yields at best unreliable and at times misleading information about the severity of the underlying disease process.

In the outpatient clinic, a rapid screening procedure is necessary to detect patients with clinically significant diabetic peripheral neuropathy, which puts them at risk for developing foot ulceration. Recently a simple neuropathy screening instrument has been developed for this purpose, which comprises a short questionnaire (15 yes-no questions) and a brief clinical assessment for foot deformity and skin abnormalities, ankle tendon reflexes, and vibration perception threshold (128 Hz tuning fork on the dorsum of the great toe). This has been shown to have both high sensitivity and high specificity. Additionally, the assessment of light touch perception using a 10 g nylon monofilament (which is the sensory threshold required to protect against the development of foot ulceration) may further enhance the clinician's ability to screen patients efficiently for clinically significant sensory deficits in the outpatient setting (Fig. 1).

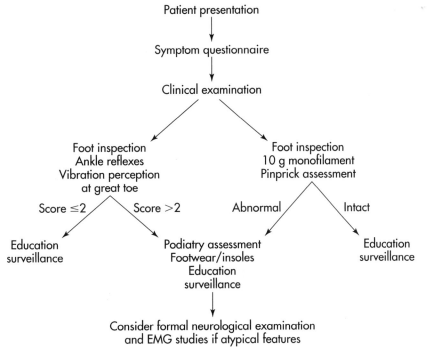

Figure 1
Clinical approaches for the diagnosis of the "at risk" diabetic neuropathic foot.

■ TREATMENT

It is useful to categorize patients with diabetic peripheral neuropathy according to the type (i.e., painful, sensory loss, motor involvement) and duration (acute versus chronic) of neuronal dysfunction when developing an approach to therapy (Table 2). Since many patients fall into more than one category, an integrated treatment approach, involving several specialty clinics, may be necessary. All types of diabetic neuropathy should be initially treated by improvement in glycemic control. Although this will uniformly improve nerve conduction velocity, its effect on clinical symptoms is less predictable.

Potential Therapeutic Role of Aldose Reductase Inhibitors

Increased activity of the aldose reductase pathway, leading to the excessive accumulation of polyols, decreased myo-inositol and taurine levels, and altered energy metabolism, has been implicated in the development of diabetic neuropathy. Questions about the possible efficacy and pathogenetic relevance of aldose reductase inhibitors to diabetic neuropathy have yet to be resolved. This failure may be the result of confusion about the rationale and expectations for early clinical intervention studies, uncertainties regarding the natural history of diabetic neuropathy, and lack of reliable clinical and clinically relevant physiologic measures of neuropathy. Alternatively, these disappointing results could indicate that aldose reductase activation has only a minor role in the pathogenesis and potential therapy of diabetic neuropathy. Recent detailed studies of nerve architecture, however, support a larger rather than a smaller role for polyol pathway activation in the processes leading to clinically evident diabetic neuropathy.

Table 2 General Therapeutic Approach to the Treatment of Diabetic Neuropathy

ACUTE PAINFUL NEUROPATHY (<6 MONTHS DURATION)
Treatment Options
Blood glucose control
Therapeutic drug trials*
Aldose reductase inhibitors
CHRONIC PAINFUL NEUROPATHY (>6 MONTHS DURATION)
Treatment Options
Blood glucose control
Therapeutic drug trials*
Consultation with pain clinic
Assess the need for psychiatric support
SENSORY IMPAIRMENT
Treatment Options
Blood glucose control
Foot care
Wound care
Physical therapy
Education and Support at Integrated Diabetic Foot Clinic
FOCAL NEUROPATHY-POLYRADICULOPATHY
Treatment Options
Physical therapy
Therapeutic drug trials

*See Table 3.

Short-term treatment with aldose reductase inhibitors in adequate doses appears to improve nerve electrophysiology in diabetic subjects but is associated with only marginal symptomatic improvement in patients with diabetic neuropathy. This most likely reflects the short duration of treatment in relationship to the advanced state of neuropathic damage (e.g., severe enough to produce foot ulcers and/or neuroarthropathy) in some patient populations. Historically, the majority of studies in humans show a trend toward, rather than clear evidence of, clinical and/or functional improvement in neuropathic patients treated with aldose reductase inhibitors. A notable exception was a study in which paired nerve biopsies were obtained before and after 12 months of treatment with the aldose reductase inhibitor sorbinol, which demonstrated consistent morphometric evidence of both nerve fiber regeneration and repair in patients with clinically evident diabetic neuropathy. This early promise has been borne out by recent studies utilizing aldose reductase inhibitors that are many times more potent than their predecessors. These studies have also demonstrated beneficial effects on both nerve function and structure, confirming the relevance of this pathogenetic pathway. A question remains, however, about the potential reversibility of neuropathic damage once more clinically advanced neuropathy has occurred.

The now confirmed regenerative and reparative responses to aldose reductase inhibitors have provided conclusive evidence that the advanced neuropathologic alterations thought to underlie chronic clinical diabetic polyneuropathy are at least partially reversible. Moreover, these studies suggest that the aldose reductase pathway may have a tonic role in the ongoing nerve fiber damage and/or the blunted nerve fiber repair and regeneration in well-established, clinically overt diabetic polyneuropathy. This would represent an effect of the aldose reductase pathway beyond its usually invoked initiating role in the pathogenesis of diabetic complications. Although the immediate clinical implications of this broad and active but early fiber regeneration and repair are uncertain, the accompanying electrophysiologic and electromyographic evidence suggests that these regenerating and remyelinating fibers are indeed physiologically functional. However, this early stage of fiber regeneration and repair is more likely to herald, rather than accompany, easily detectable clinical improvement, and extended treatment with aldose reductase inhibitors will most likely be necessary to entirely erase the characteristic morphometric (and perhaps clinical) components of diabetic neuropathy in patients afflicted with the disorder.

Painful Neuropathy

Among the symptoms associated with diabetic neuropathy, extreme pain is the most difficult to treat. In the patient with painful diabetic neuropathy, it is important to assess the predominant symptoms and their duration, together with any precipitating causes. Patients with painful neuropathy of any duration should have their glycemic control improved. Often, however, this does not result in resolution of the painful symptoms, and drug therapy becomes necessary. Patients with acute onset of symptoms that are associated (i.e., either improved or worsened) with changes in glycemic control have the best prognosis. In fact, it is not uncommon for patients with this type of pain to demonstrate spontaneous improvements. The longer the duration of pain, the less likely is improved glycemic control (or any other intervention) to be successful. Note: It is important for the physician to recognize femoral neuropathy. This distinct form of proximal motor neuropathy, which combines pain, weakness, and wasting in the thigh region, usually resolves spontaneously within 18 months.

Many different approaches have been used in the treatment of painful diabetic neuropathy, but none have proved uniformly efficacious. Table 3 summarizes the treatments that have met with at least some success. Nonsteroidal anti-inflammatory drugs may offer some relief of pain in a minority of patients. If symptoms are not improved, a trial of therapy with the tricyclic antidepressants can be instituted; approximately one out of three to four individuals will have a gratifying response. These drugs block the reuptake of nor-epinephrine, the putative neurotransmitter released by pain pathways between the brain stem and the spinal cord. This blockade prolongs the inhibitory action of norepinephrine on pain transmission by spinal cord neurons. Five drugs from this family of norepinephrine reuptake blockers have proved effective in relieving neuropathic pain in double-blind, placebo-controlled trials: amitriptyline, nortriptyline, desipramine, imipramine, and clomipramine. A useful treatment plan for patients with painful neuropathy is shown in Figure 2. If the patient has no known cardiac disease or prostatism, therapy is initiated with amitriptyline. Regardless of the patient's age, 10 mg are given a $\frac{1}{2}$ hour before bedtime. Amitriptyline is the most sedating of the tricyclics and has the greatest anticholinergic side effects. We therefore increase the drug by 10 mg increments every 3 days until the patient becomes intolerant of the side effects or until we have reached 100 mg. Although essentially all patients at this dose complain of dry mouth, the side effects are more likely to occur at lower doses in the elderly (over 65 to 70 years of age). If a patient has experienced no pain relief after 1 month on 100 mg per night, the dose should be increased, using the same paradigm, until 150 to 300 mg per night is reached or side effects become intolerable. Doses greater than 300 mg per night are not associated with increased therapeutic efficacy. Serum drug levels have not proved helpful in guiding therapy. Dosage adjustment is best gauged by the response of the patient's symptoms and side effects.

Nortriptyline is used in lieu of amitriptyline when daytime sedation becomes a problem. In elderly subjects, nortriptyline is less sedating than amitriptyline. The same paradigm can be used for instituting nortriptyline therapy as for amitriptyline therapy. Nortriptyline has the same general side effect profile as amitriptyline, but sedation, urinary retention, and orthostatic hypotension occur less frequently. The two drugs should never be used concurrently. If urinary retention becomes a problem, desipramine therapy can be instituted. Among the tricyclics, this drug has the least anticholinergic activity. If the patient has a history of cardiac arrhythmias or significant cardiac disease, doxepin may be preferred. Doxepin is only slightly less sedative than amitriptyline, but at daily doses less than 150 mg it has the least cardiotoxic effects of the tricyclics. At higher doses this advantage is lost. The same paradigm can be employed for the institution of desipramine or doxepin as for amitriptyline and nortriptyline. A clinical trial is currently in progress with tramadol hydrochloride, which is an attractive prospective treatment for painful diabetic neuropathy because it blocks the reuptake of both norepinephrine and serotonin, interacts with central opioid receptors, and is in general well tolerated.

If a patient still has significant discomfort after an adequate trial of tricyclics, capsaicin cream (0.075%) should be added. Patients are instructed to apply the cream four times a

Table 3 Specific Therapeutic Strategies in the Treatment of Painful Diabetic Neuropathy

Improved glycemic control
Nonsteroidal drugs
    Ibuprofen (600 mg q.i.d.)
    Sulindac (200 mg b.i.d.)
Tricyclic antidepressant drugs
    Amitriptyline (50 mg at night)
    Imipramine (100 mg q.d.)
Nonaddicting analgesics
    Carbamazepine (200 mg q.i.d.)
    Phenytoin (300 mg q.d.)
    Lidocaine (5 mg/kg)
    Mexiletine (10 mg/kg)
Others
    Capsaicin cream (0.075%)
    OpSite film
    Fluphenazine (1 mg t.i.d.)
    Clonidine (0.1 mg at night)
    Transcutaneous nerve stimulation

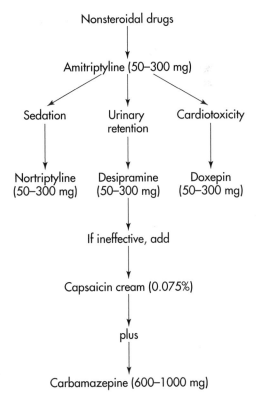

Figure 2
A management plan for painful neuropathy.

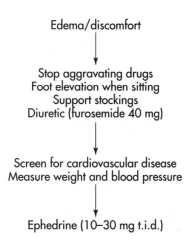

Edema/discomfort

↓

Stop aggravating drugs
Foot elevation when sitting
Support stockings
Diuretic (furosemide 40 mg)

↓

Screen for cardiovascular disease
Measure weight and blood pressure

↓

Ephedrine (10–30 mg t.i.d.)

Figure 3
Management of symptoms resulting from autonomic neuropathy.

day to the painful areas. Patients should be informed that for the first 1 to 3 days pain may actually increase. However, after 1 week of therapy a substantial percentage of patients notice pain relief. A combination of a tricyclic antidepressant and capsaicin cream provides relief in approximately two-thirds of patients with painful diabetic neuropathy. In the remaining one-third of patients, pain is still disabling. In such individuals we add a third drug to the regimen, while maintaining the tricyclic and capsaicin therapies. We most often use carbamazepine, starting at a dose of 100 mg twice daily and increasing by 100 mg increments every 3 days until the patient reaches 200 mg three times per day or becomes intolerant of side effects. The chief side effects are dizziness and/or a feeling of drunkenness. Nausea and a truncal skin rash may also occur. Leukopenia has been associated with carbamazepine therapy, and a complete blood count with differential must be checked on a weekly basis for the first month, and at monthly intervals thereafter, for 3 months. Monitoring serum carbamazepine levels is helpful in these patients.

Chronic pain is always difficult to treat, and referral to a pain clinic may be necessary. Severe contact dysesthesias, which may be particularly severe at night, are helped by providing a cradle to lift the bed covers off the legs. Techniques such as transcutaneous nerve stimulation or lumbar nerve blocks may be helpful in a limited number of patients. Recently the application of a plastic film (OpSite) to the painful region has been shown to help alleviate chronic pain, possibly by a mechanism involving desensitization.

■ PERIPHERAL AUTONOMIC DENERVATION

Although it is frequently subclinical, peripheral autonomic neuropathy is common in diabetic patients and can lead to skin and nail changes and loss of sweating. Excess callus formation, the harbinger of foot ulceration, can result from vascular denervation and excess blood flow, which are characteristic of the diabetic neuropathic foot. Destruction of the sympathetic nerve supply to the vasculature causes increased

blood flow and arteriovenous shunting, which can be documented by demonstrating raised oxygen levels in venous blood and by the rapid appearance of albumin microspheres in the venous circulation after arterial injection. This high peripheral blood flow may be manifested clinically by edema and prominent veins on the feet. Pooling of blood in the feet may exacerbate postural hypotension, and impaired venous drainage and edema can lead to skin breakdown. Sympathetic denervation of the vasculature in the lower extremities has grave prognostic implications because it indicates severe end-stage neuropathy and is often associated with cardiac denervation, which can predispose to sudden death.

The techniques available to evaluate sympathetic nerve activity in the peripheral nerves are limited. Direct recording of sympathetic nervous activity in postganglionic C fibers using microelectrodes is a highly specialized procedure and is not useful in the routine diagnosis of autonomic neuropathy. Galvanic skin responses are easily measured on the skin of the foot and correlate well with the preservation of sympathetic innervation. This technique does not allow gradation of the neuropathy, however, and therefore lacks sensitivity in milder cases. Peripheral sympathetic denervation can be detected by the finding of abnormal vascular responses in the diabetic foot. Reduced peak skin blood flow after local thermal stimulation and, in particular, paradoxical vasoconstriction responses are detectable before the characteristic finding of biphasic ankle sonograms reflecting reduced peripheral vascular tone. Peripheral autonomic neuropathy is usually found in association with evidence of other small fiber damage (i.e., thermal insensitivity), and this may afford an indirect method of assessment.

The altered vascular responses that occur in the feet during the development of Charcot's arthropathy reflect underlying bony destruction and altered blood flow distribution. These changes in foot blood flow are potentially amenable to therapy. Sympathomimetic drugs (ephedrine and midodrine) can reduce the high arteriovenous shunt flow seen in diabetic peripheral neuropathy. Ephedrine (10 to 30 mg three times a day) is an effective treatment for neuropathic edema and may be helpful in the treatment of pain and discomfort (Fig. 3). The mechanism by which ephedrine works is unclear, but it probably involves an increase in peripheral vascular tone and increased sodium excretion. This drug has the disadvantage of central nervous system (CNS) side effects, irritability, and insomnia. It may also cause tachycardia and so should be avoided in patients with a history of cardiac disease. It should be used with great caution in patients with hypertension. Midodrine (10 mg three times a day), a selective alpha-adrenergic agonist that has been shown to be useful in the management of postural hypotension, may be better tolerated because it causes fewer CNS side effects. By reducing the high bone blood flow that enhances bone resorption, these sympathomimetic drugs may have a beneficial effect in preventing the development of the Charcot foot. However, early intervention—by instigating nonweight bearing and supportive foot wear (preferably a surgical cast) at the earliest stages of the Charcot foot—remains the principal mode of therapy.

The most beneficial approach to the management of autonomic neuropathy in the diabetic foot is regular foot care, removing excess callus, and the treatment of local infections with appropriate antibiotics. (See the chapter *The*

Diabetic Foot.) Regular surveillance and educating patients to report any new foot swelling, discomfort, or infection immediately provide the best prevention of foot deformities and amputations.

Suggested Reading

American Diabetes Association, American Academy of Neurology. Report and recommendations of the San Antonio Conference on diabetic neuropathy. Diabetes Care 1988; 11:592–597.

This is the report on a conference whose purpose was to assess the state of knowledge of diabetic neuropathy, assess the performance of evaluation procedures, and recommend research guidelines for future clinical investigations.

Boulton AJM, Levin S, Comstock J. A multicenter trial of the aldose-reductase inhibitor, tolrestat, in patients with symptomatic diabetic neuropathy. Diabetologia 1990; 33:431–437.

This study assessed the effects of the aldose-reductase inhibitor tolrestat in a placebo-controlled, randomized 52-week multicenter trial and demonstrated improvements in both patient symptoms and motor nerve conduction velocity.

Capsaicin Study Group. Effect of treatment with capsaicin on daily activities of patients with painful diabetic neuropathy. Diabetes Care 1992; 15:159–165.

This article reported the results of topical capsaicin therapy in painful diabetic neuropathy in a double-blind vehicle-controlled study. Topical 0.075% capsaicin was found to be effective in reducing pain, with improvement in the patient's quality of life.

Feldman EL, Stevens MJ, Thomas PK, et al. A practical two-step quantitative clinical and electrophysiological assessment for the diagnosis and staging of diabetic neuropathy. Diabetes Care 1994; 17:1281–1289.

This article describes the Michigan Neuropathy Screening Instrument and its utility for the detection of diabetic peripheral neuropathy in the outpatient clinic.

Foster AV, Eaton C, McConville DO, Edmonds ME. Application of OpSite film: A new and effective treatment of painful diabetic neuropathy. Diabetic Med 1994; 11:768–772.

This article describes the application and effectiveness of this novel approach in the management of painful diabetic neuropathy.

Greene DA, Sima AAF, Albers JW, Pfeifer MA. Pathophysiology of diabetic neuropathy. In: Rifkin H, Porte D, eds. Ellenberg and Rifkin's diabetes mellitus. 4th ed. Connecticut: Appleton & Lange, 1990:710.

This chapter gives an extensive overview of diabetic neuropathy, including diagnosis, pathophysiology, and treatment strategies.

Max MB, Lynch SA, Muir J, et al. Effects of desipramine, amitriptyline, and fluoxetine on pain in diabetic neuropathy. N Engl J Med 1992; 326:1250–1256.

This paper reports the results of two randomized, double-blind crossover studies evaluating the success of tricyclic agents in the treatment of painful diabetic neuropathy. The authors conclude that desipramine relieves pain as well as amitriptyline, thus offering a suitable alternative. Fluoxetine was ineffective.

Spallone V, Ucciloi L, Menzinger G. Diabetic autonomic neuropathy. Diabetes Metab Rev 1995; 11:227–257.

This is a general review of diabetic autonomic neuropathy, which details diagnostic methodology, clinical manifestations, and therapeutic approaches.

AUTONOMIC NEUROPATHY

Aaron I. Vinik, M.D., Ph.D.
Sompongse Suwanwalaikorn, M.D.

■ DEFINITION

Autonomic neuropathy (AN), or dysfunction of the autonomic nervous system (ANS), is very common in both type 1, or insulin-dependent (IDDM), and type 2, or non–insulin-dependent (NIDDM) diabetic patients, and its prevalence increases with the duration of diabetes and the level of hyperglycemia. The ANS comprises an afferent and an efferent system, with long efferents in the vagus and short postganglionic unmyelinated fibers in the sympathetic nervous system (SNS). Until recently it has been acceptable to consider only the major neurotransmitters (i.e., acetylcholine, norepinephrine, and epinephrine) as mediators of autonomic function. New information on peptidergic neurotransmission dictates a revision of our thinking. Less than 10 percent of the vagus nerve is made up of cholinergic fibers; the remainder are neuropeptidergic. Peptides that exert important effects include substance P, neuropeptide K, calcitonin gene-related peptide (CGRP), and pancreatic polypeptide (PP), among others. Some of these peptides have profound vascular, smooth muscle, and metabolic effects, while others are exquisitely sensitive to autonomic activation and must clearly be considered as essential components of the ANS. Autonomic neuropathy is classified as organic or functional, with further subdivisions based upon the overt nature of the disorder.

Organic

In organic AN, there is a diffuse anatomic lesion affecting small nerve fibers of the cholinergic, noradrenergic, and peptidergic nervous system. Impaired parasympathetic (vagal), sympathetic (adrenergic and noradrenergic), and peptidergic function is accompanied by impaired warm thermal perception or sudomotor dysfunction (C fibers), impaired cold perception (A-delta fibers), and decreased neurogenic thermal flare (mediated by neuropeptides, substance P, CGRP, neuropeptide K, and others). Organic AN may be further divided into subclinical (no clinical symptoms; diagnosed by tests) and clinical (presents with symptoms and signs) categories.

Functional

In functional AN, there is no organic lesion. Functional AN may be further classified as occurring (1) after hypoglycemia, (2) after intensive diabetes control, or (3) after hyperglycemia.

■ INCIDENCE

Although AN is thought to occur most frequently in IDDM, its prevalence is actually greater among NIDDM patients. The accompaniments of NIDDM—hypertension, obesity, a greater female preponderance, raised low-density lipoprotein (LDL) cholesterol, and reduced high-density lipoprotein (HDL) cholesterol—are independent risk factors for the development of AN. Age is a more important determinant than duration of diabetes.

Although it is commonly stated that AN is a disease of lean people, AN occurs more frequently in people with a higher body mass index.

■ RISKS

The 5-year survival of diabetic patients who are free of neuropathic complications is greater than 99 percent, whereas patients with clinically overt AN have a 25 to 40 percent chance of dying within 5 years. Subtle tests of autonomic function (i.e., pancreatic polypeptide response to hypoglycemia or loss of the [R-R] variation with deep breathing) reveal minor abnormalities in almost 100 percent of even newly diagnosed diabetic patients. However, these asymptomatic findings do not constitute a risk for progression, and only those individuals with symptoms are at risk of sudden death, myocardial infarction, or renal failure.

■ DIFFERENTIAL DIAGNOSIS

The differential diagnosis of AN includes idiopathic orthostatic hypotension, Shy-Drager syndrome (orthostatic hypotension, pyramidal and cerebellar signs including tremor, rigidity, hyperreflexia, ataxia, urinary and bowel dysfunction), panhypopituitarism, pheochromocytoma, hypovolemia (due to poor glycemic control or diuretics), and medications such as insulin, vasodilators (nitrates, calcium channel blockers, hydralazine), and sympathetic blockers (methyldopa, clonidine, prazosin, guanethidine, phenotiazines, tricyclic antidepressants). Alcoholic neuropathy may also cause orthostatic hypotension.

A careful history and physical examination, family history, medication review, and clinical evaluation will usually rule out other causes. Norepinephrine responses to hypoglycemia may be of value in idiopathic orthostatic hypotension as well as Shy-Drager syndrome, and screens for heavy metals, as well as serologic tests for Chagas' disease, may be helpful. The diagnosis of diabetic AN is one of exclusion.

■ FREQUENCY OF EVALUATION

A paradigm for the evaluation of AN and a general approach to therapy are depicted in Figure 1. Autonomic neuropathy is uncommon within the first 5 years after the onset of IDDM. In contrast, the onset of diabetes in NIDDM patients occurs long before the clinical diagnosis is established, and AN may be evident at the time of initial presentation. After 5 years in IDDM and at the time of diagnosis in NIDDM, patients should be evaluated for the presence of AN (Table 1). Thereafter, individuals should be evaluated yearly. A more detailed description of each test of autonomic function is provided under each particular organ system disorder. In all diabetic patients with AN an attempt should be made to improve glycemic control. Other therapeutic interventions are specific for the organ system that is affected.

■ TESTS OF AUTONOMIC FUNCTION

The ANS is usually tested by evaluating reflex arcs. A reflex arc involves a standard stimulus, a sensor, an afferent nerve, central processing, an efferent nerve, and an end organ response. In addition to the reflex arc, there are several

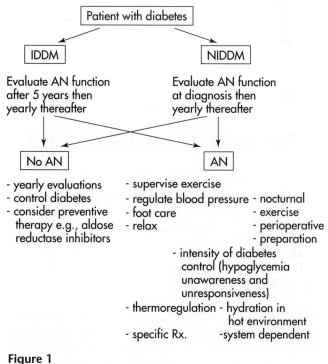

Figure 1
Suggested paradigm for management of autonomic neuropathy.

synaptic clefts involved throughout the pathway and different neurotransmitters at each synaptic cleft. It is to be noted that many organs are dually innervated, and parasympathetic and sympathetic pathways work as a check-and-balance system. Therefore, a decrease in one pathway may be followed by an increase in another. There are tests that are helpful in evaluating patients for autonomic dysfunction. Since eating, drinking coffee, smoking, volume status, upright posture, medicines, and exercise affect the cardiovascular ANS and presumably other ANS organ systems as well, the studies should be performed in the morning after an overnight (8-hour) fast, in a quiet, relaxed atmosphere following 30 minutes of supine rest. Patients should refrain from smoking and should not have performed vigorous exercise or had a recent bout of hypoglycemia. Patients should not have taken bolus short-acting insulin for at least 8 hours, and if they are on long-acting insulin or an insulin pump, they should maintain the dose or basal infusion rate to provide a normal glucose level on the morning of the test.

To define neuropathy, tests have been designed to focus upon the specific subdivision affected (Table 2).

■ SPECIFIC SYSTEM INVOLVEMENT IN AUTONOMIC NEUROPATHY (Table 3)

Pupillary Abnormalities

Failure of pupillary contraction with exposure to car headlights may interfere with night driving, and patients should be cautioned against driving after sunset. Dark-adapted pupil size and pupillometry are done in specialized research laboratories but are not available for general use. There is no treatment for disturbances of pupillary function.

Iris Abnormalities

Diabetic patients with iris AN have difficulty in pupil dilation. This allows less light to enter the eye, impairing dark vision.

Dark-adapted pupil size after total parasympathetic blockade is a useful tool for evaluating ANS function and is related to poor dark vision. Hippus and pupil latency time represent additional tests that can be performed. There is no specific treatment for iris AN.

Cardiovascular Abnormalities

Autonomic neuropathy most commonly involves the cardiovascular system. Reduced ejection fraction and systolic dysfunction, as well as decreased diastolic filling, impair exercise tolerance. The patchy loss of cardiac sympathetic innervation and prolongation of the QTc interval predisposes to bradycardia-induced arrhythmias. Reduced sympathetic vasoconstriction with peripheral pooling of blood causes orthostasis and predisposes to hypotension during anesthesia. The instability of blood pressure is common in the early morning and improves as the day progresses. Hypotension is often made worse by insulin given with the patient standing. Dizziness within minutes of an injection of insulin is not hypoglycemia.

Edema is common in diabetic patients with cardiac AN because of venous pooling and renal sodium retention due to insulin therapy or renal disease. The edema is often treated with diuretics, leading to contracted plasma volume and hypotension, with which the individual with AN cannot cope. Patients with cardiac AN suffer from sudden-death syndrome, and the mechanism(s) underlying this have yet to be adequately explained. Patients may have had a silent myocardial infarction. Arrhythmias may complicate the clinical presentation. Paroxysmal nocturnal hypertension with hypertensive crises has been reported and may compromise attempts to

Table 1 Tests of Autonomic Function

SYSTEM	CLINICAL PRACTICE	RESEARCH
Cardiovascular	Resting pulse R-R variation with respiration BP response to standing	Handgrip Cold pressor Skin blood flow
Pupillary	Pupillary size, shape, and reflexes	Dark-adapted pupil size Pupillary response
Gastrointestinal	Solid-phase gastric emptying in symptomatic subjects	Manometry IMMC Transit time PP response to hypoglycemia
Genitourinary	Cystometrogram	EMG Sphincter myography

Sexual
  Male
  Female
	Rigiscan	Sleep studies
		Vaginal
		Plethysmography

Sudomotor	—	Sweat beads, QSART, thermoregulatory reflexes
Metabolic	—	Stepped glucose insulin clamp Insulin hypoglycemia

R-R = interval recorded by electrocardiography; BP = blood pressure; PP = pancreatic polypeptide; EMG = electromyogram.

Table 2 Tests of Specific Subdivisions of the Autonomic Nervous System

SYMPATHETIC
Postural BP ≥30 mm Hg; fall in systolic BP on standing
Spectral analysis of R-R tracing of beat-to-beat variation with
    deep breathing
Impaired norepinephrine response to hypoglycemia
PARASYMPATHETIC
Abnormal R-R interval variation with breathing 5 breaths/min
Decreased PP response to insulin-induced hypoglycemia
PEPTIDERGIC
Loss of wheal and flare response to histamine (mediated by
    substance P)
Reduced cutaneous content of neuropeptides—protein S-100,
    substance P, CGRP
CENTRAL VS PERIPHERAL
Loss of the vasoconstrictive cutaneous blood flow
    response to:
        Mental arithmetic—(central)
        Cold pressor test—(peripheral)
        Sustained isometric hand grip contraction—(peripheral)

BP = blood pressure; *R-R* = interval recorded by electrocardiography *PP* = pancreatic polypeptide; *CGRP* = calcitonin gene-related peptide.

Table 3 Autonomic Neuropathy: Clinical Manifestations

PUPILLARY ABNORMALITIES
Decreased diameter of dark-adapted pupil
Argyll-Robertson type pupil
CARDIOVASCULAR ABNORMALITIES
Tachycardia, exercise intolerance
Cardiac denervation
Orthostatic hypotension
Heat intolerance
Skin temperature reversal, dry skin, and dependent edema
MOTOR DISTURBANCES OF GASTROINTESTINAL TRACT
Esophageal enteropathy
Gastroparesis diabeticorum
Constipation
Diarrhea
Fecal incontinence
GENITOURINARY TRACT DISTURBANCES
Neurogenic vesical dysfunction
Impotence
Cystopathy
Retrograde ejaculation
SWEATING DISTURBANCES
Areas of symmetrical anhidrosis
Gustatory sweating
METABOLIC DISTURBANCES
Hypoglycemia unawareness
Hypoglycemia unresponsiveness
Hypoglycemia-associated autonomic failure (HAAF)

Table 4 Cardiovascular Autonomic Neuropathy

CLINICAL EVALUATION
Symptoms
Decreased effort tolerance
Heat intolerance
Arrhythmias
Orthostasis
Signs
Tachycardia
Loss of sinus arrhythmia
Orthostasis and perioperative hypotension
Dry, scaly feet
DIAGNOSTIC TESTS
Resting heart rate >100 bpm
R-R variation >15 bpm, R-R <1.0 (Expiration/Inspiration)
Valsalva ratio <1.2
30:15 ratio <1.02
SBP fall with standing >20 mm Hg
DBP response to hand grip <16 mm Hg with 30% max for 5 min
QTc interval >440 msec
TREATMENT
Supervise exercise programs
Care with heat exposure—hydration
Perioperative—alert anesthesiologist-respiratory problems
Scrupulous foot care
Relax control (loss of warning palps)
Manage arrhythmias
Regulate—nocturnal BP

R-R = interval recorded by electrocardiography; *SBP* = systolic blood pressure; *DBP* = diastolic blood pressure; *BP* = blood pressure.

ing upon carbon dioxide as the respiratory stimulus. It is important to warn the anesthesiologist about the instability of blood pressure during anesthesia. Because patients with AN have difficulty in regulating thermogenic vascular responses, they tolerate heat poorly and are candidates for heat stroke.

Table 4 summarizes the features, differential diagnosis, and management of cardiovascular AN.

Testing for Cardiovascular Autonomic Neuropathy

A number of sensitive tests have been developed to test for the presence of cardiovascular AN.

Resting Heart Rate. A resting heart rate greater than 100 beats per minute is considered abnormal (normal is less than 100 beats per minute.)

Beat-to-Beat Heart Rate Variation. With the patient supine and breathing 6 breaths per minute, the heart rate is monitored by electrocardiography (ECG). Resting R-R variation is the difference between the influences of the SNS and the parasympathetic nervous system (PNS). A difference (maxi-mal-minimal) in heart rate of more than 15 beats per minute is normal; under 10 beats per minute is abnormal. R-R variation was once considered to be exclusively under the control of the PNS. However, a small decrease in R-R variation can result from SNS neuropathy. An abnormality in heart rate variability is a good predictor of long-term survival after acute myocardial infarction.

raise blood pressure in patients with orthostasis. This paradox often goes unrecognized, and futile attempts to raise ambulatory pressures may be associated with nocturnal hypertensive crises.

A problem for the anesthesiologist is the impaired hypoxia-induced ventilatory drive, and care must be exercised in rely-

---

Table 5 Orthostatic Hypotension

CLINICAL EVALUATION	TREATMENT
Symptoms	**Nonpharmacologic**
Dizziness	Correct or remove aggravating factors: drugs, volume depletion,
Lightheadedness	prolonged bed rest, alcohol
Dimming of vision upon standing	Head-up tilt during sleep
Syncope	Waist-high support stockings
Signs	**Pharmacologic**
Systolic blood pressure drop >30 mm Hg on standing	Mineralocorticoid: 9-alpha fluorocortisone (0.1–1.0 mg/day)
DIAGNOSTIC TESTS	Sympathomimetics: ephedrine, phenylephrine
Cardiovascular Reflexes Test	Indomethacin
Postural test	Clonidine
Expiration:Inspiration I ratio on deep breathing	Dihydroergotamine with caffeine
Valsalva ratio	
Handgrip test	
Cold pressor test	

Valsalva's Maneuver. Valsalva's maneuver has been well studied. It encompasses a complex reflex arc involving both SNS and PNS pathways to the heart, sympathetic pathways to the vascular tree, and baroreceptors in the chest and lungs. Therefore, it does not give as pure an evaluation of a specific area in the cardiovascular ANS as does R-R variation (which predominantly measures PNS). However, it provides insight into total cardiovascular ANS function.

To perform Valsalva's maneuver, the subject blows into the mouthpiece of a manometer to 40 mm Hg for 15 seconds with continuous ECG monitoring before, during, and after the procedure. Healthy subjects normally develop tachycardia and peripheral vasoconstriction during strain, and an overshoot rise in blood pressure and bradycardia on release. The ratio of longest R-R to shortest R-R is the Valsalva ratio. The normal value is 1.2 or more.

Heart Rate Response to Standing. The subject stands with continuous ECG monitoring, and the R-R interval is measured at beats 15 and 30. The normal response is tachycardia at beat 15 and bradycardia at beat 30. The 30:15 ratio is normally greater than 1.03.

Systolic Blood Pressure Response to Standing. In normal subjects the systolic blood pressure (SBP) falls by less than 10 mm Hg in 30 seconds. The response is abnormal if SBP falls more than 20 mm Hg within 2 minutes of standing. A fall of 20 to 29 mm Hg is considered borderline, but if the decline is accompanied by symptoms of orthostasis in addition to another abnormal test of autonomic function, it is taken as evidence of AN.

Diastolic Blood Pressure Response to Sustained Exercise. A handgrip dynamometer is squeezed to determine the isometric maximum. The dynamometer is then held at 30 percent of this value for 5 minutes. The normal response is a rise of diastolic blood pressure (DBP) greater than 16 mm Hg. The abnormal response is less than 10 mm Hg.

QTc Interval. Examination of the ECG may reveal a prolonged QTc interval in patients with cardiac AN. The QTc is the interval corrected for the cardiac cycle length and is normally less than 440 msec.

Treatment of Orthostatic Hypotension

Table 5 provides an approach to the treatment of orthostatic hypotension in diabetic patients with AN. The initial approach involves the use of full-length supportive stockings to increase venous return. These are taken off only when the patient goes to bed. Although effective, they can be troublesome in hot, humid climates in the summer. The patient needs to be cautioned to get out of bed slowly, to avoid hot baths (which cause vasodilation), and always to give insulin in the lying position (insulin enhances the transcapillary efflux of albumin out of the vascular compartment).

A number of drugs may be helpful in the treatment of orthostasis:

1. Clonidine (100-500 µg at bedtime). Paradoxically, the deficiency of postganglionic sympathetic neuronal alpha$_2$ receptors allows clonidine to act on the vasoconstrictive post-synaptic alpha$_2$ receptor.
2. Mineralocorticoids: 9-alpha fluorohydrocortisone (0.05-2.0 mg daily) may be used but generally causes edema before raising the blood pressure.
3. Metoclopramide hydrochloride (10 mg three times a day) has been observed to raise blood pressure in some people with orthostasis.
4. Midodrine (2.5-40 mg every 6 hours). This direct adrenergic agonist is an investigational drug that is helpful in selected cases.
5. Ergotamine (2.5-40 mg every 6 hours). When given together with caffeine, the combination can be a useful adjunct in some patients. Care must be exercised in patients with poor peripheral circulation not to induce ergotism.
6. Yohimbine (10 mg every 6-8 hours). This alpha$_2$ adrenergic antagonist, which is used for the treatment of impotence, raises blood pressure as a side effect, and this action can be embraced in the treatment of orthostasis.
7. Octreotide (0.1-0.5 µg per kilogram daily or twice daily). This is a last resort drug that may be very helpful in refractory cases. Given by injection, timing with the insulin dose in the morning is convenient.
8. Erythropoietin (50 U per kilogram three times per week). Patients with a reduced red blood cell volume may do well with volume expansion.

Motor Disturbances of Gastrointestinal Tract

Motor disturbances involving all anatomic subdivisions are very common in diabetic patients and are invariably associated with poor glycemic control.

Esophageal Enteropathy

Esophageal enteropathy is usually discovered accidentally while reviewing upper gastrointestinal (GI) studies. When symptomatic, dysphagia is the most common clinical complaint. As part of the differential diagnosis, the physician should consider achalasia, progressive systemic sclerosis (cutaneous manifestations), and esophageal candidiasis (painful dysphagia). Table 6 provides an approach to diagnosis and treatment. Eating in the upright position and drug therapy (metoclopramide, antacids, or H$_2$ receptor blockers) offer symptomatic relief.

Gastroparesis Diabeticorum

The major clinical features of gastroparesis diabeticorum are early satiety, anorexia, nausea, vomiting, epigastric discomfort, and bloating. Weight loss is uncommon. Disorders that can mimic diabetic gastroparesis include peptic ulcer disease, gastritis, gastric carcinoma, and ingestion of anticholinergic agents. A careful history of medications, including ganglionic blocking agents and psychotropic drugs, should be obtained. In addition, gastroduodenoscopy should be performed to exclude pyloric or other causes of mechanical obstruction. Almost 60 percent of patients attending a diabetes clinic have symptoms such as these, but only rarely is gastroparesis found (in under 10 percent). Paradoxically, as many as 25 percent of asymptomatic diabetic patients, and even more of those with "brittle diabetes," have been found to have some degree of gastroparesis with sophisticated testing.

Table 7 lists the clinical features, diagnostic approach, and treatment modalities. In evaluating a patient with suspected diabetic gastroparesis, the level of glycemic control should be assessed. Hyperglycemia, per se, impairs gastric emptying. After optimization of glycemic control, manometry (to detect antral hypomotility and/or pylorospasm) and double-isotope scintig-

---

Table 6 Esophageal Dysfunction

CLINICAL EVALUATION	Manometric studies
Symptoms	Decreased esophageal motor activities
Dysphagia	Reduced lower esophageal sphincter tone
Retrosternal discomfort	**TREATMENT**
Heartburn (rare)	**Nonpharmacologic**
Usually silent—discovered by accident	Dietary manipulation
Signs	Eating in upright position
None	Reducing food particle size (e.g., blenderized)
DIAGNOSTIC TESTS	Walking for 1 hr after meals
Radiologic Studies	**Pharmacologic**
Barium swallow	Metoclopramide (5–20 mg orally 3–4 times/day)
Dilatation	Antacid or H$_2$ receptor blocker
Tertiary peristalsis	
Reduced or absent primary peristalsis	
Delayed emptying	

Table 7 Gastroparesis Diabeticorum

CLINICAL EVALUATION	**TREATMENT**
Symptoms	**Nonpharmacologic**
Early satiety, anorexia	Dietary manipulation
Nausea, vomiting	Several small meals, low-fat diet, avoidance of milk, fibrous vegetables
Epigastric discomfort, abdominal bloating	Nasogastric suction
Signs	Rest stomach for 3 weeks
Epigastric or left upper quadrant tenderness	Jejunostomy feeding
Gastric succussion splash	Nocturnal nutrient supply with continuous insulin
DIAGNOSTIC TESTS	**Pharmacologic**
Radiologic Studies	Metoclopramide (5–20 mg 3–4 times/day)
Upper GI series	Bethanechol (10–20 mg 3–4 times/day)
Gastric dilatation	Domperidone (10–20 mg ½ hr before meals and at bedtime)
Prolonged retention of barium	Cisapride (10–20 mg ½ hr before meals)
Radionuclide studies	Erythromycin (250 mg ½ hr before meals)
Delayed solid phase gastric emptying time	
Manometric studies	
Decreased interdigestive myoelectric activity	
Reduced lower esophageal sphincter tone	

raphy (to measure solid and liquid phase gastric emptying times) may be indicated.

Treatment should emphasize improvement of glycemic control and correction of other metabolic abnormalities. It also includes dietary modification (small, low-fat, and/or liquid meals), gastric suction, metoclopramide (5 to 20 mg every 6 to 8 hours by IV or oral suspension), domperidone (10 to 20 mg ½ hour before meals and at bedtime), cisapride (10 to 20 mg ½ hour before meals), bethanechol (10 to 20 mg every 6 to 8 hours), or the antibiotic erythromycin (250 mg ½ hour before meals). In severe cases, jejunostomy may be needed to provide for feeding and resting the stomach.

Constipation

The extent of the evaluation in a diabetic patient complaining of constipation depends on the severity of the constipation and associated signs. It is important to exclude colonic carcinoma (positive guaiac), achalasia, and drugs that impair colonic motility. All patients should have a careful digital examination. Women should have a pelvic examination with bimanual examination. Three stool specimens should be tested for occult blood. If occult blood is detected, complete blood count, iron, total iron binding capacity, and proctosigmoidoscopy and barium enema or full colonoscopy should be performed.

Table 8 lists the clinical features, diagnosis, and management of constipation. Treatment of diabetic constipation includes improvement of glycemic control with correction of glycosuria, adequate hydration, a high-fiber diet, and psyllium. If these measures are not sufficient, trials of metoclopramide, domperidone, and cisapride may be considered.

Diarrhea

Diarrhea in AN can be sudden, explosive, paroxysmal, nocturnal or seasonal, uncontrollable, and embarrassing. Surprisingly, it does not lead to malnutrition and tends to be self-limiting. The diagnosis of diabetic diarrhea is established by excluding other causes of diarrhea and by confirming the presence of AN.

A history should be taken to rule out diarrhea secondary to ingestion of lactose, nonabsorbable hexitols, or medication.

Travel and sexual histories should be obtained, and patients should be questioned regarding similar illnesses among both household members and co-workers. History of ethanol consumption, symptomatic pancreatitis, and biliary stone diseases should be assessed. Initially stools should be tested for occult blood, enteric pathogens, ova, and parasites. Serum vitamin B_{12} and folate concentrations should be measured. Diarrhea should be quantitated with a 72-hour stool collection for volume, weight, and fat measurement.

If occult blood is detected, both upper and lower GI endoscopy should be performed to exclude Crohn's disease. If the history and examination suggest small bowel disease, the hydrogen breath test and Schilling test should be performed. The hydrogen breath test will be positive in patients with bacterial overgrowth but is also positive in individuals with lactose intolerance. Bacterial overgrowth may be inferred if, after a positive hydrogen breath test and course of broad-spectrum antibiotics (metronidazole, tetracycline, or Bactrim), symptoms resolve and the hydrogen breath test reverts to normal. Celiac disease is often accompanied by features (steatorrhea, hypoalbuminemia, anemia, and low serum B_{12} and folate levels) of more severe malabsorption than bacterial overgrowth or uncomplicated diabetic diarrhea. If celiac disease is suspected, upper GI endoscopy with small bowel biopsy should be performed. Since blunting of villi may occur in both severe bacterial overgrowth and celiac disease, determination of clinical and histologic responses to antibiotics or gluten-free diet may be the only means of distinguishing the two. If significant steatorrhea is detected, a plain film of the abdomen to assess pancreatic calcification and formal pancreatic function tests should be performed. A trial of oral pancreatic enzymes should be considered if these are abnormal.

Table 9 summarizes the diagnostic approach and management of diarrhea. Pancreatic insufficiency is managed with replacement of pancreatic enzymes (Pancrease, 2 to 4 tablets with each meal). A trial of antibiotics (tetracycline, metronidazole) is indicated for bacterial overgrowth, which may complicate diabetic intestinal AN.

The severe and intermittent nature of diabetic diarrhea makes its assessment and treatment very difficult. Since afferent denervation may contribute to the problem, a bowel program that includes insoluble fiber (psyllium and kaolin), multiple small feedings (low in fat), and regular efforts to move the bowels is indicated. Trials of cholestyramine (to chelate bile salts and reduce bile acid contribution to the diarrhea), clonidine (an alpha$_2$ agonist that may reverse adrenergic nerve dysfunction). Antidiarrheal agents (Lomotil or loperamide) should not be given, because they tend to perpetuate the problem. Metoclopramide and cholinergic agents or choline esterase inhibitors may benefit some patients, but it must be explained that diarrhea will occur before they get relief. Lastly, if all else fails, a therapeutic trial with octreotide can be instituted (see Table 9 for dosage regimen).

Fecal Incontinence

Fecal incontinence is a disturbing symptom that results from impaired function of the sacral outflow tract. In evaluating fecal incontinence, it is important to take an accurate history and to assess 72-hour stool volume and weight. Anorectal function is evaluated by anorectal manometry, which quantitates maximal basal sphincter pressure, and by the rectoanal

---

Table 8 Constipation

CLINICAL EVALUATION	Pharmacologic
Symptoms	High-insoluble fiber diet
Intermittent	supplement with a
Alternates with diarrhea	daily hydrophilic col-
Signs	loid (e.g., psyllium)
Impaction of feces	Intermittent saline or
DIAGNOSTIC TESTS	osmotic laxative
Radiologic Studies	Metoclopramide, dom-
Rule out other causes (e.g., carci-	peridone, cisapride
noma, achalasia, irritable bowel)	Fleet enemas as needed
TREATMENT	
Nonpharmacologic	
Toilet habit training	
Maintenance of adequate hydration	
Regular exercise	

Table 9 Diabetic Diarrhea

CLINICAL EVALUATION	Small bowel biopsy
Symptoms	Celiac disease, ileitis, parasites
Paroxysmal, seasonal, explosive, unpredictable	Stool exam and stool fat
Spontaneous remission, variable duration	Rule out malabsorption
Normal bowel habits between episodes	**TREATMENT**
Weight loss usually not prominent	**Nonpharmacologic**
Coincident rectal incontinence	Gluten-free, decreased lactose diet
Signs	**Pharmacologic**
Minimal—loss of anal sphincter tone	Antibiotics (tetracycline, metronidazole)
DIAGNOSTIC TESTS	Pancreatic enzymes (2–4 caps with meals)
Radiologic Studies	Psyllium (1 tsp–tbsp 1–3 times/day)
Long GI series	Cholestyramine (1 pack [4 g] 1–6 times/day)
Rule out other causes of diarrhea	Clonidine (200 µg 2–3 times/day)
Test of pancreatic function	Octreotide (50 µg 3 times/day)
Rule out steatorrhea	
Breath hydrogen test	
Bacterial overgrowth/lactose intolerance	

inhibitory reflex (inflation of a balloon in the rectum causes a reflex relaxation of the internal anal sphincter). Continence for solids and liquids is assessed directly by simulating the stress of stools with a solid sphere or rectally infused saline.

It is more difficult to retain loose than solid stools. Therefore, a combination of fiber supplement with an anti-diarrhea agent (loperamide, starting dose 2 mg twice a day) may prove useful. Sphincter strengthening exercises should be taught to the patient. Diabetic patients with intact rectal sensation and good motivation are candidates for biofeedback training.

Genitourinary Tract Disturbances
Impotence

Table 10 summarizes the clinical features of impotence in male diabetic patients. The etiology of impotence can be defined by a series of tests including medical history (libido, erectile function, ejaculatory function, and fertility), review of medications, assessment of glycemic control (glycosylated hemoglobin), measurement of nocturnal penile tumescence (snap gauge), and measurement of penile blood pressure with a Doppler probe (a penile-brachial pressure index less than 0.75 is suggestive of penile vascular disease). Integrity of the penile vasculature is assessed by quantitation of blood flow in response to the potent vasodilator prostaglandin E (alprostadil, 20 µg) given directly into the corpora cavernosa, hormonal evaluation (luteinizing hormone, testosterone, free testosterone, prolactin), and psychological evaluation (Minnesota Multiphasic Personality Inventory). Special tests of penile function include (1) Doppler ultrasound measurement of penile systolic blood pressure, (2) penile tumescence measurement by strain gauge, and (3) bulbocavernosus reflex response latency.

It is important to exclude psychological causes (which may be part of the diabetic condition or related to other associated medical conditions or stress); medications (e.g., antihypertensives, antidepressants, phenothiazines, tranquilizers, estrogens); other chronic medical conditions and vascular problems that can cause impotence; and endocrine causes (hyperprolactinemia and hypotestosteronemia).

Treatment of erectile failure should be discussed with the patient and his partner. Treatments include psychological

Table 10 Impotence

CLINICAL EVALUATION	**TREATMENT**
Symptoms	**Nonpharmacologic**
Decreased rigidity	Avoid or change to drug
Reduced frequency of erection	with lower impotence
Absence of nocturnal penile	effect
tumescence	Improve glycemic control
Normal libido	Mechanical suction device
Signs	**Pharmacologic**
Testicular anesthesia	Yohimbine (10 mg three
Delayed bulbocavernosus reflex	times a day)
response	Intracorporeal injection of
DIAGNOSTIC TESTS	prostaglandin, papaver-
Angiography/Doppler ultrasound	ine, phentolamine
Arterial/venous insufficiency	Penile prosthesis
Venous leakage	Vascular surgery
Nocturnal penile tumescence test	
Psychogenic	
Autonomic nerve dysfunction/	
vascular	

counseling, improvement in glycemic control and general health, change in medications, treatment of hypogonadism or hyperprolactinemia, noninvasive erection assistance devices, alpha adrenergic antagonists (yohimbine, 10 mg three times a day), injection of papaverine (40 to 80 mg) or alprostadil (10 to 40 µg) directly into the corpus cavernosum or introduction into the meatus (MUSE), reconstructive vascular surgery for vasculogenic impotence, and insertion of a semirigid or inflatable penile prosthesis.

Acquired ejaculatory failure due to AN is of importance if fertility is desired. Retrograde ejaculation may be diagnosed by the presence of azoospermia or the finding of sperm in the postcoital urine. If the failure is of recent onset or incomplete, the patient should be instructed to have intercourse with his bladder distended. Sometimes ejaculation can be restored with desipramine (50 mg). Alternatively, spermatozoa may be concentrated from the first urine voided after ejaculation, and these may be used for artificial insemination performed with ultrasound monitoring of ovulation.

Table 11 Bladder Dysfunction	
CLINICAL EVALUATION	**TREATMENT**
Symptoms	**Asymptomatic**
Poor urine stream	Timed voiding, double void-
Feeling of incomplete bladder	ing, abdominal straining
emptying	**Symptomatic**
Straining to void	Intermittent self-catheteri-
Hesitancy	zation
Infrequent voiding	Treat infection aggressively
Absence of nocturia with	**Reduction of Bladder**
increased volume of first	**Outlet Obstruction**
morning urine	Surgical
Signs	TURP, open prostatec-
Full bladder on percussion	tomy
DIAGNOSTIC TESTS	Nonsurgical
Radiologic Studies	Bethanechol
Increased residual urine	Balloon dilatation
Urodynamic Studies	Local hyperthermia
Increased bladder capacity	Prostatic stents
(>1000 ml)	
Impaired bladder sensation	
Increased postvoid residual urine	
(>200 ml)	
Decreased bladder contractility	
Acontractile detrusor	
Impaired urine flow (<10 ml/sec)	

TURP = transurethral prostatic resection.

Female Sexual Dysfunction

Diagnosis of female sexual dysfunction using vaginal plethysmography to measure lubrication and vaginal flushing has not been well established. It may be valuable in the future, but much in the way of standardization needs to be accomplished before it can be recommended as a routine test.

Cystopathy

Table 11 details the clinical features of bladder dysfunction. Evaluation for diabetic bladder dysfunction should be performed in any diabetic patient with recurrent urinary tract infection, pyelonephritis, incontinence, or a palpable bladder. In the male it is especially important to exclude prostatic hypertrophy. Chronic urinary tract infection, anticholinergic drugs, and spinal cord lesions need to be ruled out. Evaluation should include assessment of renal function, urinary culture, postvoid ultrasound to assess residual volume, and upper urinary tract dilatation. Cystometry and voiding cystometrogram are performed to measure bladder sensation and the volume pressure changes that accompany filling the bladder with known volumes of water and voiding. Diabetic cystopathy is evident as an increase in the threshold of occurrence of a detrusor reflex contraction. Special tests of bladder function include (1) cystometry, (2) sphincter electromyography, (3) uroflowmetry, (4) urethral pressure profile, and (5) electrophysiologic test of bladder innervation.

The principal aim of treatment should be to improve bladder emptying and to reduce the risk of urinary tract infection. The patient with a grossly overdistended bladder should undergo an initial period of catheter drainage to improve bladder contractility. Care should be taken to avoid the introduction of infection. Thereafter the patient should be instructed to void by the clock rather than waiting for the conscious sensation of bladder distention. Pressure applied to the bladder (Credé's maneuver) will often facilitate emptying. Cholinergic agents (bethanechol chloride, 10 to 20 mg orally four times a day) or clean intermittent self-catheterization may also be used to facilitate bladder emptying. Bladder neck resection in men and urethral dilatation in women should be approached with circumspection because of the risks of urinary incontinence.

Alterations in Distal Autonomic Function
Sweating Disturbances

Hyperhidrosis of the upper body, often related to eating, and anhidrosis of the lower body are characteristic features of diabetic AN. Loss of lower body sweating can lead to dry, brittle skin that cracks easily and predisposes to ulcer formation. Impaired sweating may be evaluated using simple starch, iodine, or more sophisticated measurements of iontophoresis and by electromyographic evaluation of small nerve fiber function. The latter, however, is overkill, and the clinical evaluation is usually sufficient.

QSART, sweat beads, and thermoregulatory control represent tests that have proved useful in evaluating sweat gland function. QSART is quantitative, well established, and has been validated for research. During the test a skin thermistor probe is attached to the dorsum of the left foot at midfoot level and the foot is warmed to 31° C using an infrared lamp. Four sites on the foot are used and are studied with the patient supine.

Sweat beads count the number of sweat glands that are innervated. This test is qualitative rather than quantitative, although the number of glands can be used as a quantitative index. Thermoregulatory control evaluates the amount of surface area that does not sweat after standard heating. It is less precise than the previous two tests.

Some people with gustatory sweating or hyperhidrosis have received benefit from a scopolamine patch placed behind the ear.

Alterations in Cutaneous Blood Flow

Microvascular skin flow is under the control of the ANS and is regulated by both the central and peripheral components of the ANS. Microvascular blood flow can be accurately measured noninvasively using laser Doppler flowmetry. Smooth-muscle microvasculature in the periphery reacts sympathetically to a number of stressor tasks. These may be divided into those dependent upon the integrity of the central nervous system (orienting response and mental arithmetic) and those dependent upon the distal sympathetic axonal response (handgrip and cold pressor tests).

At present there are no therapeutic interventions that specifically reverse autonomically mediated abnormalities in microvascular blood flow.

Metabolic Disturbances

Clinical features of the hypoglycemia-associated syndromes are given in Table 12. Before attributing the problem to diabetes, other causes of autonomic dysfunction need to be considered. Endocrine deficiencies, including hypopituitarism and hypoadrenalism, and organic causes of hypoglycemia must be excluded. Beta-blockers promote hypoglycemia, cause hypoglycemic unawareness, and impair recovery from hypoglycemia.

Hypoglycemia Unresponsiveness

An acquired selective deficiency of the glucagon secretory response to hypoglycemia is a characteristic finding in patients with long-standing IDDM. Patients with AN have a combined deficiency of their glucagon and epinephrine secretory response to plasma glucose decrements. This results in defective glucose counter-regulation and an inability to restore blood glucose concentrations to normal levels. When IDDM patients with combined glucagon/epinephrine deficiency are compared with patients who have deficient glucagon response alone, they have been shown to be at an increased risk (approximately twenty-five fold or greater) for severe clinical hypoglycemia during intensive insulin therapy for diabetes.

Hypoglycemia Unawareness

Patients with hypoglycemia unawareness lose the warning neuroglycopenic symptoms of developing hypoglycemia and fail to compensate by eating to prevent progression to severe hypoglycemia. The syndrome is thought to be the result of deficient sympathetic neural (norepinephrine) and adrenomedullary (epinephrine) responses to falling glucose levels.

Hypoglycemia-Associated Autonomic Failure in IDDM

In IDDM patients, three hypoglycemia-associated clinical syndromes have much in common: defective glucose counter-regulation, hypoglycemia unawareness, and elevated glycemic thresholds for symptoms and activation of counter-regulatory systems during intensive insulin therapy. They segregate together, are associated with an increased frequency of severe iatrogenic hypoglycemia, and share several pathophysiologic features. These include reduced ANS responses during hypoglycemia, such as reduced sympathetic (elevated glycemic thresholds for epinephrine) and parasympathetic (pancreatic polypeptide) responses. In the setting of reduced (often absent) glucagon responses, the reduced epinephrine response plays a key role in the pathogenesis of iatrogenic hypoglycemia in diabetic patients. These syndromes are examples of hypoglycemia-associated autonomic failure (HAAF) in IDDM, a disorder distinct from classic diabetic AN. Short-term antecedent hypoglycemia results in reduced symptomatic and autonomic, including epinephrine, responses to subsequent hypoglycemia. Therefore, recent antecedent iatrogenic hypoglycemia, which reduces both symptoms of and defenses against developing hypoglycemia, predisposes to recurrent severe hypoglycemia, creating a vicious cycle.

HAAF is distinct from classic diabetic AN in several ways. First, the two disorders tend to occur in different patients. Second, in HAAF the deficient autonomic responses appear to be specific for the stimulus of hypoglycemia, whereas reduced sympathetic and parasympathetic responses to multiple stimuli characterize classic diabetic AN. Third, reduced epinephrine responses to hypoglycemia are a central feature of HAAF, whereas plasma epinephrine responses are reduced little, if at all, in classic diabetic AN. Fourth, there is now good evidence that classic diabetic AN does not cause excessive iatrogenic hypoglycemia in IDDM. Fifth, recent data suggest that HAAF is at least in part reversible (see subsequent discussion). In contrast, there is no evidence that classic diabetic autonomic failure is reversible, although responses to treatment with growth factors suggest that recovery may be possible.

Lowered Glycemic Thresholds with Intensive Therapy

The results of the Diabetes Control Complications Trial have provided an impetus for intensified insulin therapy to achieve lower blood glucose levels in people with IDDM. However, it is now clear that such tight glycemic control with insulin lowers the threshold at which counter-regulatory hormones are released, maintains brain glucose utilization, and causes hypoglycemia unawareness because the brain perceives that it is receiving glucose. There is a poor correlation between altered counter-regulatory hormone thresholds, unawareness of hypoglycemia, and the presence of diabetic AN. Defective glucose counter-regulation, hypoglycemia unawareness, and elevated glycemic thresholds during effective therapy cosegregate in the same patient and are associated with a high frequency of iatrogenic hypoglycemia. These factors have recently been grouped together by Cryer and colleagues as HAAF. In contrast to HAAF, there is little evidence that AN contributes to iatrogenic hypoglycemia. It appears that the vicious cycle of HAAF is initiated by repeated episodes of hypoglycemia, which reset the threshold for the response, thereby generating further episodes of hypoglycemia and failure of the normal counter-regulatory response.

In normal subjects, autonomic symptoms (anxiety, palpitations, sweating, irritability, and tremor) begin at a blood glucose concentration of 58 plus or minus 2 mg per deciliter. This is significantly higher than the threshold for neuroglycopenic symptoms (hunger, dizziness, tingling, blurred

---

Table 12 Hypoglycemic Unawareness and Unresponsiveness (Hypoglycemia-Associated Autonomic Failure)

CLINICAL EVALUATION	DIAGNOSTIC TESTS
Symptoms	Stepped hypoglycemic clamp (insulin 1.0 mU/kg/min, glucose level of
Hyperadrenergic	5.0, 4.4, 3.9, 2.8, 2.2 mmol/L)
Palpitation, anxiety, tremor, diaphoresis, irritability	Insulin infusion test (overnight normalization of plasma glucose, insulin
Neuroglycopenic	0.67 mU/kg/min, plasma glucose 2.0 mmol/L $\pm$ neuroglycopenia)
Headache, hunger, dizziness, tingling, blurred vision, difficulty	**TREATMENT**
thinking, faintness	Scrupulous avoidance of hypoglycemia
Signs	Less stringent blood glucose control
Convulsions, loss of consciousness	

vision, difficulty thinking, and faintness), which begin at blood glucose levels of 51 plus or minus 3 mg per deciliter and for deterioration in cognitive function tests, which begin at 49 plus or minus 2 mg per deciliter. The release of glucagon and epinephrine occurs at plasma glucose concentrations between 65 and 70 mg per deciliter. In IDDM patients who are intensively treated with insulin, the thresholds for autonomic symptoms and counter-regulatory hormonal release are significantly reduced, and altered cognitive function and coma may occur without premonitory symptoms.

Testing for the presence of these syndromes requires elaborate and expensive equipment and is best done in a research environment. Using the stepped hypoglycemic clamp technique, insulin is infused at a continuous rate and the plasma glucose concentration is allowed to decline gradually at stepped intervals. Symptoms, cognitive function, and hormone responses are assessed at the end of each hypoglycemic step. Individuals in whom recognition of sympathetic autonomic symptoms and epinephrine/glucagon release are impaired are at high risk for severe hypoglycemic reactions, and the use of intensified insulin therapy in this group should be re-evaluated.

Suggested Reading

Amiel SA, Tamborlane WV, Simonson DC, Sherwin RS. Defective glucose counter-regulation after strict control of insulin-dependent diabetes mellitus. N Engl J Med 1987; 316:1376–1383.

These authors show that intensive control of IDDM leads to defective glucose counter-regulation not unlike that found in people with defective autonomic function.

Brown CK, Khanderia U. Use of metoclopramide, domperidone, and cisapride in the management of diabetic gastroparesis. Diabetic Med 1990; 9:357–365.

These authors discuss the use of metoclopramide, domperidone, and cisapride in the management of diabetic gastroparesis.

Cryer PE, Binder C, Bolli GB, et al. Hypoglycemia in insulin dependent diabetes mellitus. Diabetes 1989; 38:1193–1199.

This is an excellent overview of glucose counter-regulation, hypoglycemia unawareness, and hypoglycemia unresponsiveness.

De Tejada IS, Goldstein I, Kazem A, et al. Impaired neurogenic and endothelium-mediated relaxation of penile smooth muscle from diabetic men with impotence. N Engl J Med 1989; 320:1025–1030.

This article reports on a sophisticated investigation of the role of endothelium-mediated relaxation of penile smooth muscle as an important determinant of impotence in diabetic AN.

Diabetes Control and Complications Trial Research Group. Epidemiology of severe hypoglycemia in the diabetes control and complications trial. Am J Med 1991; 90:450–459.

This report presents the epidemiology of severe hypoglycemia and identifies patient characteristics or behaviors associated with severe hypoglycemia. Predictors are previous episodes of severe hypoglycemia, longer duration of IDDM, higher baseline glycosylated hemoglobin (HbA$_{1c}$) levels, and a greater reduction of HbA$_{1c}$.

Kahn JK, Sisson JC, Vinik AL. QT interval prolongation and sudden cardiac death in diabetic autonomic neuropathy. J Clin Endocrinol Metab 1987; 64:751–754.

This is a description of the poor man's test of autonomic function, indicating that a prolonged QT interval on ECG is diagnostic and a predictor of sudden cardiac death.

Maser RE, Pfeifer MA, Dorman JS, et al. Diabetic autonomic neuropathy and cardiovascular risk. Pittsburgh Epidemiology of Diabetes Complication Study III. Arch Intern Med 1990; 150:1218.

The study uses logistic analysis, in which heart rate response to deep breathing as an independent variable is shown to correlate with hypertension, LDL cholesterol, HDL cholesterol, and female gender as independent determinants of diabetic AN. That is, these traditional cardiovascular risk factors are important correlates of diabetic AN and may relate to both its cause and prognosis.

McLeod JG, Tuck RR. Disorders of the autonomic nervous system: I. Pathophysiology and clinical features, II. Investigation and treatment. Ann Neurol 1987; 21:419–430, 519–529.

Part 1 of this paper presents the notion that autonomic dysfunction may result from diseases that affect primarily the central nervous system or the peripheral ANS. Part 2 is a detailed examination of invasive measurements of vasomotor function compared with noninvasive tests of sympathetic and parasympathetic pathways, including the response of blood pressure to change in posture and isometric contraction, heart rate response to standing, variation in heart rate with respiration, Valsalva ratio, sweat tests, and plasma nonadrenaline measurements. The treatment of orthostatic hypotension is also discussed.

Niakan E, Harati Y, Comstock JP. Diabetic autonomic neuropathy. Metabolism 1986; 35:224–234.

This article reviews the clinical presentation of diabetic AN.

Rendell M, Bergman T, O'Donnell G, et al. Microvascular blood flow, volume, and velocity measured by laser Doppler techniques in IDDM. Diabetes 1989; 38:819–824.

These authors demonstrate that laser Doppler techniques can be used to assess microvascular changes in the skin of diabetic patients. Flow is generally reduced in diabetic patients because of a reduction in both microvascular volume and velocity.

Sampson MJ, Wilson S, Karaginnis P, et al. Progression of diabetic autonomic neuropathy over a decade in insulin-dependent diabetics. Q J Med 1990; 278:635–646.

This study examines young IDDM patients tested between 1972 and 1977 and again 10 to 15 years later. Patients with abnormal autonomic function and symptomatic AN with abnormal heart rate availability had the highest mortality, due predominantly to renal failure, myocardial infarction, and sudden unexpected death.

Tsai ST, Vinik AL, Brunner JF. Diabetic diarrhea and somatostatin. Ann Intern Med 1986; 104:894.

These authors demonstrate that diabetic diarrhea can be controlled by octreotide.

Veglio M, Carpano-Maglioli P, Tonda L, et al. Autonomic neuropathy in non–insulin-dependent diabetic patients: Correlation with age, sex, duration and metabolic control of diabetes. Diabetes Metab Rev 1990; 16:200–206.

These authors present data on the frequency of AN in non–insulin-dependent diabetes and its cosegregation with age, female sex, duration, and metabolic control of diabetes, as well as obesity, hypertension, and dyslipidemia.

Vinik AL, Glowniak JV. Hormonal secretions in diabetic autonomic neuropathy. N Y State J Med 1982; 82:871–878.

These authors give a detailed presentation of all the GI hormonal secretions that are abnormal in patients with diabetic AN, including catecholamine responses to hypoglycemia and to standing; pancreatic polypeptide–induced hypoglycemia as a marker for loss of vagal integrity; impairment of GIP responses to ingestion of a mixed meal in AN; and lack of effect of fiber ingestion on glucose, insulin, and GI hormone responses to meal ingestion.

Vinik AK, Holland MT, LeBeau JM, et al. Diabetic neuropathies. Diabetes Care 1992; 15:1926–1975.

This paper describes a classification and clinical presentations of somatic and autonomic neuropathies in diabetes and their distinction from other forms of neuropathy.

Vinik AL, Newlon PG, Lauterio TJ, et al. Nerve survival and regeneration in diabetes. Diabetes Rev 1995; 3:139–157.

This paper discusses current views on the pathogenesis of diabetic neuropathy with emphasis on factors effecting nerve damage, as well as new views on the ability of nerves to regenerate and the defects that are found in diabetes.

White NH, Skor DA, Cryer PE, et al. Identification of type 1 diabetic patients at increased risk for hypoglycemia during intensive therapy. N Engl J Med 1983; 308:485–491.

An IV insulin infusion tests the ability to counter-regulate to hypoglycemia with deficient glucagon and epinephrine responses and identifies patients who are at increased risk for severe hypoglycemia during intensive therapy.

Zola B, Kahn JK, Juni JE, and Vinik AL. Abnormal cardiac function in diabetics with autonomic neuropathy in the absence of ischemic heart disease. J Clin Endocrinol Metab 1986; 63:208–214.

About one-third of a randomly selected group of patients with long-standing insulin-dependent diabetes without clinical ECG or tomographic thallium scan evidence of heart disease have depressed ventricular function, which is related to the severity of cardiac AN. Therefore cardiac AN may be a contributor to cardiac dysfunction in diabetes mellitus.

ATHEROSCLEROTIC CARDIOVASCULAR DISEASE

David A. Escalante, M.D.

Duk Kyu Kim, M.D.

Alan J. Garber, M.D., Ph.D.

Atherosclerotic macrovascular disease accounts for more than 80 percent of the mortality in the diabetic population. Ischemic coronary heart disease alone produces 60 percent of total mortality and 77 percent of the total diabetic patient hospitalizations. However, it is clear that diabetes is not unique as a cause of accelerated atherosclerosis, nor is it the most potent accelerator of that pathologic process. The most important aspects of diabetes that account for the increased prevalence of atherosclerosis include dyslipidemia, hyperglycemia, hypertension, and obesity. All of these factors may be linked by a common element; namely, insulin resistance. It is therefore not surprising that the incidence of coronary heart disease in adult diabetic patients is two- to fourfold greater than in age, weight, and sex matched nondiabetic controls. Furthermore, the hormonally mediated cardioprotection is obliterated in premenopausal diabetic women, who have the same coronary artery mortality as matched diabetic males.

■ PATHOGENESIS

Although various mechanisms have been postulated in the pathogenesis of atherosclerosis, it seems evident that an initial "response to injury" at the endothelial cell level is an essential early element. Chronic injury from chemical toxins and biomechanical forces, such as dyslipidemia, carbon monoxide, hyperglycemia, and hypertension, are necessary to damage the endothelial-basement permeability barrier. Thereafter, an accumulation of low-density lipoprotein (LDL) deposits occurs in the subendothelial intima, followed by uptake by macrophages and fibroblasts, and then a reactive proliferation of smooth muscle and deposition of collagen and elastin. The early stages of atherosclerosis can be identified grossly by the appearance of fatty streaks, which are subendothelial intimal lesions filled with lipid-laden macrophages or foam cells. After a period of time, fibrous tissue deposition and smooth muscle proliferation develop, in part as the tissue result of the hyperinsulinemia of an insulin-resistant state. Other growth factors also encourage smooth muscle proliferation; important among them are platelet-derived growth factor and other advanced products of glycosylation. Ultimately, the core of atheromatous lipid is surrounded by necrotic debris and fibromuscular cap, protruding from the arterial wall and leaving a narrow residual lumen.

In the diabetic patient, hyperglycemia itself functions as an independent risk factor for atherosclerosis. In part, this effect results from the nonenzymatic glycosylation of many arterial proteins including basement membrane protein. Such a reaction produces a membrane with increased permeability to many proteins and lipoproteins, particularly LDL. Glycosylation of the glycoprotein ground substance of the arterial matrix leads to advance glycosylation end products (AGEs), which induce transendothelial chemotaxis of mononuclear leukocytes and the secretion of platelet-derived growth factor (PDGF), cytokines such as tumor necrosis factor (TNF), cachectin, interleukin 1, and insulin-like growth factors (IGF I and IGF II).

Glycation also induces modification of apolipoprotein metabolism such as LDL-Apo B-100. This glycosylation increases LDL binding affinity and renders a LDL lipid more susceptible to oxidation, thereby augmenting LDL uptake in macrophages through the scavenger pathway. LDL glycation also is associated with increased thrombin levels, enhanced platelet aggregation, and accelerated thromboxane B2 (TxB2) elaboration, as well as decreased endothelial antithrombotic properties, including decreased production of prostaglandin F 1 alpha.

High-density lipoprotein (HDL) is the key lipoprotein catalyzing the process of reverse cholesterol transport. Both the circulating level and metabolic functions of HDL are affected by changes produced by diabetes in the metabolic milieu. Decreased levels of HDL are twice as common in diabetic as compared to nondiabetic patients. Glycation of HDL decreases its binding to the receptor, decreases apoprotein C catalytic activity, and may increase its rate of catabolism. Furthermore, glycation reduces by one-half rates of reverse cholesterol transport as measured by crude in vitro assays. Lipid profiles also change as the result of insulin resistance. For example, diabetic dyslipidemia increases very-low–density lipoprotein (VLDL) triglyceride. Decreased HDL cholesterol may precede by years the clinical appearance of hyperglycemia and may therefore reflect the insulin-resistant state.

■ DIAGNOSIS OF ATHEROSCLEROSIS

Although there is angiographic evidence that the extent of atherosclerotic disease is greater in diabetic than in nondiabetic patients, classic ischemic symptomatology of coronary insufficiency is often not present in the diabetic patient. In approximately 30 percent of cases, coronary insufficiency may present without any pain whatsoever. More frequently, there may be highly atypical features such as epigastric, jaw, neck, or arm discomfort with or without concomitant chest symptoms. Congestive heart failure alone may be the presenting symptom, in which case intermittent exertional congestive failure should always arouse suspicions of silent ischemia. In the long-standing diabetic patient, a presentation of unexplained severe heart failure, cardiogenic shock, and/or malignant arrhythmias may indicate a silent acute myocardial infarction. On the other hand, acutely uncontrolled blood sugars or even diabetic ketoacidosis might be the only presenting finding of a silent myocardial infarction.

■ DYNAMIC TESTING FOR DIAGNOSIS OF CORONARY ARTERY DISEASE

In most, if not all, diabetic patients with significant coronary artery disease, electrocardiographic (ECG) evidence of ischemia in terms of changes in the ST segment will be present upon adequate exercise cardiac stress testing. Thallium stress testing is more sensitive and specific for the diagnosis of coronary insufficiency in diabetic patients than routine treadmill ECG exercise tests, particularly in cases of underlying abnormalities of the resting ECG. Because of obesity, severe neuropathy, diabetic foot ulcers, degenerative joint disease, claudication, or amputations, a relatively large number of diabetic patients will not be capable of achieving an adequate exercise stimulus to the heart rate. Therefore, pharmacologic stress testing with adenosine, dipyridamole, or dobutamine should be used to produce adequate evaluation of the coronary circulation.

Patients who are refractory to routine medical therapy, those who present with unstable angina, and diabetic patients with multiple risk factors should undergo selective coronary angiography to characterize the distribution and extent of atherosclerosis. Candidates for organ transplantation or patients undergoing peripheral vascular surgery also require coronary arteriography.

Coronary cineangiography should be performed in all diabetic patients with suspected coronary artery disease because comparison studies on diabetic and nondiabetic patients undergoing consecutive catheterizations have shown that the incidence of progressive multiple vessel disease and the degree of involvement of intermediate-sized coronary branches are higher in diabetic than in nondiabetic patients.

Steps to prevent the renal complications of dye infusions are always required, even with the use of low ionic contrast media. All patients should be well hydrated before the procedure, and the use of hyperosmolar diuretics like mannitol could be considered in the presence of any degree of underlying nephropathy. Intravenous therapy should be continued for 12 to 24 hours after catheterization.

■ MYOCARDIAL INFARCTION

Diagnosis

An absence of pain characteristic of acute myocardial infarction is described in 30 percent of diabetic patients, as compared to 5 to 10 percent of nondiabetic patients admitted to a coronary intensive care unit. Equally distinctive is the fact that most diabetic patients present with the first myocardial infarction at a younger age than nondiabetic patients. This disparity is even more apparent with type 1 than with type 2 diabetic patients.

Compared with nondiabetic patients, diabetic patients have higher rates of complication development in the peri-infarction period. These include an increased propensity to malignant arrhythmias, reduced diastolic ventricular compliance, and greater extent of infarction and repeated recurrent infarctions, all of which lead to a high frequency of congestive heart failure. Patients with diabetes have a twofold increase of non–Q wave infarction; these tend to be multiple in nature, frequent in occurrence, and atypical in presenting symptoms. Each of these factors significantly increases in-hospital mortality for diabetic patients. In a prospective study comparing diabetic and nondiabetic patients with acute myocardial infarction matched for Holter monitoring scores, submaximal treadmill test, and ejection fractions, postinfarct mortality was more than double in the diabetic population over a 2-year period. The leading causes of this excess mortality were progressive heart failure and sudden death. For unknown reasons, women with diabetes appear to have a worse prognosis than men. The MILIS study (Multicenter Investigation of the Limitation of Infarct Size) showed a twofold greater in-hospital mortality in females than in males with diabetes. This survival difference persisted throughout the 4-year postinfarction period studied.

Patients with suspected myocardial infarction must be admitted to the coronary care unit, which should be a pleasant and quiet environment where the patient can rest. All patients should be under continuous ECG monitoring; early detection of the increased frequency of malignant arrhythmias may help to decrease the excess mortality in diabetics. In view of the high prevalence of non–Q wave infarction in diabetic patients, serial creatine kinases with MB fractionation done at 8-hour intervals are the most reliable method of diagnosing acute myocardial infarction.

In nondiabetic patients, thrombolytic therapy within 6 hours of acute infarction has reduced in-hospital mortality. Agents available include streptokinase, anisoylated plasminogen streptokinase activator complex (APSAC), recombinant alteplase, and recombinant tissue plasminogen activator (RTPA). Major side effects of such therapy are bleeding from multiple sites, including intracranial locations, and reperfusion arrhythmias. In diabetic patients with proliferative (nonbackground) retinopathy, these thrombolytic activators are contraindicated because retinal bleeding may be produced, which generally leads to blindness. Once reperfusion of the acute coronary obstruction is established, an unstable and frequently critical stenosis is left behind. Therefore a coronary angiogram is indicated to decide on more definitive intermediate term therapies. Percutaneous transluminal coronary angioplasty (PTCA) may be effective for the single or several critical lesions in the coronary circulation. However, coronary revascularization with multiple bypasses using internal mammary artery supplementation may be preferred because of the frequency of multiple lesions, particularly in the distal vessels.

Additional considerations in non–insulin-treated diabetic patients include a bland diet with sufficient maintenance calories. Sulfonylureas should be discontinued and low-dose continuous intravenous insulin infusion therapy started. Since insulin resistance is substantially augmented by the many stressors of the illness and environment, frequent blood glucose monitoring is necessary to prevent hyperglycemia or ketoacidosis.

Cardiac rehabilitation should be started after the patient is transferred out of the intensive care unit, usually after 72 hours, assuming an uncomplicated infarction. The initial rehabilitation efforts involve only assisted sitting and walking to progressive self-ambulation; there should be no weight lifting or pulling exercises for the first 6 weeks of recovery.

Prior to hospital discharge, a submaximal exercise test should be done in all patients with Q wave infarction, and if the results are positive, one should proceed with a coronary angiogram. In the patient with a negative submaximal exercise test, a maximal stress test should be done 6 weeks later. All patients with non–Q wave infarction should have coronary angiograms performed prior to any disposition regarding long-term posthospital therapy.

■ THERAPEUTIC MODALITIES FOR ATHEROSCLEROSIS IN DIABETES

A balance between diet, exercise, and appropriate life-style changes is the first objective of management; pharmacologic therapies are essential secondary modalities of treatment. The goal of therapy is not only to prevent progression, but also to produce regression of established atherosclerotic disease. Though many aspects of the therapeutic program in diabetic patients are similar to the treatment of established atherosclerosis in the nondiabetic population, certain key points are of considerable concern to diabetic patients.

Surgical Management

Patients refractory to medical therapy for ischemic heart disease should be considered for invasive management, such as PTCA or alternatively, coronary artery bypass graft.

Percutaneous Transluminal Coronary Angioplasty

Percutaneous transluminal coronary angioplasty is a well-tolerated procedure associated with lower mortality and morbidity than the surgical alternatives and has become an attractive choice; there is an in-hospital mortality as low as 0.2 percent in some centers. Good candidates for the procedure are patients with angiographic evidence of single vessel disease, proximal multiple coronary lesions, or stenotic areas of prior grafts and high-risk patients with other comorbid illnesses. Restenosis rates at 6 months are 30 to 40 percent. Higher restenosis rates and mortality are expected in patients with diabetes, unstable angina, male sex, and longer or narrower lesions (Table 1). If restenosis occurs, a second procedure may be done with even better results. Complications include perforation, dissection, aneurysmal formation, and acute obstruction of a coronary artery precipitating an ischemic event. Proper patient preparation and the precautions described for coronary angiograms also apply to this therapeutic maneuver.

Table 1 Characteristics of Patients at Risk for Restenosis after Percutaneous Transluminal Coronary Angioplasty

Diabetes
Unstable angina
Male
Larger and narrower lesions

Coronary Artery Bypass Surgery

A high incidence of silent ischemia or atypical features in the clinical presentation of ischemic heart disease in diabetes requires a high index of suspicion for ischemic heart disease on the part of the physician. The greatest benefit from coronary artery bypass surgery has been seen in the survival and quality of life of patients with documented left main coronary stenosis, patients with low ejection fractions and triple vessel disease, and patients in whom two vessels marginally irrigate large amounts of the myocardium (Table 2).

Recent studies have shown no significant differences in perioperative mortality between diabetic and matched nondiabetic patients. However, there is significantly higher perioperative morbidity, especially because of infections in graft harvest areas of the legs and in the sternotomy site. There is also an increased risk of renal insufficiency and a longer hospital stay in diabetic patients.

Short-term follow-up has shown no differences in patency of the bypass vessels and symptom relief, but long-term (10 to 15 years) studies have shown lower survival rates, mainly in the poorly controlled or insulin-requiring diabetic. Well-controlled patients treated with insulin and those treated with oral agents or diet have a 15-year survival similar to the nondiabetic population.

Of greatest importance is establishing metabolic control before surgery to minimize perioperative morbidity. Adequate insulin regimens must be tailored to the individual patient. Hypoglycemia must be avoided because hypoglycemia may precipitate a myocardial infarction. Because of the resistance to insulin action that results from the stress of surgery, the stay in the intensive care unit, and the use of pressors, frequent blood sugar monitoring is recommended during the surgery and perioperative period to prevent uncontrolled diabetes and ketoacidosis. Intensive insulin therapy, often including a continuous insulin infusion, is required. Because protamine is a component of neutral protamine Hagedorn (NPH) insulin, diabetic patients on NPH have been sensitized to the drug. Intravenous use of protamine to reverse heparinization during surgery may precipitate an anaphylactic reaction; this can be reversed easily in most cases.

Pharmacologic Treatment
Insulin and Sulfonylureas

Although numerous large-scale prospective studies have found that cardiovascular mortality correlates to some extent with fasting hyperglycemia and perhaps better with postprandial hyperglycemia, it is currently unproved whether or not tight glucose control will prevent or retard the evolution of atherosclerotic macrovascular disease. Studies that have addressed this issue so far are inconclusive. Typically, the poorly controlled diabetic patient is highly dyslipidemic, having extremely low levels of HDL cholesterol and high VLDL triglycerides and perhaps some increase in LDL cholesterol. All of these changes are risk factors associated with increased cardiovascular mortality.

In the patient with severe hypertriglyceridemia (greater than 1,000 mg per deciliter) there may be therapeutic advantages to the use of insulin owing to the induction of lipoprotein lipase. This will positively impact triglyceride and HDL cholesterol metabolism.

Care should be taken in the peri-infarct period to avoid both extremes of blood glucose. Both hypoglycemia and significant hyperglycemia are associated with augmented adrenergic responses, which may cause increased cardiac work, thus precipitating an ischemic attack if residual lesions remain.

Sulfonylureas have no role in the hospital setting of unstable or crescendo angina or in treating the diabetic patient with an acute myocardial infarction. Insulin requirements are greatly augmented by the many added stressors of the situation. Insulin becomes the first-line therapy for glucose control because frequent adjustments are needed; Regular insulin by intravenous continuous infusion should be started at a basal rate of 0.5 to 1.0 U per hour and should be adjusted according to the individual response as monitored by blood glucose. Insulin boluses are added to the regimen before any meal in order to avoid postprandial hyperglycemia. Postdischarge stable type 2 diabetic patients may be returned to sulfonylureas provided adequate glucose and lipid control is maintained.

Aspirin

The antiaggregation properties of this pharmacologic agent make this inexpensive medication potentially quite valuable. Independent of other medications, various studies have demonstrated a 50 percent risk reduction in the rate of myocardial infarction in patients with unstable angina. In the acute infarction, combination therapy with thrombolytic agents further reduces mortality. Studies in the nondiabetic population have shown that daily use of aspirin reduces cardiovascular mortality. In diabetic patients, the number of transient ischemic attacks and amount of cerebrovascular disease fall significantly with aspirin, but whether coronary events will decrease is as yet unknown. A complete funduscopic examination has to be done before instituting this therapy in order to avoid retinal bleeds in patients with diabetic retinopathy.

Nitrates

Nitrates have been important elements in the treatment of acute and chronic coronary insufficiency. The vasodilation of the vascular venous bed, epicardial coronary vessels, and to a lesser extent the arterial bed results in a net decrease in the oxygen consumption of the myocardium by decreasing both the preload and afterload. In addition, nitrates do not interfere significantly with carbohydrate or lipid metabolism in the diabetic patient, in either the acute setting or chronic therapy.

Adverse effects frequently seen include headaches, palpitations, and reflex tachycardia, but it is the hypotension per se that limits its clinical usefulness. In long-standing diabetic patients with marked autonomic neuropathy, a small dose of nitrates may cause severe orthostatic hypotension. Another adverse feature of nitrates is the patient's tendency to develop tolerance, thereby rendering them therapeutically ineffective. However, shorter acting congeners might

---

Table 2 Indications for Revascularization

Left main coronary stenosis
Triple vessel disease, especially lower ejection fractions
Two vessel stenosis in the patient with peculiar anatomy that leaves a large portion of the myocardium at risk

Table 3 Characteristics of Common Drugs Used for Ischemic Heart Disease

AGENT	DOSAGE	ADVANTAGES/DISADVANTAGES
NITRATES		
Nitroglycerin	0.4 mg as required; maximum of 3 doses every 5 min	Immediate action, short action, about 30 min headache, sublingual or IV infusion, orthostatic hypotension
Ointment	0.5–2.0 inches every 4–6 hr	Long acting, might develop tolerance
Transdermal patch	2.5–15 mg q.d.	Long acting, might develop tolerance
BETA-BLOCKERS **Nonselective**		
Propranolol	40–120 mg PO q.i.d.	Antiarrhythmic effects, hyperlipidemia, glucose intolerance, cardiodepressive bronchoconstriction
Cardioselective Atenolol	50–100 mg PO b.i.d.	Less metabolic disturbance, low antiarrhythmic potential
Metoprolol	50–200 mg PO b.i.d.	Less metabolic disturbance
CALCIUM CHANNEL BLOCKERS Nifedipine	10–30 mg PO every 8 hr	Marked vasodilation, flushing, hypotension, increased proteinuria, fluid retention
Diltiazem	30–120 mg PO q.i.d.	Probable renoprotective effects, moderate vasodilation, bradycardia
Verapamil	80–120 mg PO q.i.d.	Moderate vasodilation, bradycardia
SALICYLATES Aspirin	80–650 mg PO q.d.	Antiplatelet effect, inexpensive, bleeding tendency

be somewhat more advantageous than transdermal nitrate delivery systems (Table 3).

Beta-Blockers

Two clinically important beta receptors have been identified: B1 receptors are primarily found in heart tissue, in renin releasers, and in lipolysis-stimulating sites. Stimulation of B2 receptors results in vasodilation, glycogenolysis, and relaxation of smooth muscle in the uterus and the bronchial walls. The prototypical beta-blocker, propranolol, is a nonselective agent that blocks both receptors. A subclass of newer agents, when used at only low doses, impacts primarily the B1 receptors, giving these agents a theoretical advantage over the nonselective beta-blockers. Clinically, both subclasses are effective in the treatment of coronary artery insufficiency.

Despite a myriad of undesirable effects, this family of medications maintains an undisputed efficacy for prevention of reinfarction in patients who have suffered a Q wave myocardial infarction. Multiple studies of cardioselective and nonselective beta-blockers conducted in nondiabetic patients and a subgroup of diabetic patients have proved this point. These agents are the only medical therapy prolonging survival. They may also have potential use in refractory angina pectoris. Beta-blockers should not be used as first-line therapy in diabetics with mild angina or essential hypertension, because other pharmacologic agents of equal or greater efficacy may be without many of the adverse effects of this class of antagonist.

The major issue is the clear potential for increasing insulin resistance and diminishing glucose tolerance. Hypoglycemia may also occur with greater frequency and severity in the presence of beta-blockers secondary to an interference in glycogenolysis and an inhibition of gluconeogenesis with a prolonged period of recuperation from hypoglycemia. There is also blunting of the adrenergic response to hypoglycemia. The underlying sympathetic neuropathy in many long-standing diabetic patients complicates this effect even more. Finally, hyperkalemia may occur in predisposed patients and is seen frequently as a contributing factor in hyporeninemic hypoaldosteronism.

Other major adverse effects of beta-blockers include worsening of congestive heart failure because beta-blockers can depress myocardial contractility, particularly in the patient with a low ejection fraction; bronchial asthma, which may be precipitated by blocking the B2 receptors (this may be avoided by using low-dose cardioselective agents); and cardiac conduction defects, which makes these agents relatively undesirable in patients with high degree blocks or bradyarrhythmias (Table 3).

Calcium Channel Blockers

The effects of these agents—to decrease blood pressure, myocardial contractility, and heart rate and to increase coronary blood flow—make this therapeutic class unique, not only in the treatment of hypertension but also as an excellent antianginal therapy. Diltiazem has been used as adjunctive therapy in uncomplicated non–Q wave myocardial infarction with improved survival. The first three members of this family in clinical use, verapamil, nifedipine, and diltiazem, have been utilized in classic as well as variant, or Prinzmetal's, angina. From these original calcium slow channel entry blockers, with molecular structures totally unrelated to each other, have evolved a host of derivatives, particularly in the dihydropyridine class.

Undesirable adverse effects of these agents include hypotension as a major concern in the diabetic patient with autonomic neuropathy. Atrioventricular block, seen in particular with verapamil and to a lesser extent with diltiazem, may progress to a complete heart block. Negative inotropic effects are seen with all of the calcium channel blockers. Therefore, patients with heart failure should be treated very carefully, in particular if these agents are prescribed in combination with beta-blockers, which may potentiate this side effect. This combination should be used only in the treatment of patients who are refractory to calcium channel blockers and nitrates alone or in combination.

In diabetic patients, nifedipine as well as other dihydropyridine antagonists appear to increase fasting blood sugar and worsen the proteinuria of diabetic nephropathy. Verapamil has also been reported to worsen hyperglycemia (Table 3).

Risk Factor Modification to Prevent Reinfarction
Smoking
Smoking per se increases the risk of sudden death and myocardial infarct by 70 percent over the general population and probably accounts for an estimated 30 to 40 percent of all cardiovascular deaths. The degree is proportional to both the duration and quantity of cigarette smoke exposure. Large amounts of tobacco usage will also lower HDL cholesterol and enhance thrombotic states by increasing the levels of fibrinogen. Although there has been a decline in the use of tobacco in the general population over the last half-century, the incidence of tobacco use is rising in unique groups like adolescents and young women. Smoking is synergistic with diabetes mellitus as an amplifier of coronary and peripheral atherosclerosis. In the Framingham population, smoking is the best predictor of coronary heart disease.

Education encouraging smoking cessation should be greatly emphasized. The excess coronary artery risk is lowered by as much as 50 percent over a period of 1 year smoke-free. Over time the detrimental effects gradually disappear, and they are almost eliminated after 3 smoke-free years.

Obesity
Careful analysis of all risk factors has isolated obesity as an independent risk factor. Importantly, one aspect of obesity is the body fat distribution; truncal obesity (abdominal or male pattern) produces greater coronary heart disease than other patterns of fat distribution. With weight loss, favorable changes can be seen in the lipid profile, glucose tolerance, and insulin resistance.

Education, behavior modification, and exercise in conjunction with a low-fat, low-cholesterol, low-calorie diet is the ideal therapy. Support groups often enhance patient motivation and compliance and need to be encouraged.

Exercise
Substantial benefits can be obtained from a regular, supervised exercise program. Prior to the initiation, all patients should undergo a complete clinical evaluation including an ophthalmologic, renal, and cardiovascular assessment. Planning is the key to prevention of many complications. The most commonly encountered complications are hypoglycemia, due to an increased sensitivity to insulin, and changes in the pharmacokinetics at the sites of injection, such as exercising the limb where insulin is injected. This will hasten the peak of insulin action. Exercising before meals can also lead to hypoglycemia. Increased intravascular pressure can occur in the retinal vessels; this is sometimes seen in weight bearing or lifting exercises and may lead to retinal hemorrhage and damage. Lower extremity skin breakdown may serve as a port of entry to infection of the surrounding soft tissue and adjacent bones, mainly as innervation and blood supply are decreased. Charcot's joint with its complications could be a problem in the stressed insensible joint. Important exercise-associated increments in proteinuria may aggravate underlying diabetic nephropathy.

Daily exercise improves insulin sensitivity. Even in the absence of weight loss, this may lead to reduction in the doses of oral hypoglycemic agents or exogenous insulin. Increased energy expenditure can reduce obesity, thus modifying this risk factor. Other important effects include an improvement in the lipid profile, namely a decline in triglycerides and a significant increase in HDL cholesterol. Indeed, exercise is one of the few therapies for the low HDL cholesterol syndromes.

A structured program should be tailored to the needs of every patient. Minimum requirements include (1) a schedule of 5 to 7 exercise sessions a week, (2) aerobic duration of 20 minutes minimum, (3) adequate time to warm up and cool down (10 minutes each), and (4) submaximal effort (no more than 70 percent of maximal capacity).

Diet
Diet plays a very important role in the modification of various risk factors. Blankenhorn et al have demonstrated the beneficial effects of colestipol and niacin in combination with a diet containing less than 125 mg of cholesterol per day and 22 percent of the total energy provided as fat (10 percent as polyunsaturated and 4 percent as saturated). Other pertinent aspects include the following: (1) A caloric restriction that allows improvement in glucose homeostasis and decrements in insulin requirements. Normalization of blood sugars will also lower but not normalize VLDL and LDL cholesterol levels. (2) High-fiber diets may result in lower serum cholesterol because they bind bile salts and a decrease in enteric transit will prevent a sharp postprandial glucose rise. (3) A low-salt diet in the case of hypertensives or those with complicated congestive heart failure is very helpful when used in conjunction with pharmacologic intervention. (4) A low-protein diet lowers the load of nitrogen waste products and delays the onset of end-stage renal disease. A protein-restricted diet might be appropriate for the diabetic patient with both nephropathy and atherosclerotic heart disease. (5) Alcohol is a common preventable cause of hypertension and dyslipidemia. The effect of alcohol in raising the levels of HDL cholesterol may be offset by the hypertension and triglyceride elevations seen. Therefore the recommendation of abstinence or limitations on ingestion of alcoholic beverages seems warranted.

Hypolipidemic Agents

The therapeutic role for this category of pharmacologic agents has expanded from simply reducing lipids, thereby preventing coronary events, to a totally new area of treatment, namely the regression of established atheromatous disease. Studies on regression have thus far included primarily nondiabetic patients. Those involving diabetic patients have been limited to small subgroups of patients in primary prevention trials.

This form of therapy is no doubt where the future focus in the medical management of atherosclerosis will evolve, particularly in the combination of lipid lowering agents.

Suggested Reading

Blakenhorn DH, Nessim SA, Johnson RL, et al. Beneficial effects of combined calestipol-niacin therapy and coronary atherosclerosis and coronary venous bypass grafts. JAMA 1987; 257:3233.

Despres JP, Lamarche B, Mauriege P, et al. Hyperinsulinemia as an independent risk factor for ischemic heart disease. N Engl J Med 1996; 334:952–957.

In the Quebec Heart Study, fasting insulin levels were found to be higher in patients with ischemic heart disease than in patients without ischemic heart disease. The odds ratio for ischemic heart disease associated with hyperinsulinemia was a significant predictive factor.

Haffner SM, Stern MP, Hazuda HP, Mitchell BD, Patterson JK. Cardiovascular risk factors in confirmed prediabetic individuals: Does the clock for coronary heart disease start ticking before the onset of clinical diabetes? JAMA 1990; 263:2893–2898.

This paper demonstrates that a dyslipidemia is clearly evident in hyperinsulinemic prediabetic individuals long before the hyperglycemia is apparent. This dyslipidemia may be the principal mechanism by which insulin resistance per se produces accelerated atherosclerosis before carbohydrate intolerance appears.

Levine GN, Keaney JF Jr, Vita JA. Cholesterol reduction in cardiovascular disease. N Engl J Med 1995; 332:512–521.

This article is the most recent and comprehensive review of the issue of atherosclerotic cardiovascular disease and the role of lipids in the progression as well as regression of that disorder.

Pedersen TR, Kjekshus J, Berg K, et al. Cholesterol lowering and the use of healthcare resources: Results of the Scandinavian Simvastatin Survival Study. Circulation 1996; 93:1796–1802.

In this study, secondary prevention in individuals with very high LDL concentrations (187 mg per deciliter) were investigated and the cost-effectiveness quantitated. Secondary prevention is clearly beneficial.

Reaven GM, Ida Chen YD, Jeppesen J, Maheux P, Krauss RM. Insulin resistance and hyperinsulinemia in individuals with small, dense, low density lipoprotein particles. J Clin Invest 1993; 92:141–146.

In this study, the authors demonstrate that insulin resistant individuals have a predominance of smaller, denser LDL particles. These particles have approximately three times the atherogenic potential of phenotype A or larger, less dense LDL particles.

Sacks FM, Pfeffer MA, Moye LA, et al. The effect of pravastatin on coronary events after myocardial infarction in patients with average cholesterol levels. N Engl J Med 1996; 335:1001–1009.

In this study with patients having a more normal mean LDL cholesterol of 139 mg per deciliter, secondary prevention was demonstrated to be safe and effective. The degree of efficacy of secondary prevention was in part related to initial LDL concentrations. In a diabetic subpopulation, statistically significant, meaningful prevention of recurrent events was produced by pravastatin.

HEART FAILURE

Robert DiBianco, M.D.

Already of staggering proportions in modern societies, the incidence and prevalence of heart failure are growing dramatically and consuming an increasing share of health care resources. This is especially true for elderly patients, who have an increased incidence of both non–insulin-dependent diabetes mellitus (NIDDM) and heart failure. In the United States, each year, 3 cases of heart failure develop for each 1,000 persons under 65 years of age. This incidence increases to more than 10 cases per 1,000 persons in those over age 65. Heart failure afflicts 1 percent of all persons under age 50 and more than 10 percent of those over age 80. The prevalence of heart failure approximately doubles for each decade of life. For the diabetic patient, the incidence of heart failure is increased two- to sixfold compared to the nondiabetic individual, apparently a result of the higher frequency of both coronary heart disease and hypertension (Fig. 1).

Unfortunately, despite the best medical efforts, the clinical course of the patient with heart failure today remains progressively limiting. Life-style is compromised by symptoms of dyspnea, fatigue, and exercise intolerance, and there is a markedly shortened survival from deteriorating pump performance or sudden cardiac death. For the diabetic patient, especially those with nephropathy, the severity of symptoms, complications, and mortality are particularly high.

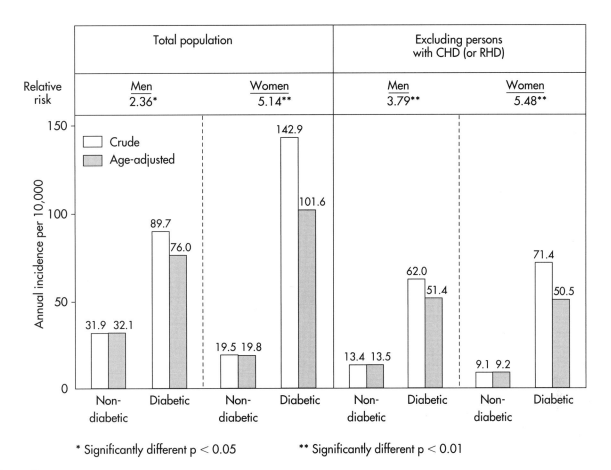

Figure 1
Risk of heart failure according to diabetic status in men and women 45 to 74 years of age. Framingham Study: 18-year fol-low-up. *(From Zoneraich S. Diabetes and the heart. Springfield, Ill: Charles C Thomas, 1978; with permission.)*

Recently much has been learned about the pathophysio-logic derangements leading to heart failure. Multiple neuroen-docrine systems, including the sympathetic system and renin-angiotensin-aldosterone system, have been implicated (Fig. 2).

Cardiac structure (Fig. 3) forms the basis for recommen-dations about the treatment of heart failure. In the diabetic patient, heart failure is most often secondary to macrovas-cular disease of the coronary arteries, resulting in ischemic heart disease and myocardial infarction with or without myocardial aneurysm. In these patients, cardiac structure typically demonstrates a dilated left ventricle with segments of poor noncontracting muscles. Heart failure may also result from hypertensive heart disease producing left ven-tricular hypertrophy, which, in the absence of critically obstructed coronary arteries, usually produces a nondilated left ventricle with thickened walls and maintained contrac-tility (i.e., normal ejection fraction). Contrasting with both coronary and hypertensive heart disease is so-called "dia-betic cardiomyopathy," which represents a distinct patho-logic process resulting in myocardial hypertrophy, increased interstitial connective tissue, and associated microvascular pathology. Diabetic cardiomyopathy has been associated with ventricular dysfunction of both systolic (contractility) and diastolic (relaxation) types.

■ MAKING THE DIAGNOSIS OF HEART FAILURE (Table 1)

History
Heart failure patients most often complain of fatigue and dys-pnea on exertion. In its most severe form, symptoms of breathlessness and profound fatigue occur even at rest. Some patients describe exercise intolerance and may, because of the insidious onset of symptoms, attribute the lack of stamina to growing old or being "out-of-shape". Other symptoms com-monly seen in heart failure include orthopnea, paroxysmal nocturnal dyspnea, nocturia, and weight gain secondary to salt and water retention.

Physical Examination
The physical findings in heart failure include sinus tachycar-dia, elevation of venous pressure (most easily assessed at the internal jugular pulse), pulmonary rales with pleural effu-sions, a ventricular gallop or third heart sound, hep-atomegaly, and peripheral (dependent) edema. The clinical findings may suggest low output heart failure in a diabetic patient with renal failure; however, an underlying high car-diac output may be present. Patients are clinically congested, and treatment is based on reducing intravascular volume

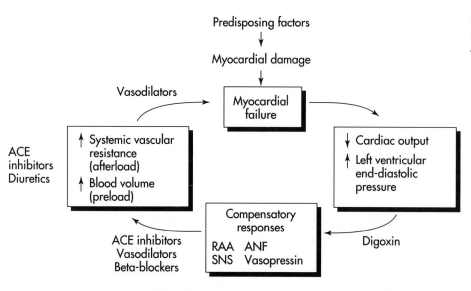

Figure 2
Pathophysiology of heart failure
with general effects of treatments.

RAA = Renin-angiotensin-aldosterone system
SNS = Sympathetic nervous system
ANF = Atrial natriuretic factor

Table 1 Descriptors of the Clinical Diagnosis of Heart Failure

HISTORY	**ELECTROCARDIOGRAM**
Dyspnea on exertion or at rest	Left atrial overload pattern
Fatigue	Ventricular hypertrophy
Weight gain	Prior myocardial infarction
PHYSICAL	**ECHOCARDIOGRAM**
Sinus tachycardia	Enlarged left atrium
Elevated jugular venous pressure	Systolic failure
Pulmonary rales	Enlarged left ventricular chamber size
Cardiomegaly	Variable left ventricular wall thickness
Ventricular gallop (third heart sound)	Poor contractility (low ejection fraction)
Peripheral (dependent) edema	Diastolic failure
CHEST RADIOGRAPH	Normal left ventricular chamber size
Increased pulmonary vascularity	Increased left ventricular wall thickness
Pleural effusion	Normal or increased contractility
Cardiac silhouette enlargement	(Normal or increased ejection fraction)

---

and cardiac filling pressures with diuretics (or dialysis) and increasing oxygen-carrying capacity by correcting the usual concomitant anemia.

Chest Radiograph and Electrocardiogram

Confirmatory evidence of elevated pulmonary venous pressures (left ventricular filling pressures) are available from the typical pattern of interstitial and/or alveolar pulmonary edema on the chest radiograph, which may be accompanied by left atrial enlargement. An electrocardiogram (ECG) may indicate an atrial overload pattern, ventricular hypertrophy, or evidence of prior myocardial infarction.

Echocardiogram

The most informative noninvasive test for patients suspected of having heart failure is the two-dimensional echo-

cardiogram. The "echo" will confirm that heart failure is present. This is most easily identified by evidence of increased left atrial size because this thin-walled chamber is an excellent "manometer" of chronic left ventricular filling pressure. The left atrium is virtually always increased in size in chronic left ventricular failure; therefore, the diagnosis of heart failure must be placed in serious doubt without left atrial enlargement.

Since the appropriate drug treatment of heart failure depends upon the type of ventricular function abnormality present, it is necessary in all patients to determine whether there is a failure of contractility (systolic failure: 70 to 90 percent of patients) or relaxation (diastolic failure: 10 to 30 percent of patients) (see Table 1). The echo provides the best and most easily applied discriminator between patients with systolic and diastolic heart failure (Fig. 4).

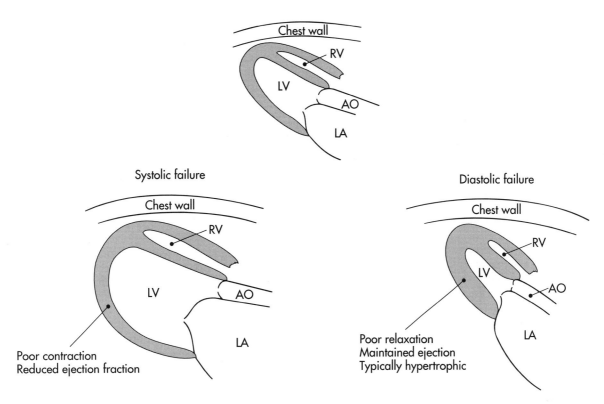

Figure 3
Cardiac structure as displayed on the echocardiogram.

Table 2 Structural Causes of Heart Failure	
Myocardial Damage	Volume
Ischemic heart disease (myocardial infarction, aneurysm)	Mitral regurgitation*
Nonischemic cardiomyopathy	Aortic regurgitation*
Idiopathic	Compromised Ventricular Filling
Postviral infection	Pericardial restriction or constriction*
Toxic (alcohol, Adriamycin)	Mitral stenosis*
Ventricular Overload	Hypertrophic cardiomyopathy (obstructive,* unobstructive)
Pressure	Restrictive cardiomyopathy
Hypertension	Pure diastolic dysfunction
Aortic stenosis*	Infiltrative cardiomyopathy (amyloid, sarcoid, hemochromatosis)

*Consider for surgical evaluation and possible correction.

The echocardiogram elucidates cardiac structure and thus guides possible consultation with the specialist toward consideration of surgical correction or appropriate pharmacologic care (Table 2). It is strongly recommended that the physician have this information early in the evaluation of all patients with heart failure.

■ PREVENTING HEART FAILURE (Table 3)

Risk factors for developing coronary heart disease and indirectly heart failure include age, hypertension, elevated cholesterol, glucose intolerance (especially overt diabetes), cigarette smoking, left ventricular hypertrophy, low level of high-density lipoprotein (HDL) cholesterol, and obesity. Coronary heart disease produces a fourfold increase in the risk of developing heart failure; hypertension alone triples the risk. Hypertension and coronary heart disease are the predominant causes of heart failure in westernized society, accounting for 80 percent of all cases. Controlling modifiable risk factors must be emphasized in the presence of diabetes.

It is notable that "silent" myocardial infarctions are just as common a predisposing cause of heart failure as are symptomatic myocardial infarctions in patients that survive 1 year. It is estimated that up to 25 percent of infarctions in the general population are silent or atypical in presentation. Silent myocardial infarctions are more common in females, the elderly, and the diabetic patient—especially when neuropathy is present.

■ MANAGING THE PATIENT WITH HEART FAILURE

Nondrug Treatment (Fig. 5)

In both the diabetic and nondiabetic individual, management of heart failure of either the systolic or diastolic type should begin with "patient education" directed toward the disorder itself, compliance with dietary restrictions of sodium, exercise recommendations, and advice on when to seek additional medical attention. Commonly, a lack of understanding of heart failure and the effects of noncompliance coupled with denial mechanisms contribute greatly to the observed clinical deterioration and the need for urgent medical care and repeated hospitalizations. A clinical parallel exists in the management of diabetes itself, where patient participation and education are paramount to the best care.

Restricting sodium intake and avoiding excess weight should be stressed to all patients. An active life-style is beneficial, although strenuous physical activity that causes ischemic symptoms or hemodynamic instability should be avoided.

Noncompliance with medications, diet, inadequate discharge planning or follow-up, and failed social support systems, as well as delay in seeking medical attention, are major factors contributing to hospitalizations for decompensated heart failure. These facts underscore the importance of educating the patient and family about heart failure as completely as possible and emphasizing their role in the management of their serious but manageable disease.

Drug Treatment (see Fig. 2, Table 4)

The pathophysiology of heart failure primarily involves a reduced cardiac output associated with multiple neuroendocrine disturbances, resulting in increases in systemic vascular resistance and sodium and water retention. Treatment is aimed at controlling intravascular volume, improving the contractile state of the myocardium when systolic function is impaired, and reducing impedance to left ventricular ejection. The individual and additive effects of combined drug treatments as they antagonize the continuing pathophysiologic cycle are summarized in Figure 2. Pharmacologic therapy is required for virtually all patients with heart failure, perhaps reflecting the mild overall benefit of nonpharmacologic measures and the identification of patients relatively late in the natural history of heart failure. Even patients with mild symptoms often have advanced left ventricular dysfunction.

Diuretics: First-Line Treatment Regardless of Heart Failure Etiology

Diuretics are the most commonly prescribed agents for heart failure. These agents decrease salt and water retention, thereby decreasing pulmonary and systemic congestion. Diuretics produce favorable effects in heart failure secondary to either systolic or diastolic dysfunction. Although recognized to have adverse metabolic effects, including electrolyte (Na^+, K^+, Mg^{++}, Cl^-) depletion with associated alkalosis, they are generally well tolerated.

Furosemide is preferred to thiazide diuretics because of the more clearly defined onset, magnitude, and duration of action. When a patient fails to diurese with up to 80 mg of furosemide twice daily, addition of low-dose thiazide

---

Table 3 Stepped-Care Approach to the Management of Heart Failure

PRIMARY PREVENTION
Control risk factors for coronary heart disease, especially hypertension, the major causes of heart failure
    Systolic blood pressure
    Total cholesterol (and LDL cholesterol)
    Glucose intolerance and diabetes mellitus
    Cigarette smoking
    Obesity and sedentary life-style
SECONDARY PREVENTION
Following myocardial infarction
    Control ischemia (beta-blocker, aspirin)
    Control remodeling (nitrates, captopril)

LDL = low-density lipoprotein.

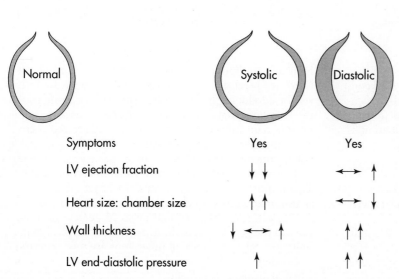

	Systolic	Diastolic
Symptoms	Yes	Yes
LV ejection fraction	↓↓	↔ ↑
Heart size: chamber size	↑↑	↔ ↓
Wall thickness	↓ ↔ ↑	↑↑
LV end-diastolic pressure	↑	↑↑

Figure 4
Differentiating systolic from diastolic heart failure.

(12.5 or 25 mg twice daily) or metolazone (2.5 or 5 mg twice daily) will often effect an excellent diuresis. One must assess potassium and magnesium levels frequently on this regimen because profound electrolyte shifts may occur. It is also recommended that the total daily diuretic dose be reassessed and high-dose diuretics terminated as soon as possible. In the patient with heart failure, it is extremely important not to deplete intravascular volume excessively. This can produce hypotension, reduce cardiac output, and exacerbate orthostatic symptoms already common in heart failure patients. The beneficial effects of diuretics may be ameliorated by their tendency to activate vasoconstriction. Although diuretics are a necessary component of the treatment of heart failure, as shown by the high recurrence rate of decompensation when they are withdrawn, the controlled studies to date support that diuretics fail in many ways when used as monotherapy to control heart failure. Diuretic monotherapy with furosemide has been compared individually and directly with the combination of diuretic and digoxin, angiotensin converting enzyme (ACE) inhibitor (captopril), phosphodiesterase inhibitor (milrinone), and partial beta agonist (xamoterol). Furosemide monotherapy

was inferior to these regimens, resulting in higher dropout rates secondary to decompensated heart failure and little or no improvement in exercise capacity or symptoms.

One comparative study assessed the dosage of diuretic after 6 months to find that one-third of patients on diuretic monotherapy had an increased diuretic need despite no significant improvement in exercise capacity or symptoms. This finding was not observed when diuretic treatment was augmented by ACE inhibitor or inotropic therapy. The diuretic and ACE inhibitor (captopril) combination group showed favorable and significant increases in exercise capacity and symptom control without associated increases in diuretic dosages. Diuretic monotherapy in this study was associated with a higher frequency of ventricular arrhythmias assessed by ambulatory ECG recordings and more frequent emergency room visits and hospitalizations to control decompensated heart failure than the combination of diuretic and ACE inhibitor. Diuretic treatment often necessitates potassium and magnesium supplementation to control excessive losses of these electrolytes, especially in the patient with diabetes in whom depletion of potassium may inhibit insulin action.

Table 4 Drug Treatment of Systolic and Diastolic Heart Failure

SYSTOLIC FAILURE	DIASTOLIC FAILURE
Diuretics*	Diuretics*
Furosemide	Furosemide
ACE inhibitors	Cautious use of all vasodilators
Nitrates, hydralazine	ACE inhibitors
Avoid calcium channel blockers	Calcium channel blockers
Digoxin	Nitrates, hydralazine
	No digoxin†

*For diabetic patients cautious use of potassium-sparing diuretics is recommended because of the risk of serious hyperkalemia.
†Digoxin may be considered for heart rate control in patients with tachycardia secondary to atrial flutter or fibrillation when other treatments such as beta-blockade, verapamil, or diltiazem have been unsatisfactory.
ACE = angiotensin converting enzyme.

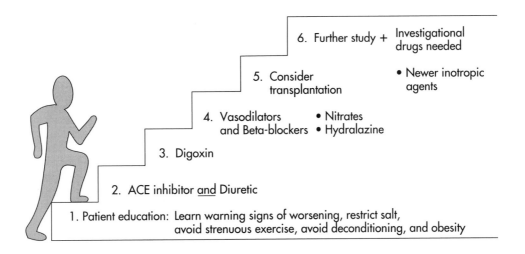

Figure 5
A stepped-care approach to the treatment of systolic heart failure.

ACE Inhibitors: Vasodilators of Choice After Diuretics in Systolic Failure

Vasodilators are agents capable of improving cardiac performance that have been used to supplement therapeutic regimens when patients remained symptomatic with fatigue, dyspnea, edema, or reduced exercise tolerance resulting from systolic failure. Recent studies using the ACE inhibitor captopril have shown hemodynamic, symptomatic, and exercise-related improvements and a reduction in cardiac end points in patients with heart failure. These benefits are not dependent on concomitant therapy with digoxin.

Initiating ACE Inhibitors (Table 5). ACE inhibitor therapy is acceptable for routine treatment of heart failure because of its established safety and efficacy. The incidence of adverse effects, primarily involving renal function, is higher in the diabetic than in the nondiabetic patient despite similar efficacy. Initiation of ACE inhibitor therapy follows diuretic treatment, with or without digoxin. It is recommended that treatment be initiated with low doses: 6.25 mg of captopril twice or three times daily or 2.5 mg of enalapril once or twice daily. Less than 5 percent of patients are expected to be withdrawn from treatment. The most common side effects are lightheadedness and dizziness secondary to hypotension. These can usually be alleviated by reduced diuretic dosages or liberalization of fluid intake.

Comparing the results of studies with vasodilators such as nitrates, hydralazine, minoxidil, and prazosin with those of studies with ACE inhibitors reveals that the improvements in symptoms and exercise capacity with ACE inhibitors are of greater magnitude and more predictable. The lower side effect profile of ACE inhibitors compared with agents such as hydralazine and minoxidil provides an additional incentive for use. Direct controlled comparisons have confirmed that the improvements associated with ACE inhibitors are greater than those produced by other presently available agents, including prazosin and nifedipine.

In preliminary and limited trials comparing captopril with other ACE inhibitors, similar benefits have been observed (Table 6).

Digoxin: Use Substantiated by Studies of Systolic Failure

The prospective controlled evaluations of digoxin conducted to date have affirmed the efficacy of chronic digoxin therapy for enhancing exercise capacity and reducing symptoms of heart failure. This has been demonstrated in the setting of sinus rhythm as well as atrial fibrillation. The benefit of digoxin therapy may relate to its favorable effect on decreasing neurohumoral activation of the renin-angiotensin-aldosterone and sympathetic systems. The cur-

---

Table 6 Beneficial Clinical Actions of ACE Inhibitors in Patients with Heart Failure

Improved cardiac performance
   Increased cardiac output
   Reduced ventricular end-diastolic pressures
   Reduced systemic vascular resistance
   Improved NYHA functional class
      Less dyspnea and fatigue
      Increased exercise capacity
Conservation of potassium and magnesium
Correction of hyponatremia (when combined with furosemide)
Reduction in ventricular arrhythmias
Reductions in emergency interventions and hospitalizations
Reduced myocardial oxygen requirement in coronary disease
Improved survival
Reduced remodeling following myocardial infarction with captopril
Reduced total and cardiovascular mortality
Reduced heart failure and hospitalization
Reduced recurrent myocardial infarction

NYHA = New York Heart Association.

Table 7 Results of the Survival and Ventricular Enlargement (SAVE) Study

STUDY GROUP
2231 survivors of acute myocardial infarction
Confirmed left ventricular ejection fraction ≤40%
Ages 27–79 years (mean 59.5 years)
Incidence of diabetes: 25%
TREATMENT
Conventional care as necessary (including thrombolysis, aspirin, beta-blockade)
On days 3–16 additional treatment with either placebo or captopril titrated from 6.25 mg test dose to 50 mg t.i.d.
RESULTS
<5% of patients discontinued captopril because of cough, dizziness, taste disturbance, diarrhea
Captopril reduced total mortality 17% and cardiovascular mortality 19% ($p<0.02$ and $p<0.015$, respectively)
Secondary end points including severe heart failure, hospitalization for heart failure, and recurrent myocardial infarction in 40% of the placebo-treated patients despite conventional care
Captopril reduced secondary end points collectively 21% including:
   Occurrence of severe heart failure, 36% $p = 0.001$
   Hospitalization for heart failure, 19% $p = 0.031$
   Recurrent myocardial infarction, 24% $p = 0.042$

*From Pfeffer Ma, et al. N Engl J Med 1992; 327: 669–677; with permission.

Table 5 Guidelines for Initiating ACE Inhibitor Therapy

PATIENT SELECTION
Confirm dilated left ventricle
Avoid hypovolemia
Stop potassium supplements or sparing diuretics
ACE INHIBITOR DOSAGE
Low initial dose
   Captopril: 6.25 mg b.i.d. or t.i.d. for 1 week
   Enalapril: 2.5 mg q.d. or b.i.d. for 1 week
Titrate slowly
   Captopril: 12.5 mg b.i.d. or t.i.d. for 1 week
   Enalapril: 5.0 mg q.d. or b.i.d. for 1 week
Maintenance dosage
   Captopril: 25 or 50 mg b.i.d. or t.i.d.
   Enalapril: 10 mg q.d. or b.i.d.
ABSOLUTE STOP POINTS
Limiting side effects (e.g., cough, rash)
Orthostatic hypotension not alleviated by diuretic reduction
Progressive azotemia not alleviated by diuretic reduction

rent value and proved efficacy are countered by limitations of information regarding the effect of digoxin on survival and the lack of a dose-response relationship to allow identification of optimal dose for each patient. Digoxin should be administered such that blood levels at steady state are above 0.7 ng per milliliter and do not exceed 2 ng per milliliter. This can be accomplished with 0.25 mg per day of digoxin for most patients under 60 years of age with serum creatinine levels of 1.4 mg per deciliter or less. In older patients or those with impaired renal function, dosages should be 0.125 mg per day or less. The presence of changing renal function or severe degrees of renal impairment seen in diabetic nephropathy heighten the risk of digitalis toxicity and may compromise the value of continued use of digoxin. Digoxin's beneficial inotropic effect and the vasodilating and neurohumoral benefits of ACE inhibition are independent mechanisms, which are favorable and additive in the patient with systolic heart failure.

■ REDUCING HEART FAILURE RISK FOLLOWING MYOCARDIAL INFARCTION

The goal of medical therapy following myocardial infarction is to limit ventricular damage (or remodeling) and reduce the subsequent risk of heart failure. During the acute phase of a myocardial infarction it is beneficial to re-establish coronary perfusion with thrombolytic agents and control hypertension, wall stress, and ischemia. Between day 3 and day 16 after a myocardial infarction, initiation of ACE inhibition with captopril has produced 17 to 36 percent reductions in total mortality, cardiovascular mortality, occurrence of severe heart failure, hospitalization for heart failure, and recurrent myocardial infarction. These are findings of the Survival and Ventricular Enlargement (SAVE) study, in which 25 percent of the study population had diabetes (Table 7). Use of captopril was additive to the proved benefits of thrombolysis, aspirin use, and beta-blockade after myocardial infarction. It is recommended that each patient found to have a left ventricular ejection fraction less than 40 percent after myocardial infarction be considered for ACE inhibitor treatment. ACE inhibitor treatment is recommended whether or not heart failure symptoms are evident.

■ EFFECTS OF TREATMENTS ON SURVIVAL

It is well recognized that the natural history of patients with heart failure includes an increased annual mortality. The ability of pharmacologic treatments to improve symptoms of heart failure has until recently failed to show a corresponding improvement in survival. The Veterans Administration Cooperative Vasodilator Heart Failure Trial (VHeFT) found that the combination of hydralazine (300 mg per day) and isosorbide dinitrate (160 mg per day) when added to baseline treatment of digoxin and diuretics could improve 1-year mortality by 38 percent, 2-year mortality by 25 percent (p<.03), and 3-year mortality by 23 percent in patients with moderate heart failure. The confirmation that enhanced sur-

vival occurs with ACE inhibition has been adequately demonstrated by the Cooperative North Scandinavian Enalapril Survival Study (CONSENSUS) trial study group, and survival results from the Studies Of Left Ventricular Dysfunction (SOLVD) treatment trial and the Munich Mild Heart Failure trial. The SOLVD treatment trial demonstrated a 16 percent reduction in total mortality and an 18 percent reduction in cardiovascular mortality during enalapril treatment (average dose 17 mg per day) for 3.5 years compared to placebo (both p <0.01). The Munich Mild Heart Failure trial reported by Kleber et al found that ACE inhibition with captopril is associated with reduced frequency of progressive pump failure and death in patients with mild heart failure. The captopril dosage of 25 mg twice daily is lower than in previous trials. The newest data comparing ACE inhibitors with the direct-acting vasodilators nitrates and hydralazine show better survival with ACE inhibitor use in male veterans with moderately severe heart failure and patients with severe heart failure awaiting transplantation.

■ DRUG TREATMENT OF DIASTOLIC HEART FAILURE—A PROBLEM

Clinical studies of patients with diastolic heart failure are presently inadequate to direct the physician in the routine management of these patients. It is generally accepted that all guidelines for prevention of hypertension and coronary heart disease apply to these patients. Hypertension and obesity should be controlled because each produces a strong stimulus to left ventricular hypertrophy and can be modified successfully. Reductions in hypertrophy would be expected to reduce relaxation abnormalities and improve diastolic function. The use of ACE inhibitors, calcium channel blockers, selective alpha-1 blockers and beta-blockers is acceptable. One must avoid excessive heart rate lowering because this may compromise cardiac output and be poorly tolerated. Diuretics should be used to control pulmonary and systemic congestion without depleting intravascular volume. Digoxin should be avoided unless its use is mandated by the presence of a supraventricular tachyarrhythmia with a rapid ventricular response that is unresponsive to other treatments (verapamil, diltiazem, or beta-blocker). Control of ischemia is important because muscle relaxation, an active metabolic process, is worsened during ischemia. The usual inability of the hypertrophied and stiff ventricle found in diastolic heart failure to increase cardiac output in response to peripheral vaso- dilatation makes the use of direct-acting vasodilators such as hydralazine and high-dose nitrates problematic. Arterial vasodilatation accompanying the use of these agents may be associated with hypotension.

Suggested Reading

Packer M, Lee WH, Medina N, et al. Influence of diabetes mellitus on changes in left ventricular performance and renal function produced by converting enzyme inhibition in patients with severe chronic heart failure. Am J Med 1987; 82:1119–1126.

This excellent study provides a background for understanding how and to what extent the diabetic state modifies the efficacy and safety of ACE inhibitors when used to manage heart failure. Since the study population has severe heart failure, the risks are perhaps slightly higher than in diabetic patients with milder and less symptomatic levels of heart failure. The results emphasize that ACE inhibitors are the vasodilators of choice in heart failure and should not be withheld from the diabetic patient but do require closer monitoring than in the nondiabetic patient.

Perez JE, McGill JB, Santiago JV, et al. Abnormal myocardial acoustic properties in diabetic patients and their correlation with the severity of disease. J Am Coll Cardiol 1992; 19:1154–1162.

Accompanying editorial comments:

Regan TJ, Weisse AB. Diabetic cardiomyopathy. J Am Coll Cardiol 1992; 19:1165–1166.

Skorton DJ, Vandenberg B. Ultrasound tissue characterization of the diabetic heart: Laboratory curiosity or clinical tool? J Am Coll Cardiol 1992; 19:1163–1164.

The authors offer a possible technique for the early identification of structural changes associated with diabetic cardiomyopathy using echocardiography. Although very preliminary, these data suggest an exciting opportunity to investigate the changes in ventricular function that accompany diabetes that is independent of coronary disease, hypertension, and other causes of heart failure. If successful, it may lead the way to studying treatments aimed at modification of these myopathic processes.

PERIPHERAL VASCULAR DISEASE

Marvin E. Levin, M.D.
Gregorio A. Sicard, M.D.

Peripheral vascular disease (PVD) is extremely common in patients with diabetes. About 8 percent of the diabetic population have PVD at the time of diagnosis; 10 years after diagnosis, 15 percent have PVD; and after 20 years, 45 percent have PVD. Of the 20 percent of diabetics who enter the hospital because of foot problems, 30 percent have symptomatic PVD and 7 percent require vascular surgery and/or amputation.

Peripheral vascular disease contributes to amputation by arterial occlusion or by impeding the delivery of antibiotics, oxygen, and nutrients which causes delayed wound healing and an inability to fight infection. Clearing of infection and wound healing are unlikely if the ankle brachial index is below 0.45 or the transcutaneous oxygen pressure (TcPo$_2$) is under 30 mm Hg.

Of all nontraumatic amputations, 50 percent occur in diabetics. It was recently reported that there were 51,605 diabetic lower extremity amputations from the data of the National Hospital Discharge Summary.

Bild and colleagues have reviewed a number of epidemiologic factors that contribute to amputation in diabetic patients. Race may play a significant role. A 1.4 to 2.3 times greater incidence of amputation has been shown to occur in blacks compared to whites. The increased prevalence of hypertension and smoking in blacks may be a significant contributing factor. The Pima Indians in the Southwest have

an exceptionally high rate of amputation, a 3.7 times greater incidence than whites. Age is also a significant factor: 96 percent of all lower extremity amputations occur in those over age 45. The amputation rate in the 45- to 64-year-old group is two to three times greater in the diabetic population than in the nondiabetic population. In those over 65 years of age, it is seven times greater. Diabetes is an equalizer between the sexes when looking at PVD. The incidence of PVD is much more prevalent in nondiabetic men than in nondiabetic women, whereas in diabetic men and women, the ratio is almost equal.

■ PATHOGENESIS

The deposits of lipids, cholesterol, calcium, smooth muscle cells, and platelets in the atherosclerotic plaque are qualitatively the same in the diabetic as in the nondiabetic. Differences in the clinical presentation of PVD in diabetic and nondiabetic patients are listed in Table 1. A most important difference is which vessels are involved. In the diabetic patient, the vessels involved are primarily those below the knee: the tibials and the peroneals.

Risk Factors
Aggressive efforts to control risk factors associated with the development of PVD are extremely important in preventing macrovascular disease (Table 2).

Smoking
Beach and Strandness found smoking to be one of the most important risk factors for atherosclerosis and have shown that cessation of smoking is associated with a decrease in the progression of atherosclerotic disease. Interestingly, smoking low-nicotine cigarettes has not been shown to reduce the incidence of myocardial infarction. Smoking may lead to PVD in at least four different ways:

1. Smoking causes vasospasm; smoking just one cigarette can cause vasospasm for several hours;

2. Smoking increases the production of carboxyhemoglobin and carbon monoxide, which may lead to endothelial injury;
3. Smoking worsens diabetes dyslipidemia by increasing low-density lipoprotein (LDL) cholesterol and triglyceride levels and lowering the high-density lipoprotein (HDL) cholesterol concentration; and
4. Smoking increases thrombogenesis by decreasing prostacyclin and increasing blood viscosity and clotting factors.

Dyslipidemia

A study by Laakso and Pyorala found that total LDL cholesterol and very–low-density lipoprotein (VLDL) triglycerides tended to be higher and HDL and HDL2 cholesterol to be lower in type 1 and type 2 diabetic patients with claudication. Therefore, control of cholesterol and lipid abnormalities should be as vigorous in patients with PVD as in those with coronary artery disease.

Hypertension

Hypertension, both systolic and diastolic, is a risk factor for PVD. The initial treatment of hypertension is with a low-salt diet, weight reduction, and exercise. When these approaches are unsatisfactory, pharmacologic treatment is indicated. The antihypertensives of choice for diabetic patients are calcium channel blockers and angiotensin converting enzyme inhibitors. The older antihypertensive drugs, beta-blockers and diuretics, especially thiazides, may have an adverse effect on atherosclerosis. Beta-blockers have been shown to increase fasting blood sugars, HbA_{1c} levels, insulin levels, VLDL, and triglycerides and to lower HDL. Thiazides increase blood glucose, cholesterol, LDL cholesterol, triglycerides, and insulin resistance. Warram et al showed that diuretic use was associated with a fourfold increased risk for cardiovascular mortality in patients without proteinuria and a tenfold increased risk for those with proteinuria. Multivariant analysis revealed that diuretic therapy alone as a treatment for hypertension was associated with an increased risk for CVD mortality in both the proteinuric and nonproteinuric groups. When thiazides are indicated as an adjunct in the treatment of hypertension, the dose should not exceed 12.5 mg to 25 mg per day.

Obesity

Obesity, especially truncal, is a proved macrovascular risk factor. Björntorp has reviewed the multiple metabolic implications of body fat distribution and how it contributes to atherogenesis. Fat distribution is genetically determined to a major degree. However, weight loss can ameliorate the atherogenic risk factors related to truncal obesity. Smoking has also been shown to increase the waist-hip ratio, another reason to stop smoking.

Renal Transplantation

An additional risk factor for PVD and amputation is renal transplantation. This effect is more common in diabetic than in nondiabetic patients. Lemmers and Barry reported peripheral arterial events to have occurred in 36 percent of subjects after renal transplantation, with 25 percent requiring at least one amputation. The exact mechanism for this finding needs to be clearly identified.

■ SIGNS AND SYMPTOMS OF PERIPHERAL VASCULAR DISEASE

Intermittent Claudication

The word *claudication* comes from the Latin, meaning "to limp." Patients with claudication may limp, but more characteristically, they stop to rest. In the Framingham study, diabetes was associated with two- to threefold excess risk of intermittent claudication for both sexes. Diabetics with intermittent claudication were at especially high risk for cardiovascular events. The pain or discomfort is usually localized to the calf. The pain is characteristically associated with walking and is relieved by cessation of walking without the need to sit down. The discomfort associated with intermittent claudication must be distinguished from pain resulting from degenerative arthritic changes, disk disease, tumors of the spinal cord (particularly the cauda equina), thrombophlebitis, anemia, and even myxedema. Pain with walking due to these causes is referred to as pseudoclaudication. One can usually differentiate ischemic claudication from pseudoclaudication by taking a careful history. Patients with claudication due to ischemia simply need to stop walking and rest

Table 1 Differences in Diabetic and Nondiabetic Peripheral Vascular Disease		
	DIABETIC	**NONDIABETIC**
Clinical	More common	Less common
	Younger patient	Older patient
	More rapid	Less rapid
Male:Female	M = F	M > F
Occlusion	Multisegmental	Single segment
Vessels adjacent to occlusion	Involved	Not involved
Collaterals	Involved	Usually normal
Lower extremities	Both	Unilateral
Vessels involved	Tibials	Aortic
	Peroneals	Iliac
		Femoral

From Levin ME, Bowker JH. The diabetic foot: Pathophysiology, evaluation and treatment. In: Levin ME, O'Neal LW, eds. The diabetic foot. 5th ed. St Louis: Mosby–Year Book, 1993, p 17; with permission.

for a minute or two and can then proceed. Patients with pseudoclaudication usually require 15 to 20 minutes of rest and frequently have to sit down, change position, and/or flex or extend their back to get relief. Symptoms of intermittent claudication depend upon ischemia in the muscle. Because of the small muscle mass in the foot, some investigators believe that claudication of the foot is infrequent or does not occur. Higher vascular obstruction (e.g., in the aorta) will cause claudicatory pain in the upper thighs and buttocks and may be accompanied by impotence.

Some diabetic patients, despite significant PVD, may not have symptoms of intermittent claudication because of their loss of pain sensation. This emphasizes the need for routine examination of the diabetic patient's lower extremities for signs of PVD, even though the patient has no symptoms.

Examination of the patient with intermittent claudication involving the calf muscles may reveal both a femoral and pedal pulse but no popliteal pulse. Pedal pulses are present because of the development of collaterals around the knee. However, after a brisk walk the foot will pale and become pulseless. Therefore, treadmill testing is indicated in patients with a good history for claudication but detectable peripheral pulses. Exercise will lead to a diminution or disappearance of peripheral pulses because of decreased pulse pressure. Patients with normal circulation have no drop in ankle pulses with exercise. Intermittent claudication usually begins when the ankle brachial index falls to 0.75 or below. The cornerstones for the treatment of intermittent claudication are smoking cessation and exercise. Gardner and Poehlman in a meta-analysis found that the optimal exercise program for improving claudication pain distances in patients with PVD uses intermittent walking to near-maximal pain during a program of at least 6 months. Bicycle riding is probably less beneficial because it exercises the thigh muscles and not the calf muscles.

The hemorrheologic agent pentoxifylline (Trental) has been demonstrated to be helpful in a significant number of patients with intermittent claudication. It does not dilate the vessels, but by improving red blood cell flexibility decreases blood viscosity and therefore increases blood flow. It must be

---

Table 2 Risk Factors for Diabetic Macrovascular Disease

Smoking
Dyslipidemia
Hypertension
Obesity (truncal)
Renal transplantation

From Levin ME, Bowker JH. The diabetic foot: Pathophysiology, evaluation and treatment. In: Levin ME, O'Neal LW, eds. The diabetic foot. 5th ed. St Louis: Mosby–Year Book, 1993, p 17; with permission.

Table 3 The Five P's of Acute Arterial Occlusion in the Lower Extremity

Pain: sudden onset
Pallor: waxy
Paresthesia: numbness
Pulselessness: no pulse below block
Paralysis: sudden weakness

---

kept in mind that pentoxifylline should be given for at least 2 to 3 months to establish whether or not it is effective. There is debate about the efficacy of another hemorrheologic agent, ketanserin, a serotonin antagonist, in improving exercise tolerance in patients with intermittent claudication. Its use is still experimental. Vascular surgery is rarely indicated in the treatment of intermittent claudication and then only if the patient is severely disabled, being able to walk less than 1½ blocks, or for those whose livelihood depends upon walking.

Beta adrenergic receptor blockage has been considered a relative contraindication in patients with intermittent claudication. However, a report by Radack and Deck found that beta-blockers do not adversely affect walking capacity or symptoms of intermittent claudication in patients with mild to moderate peripheral arterial disease. They felt that beta-blockers could probably be used safely in such patients. Nevertheless, patients with intermittent claudication and severe PVD who are taking beta-blockers should be watched carefully for symptoms of increased claudication.

The long-term outlook for patients with intermittent claudication is relatively good with conservative management. Most patients who have been followed for long periods of time stay the same or actually improve if they stop smoking and continue an exercise program.

Rest Pain and Night Pain

Rest pain indicates at least two hemodynamically significant arterial blocks in a series. Rest pain is caused by nerve ischemia and is persistent with peaks of intensity. It is worse at night and may require narcotics for relief. Rest pain is decreased by dependency of the legs. Therefore, the patient often sleeps in a chair, and edema of the leg, secondary to constant dependency, is common.

Nocturnal ischemic pain is a form of neuritis that usually precedes rest pain. It occurs at night when perfusion of the extremities is decreased and disrupts sleep. Patients invariably gain relief by standing up, dangling their feet over the edge of the bed, and/or walking a few steps. This activity increases cardiac output, leading to improved perfusion of the lower extremities and relief of the ischemic neuritis. If vascular lesions that produce rest and nocturnal pain are not corrected by vascular surgery, gangrene almost always develops, necessitating amputation. Rest pain and nocturnal pain are therefore indications for consultation with a vascular surgeon. Diabetics with severe PVD and ischemia may not experience rest pain or night pain because of peripheral neuropathy and loss of sensation. You may test for PVD in these patients by raising the legs 45 degrees until they blanch. The patient is then asked to sit with the legs dependent. Normally, venous filling will occur within 15 seconds. Severe ischemia is present if filling requires more than 25 seconds.

Acute Occlusion

Sudden occlusion from emboli or acute complete thrombosis can occur. Most emboli (over 70 percent) originate in the heart. The most common cardiac pathology is atrial fibrillation. Myocardial infarction with mural thrombi is the second most common. Acute thrombosis has atherosclerosis as the underlying cause. The signs and symptoms of sudden arterial occlusion are usually referred to as the five P's (Table 3).

With embolism, the affected extremity is waxlike and lemon yellow in color. With thrombosis, the extremity is less cadaverous in appearance and tends to be somewhat cyanotic. Most sudden occlusions are the result of emboli. The extent of ischemia and final outcome depend on collateral circulation, size, location of the clot, and time elapsing from the onset of acute occlusion to treatment. These occlusions must be treated as soon as possible because peripheral nerve and skeletal muscles have less resistance to ischemia than do skin and bone. Irreversible changes of skeletal muscle and peripheral nerves may occur after 4 to 6 hours of severe ischemia. The skin may tolerate severe ischemia for 10 hours. Treatment of acute arterial occlusion requires either emergent surgical intervention or, in selected cases, thrombolytic therapy and adjunctive endoluminal treatment (angioplasty or atherectomy).

Blue Toe Syndrome

Ischemia or gangrene of the toes can results from four possible causes: (1) atherosclerosis with thrombosis, (2) microthrombi formation resulting from infection, (3) drugs that cause decrease in blood flow, such as pressor agents, and (4) cholesterol emboli. Embolization of the digital arteries results in the blue or purple toe syndrome, in which the toe takes on a deep purplish discoloration, and gangrene can develop. Cholesterol emboli to the foot result in sudden onset of painful toes and petechiae. A livedo reticular pattern is usually present due to embolization of cutaneous arterioles. Sharp demarcation frequently occurs between the normally perfused skin and the ischemic areas. It should be noted that many of these patients have received anticoagulant therapy with warfarin. The blue toe syndrome has also been associated with thrombolytic therapy. Therefore, it is extremely important to periodically check the toes and feet of patients receiving anticoagulants and thrombolytic therapy. If the symptoms are bilateral, ulceration of an aortic plaque is likely. Surgical intervention with removal of the ulcerated plaque by endarterectomy or by aortobifemoral bypass is required (see the section *Vascular Surgery*).

Vasospasticity

Vasospasm of the extremities such as occurs with Raynaud's phenomenon may affect the toes as well as the fingers. Raynaud's phenomenon may occur as a primary disease or as a result of underlying conditions such as systemic rheumatic disorder, drugs, hyperviscosity disease, and a variety of miscellaneous conditions. The primary treatment is to avoid cold by wearing warm gloves and socks and to stop smoking. Treatment of the underlying disease and/or removal of offending drugs are important approaches. The most common agents for treating vasospasm are calcium entry blockers or sympatholytic drugs. Nifedipine (Procardia) is the calcium entry blocker with the most potent peripheral vasodilatory action. The use of topical nitroglycerin has given variable results. Lumbar sympathectomy for Raynaud's phenomenon of the toes has been reported to be relatively successful.

■ IMPROVING BLOOD FLOW

Vasodilators

Vasodilators are ineffective in the treatment of diabetic PVD. Vasodilators may worsen ischemia by the "steal effect." In this instance, dilatation of the healthy vessels steals blood away from the ischemic areas and worsens the situation.

Sympathectomy

Sympathectomy has no role in the improvement of diabetic PVD. The arteries in diabetic patients are primarily sclerosed vessels with very little capacity for dilatation after sympathectomy. In addition, many diabetic patients have autonomic neuropathy and an "auto sympathectomy."

Vascular Surgery

Vascular surgery may be necessary to improve blood flow. Indications for vascular surgery are significant signs and symptoms of PVD with confirmation by the vascular laboratory.

The evaluation of segmental pressures, as well as Doppler wave forms of the femoral, popliteal, ankle, and distal pressures, is an excellent noninvasive way to diagnose lower extremity vascular occlusive disease accurately. Unfortunately, segmental pressures may not provide accurate information in assessing occlusive disease in some diabetic patients, because the prominent medial calcification of diabetic lower extremity arteries can give falsely elevated pressures. On the other hand, Doppler wave form analysis at the femoral, popliteal, posterior tibial, and dorsalis pedis arteries will identify the level of obstruction.

Before vascular surgery can be carried out, angiography is required to establish operability and the location of the block or blocks. Because diabetic patients frequently have renal disease, and because contrast material can result in renal shutdown, as little dye as possible should be used in these patients. The use of digital imaging technique has helped in diminishing the dye load in diabetic patients. If vascular insufficiency is unilateral, only the affected side should have angiography. If a short segmental lesion is found in the iliac or femoropopliteal area, percutaneous balloon angioplasty can be performed with excellent results. Unfortunately, occlusive vascular disease in diabetics most often affects the infrapopliteal vessels, where the results with angioplasty are poor.

When to Refer

Patients with rest pain, night pain, or evidence of acute occlusive disease should be urgently referred for vascular surgical consultation. Other indications for surgery include nonhealing ulcers, infections resistant to standard treatment, or increasing symptoms and signs of PVD.

Suggested Reading

Beach KW, Strandness DE Jr. Arteriosclerosis obliterans and associated risk factors in insulin-dependent and non–insulin-dependent diabetics. Diabetes 1980; 29:882–894.

This is an excellent discussion of the various risk factors associated with arteriosclerosis obliterans.

Bild DE, Selby JV, Sinnock P, et al. Lower-extremity amputation in people with diabetes: Epidemiology and prevention. Diabetes Care 1989; 12:24–31.

This is an extremely detailed discussion of the multiple epidemiologic risk factors associated with lower extremity amputation.

Björntorp P. Metabolic implications of body fat distribution. Diabetes Care 1991; 14:1132–1143.

Truncal obesity is an accepted risk factor for atherosclerosis. This article discusses the implications of body fat distribution.

Brand FN, Abbott RD, Kannel WB. Diabetes, intermittent claudication, and risk of cardiovascular events: The Framingham study. Diabetes Care 1989; 38:504–509.

The Framingham study brings us up to date on the risk factors associated with intermittent claudication.

Centers for Disease Control. Diabetes surveillance, 1980–1987, Policy Program research, annual 1990 report. U.S. Department of Health and Human Services, Atlanta: Division of Diabetes Translation, 1990, 23–25.

Diabetes Surveillance is an ongoing program being carried out by the Centers for Disease Control. This particular surveillance updates the current statistics associated with amputation.

Gardner AW, Poehlman ET. Exercise rehabilitation programs for the treatment of claudication pain: A meta-analysis, JAMA 1995; 274:975–980.

This meta-analysis points out the importance of a supervised exercise program in the treatment of intermittent claudication.

Harris KG, Smith TP, Cragg AH, Lemke JH. Nephrotoxicity from contrast material in renal insufficiency: Ionic versus non-ionic agents. Radiology 1991; 179:849–852.

There is a great deal of discussion regarding the value of nonionic contrast material. This article reviews a recent study of diabetics and nondiabetic patients and discusses the advantages of nonionic versus ionic contrast material.

Hiatt WR, Regensteiner JG, Hargarten ME, Wolfel EE, Brass EP. Benefit of exercise conditioning for patients with peripheral arterial disease. Circulation 1990; 81:602–609.

This article points out that it is not the increase in collaterals but metabolic changes following exercise that explain the etiology of the pain of intermittent claudication.

Laakso M, Pyorala K. Lipid and lipoprotein abnormalities in diabetic patients with peripheral vascular disease. Atherosclerosis 1988; 74:55–63.
This article discusses some of the lipid and lipoprotein abnormalities in diabetic patients with PVD.

Lemmers MJ, Barry JM. Major role for arterial disease in morbidity and mortality after kidney transplantation in diabetic recipients. Diabetes Care 1991; 14:295–301.

Although usually not thought of as a risk factor for PVD, renal transplantation is associated with an increased frequency of ischemic disease in both the upper and lower extremities. The reason for this is unknown.

Levin ME, Sicard GA, Rubin B. Peripheral vascular disease in the patient with diabetes. In: Rifkin H, Porte D Jr, eds. Ellenberg and Rifkin's diabetes mellitus: Theory and practice. 5th ed. Stamford, Conn: Appleton and Lange, 1997.

This chapter provides a detailed discussion of peripheral arterial disease in the patient with diabetes.

O'Keefe St, Woods BB, Reslin DJ. Blue toe syndrome: Causes and management. Arch Intern Med 1992; 152:2197–2202.

The blue toe syndrome may lead to amputation. This comprehensive review describes the syndrome and its differential diagnosis in detail.

Radack K, Deck C. B-adrenergic blocker therapy does not worsen intermittent claudication in subjects with peripheral arterial disease: A meta-analysis of randomized controlled trials. Arch Intern Med 1991; 151:1769–1776.

It has been thought for a long time that beta-blockers were contraindicated in patients with intermittent claudication. This article demonstrates that beta-blockers are in fact not contraindicated in patients with mild to moderate intermittent claudication.

Reiber GE, Boyko EJ, Smith DG. Lower extremity foot ulcers and amputation in individuals with diabetes. In: Harris MI, Cowie CC, Stern MP, eds. 2nd ed. Washington, DC: U.S. Government Printing Office (DHHS publ. no. 95-1468), 1995, 408–428.

Understanding the epidemiology of factors leading to amputation of the diabetic lower extremity can help lower amputation rates.

Steinberg D, Witztum JL. Lipoproteins and atherogenesis: Current concepts. JAMA 1990; 264:3047–3052.

This is an up-to-date discussion of lipoproteins and atherogenesis.

Taylor LM Jr, Porter JM. The clinical course of diabetics who require emergent foot surgery because of infection or ischemia. J Vasc Surg 1987; 6:454–459.

This is a very important article because it stresses the importance of radical debridement and improving blood flow in the treatment of resistant infection in the diabetic lower extremity.

Warram JH, Laffel LMB, Valsania P, Christlieb AR, Krolewski AS. Excess mortality associated with diuretic therapy in diabetes mellitus. Arch Intern Med 1991; 151:1350–1356.

Hypertension is common in the diabetic. Based on Hippocrates' statement "Thou shalt do no harm," this article discusses the harm that can occur in treating diabetic patients with diuretics.

Young JR, Graor RA, Olin JW, Bartholomew JR, eds. Peripheral vascular disease. St Louis: Mosby–Year Book, 1991.

This is a superb book, which covers every aspect of PVD. It is highly recommended for those who desire further information.

THE DIABETIC FOOT

Lawrence Harkless, D.P.M.
Andrew J.M. Boulton, M.D.

Foot problems are the most common reason for hospital admission of diabetic patients. In-patient stay is often prolonged and usually requires multiple interventions including antibiotic therapy, surgical treatment, and input from other departments such as physical medicine, podiatry, and vascular surgery. Direct hospital costs for the diabetic foot have been estimated to be in excess of $500 million per annum. Moreover, foot disease has a devastating medical and social impact. The most important aspect of clinical management of the diabetic foot syndrome is the early identification of patients who are at risk to develop ulceration, so that progression to ulceration and gangrene can be prevented. If the practicing physician understands the basic etiologic factors responsible for foot ulceration and gangrene, these foot complications should be largely preventable.

■ ETIOLOGY OF DIABETIC FOOT PROBLEMS

The main etiologic factors leading to ulceration are neuropathy and peripheral vascular disease (Fig. 1). Because the development of these complications is gradual, they may go unnoticed by both the patient and the attending physician. Superimposed infection and trauma often contribute to the development of foot ulcers.

Neuropathy is one of the most common long-term complications of diabetes. At least one-half of older patients with non–insulin-dependent diabetes mellitus (NIDDM) have some insensitivity of the feet secondary to neuropathy. It is important to emphasize that many patients with insensitive feet give no history of any neuropathic symptoms. Conversely, many patients with symptomatic sensorimotor neuropathy never develop the insensitivity in the feet that renders them susceptible to trophic ulceration. Reduced pain sensation and disturbed proprioception contribute to the risk of foot injury by altering the dynamic pressures under the foot during standing and walking. Motor neuropathy, leading to wasting and weakness of the small muscles of the foot, contributes to the development of abnormal foot pressures, while imbalance between the long flexors and extensors of the toes leads to the claw toes and prominent metatarsal heads that are pathognomonic of the high-risk neuropathic foot. These muscle changes increase the pressure under the foot during walking. Therefore, intrinsic neuropathic foot ulceration results from a combination of insensitivity, reduced proprioception, and foot pressure abnormalities.

Limited joint mobility, which occurs secondarily to alterations in biochemical structure of collagen (cheiroarthropathy), represents another risk factor for the development of foot ulcers. Altered joint mobility contributes to elevated foot pressure. The last permissive factor in the pathogenesis of trophic foot ulcers is autonomic dysfunction. Sympathetic peripheral neuropathy causes decreased sweating and altered blood flow. Repetitive pressure under dry skin from walking leads to callus formation, and ulceration follows from the callus acting as a foreign body. This is the intrinsic neuropathic ulcer. Extrinsic neuropathic ulcers develop in the insensitive foot that is subject to external pressures (e.g., an inappropriately small shoe or a foreign body such as a nail or pebble in the shoe). It is important to remember that both intrinsic and extrinsic ulceration may occur in the presence of a normal peripheral circulation. The warm but insensitive foot is at very great risk of ulceration.

The diabetic patient is also at risk of ischemic peripheral vascular disease. The combination of peripheral ischemia and insensitivity is particularly dangerous because the neuroischemic ulcer is more likely to require an amputation than the pure neuropathic ulcer. Local infection may initiate the development of the diabetic foot ulcer but more commonly plays a contributory role after it has developed.

■ IDENTIFICATION OF THE AT-RISK FOOT

Not every diabetic patient is at increased risk of foot ulceration. Therefore, not all patients need the same level of education that is required for individuals who are at high risk. It is the task of the practicing physician to identify those patients who are at increased risk (Table 1). Diabetic patients with clinically manifest neuropathy and vascular disease are at high risk to develop foot ulceration. Individuals with a prior history of foot ulcers are particularly prone to develop subsequent ulcers. Foot deformity, callus formation, and skin changes represent important risk factors, as do the presence of diabetic retinopathy and nephropathy. Elderly patients, especially if living alone and have arthritis, have an increased likelihood of developing a foot ulcer. An algorithm for the identification and further management of diabetic patients based upon the presence or absence of risk factors is provided in Figure 2.

Table 1 Potential Risk Factors in the Diabetic Foot

Absent protective sensation
Vascular insufficiency
Foot deformity causing foci of high pressure
Autonomic neuropathy causing fissuring of integument and osseous hyperemia
Limited joint mobility
Obesity
Impaired vision
Poor glucose control causing advanced glycosylation and impaired wound healing
Poor footwear causing or providing inadequate protection from tissue breakdown
History of lower extremity amputation
History of foot ulceration

Table 2 Checklist for Examination of the Diabetic Foot

SENSORY	SHAPE
Vibration (128 Hz tuning fork)	Claw toes
Pin prick	Prominent metatarsal heads
Joint-position sensation	**VASCULAR**
MOTOR	Skin temperature
Small muscle wasting	Capillary circulation
Ankle reflexes	
AUTONOMIC	
Skin texture	
Callus	

All new patients, whether recently diagnosed with diabetes or newly referred to the clinic, should be screened for increased risk of foot problems (Fig. 2). A checklist for examination of the foot (Table 2) is simple and effective and does not require expensive equipment. However, the use of simple semiquantitative instruments such as the Semmes-Weinstein monofilaments or biothesiometer may aid the clinical examination. Evidence of neurologic dysfunction should be sought: reduced pin-prick sensation or absent perception to a vibrating 128 Hz tuning fork over the great toe places the patient into a high-risk category. Clinical evidence of motor or autonomic dysfunction in the foot categorizes the patient as high risk. Earlier diagnosis of neuropathy may be achieved by more detailed objective testing of electrophysiology or quantitative sensory testing, although the impact of such early diagnosis on the incidence of foot lesions is unknown.

Clinical examination should assess the shape of the foot and its vascular status. A cool foot with poor capillary circulation and reduced or absent foot pulses is at increased risk for ulceration. Claw toes, atrophied muscles, and prominent metatarsal heads are additional high-risk features. Although quantitative assessment of foot pressures can identify high-risk areas, the equipment needed for such measurements is expensive and not generally available in clinical practice. A useful semiquantitative assessment can be achieved using a Harris-Beath mat.

If the algorithm outlined in Figure 2 is adhered to, all high-risk patients will be identified and should receive appropriate education and management as outlined below. Diabetic individuals with healthy feet should be examined in detail at least annually to ensure that their risk status has not changed. During each visit the patient's socks should be removed and the patient's feet should be examined by the physician or skilled assistant.

■ PREVENTION OF FOOT ULCERATION

All patients with high-risk feet should receive specific education in the form of a structured program. The success of foot care education programs in reducing ulceration and preventing amputation has been confirmed in prospective studies. Patients with healthy feet should receive basic foot care advice about hygiene, footwear, and care of skin and nails. Foot care education programs should employ visual aids such as leaflets and/or a slide presentation. Brief verbal instruction by the physician has been shown to be ineffective. Small group discussions with patients and their partners, conducted by a nurse educator, is most likely to succeed. Such sessions should start with a video on diabetic foot care, followed by a practical demonstration. If patients cannot feel a cold tuning fork that is easily felt by their partners, they are less likely to deny that the problem exists. Educational material on diabetic foot care is widely available from organizations such as the American Diabetes Association and from numerous pharmaceutical companies. The advice usually takes the form of "do's and dont's" and should include the need for daily foot inspection, care in footwear purchase, regular visits to the podiatrist, avoidance of barefoot gait, corn cures, and self-treatment.

The objectives of any foot care program must be carefully planned and matched to the educational and social background of the patient. Health care professionals must set an example for high-risk patients by insisting that shoes and socks be removed at every clinic visit and that the feet be carefully checked. The doctor who fails to remove the patient's shoes in order to inspect the feet when the patient visits the office every few months cannot expect the patient to do this every day at home.

Finally, all high-risk patients must be taught that any foot problem they detect, however minor it may appear to them, is potentially serious and requires that immediate medical attention be sought.

If the physician and patient closely adhered to the diagnostic outline described above, the now unacceptably high rate of foot ulceration and amputation in diabetic patients would be reduced dramatically.

The Role of the Podiatrist

The podiatrist plays a critical role in the management of the diabetic foot. In patients with high-pressure areas demonstrated by heavy callus formation, debridement of the callus and shoe gear modifications can prevent future ulcer formation by redistributing the pressure. Knowledge of the biomechanics of the foot allows the podiatrist to predict high-pressure areas simply by performing a routine biochemical foot examination. If the examination demonstrates excessive internal pressure, appropriate shoe gear modifications with polypropylene inlays can alleviate the problem. In established neuropathic ulcers, relief or reduction of pressure has been shown to be essential to allow proper healing. The ideal solution is total relief of pressure by complete bed rest. However, this is often impractical and may lead to poor patient compliance if recommended for outpatients.

Many modalities have been used in the treatment of neuropathic ulcers. A walking plaster cast is one suitable approach, which allows the patient to remain ambulatory while relieving pressure on the infected ulcerated area and preventing the foot from any future damage. Several studies have shown that walking casts heal plantar ulcers more quickly and ulcers are less likely to become infected than those treated with traditional dressings and rest. Another technique that has proved useful is the Scotch cast boot, in which the wound is lightly padded and the foot is enclosed by a shell of fiberglass. In this boot the ankle is not fixed. This particular casting technique is contraindicated in the presence of severe infection or periph-

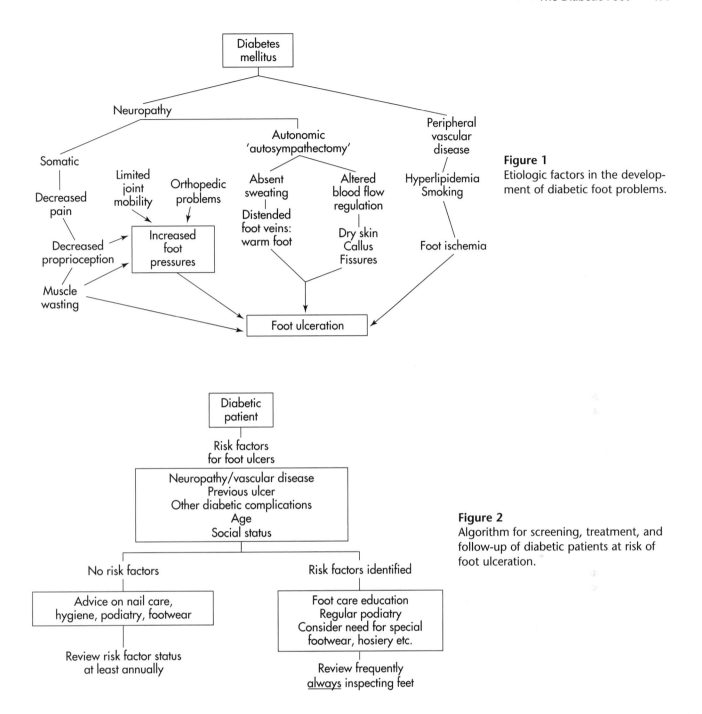

Figure 1
Etiologic factors in the development of diabetic foot problems.

Figure 2
Algorithm for screening, treatment, and follow-up of diabetic patients at risk of foot ulceration.

eral vascular disease. Some patients find it difficult to ambulate with this cast, especially if they have a prosthesis on the contralateral limb or severe obesity.

In diabetic patients with peripheral vascular disease, cessation of smoking, increased exercise, blood pressure reduction, improved lipid control, and weight loss should be advocated to reduce known cardiovascular risk factors. Since most of these patients already have autosympathectomy, surgical sympathectomy to improve limb perfusion is rarely a consideration. In situ bypass surgery should be considered in the patient with claudication, rest pain, ischemic ulcers, and gangrene. Diabetes itself is not a contraindication to surgery, and graft patency does not differ significantly between diabetic and nondiabetic individuals. In patients with purely ischemic

necrosis, amputation of a toe is usually deferred until revascularization has been performed. This may allow complete salvage of the foot or limit the level of amputation. Prophylactic surgery can play an important role in patients with areas of high foot pressure and ulceration that have not responded to traditional or conservative therapy. In these patients there is often too much bone and too little skin. Therefore, a combination of surgery and shoe modification is better than either one alone. Before any prophylactic surgery is attempted to correct anatomic deformities, the foot must be adequately vascularized to allow proper healing. In the presence of adequate blood supply, procedures such as sesamoidectomies and metatarsal head resections have demonstrated excellent success with minimal recurrence.

Treatment-Based Diabetic Foot Classification System

Appropriate care of the diabetic foot requires a clear descriptive assessment of risk that may be used to direct appropriate therapy and predict outcome. A diabetic foot classification system encompassing the major risk factors leading to amputation as well as all major neuropathic sequelae was introduced by Armstrong, Lavery, and Harkless in 1996. The classification system is divided into seven categories with the objective of reducing patients to the lowest foot risk category. Although numerous descriptive terms are given to define neuropathy and vascular disease clinically, the overall goal is to provide a common language and diagnostic-therapeutic approach for a multidisciplinary diabetic foot care team (Tables 3 and 4).

Diabetic Foot Category 0: Minimal Pathology Present

The patient in diabetic foot category 0 has intact sensation, no evidence of vascular disease, and no history of ulceration. Although this patient may have deformity present, the foot is "protected by pain." Treatment for diabetic foot category 0 includes thorough patient education, possible shoe gear accommodations if a deformity exists, and triannual visits to assess neurovascular status, dermal thermometry, and foci of stress.

Diabetic Foot Category 1: The Insensitive Foot

This patient has lost protective sensation and is therefore at higher risk for potential ulceration than is the patient in foot category 0. This patient has no history of previous pedal ulceration or neuropathic osteoarthopathy (Charcot's joint). Additionally, there is no apparent foot deformity present. Treatment for category 1 is the same as for category 0 plus possible in-shoe accommodation to reduce the magnitude of vertical and shear stress. Patients in category 1 may return every 2 to 3

Table 3 Classification of Diabetic Foot Ulcers

GRADE 0
Preulcerative lesion
  ± Cellulitis
  ±Vascular disease
GRADE 1
Superficial ulcer
  ± Cellulitis
  ± Vascular disease
GRADE 2
Deep ulcer—no tendon or bone involvement
  ± Cellulitis
  ± Vascular disease
GRADE 3
Deep ulcer—extending to tendon or bone
  ± Cellulitis
  ± Vascular disease
GRADE 4
Deep ulcer with gangrene
  ± Cellulitis
  ± Vascular disease

From Lavery LA, Armstrong DG, Harkless LB. Classification of diabetic foot wounds. J Foot Ankle Surg, 1996; (35) 35 (6):528–531.

---

months for general assessment, palliative care, and dermal thermometry. Because peak plantar pressures may increase with time under the neuropathic foot, patients in this category should receive yearly dynamic pressure analysis to evaluate trends in plantar stress.

Diabetic Foot Category 2: The Insensitive Foot with Deformity

This patient is identical to the category 1 patient but has the added risk factor of foot deformity. Treatment for this category includes those measures instituted in category 1 plus possible consultation with a prescription footwear specialist, such as a certified pedorthist or orthotist, for possible custom molded or extra depth shoe gear accommodation. If shoe gear accommodation is problematic, prophylactic surgery may be indicated to alleviate foci of stress.

Diabetic Foot Category 3: Demonstrated Pathology

This category is identical in nearly every respect to category 2. These patients are generally insensitive with deformity. However, foot category 3 patients present with a past history of pathology including ulceration and/or Charcot's arthropathy, clearly placing them at higher risk for ulceration and amputation. Treatment for this category is similar to that for category 2, but these patients may be seen more frequently as needed. Additionally, more aggressive shoe gear accommodation may be necessary to reduce the risk of pathology recurring.

Diabetic Foot Category 4: Insensitive Injury

The two major injuries stemming from injury to the insensitive foot, neuropathic ulceration and acute neuropathic osteoarthropathy (Charcot's joint), are subdivided in this foot risk category.

Category 4a: Neuropathic Ulceration. This category includes subjects with noninfected neuropathic ulcerations with no evidence of vascular insufficiency. Treatment for this category is the same as for category 3 with two additions. An off-weighting program (i.e., total contact casting) is instituted, and weekly to biweekly dressing change and debridement sessions are initiated as required.

Category 4b: Acute Charcot's Arthropathy. Category 4b incorporates the patient population diagnosed with acute neuropathic osteoarthropathy. We classify Charcot's arthropathy into two treatment-oriented phases based on radiographic, dermal thermographic, and clinical signs, acute and postacute. Treatment for this category includes prompt institution of an off-weighting program. If a grade 1A ulcer is present (using the University of Texas Wound Classification System, Table 5), treatment varies only in that more frequent cast changes may be required for inspection and debridement of the ulcer. Ulcers with deeper involvement may require further debridement; therefore total contact casting may be contraindicated. Upon quiescence of arthropathy, patients are gradually reintroduced to protected weight-bearing. Following return to prescription shoe gear, these patients are most appropriately classified in category 3.

Diabetic Foot Category 5: The Infected Diabetic Foot

Diabetic foot infection is often limb-threatening and occasionally life-threatening. Limb-threatening infections should be debrided and sepsis controlled before attempting revascularization, even in the most vascularly compromised extremity. If vascular compromise is present, a vascular consultation should be ordered concomitantly with prompt debridement of nonviable tissue. Following control of sepsis, the patient may be converted to the corresponding lower category.

Table 4 Treatment-Based Diabetic Foot Classification

Objectives of treatment are to convert patients to the lowest possible category. Prophylactic surgery is generally performed if foot cannot be safely accommodated in prescription shoe gear.

CATEGORY 0: MINIMAL PATHOLOGY PRESENT
Patient diagnosed with diabetes mellitus
Sensation intact (Semmes-Weinstein 5.07 wire detectable and/or VPT <25V)
ABI >0.80 and toe systolic pressure >45 mm Hg
Foot deformity may be present
No history of ulceration
Treatment for Category 0
Triannual visits to assess neurovascular status, dermal thermometry, and foci of stress
Possible shoe accommodations
Patient education

CATEGORY 1: THE NEUROPATHIC FOOT
Patient diagnosed with diabetes mellitus
Sensorium absent (Semmes-Weinstein 5.07 wire not detectable and/or VPT >25V)
ABI >0.80 and toe systolic pressure >45 mm Hg
No history of neuropathic ulceration
No history of diabetic neuropathic osteoarthropathy (Charcot's joint)
No foot deformity
Treatment for Category 1
Same as for category 0 plus:
 Possible shoe gear accommodation (pedorthist-orthotist consultation)
 Dermal thermometric monitoring every 2–3 months
 Yearly dynamic plantar pressure updates

CATEGORY 2: NEUROPATHY WITH FOOT DEFORMITY
Patient diagnosed with diabetes mellitus
Sensation absent
ABI >0.80 and toe systolic pressure >45 mm Hg
No history of neuropathic ulceration
No history of Charcot's joint
Foot deformity present (focus of stress)
Treatment for Category 2
Same as for category 1 plus:
 Pedorthist-orthotist consultation for possible custom molded-extra depth shoe accommodation
 Possible prophylactic surgery to alleviate focus of stress

CATEGORY 3: DEMONSTRATED PATHOLOGY
Patient diagnosed with diabetes mellitus
Sensation absent
ABI >0.80 and toe systolic pressure >45 mm Hg
History of neuropathic ulceration
History of Charcot's joint
Foot deformity present (focus of stress)
Treatment for Category 3
Same as for category 2 plus:
 Pedorthist-orthotist consultation for custom molded-extra depth shoe accommodation
 Possible prophylactic surgery to alleviate focus of stress
 More frequent visits may be indicated for monitoring

CATEGORY 4A: NEUROPATHIC ULCERATION
Patient diagnosed with diabetes mellitus
Sensation absent
ABI >0.80 and toe systolic pressure >45 mm Hg
Foot deformity normally present
Noninfected neuropathic ulceration
No acute diabetic neuropathic osteoarthropathy (Charcot's joint) present
Treatment for Category 4A
Same as for category 3 plus:
 Off-weighting program instituted: possible total contact cast
 Dressing change program instituted
 Debridement program instituted
 Weekly to biweekly visits as needed

CATEGORY 4B: ACUTE CHARCOT'S JOINT
Patient diagnosed with diabetes mellitus
Sensation absent
ABI >0.80 and toe systolic pressure >45 mm Hg
Noninfected neuropathic ulceration may be present
Diabetic neuropathic osteoarthropathy (Charcot's joint) present
Treatment for Category 4B
Same as for category 3 plus:
 Off-weighting program instituted: possible total contact cast
 Weekly to biweekly visits (as per contact casting regimen)
 Dermal thermometric and radiographic monitoring
 If ulcer is present, treatment same as for category 4a

CATEGORY 5: THE INFECTED DIABETIC FOOT
Patient diagnosed with diabetes mellitus
Sensation may or may not be intact (+/−)
Infected wound
Charcot's joint may be present
Treatment for Category 5
Same as for category 4 plus:
 Debridement of infected, necrotic tissue and/or bone
 Possible hospitalization
 Antibiosis
 Medical management
 Contact casting generally contraindicated until diabetic foot category drops to 4

CATEGORY 6: THE DYSVASCULAR FOOT
Patient diagnosed with diabetes mellitus
Sensation may or may not be intact
ABI <0.80 or toe systolic pressure <45 mm Hg or pedal transcutaneous oxygen tension <40 mm Hg
Ulceration may be present
Treatment for Category 6
Vascular consult, possible revascularization
If infection present, treatment same as for category 5; vascular consultation concomitant with control of sepsis
Contact casting generally contraindicated

VPT = gyibration; *ABI* = ankle brachial index.

Table 5 University of Texas Wound Classification System

	GRADE			
	0	**I**	**II**	**III**
A	Pre- or postulcerative lesion, completely epithelialized	Superficial wound, not involving tendon, capsule, or bone	Wound penetrating to tendon or capsule	Wound penetrating to bone or joint
B	Pre- or postulcerative lesion, completely epithelialized with infection	Superficial wound, not involving lesion, capsule, or bone, with infection	Wound penetrating to tendon or capsule, with infection	Wound penetrating to bone
C	Pre- or postulcerative lesion, completely epithelialized with ischemia	Superficial wound, not involving tendon, capsule, or bone, with ischemia	Wound penetrating to tendon or capsule, with ischemia	Wound penetrating to bone or joint, with ischemia
D	Pre- or postulcerative lesion, completely epithelialized with infection and ischemia	Superficial wound, not involving tendon, capsule, or bone, with infection and ischemia	Wound penetrating to tendon or capsule, with infection and ischemia	Wound penetrating to bone or joint, with infection and ischemia

Diabetic Foot Category 6: The Dysvascular Foot

Critical vascular compromise represents a direct threat to the patient's limb. For this reason, a prompt vascular surgery consultation is essential, followed by possible revascularization. If revascularization is successful, the patient is automatically converted to a corresponding lower category.

■ RECOMMENDATIONS

Care of the diabetic foot is not the purview of any one specialty. Routine collaboration with internists, endocrinologists, podiatrists, vascular surgeons, physiatrists, physical therapists, infectious disease specialists, and nurse-specialists is essential. All subspecialty groups have significantly different backgrounds but one common focus: prevention of diabetic foot ulceration and limb amputation. The diagnostic and therapeutic classification provided in this chapter provides a common language that allows effective communication among subspecialty groups.

Suggested Reading

Armstrong DG, Lavery LA, Harkless LB. Treatment-based classification system for assessment and care of diabetic feet. J Am Podiatr Med Assoc 1996; 86:311–316.

An efficient review of the treatment of the diabetic foot based upon a simple yet comprehensive classification of its status.

Bakker K, Nieuwenhuijzen Kruseman AC, eds. The diabetic foot. Amsterdam: Excerpta Medica, 1991.

A concise clinical overview of the diabetic foot, including a simple new proposed classification system.

Boulton AJM. The diabetic foot. Med Clin North Am 1988; 72:1513–1530.

A practical discussion of the diagnosis and management of diabetic foot problems.

Boulton AJM, Connor H, Cavanagh P, eds. The foot in diabetes. 2nd ed. Chichester, UK: John Wiley, 1994.

An updated practical guide to the evaluation and management of diabetic foot problems by the leading authorities in their subject area.

Connor H, Boulton AJM, Ward JD, eds. The foot in diabetes. Chichester, UK: John Wiley, 1987.

A very practical guide to the etiology, diagnosis, and management of diabetic foot problems, including a chapter on establishing a combined foot clinic.

Flynn MD, Tooke JE. Aetiology of diabetic foot ulceration: A role for microcirculation? Diabetic Med 1992; 320–329.

Further contributions to the ongoing debate on the importance of microvascular disease in diabetic foot ulceration.

Frykberg R, ed. The high risk foot in diabetes. New York: Churchill Livingstone, 1991.

A comprehensive, up-to-date textbook on diabetic foot problems.

Lavery LA, Armstrong DG, Harkless LB. Classification of diabetic foot wounds. J Foot Ankle Surg, 1996; (35)35 (6):528–531.

Litzelman DK, et al. Reduction of lower extremity clinical abnormalities in patients with noninsulin dependent diabetes mellitus. Ann Intern Med 1993; 119:36–41.

Selby JV, Hang D. Risk factors for lower extremity amputation in persons with diabetes. Diabetes Care 1995; 18:509–516.

Excellent summary of the major etiologic factors responsible for the diabetic foot.

HYPERTENSION IN PATIENTS WITH DIABETES

Norman M. Kaplan, M.D.

This chapter considers treatment of hypertension in patients with diabetes. In view of the extensive coverage of diabetic nephropathy elsewhere in the text, I do not go into detail about the management of this major hypertension-related complication of diabetes.

Hypertension is both more common in patients with diabetes and more dangerous. Hypertension and diabetes coexist more frequently than would be expected by chance alone. Although many studies of the prevalence of the two conditions suffer from multiple biases, the majority indicate that hypertension is more common among diabetic patients and that diabetes is more common among hypertensive patients than would be predicted based on the prevalence of the other condition.

Not only is the prevalence of overt hypertension increased among patients with diabetes, but even those who are normotensive by routine office sphygmomanometry may have high readings recorded by ambulatory monitoring both during the day but particularly at night. When 24-hour ambulatory monitoring was performed on 25 insulin-dependent diabetics and 21 healthy normotensive subjects of similar age and gender, the casual office blood pressures in the two groups differed little, averaging 128/74 in the diabetic patients and 122/73 in the nondiabetic patients. However, the diabetic patients had distinctly higher readings by ambulatory monitoring during the daytime and even more so during the night (Fig. 1). Such higher nocturnal readings have been correlated with the presence of more advanced cardiac and retinal damage. Therefore, diabetic patients may be more vulnerable to hypertensive complications than their casual blood pressures would suggest.

The dangers of coexisting diabetes and hypertension are reflected in the higher rates of morbidity and mortality from hypertension-related cardiovascular diseases described in prior chapters in this book. The leading causes of premature mortality in patients with diabetes, coronary disease, stroke, and nephropathy are directly induced by hypertension. The more effective control of hypertension—the objective of this chapter—is one of the few measures that are of proved benefit in slowing the progress of the degenerative complications of diabetes.

■ LIFE-STYLE MODIFICATIONS

The foundation for the treatment of hypertension in patients with diabetes is the modification of harmful life-styles: smoking; excessive intake of calories, saturated fat, sodium, and alcohol; insufficient amounts of exercise and dietary potassium (Table 1). Vigorous pursuit of an improved life-style provides relief not only of hypertension but also of many concomitant risk factors commonly found in diabetic subjects. As noted earlier, weight loss and exercise may literally cure non–insulin-dependent diabetes. The benefits of life-style modification relative to hypertension may be less dramatic, but they should never be forsaken in the rush toward active drug therapy.

Smoking

As one of the major three risk factors for premature cardiovascular disease, smoking is often the hardest to overcome, but once overcome, its cessation is followed by the greatest immediate benefit to cardiovascular health. Therefore, the first move in managing a smoker is to demand that smoking be stopped while offering all the help available to do so. The more severe the diabetes and the hypertension, the greater is the need for immediate cessation of smoking. Although smoking has been shown to be directly associated with microalbuminuria and glomerular hyperfiltration in young insulin-dependent diabetic patients, the threat is far greater for coronary ischemia.

Smokers should be identified and given as much support as possible to quit. As documented in a series of papers in the December 11, 1991 issue of the *Journal of the American Medical Association,* fewer than one-half of U.S. physicians bother to ask their patients if they smoke and fewer than 4 percent of smokers who successfully quit identify a physician as a source of help in their having done so. The pernicious enticement of young children by cigarette advertising directly aimed at them (e.g., Old Joe the Camel) must be countered by equally aggressive campaigns to keep children from starting to smoke. The tobacco companies' need to replenish the stock of 500,000 smokers who die prematurely each year because of their smoking must be met head on by health care providers. Those who treat young diabetic patients must be particularly sensitive and aggressive about the problem.

Numerous aids are available to help patients quit smoking. In particular, the use of nicotine patches has been shown to more than double the number of successful quitters. In the process of quitting, patients need all the psychological support they can get. In addition, they should be helped to overcome the tendency to gain weight that accompanies the withdrawal of nicotine-induced thermogenesis. Such weight gain may interfere with control of both blood pressure and diabetes and can best be countered by increased physical activity.

Weight Reduction

Almost all non–insulin-dependent diabetic patients are overweight. Their obesity plays a major contributing role in the development of hypertension in these patients. Weight loss, by whatever means, will often help reverse both the diabetes and the hypertension, along with the dyslipidemias that usually accompany the other two conditions. The multiple benefits of weight reduction were nicely documented when 80 obese patients with significant glucose intolerance were followed for 55 weeks on a lower calorie–increased exercise regimen. As shown in Table 2, the overall impact of an average weight loss of only 6.8 kg was quite dramatic.

The manner by which weight is lost may be relevant, particularly in the presence of diabetes. A very low calorie diet (e.g., 400 to 800 calories per day) has been recommended for more rapid and greater weight loss, but the improved glycemic control that accompanies use of a very low calorie diet has been related to increased insulin secretion, an effect that may not be desired. The additional rise in insulin could reflect the relatively high carbohydrate content of a diet that is markedly restricted in fat content in order to achieve such a low calorie level.

On the other hand, increased consumption of saturated fat was associated with higher fasting insulin concentrations in a cross-sectional study of 215 nondiabetic men with angiographically proved coronary artery disease. This relation was independent of body weight and the pattern of fat distribution. Therefore, the most effective way to reduce calories in obese diabetics with hypertension may be with a diet more modestly reduced in calories, following the "prudent diet" proportions of 20 to 30 percent of calories from fat and 50 percent of calories from complex carbohydrates.

Physical Activity

Weight loss can rarely be achieved by diet alone without concomitant increased physical activity. Such exercise will almost certainly improve glycemic control, reduce insulin resistance, and lower blood pressure while also improving the blood lipid profile—effects that may be independent of weight loss but that certainly complement and enhance it. Most con-

trolled studies have shown that reductions of blood pressure and increased sensitivity to insulin are both immediate and persistent for days after the exercise. These short-and long-term effects may reflect the decrease in sympathetic nervous system activity that has been shown to accompany repetitive aerobic (isotonic) exercise. On the other hand, isometric (body building) exercise most likely has little if any beneficial effect on either blood pressure or diabetic control.

There may be a threshold for the beneficial effects of aerobic exercise. For example, bicycling 40 minutes three times a week has been shown to lead to the same fall in blood pressure as bicycling seven times a week, with a greater increase in insulin sensitivity (Jennings, 1986).

Those patients who need antihypertensive drugs may have some difficulty in performing exercise: diuretic-induced hypokalemia may reduce muscle blood flow; beta-blockers may reduce exercise ability by limiting the needed increase in cardiac output. To obtain the desired blunting of the usual rise in blood pressure during exercise but avoid interference with exercise ability, the use of either alpha-blockers or calcium entry blockers may be preferable.

Sodium Restriction

Most diets reduced in calories are also lower in sodium content, and some find that the fall in blood pressure with weight loss is related more to the decrease in sodium than the decrease in weight. However, the two are almost certainly independently capable of lowering blood pressure, and their effects are additive.

Despite the preachings of some contrarians, evidence for a significant effect of only modestly reduced sodium intake is consistent and considerable. A review of 78 controlled trials found that those patients who reduced daily sodium intake by 50 mmol for 5 weeks or longer had an average fall in systolic blood pressure of 7 mm Hg, the fall tending to be greater in elderly patients with higher levels of blood pressure (Law, 1991). Restrictions of 100 mmol per day provided an average fall in blood pressure of 10 mm Hg.

Table 1 Life-Style Modifications for Patients with Hypertension
Stop smoking for overall cardiovascular health
Lose weight, particularly for upper body obesity
Reduce sodium intake to less than 100 mmol/day
(2.5 g sodium or 6 g sodium chloride)
Moderate alcohol intake (no more than 2 usual portions/day)
Exercise (isotonic) regularly
Maintain adequate potassium, calcium, and magnesium intake

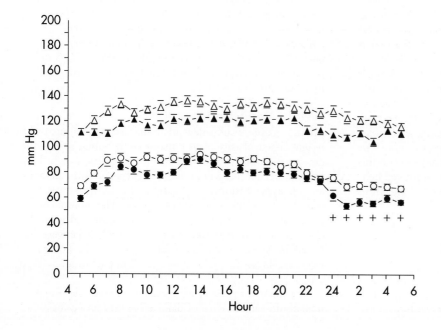

Figure 1
Hourly comparison of systolic (*triangles*) and diastolic (*circles*) blood pressure in subjects with (*open symbols*) and without (*solid symbols*) insulin-dependent diabetes mellitus. Values are mean ± standard deviation. P <0.05 between groups. (*From Wiegmann TB, Herron KG, Chonko AM, et al. Recognition of hypertension and abnormal blood pressure burden with ambulatory blood pressure recordings in type 1 diabetes mellitus. Diabetes 1990; 39:1556–1560; with permission.*)

Almost all patients can easily reduce their sodium intake by 50 mmol per day, considering that the average sodium content of the U.S. diet is around 175 mmol per day. Because almost 80 percent of the sodium in the U.S. diet is added in the processing of canned and other prepared foods the simplest way to achieve a modest decrease in sodium intake is to substitute natural foods (all low in sodium, most high in potassium) for processed foods (most high in sodium and lower in potassium). The new requirements for food labeling promulgated in early 1993 have made it much easier for the average consumer to avoid hidden salt mines (e.g., tomato juice, with 30 mmol per 6 oz) and to choose foods much lower in sodium content (e.g., orange juice, with less than 1 mmol per 6 oz).

There is absolutely no potential danger from a moderately restricted sodium intake. Those who raise the specter of impaired growth and hypotensive crises with heat stress in rats given virtually no dietary sodium are purposely invoking irrelevant basic research to obfuscate the management of a major clinical problem. The proved benefits of moderate sodium restriction are particularly beneficial to diabetic hypertensive patients because sodium retention almost certainly plays a major role in the pathogenesis of hypertension. The central role of sodium in the hypertension seen in diabetic patients most likely reflects the sodium-retaining effect of the hyperinsulinemia present in all diabetic patients, as well as the initial hyperfiltration and later glomerulosclerosis common in such patients.

The beneficial effects of moderate sodium restriction in non–insulin-dependent diabetic hypertensive patients was documented in a randomized, controlled 3-month study involving 34 elderly patients (mean age 62) (Table 3). Note that a mean reduction of 60 mmol per day of sodium effected a significant reduction of both supine and standing systolic pressures.

Potassium Supplements

A majority of studies show a significant antihypertensive effect, averaging about 5 mm Hg, with potassium supplements of 40 to 80 mmol per day. However, such large doses of potassium supplements cost too much and may cause considerable gastric distress. Far better would be the substitution of high-potassium natural foods for low-potassium processed foods, which can easily add 40 or more mmol per day to the diet.

Once hypokalemia is noted, usually from diuretic use, correction of the deficit will almost certainly require potassium supplements. By that means, the blood pressure may come down and the disturbed glucose tolerance frequently noted in diuretic-induced hypokalemia will most likely improve.

Caution is needed in giving potassium supplements to diabetic patients with renal damage. Some may have had enough loss of juxtaglomerular cell function to become hyporeninemic and thereby unable to secrete aldosterone. The majority of those with hyporeninemic hypoaldosteronism are elderly diabetic patients with mild renal insufficiency.

Moderation of Alcohol

Either too much or too little alcohol may be harmful. Alcohol abusers suffer multiple consequences, including a rise in

---

Table 2 Effects of Weight Reduction in Obese Patients with Impaired Glucose Tolerance

	INITIAL	END OF 55 WEEKS
Body weight (kg)	81.3	74.5
Fasting blood glucose (mmol)	6.3	5.9
Glucose at 2 hr of OGTT (mmol)	11.2	10.6*
Fasting serum insulin (PM)	101	68
Insulin at 1 hr of OGTT	524	291
Blood pressure (mm Hg)	140/80	120/65
Triglycerides (mg/dL)	151	116
Cholesterol:HDL cholesterol ratio	4.8	4.5

From Calle-Pascual AL, Rodriguez C, Martin-Alvarez PJ, et al. Effect of weight loss on insulin sensitivity and cardiovascular risk factors in glucose tolerant obese subjects. Diabetes Metab 1991; 17:404–409; with permission.
OGTT = oral glucose tolerance test; *HDL* = high-density lipoprotein.
*Performed at week 35.

Table 3 Sodium Restriction in Hypertensive Non–Insulin-Dependent Diabetic Patients

	CONTROL		SODIUM RESTRICTION	
	START	3 MO	START	3 MO
Urine sodium (mmol/24 hr)	183	181	199	137
Body weight (kg)	80	81	77	77
Supine blood pressure (mm Hg)	174/92	168/90	180/91	160/88
Standing blood pressure (mm Hg)	176/101	166/95	182/95	160/92
Glycosylated hemoglobin (%)	10.4	10.9	10.2	10.0

From Dodson PM, Beevers M, Hallworth R, et al. Sodium restriction and blood pressure in hypertensive type 2 diabetics: Randomised, blind, controlled, and crossover studies of moderate sodium restriction and sodium supplementation. BMJ 1989; 298:227–230; with permission.

blood pressure that is responsible for perhaps 10 percent of the hypertension seen in men. Diabetic patients are certainly not immune to alcohol abuse and may suffer even more from some of the metabolic mischief it induces, including interference with hepatic gluconeogenesis, hypertriglyceridemia from the increased secretion of very–low-density lipoprotein (VLDL), and pancreatic damage.

On the other hand, multiple studies have shown an impressive protection against coronary disease by regular intake of $\frac{1}{2}$ to 2 drinks per day. The protection provided by small amounts of ethanol most likely reflects a stimulation of high-density lipoprotein (HDL) cholesterol synthesis, the antithesis of the acute rise in VLDL seen with alcohol abuse.

There is no reason that diabetic hypertensive patients should not share in the benefits of regular consumption of from $\frac{1}{2}$ to as much as 2 drinks per day, and in view of their increased risk of coronary disease, there is good reason that they should. The number of calories, averaging 150 per drink, can be subtracted from the daily allowance of carbohydrates. There should be no aggravation of hypertension or diabetes by such a moderate amount of alcohol, so the potential benefit clearly outweighs the possible risks.

Other Dietary Factors

Fish oils have been found to have a slight but fairly consistent effect on blood pressure both in diabetic and nondiabetic hypertensive patients (Table 4). In the insulin-dependent diabetic patients studied by Jensen et al, lipid levels improved and glycemic control was unchanged. However, in studies by Kasim et al and other investigators, lipid and glucose levels were seen to deteriorate. Therefore, fish oil supplements should not be given to diabetic hypertensive patients, particularly since a few portions of fish per week will most likely provide all of the beneficial effects on cardiovascular health that the fish oil supplements provide.

Increased amounts of fiber have been found to lower the blood pressure and increase glycemic control in diabetic hypertensive patients by some investigators but not by others. As an example of the positive data, a high-fiber, low-fat, and low-sodium diet was given to 25 such patients while another

---

Table 4 Trials of Fish Oil on Blood Pressure in Hypertension and Diabetes

| | | | | BP (MM HG) | | CHANGE IN PLASMA LIPIDS (MM) | | |
REFERENCE	PATIENTS (N)	DAILY OF ω-3 FATTY ACID (G)	TIME OF STUDY (WEEKS)	BEFORE	AFTER	TOTAL CHOLESTEROL	HDL CHOLESTEROL	TRIGLYCERIDES
Knapp and Fitzgerald, 1989[1]	32 HT	15.0	4	134/94	132/90			
Bønaa et al, 1992[2]	78 HT	6.0	10	145/95	140/92			
Kasim et al, 1988[3]	22 DM	2.7	8	143/85	129/80	−0.03	−0.5	−0.11
Jensen et al, 1989[4]	18 DM	4.6	8	146/90	139/85	+0.07	+0.14	−0.12

From Tjoa HI, Kaplan NM. Nonpharmacological treatment of hypertension in diabetes mellitus. Diabetes Care 1991; 14:449–460; with permission.
[1]Knapp HR, FitzGerald GA. The antihypertensive effects of fish oil. A controlled study of polyunsaturated acid supplements in essential hypertension. N Engl J Med 1989; 320:1037–1043.
[2]Bønaa KH, Bjerve KS, Straume B, Gram IT, Thelle D. Effects of eicosapentaenoic and docosahexaenoic acids on blood pressure in hypertension. A population-based intervention trial from the Tromsø Study. N Engl J Med 1990; 322:795–801.
[3]Kasim SE, Stern B, Khilnani S, McLin P, Baciorowski S, Jen K-LC. Effects of ω-3 fish oils on lipid metabolism, glycemic control, and blood pressure in type 2 diabetic patients. J Clin Endocrinol Metab 1988; 67:1.
[4]Jensen T, Stender S, Goldstein K, Holmer G, Deckert T. Partial normalization by dietary cod-liver oil of increased microvascular albumin leakage in patients with insulin dependent diabetes and albuminuria. N Engl J Med 1989; 321:1572–1577.
BP = blood pressure; *DM* = diabetic; *HDL* = high density lipoprotein; *HT* = hypertensive.

Table 5 Changes After 3 Months of Therapy with Diuretic or Diet, Each Given to 25 Diabetic Hypertensive Patients

	WEIGHT (KG)	BLOOD PRESSURE (MM HG)	TOTAL CHOLESTEROL (MG/DL)	HIGH-DENSITY LIPOPROTEIN CHOLESTEROL (MG/DL)	GLYCOSYLATED HEMOGLOBIN (%)
DIURETIC					
Bendrofluazide (10 mg)	−1.6	−20.9/-6.4	+8	+4	+0.9
DIET					
High fiber (30–45 g), low fat (15%), low sodium (40–50 mmol)	−2.9	−15.5/-8.6	−4	+8	−1.6

From data reported by Pacy PJ, Dodson PM, Kubicki AJ, et al. Comparison of the hypotensive and metabolic effects of bendrofluazide therapy and a high fiber, low fat, low sodium diet in diabetic patients with mild hypertension. J Hypertens 1984; 2:215–220; with permission.

25 diabetic hypertensive patients were treated with a rather large dose of a thiazide diuretic (Table 5). The multiple benefits of the diet versus the deleterious effects of the high dose of diuretic are obvious. The persistent antihypertensive effect of a similar diet was noted over a 4-year follow-up period in 19 of 32 nondiabetic patients with primary hypertension.

Calcium supplements have been claimed to lower blood pressure in nondiabetic hypertensive patients but in meta-analyses of all the controlled trials, the effect has been unimpressive: about a 2 mm Hg fall in systolic pressure and no fall in diastolic pressure.

Magnesium supplements have been studied much less vigorously than potassium, but the majority of data show no effect on blood pressure in nondiabetic hypertensive patients.

Garlic and onions have been touted in the nonmedical literature and by a few health gurus. There are a few properly controlled studies in the literature of the benefits of garlic but none of onions.

Relaxation

Most patients experience a fall in blood pressure while relaxed and even more so while asleep. However, the majority of properly controlled studies show no lasting benefit from any type of relaxation therapy.

Comments

When all the evidence about the value of life-style modification—usually referred to as "nondrug therapy"—is considered, it adds up to a most impressive body of data strongly documenting its beneficial effects on lowering blood pressure and improving glycemic control. In practice, such maneuvers are much less successful than what would be expected from controlled clinical trials. The inability or unwillingness of patients to respond to them is usually given as the reason, but physician nonacceptance is most likely as important.

Physicians often do not have confidence in either the potency of life-style modifications or the ability of their patients to follow them. Therefore, they mention them as an aside and rush to more powerful drug therapies before giving them a chance. With a busy practice, the time and energy required to instruct, motivate, and follow patients so that they will make meaningful modifications in life-style seems to be much less cost-effective than antihypertensive and antidiabetic drugs. However, the use of such drugs as initial therapy before life-style modifications have been given an adequate chance almost certainly reduces the patient's already borderline motivation to adopt the changes in life-style. Why bother to lose weight, exercise more, or modify alcohol intake when a pill or two a day will lower the blood pressure and the levels of lipid and glucose?

The entire medical care system often works against the success of life-style modifications before and instead of drug therapy. Third party payers provide the physician with the same amount of money for an office visit for the diagnoses of hypertension and diabetes if that visit takes 3 minutes or 30 minutes. Most will not pay for the services of dieticians and other professionals who can relieve the physician and often do an even better job of instructing and following the patient.

We must recognize the value of life-style modifications, not only for managing hypertension and diabetes but also for reducing the high-risk status of many patients for premature cardiovascular disease.

■ DRUG THERAPY

Once the decision has been made to use drugs to treat hypertension, the coexistence of diabetes should have a major impact upon the manner in which these drugs are used. In the not-so-distant past, diabetic hypertensive and nondiabetic hypertensive patients were treated just alike. Although such therapy may have protected them both from stroke morbidity and mortality, it was most likely not as protective against coronary disease and renal disease for the diabetic patient as was expected from the degree of blood pressure reduction achieved. Unfortunately, there are no large-scale clinical trials of the effect of antihypertensive therapy upon morbidity and mortality in diabetic hypertensive patients.

In the absence of data from controlled trials, we cannot be sure that diabetic hypertensive patients will do better by the modifications in the traditional diuretic-first, step-care approach that will be described. The argument has been made that because stroke morbidity and mortality have *only* been shown to be improved by therapies based on diuretics and beta-blockers (the only agents that have been tested), these agents should continue to be the choice for initial therapy unless there are clear contraindications to their use, particularly since they are so much cheaper than the newer agents.

Table 6 Hypertension and Diabetics: A Therapeutic Challenge

THE PROBLEMS	THE SOLUTIONS
The two coexist more than by chance alone.	To minimize interference with treatment of hypertension:
The therapy of diabetes may interfere with the treatment of hypertension.	Encourage weight loss and exercise.
Hyperinsulinemia may raise blood pressure.	Give least possible doses of insulin.
Hypoglycemia will cause acute hypertension.	Use metformin or troglitazone in place of insulin/oral
The therapy of hypertension may interfere with the treatment of diabetes.	hypoglycemics.
Diuretics and beta-blockers worsen insulin resistance and glucose	To minimize interference with therapy of diabetes:
tolerance.	Minimize use of diuretics and beta-blockers.
Diuretic-induced hypokalemia may worsen glucose tolerance.	Avoid and correct hypokalemia.
Beta-blockers mask and prolong insulin-induced hypoglycemia.	Reduce blood pressure slowly and gently.
Postural hypotension and impotence may be precipitated by antihypertensive drugs.	Use vasodilatory agents, particularly those shown to
Absorption of insulin may be influenced by different drugs.	improve insulin sensitivity.

Diabetes, per se, is not a clear contraindication to the use of either diuretics or beta-blockers. However, the many challenges to the therapy of hypertension in diabetic patients that are associated with diuretic and beta-blocker therapy lead me among others to recommend a different approach (Table 6).

The validity of this different approach may not ever be proved by proper large-scale clinical trials comparing older to newer therapies. Rather, we may have to depend upon surrogate end points such as protection against the progression of renal damage, congestive heart failure, and carotid atherosclerosis, which are being examined in large groups of hypertensive patients, including those with diabetes.

Problems with Diuretics and Beta-Blockers

As noted before, all of the data now available concerning the effect of antihypertensive therapy on morbidity and mortality have been obtained with diuretics as initial therapy (except in half of the drug-treated patients in the Medical Research Council trial, who received a beta-blocker first). In most of these trials, a beta-blocker was the second drug and a direct vasodilator the third. In the nine trials involving middle-aged patients with mild to moderate degrees of hypertension (i.e., diastolic blood pressures from 90 to 115 mm Hg), the mortality from strokes was reduced by 38 percent but mortality from coronary disease by only 8 percent. However, better coronary protection was seen in the three

more recent trials in the elderly, perhaps because much lower doses of diuretics were used.

Among many possible explanations for the lesser effect upon coronary disease, one stands out: unintended and usually unrecognized metabolic side effects (i.e., hypokalemia, insulin resistance, glucose intolerance, and dyslipidemia). These adverse metabolic effects obviously could worsen coronary risk, ablating much of the benefit provided by the reduction in blood pressure. The development of these adverse effects may reflect the use of what are now known to be excessively large doses of diuretics and, to a lesser degree, the use of noncardioselective beta-blockers.

The majority of the patients in these trials received the equivalent of 50 to 100 mg per day of hydrochlorothiazide. As shown in a controlled trial in which groups of about 50 hypertensive patients each received either a placebo or progressively larger doses of bendrofluazide, the use of 1.25 mg per day (equivalent to about 12.5 mg of hydrochlorothiazide) provided the full antihypertensive effect of the 10 mg dose but with none of the attendant metabolic adverse effects (Table 7). In other words, diuretics, given in appropriately lower doses than they are being used in the present, may be safer than they seemed to be in the past.

However, diuretics in relatively high doses, as they have commonly been used, may pose additional problems for diabetic hypertensive patients. Testimony comes from a retro-

Table 7 Effect of Varying Doses of the Diuretic Bendrofluazide

DOSE (MG/DAY):	0	1.25	2.5	5.0	10.0
Change after 10 weeks					
Blood pressure (mm Hg)	−3/3	−13/10	−14/11	−13/10	−17/11
Potassium (mmol/L)	+0.9	−0.16	−0.20	−0.33	−0.45
Glucose (μmol/L)	−.08	−0.19	0.14	0.04	0.27
Cholesterol	−0.6	−0.3	.00	0.12	0.25

From Carlsen JE, Kober L, Torp-Pedersen C, Johansen P. Relation between dose of bendrofluazide, antihypertensive effect, and adverse biochemical effects. BMJ 1990; 300:975–978; with permission.

Table 8 Mortality and Cardiovascular Risk Factors According to Type of Antihypertensive Treatment at First Annual Follow-Up Visit

			HYPERTENSION TREATED WITH		
	NORMAL BLOOD PRESSURE	UNTREATED HYPERTENSION	OTHER AGENTS	DIURETICS ONLY	BOTH
PROTEINURIA ABSENT					
N	264	81	59	53	39
Mortality per 1,000 person-years					
Cardiovascular disease	18	30	28	66	31
All	29	41	39	78	39
Blood pressure with treatment, mm Hg*	137/79	155/92	155/87	151/82	160/90
PROTEINURIA PRESENT					
N	90	60	34	36	43
Mortality per 1,000 person-years					
Cardiovascular disease	21	27	82	186	107
All	35	64	133	261	187
Blood pressure with treatment, mm Hg*	144/80	159/94	165/89	156/85	163/90

From Warram JH, Laffel LMB, Valsania P, et al. Excess mortality associated with diuretic therapy in diabetes mellitus. Arch Intern Med 1991; 151:1350–1356; with permission.
*Average of the blood pressures recorded at entry to the study and at the first and second annual follow-up examinations.

spective analysis of the mortality experience among 759 diabetic patients treated at the Joslin Clinic between 1972 and 1979 over a 4.5-year median follow-up period. Most of these patients were on insulin and their mean duration of diabetes was 18 years. Mortality from cardiovascular disease and from all causes was analyzed separately for those with or without 1+ or more proteinuria by dipstick on a random urine sample (Table 8). Those who were given only diuretics for treatment of hypertension had significantly higher mortality rates than those treated with other agents, even though the diuretic-treated group had the lowest blood pressure of the treated patients. The diuretic-treated groups were not afflicted with increased degrees of other cardiovascular risk factors, and the authors of this study could find no cause beyond the provision of diuretics to explain their findings. They conclude that "there is urgent need to reconsider the continued usage of diuretics in this population."

Potential Advantages of Other Agents

Three classes of vasodilating drugs—alpha-blockers, angiotensin converting enzyme (ACE) inhibitors, and calcium entry blockers (CEBs)—can be used as initial or subsequent therapy in place of either diuretics or beta-blockers. Each class offers special benefits and problems for diabetic hypertensive patients (Table 9).

The use of beta-blockers in insulin-dependent diabetic hypertensive patients produces another set of potential problems beyond their adverse effects on lipids and insulin sensitivity, namely their masking of the symptoms of hypoglycemia (except for sweating) and delaying the return of the blood glucose toward normal. Unless they are specifically needed for management of other conditions, beta-blockers should not be used in diabetic patients.

One particular effect of these various classes of antihypertensive drugs that may have particular relevance for diabetic hypertensive patients is their effect on insulin sensitivity. Results of a systematic study of the effects of various antihypertensive drugs on insulin sensitivity as measured by the euglycemic insulin clamp in different groups of nondiabetic hypertensive patients are shown in Figure 2. With all four beta-blockers and hydrochlorothiazide, insulin sensitivity was reduced, whereas with the ACE inhibitor captopril and the two alpha-blockers, insulin sensitivity was improved.

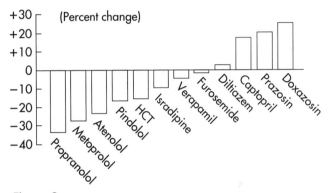

Figure 2

Percent of change in insulin sensitivity as measured by the euglycemic hyperinsulinemia clamp procedure in variable numbers of hypertensive patients given the single antihypertensive agents as indicated for 3- to 6-month intervals. *(Data from Lithell HOL. Effect of antihypertensive drugs on insulin, glucose, and lipid metabolism. Diabetes Care 1991; 14:203–209; with permission.)*

Table 9 Antihypertensive Drugs in Patients with Diabetes

CLASS	BENEFIT	PROBLEMS
Diuretics	Overcome volume expansion	Increase insulin resistance
		Worsen glucose tolerance
	Enhance efficacy of other drugs	Raise serum cholesterol
		Impotence
Beta-blockers	Treat coronary artery disease	Increase insulin resistance
		Mask and prolong hypoglycemia
		Raise serum triglycerides
		Lower HDL cholesterol
		Interfere with exercise ability
Central alpha-agonists	Lipid, glucose neutral	Sedation
Alpha-blockers	Improve lipids and insulin resistance	Postural hypotension
	Relieve prostatism	
ACE inhibitors	Renal protection	Cough
	Lipid, glucose neutral or positive	Hyperkalemia
Calcium blockers	Lipid, glucose neutral	Constipation (verapamil)
	Treat coronary disease	Conduction disturbances
	Renal protection (?)	(verapamil, diltiazem)
		Pedal edema (dihydropyridine)
Direct vasodilators	Effective with renal insufficiency	Reflex sympathetic activation
		No regression of left
	Lipid, glucose neutral	ventricular hypertrophy
		Reactive volume retention

HDL = high-density lipoprotein; *ACE* = angiotensin converting enzyme.

Table 10 Concurrent Medical Conditions in Diabetic Patients That May Influence Choice of Antihypertensive Drug Selection

CONDITION	DRUGS OF CHOICE	DRUGS TO AVOID
CARDIAC		
Coronary heart disease	ACE inhibitor, calcium channel blockers, cardioselective β-blocker; diuretic	None
Heart failure	ACE inhibitor, diuretic, vasodilator	β-blocker, calcium channel blocker
Left ventricular hypertrophy	ACE inhibitor, α-blocker, cardioselective β-blocker	Hydralazine
METABOLIC		
Frequent hypoglycemia	ACE inhibitor, calcium channel blocker	β-blocker
Hyperlipidemia	ACE inhibitor, α-blocker, calcium channel blocker	β-blocker, diuretic
Hypoaldosteronism	Calcium channel blocker, α-blocker	ACE inhibitor, β-blocker, potassium-sparing diuretic
NEUROPATHIC		
Impotence	ACE inhibitor, α-blocker channel blocker, vasodilator inhibitor, diuretic	β-blocker, central or peripheral adrenergic
Orthostatic hypotension	ACE inhibitor, calcium channel blocker, vasodilator	α-blocker, central or peripheral adrenergic inhibitor
RENAL		
Nephropathy	ACE inhibitor, calcium channel blocker	None
VASCULAR		
Peripheral vascular disease	ACE inhibitor, α-blocker, calcium channel blocker	β-blocker

From Christlieb AR. Treatment selection considerations for the hypertensive diabetic patients. Arch Intern Med 1990; 150:1167–1174; with permission.

The explanation for these varying effects of different classes of drugs is not obvious. Those drugs that reduce blood flow to the muscles—diuretics and beta-blockers—reduce insulin sensitivity; two classes that increase blood flow to muscles—ACE inhibitors and alpha-blockers—increase insulin sensitivity. Before assuming that the changes in peripheral blood flow could explain the effects on insulin sensitivity recall that calcium entry blockers—also vasodilators—were largely neutral in their action.

Regardless of the explanation, these effects of antihypertensive drugs on insulin sensitivity may or may not make a clinical difference to their use in diabetic hypertensive patients. Nonetheless, in a manner similar to their differing effects on other cardiovascular risk factors, we should give high-risk patients all the help we can to reduce their cardiovascular risk status. Therefore, the use of vasodilatory agents will most likely continue to expand in the treatment of diabetic hypertensive patients.

Basis for the Choice of Therapy

The most logical way to choose the initial drug for therapy of hypertension in diabetic patients is to consider the concomitant conditions that are commonly seen in such patients and then choose from those drugs that favorably influence the most important of these conditions and avoid drugs that may make them worse (Table 10). Such an approach translates into much more use of ACE inhibitors, calcium entry blockers, and alpha-blockers and less use of diuretics and beta-blockers.

If the first choice does not work well or causes bothersome side effects, it should be stopped and a drug of another class substituted. If the first choice works only partially, additional drugs may be added in a step-wise manner. A low dose of a diuretic will often prove to be an appropriate choice for the second drug, but if the potential problems from diuretic use seem to outweigh the benefits, two or three nondiuretic drugs can certainly be chosen.

Non–insulin-dependent diabetic patients may be relatively resistant to antihypertensive drug therapy. In a cross-sectional study of 559 randomly selected hypertensive patients in Israel, increasing degrees of obesity, glucose intolerance, and hyperinsulinemia—characteristics typical of non–insulin-dependent diabetes—were associated with the need for larger numbers and doses of antihypertensive drugs (Modan, 1991).

Systolic Hypertension in the Elderly

Many elderly diabetic patients have isolated systolic hypertension. Until recently, there was no evidence that reducing systolic pressure would be helpful. However, the results of the Systolic Hypertension in the Elderly Program (SHEP), published in mid-1991, clearly document the significant benefits of antihypertensive therapy in a population whose mean age was 72 years and whose mean pretreatment blood pressure was 177/77 mm Hg. Of these subjects 10 percent had a history of diabetes, but they were almost all free of any limitation of activities of daily living. Therefore, the benefits of therapy seen in this fairly healthy older population might not be applicable to those afflicted with other chronic diseases. In particular, the presence of significant postural hypotension or coronary artery disease could make therapy more hazardous.

Goal of Therapy

Once drug therapy is begun, the desired goal of therapy should be ascertained. In most hypertensive populations, that goal should most likely be around 145/85 mm Hg. Thereby, the potential for inciting coronary ischemia by reducing perfusion pressures below the critical level needed to maintain myocardial blood flow—the J curve—should be avoided. Certainly this caution is advisable for those hypertensive patients with known coronary disease.

However, lower levels of pressure may be needed to protect hypertensives from the other two major threats they face: stroke and renal damage. There does not appear to be a J curve for either of these target organs, and lower pressures may protect them better. In particular, the progression of nephropathy in diabetic hypertensive patients may require considerably lower systemic pressures than typically provided, an issue discussed in earlier chapters in this book.

■ OTHER THERAPIES

Diabetic hypertensives may be helped by the availability of metformin. This agent increases insulin sensitivity and lowers plasma insulin levels in non–insulin-dependent diabetics. In short-term studies, its use has been accompanied by lowering of blood pressure and plasma cholesterol levels.

Since hyperinsulinemia may exert a direct prohypertensive effect, the least amounts of exogenous insulin needed to maintain glycemic control should be given.

Suggested Reading

Christlieb AR. Treatment selection considerations for the hypertensive diabetic patients. Arch Intern Med 1990; 150:1167–1174.

The most reasonable set of guidelines for treatment of hypertension in diabetic patients written by a life-long worker in this area.

Jennings G, Nelson L, Nestel P, et al. The effects of changes in physical activity on major cardiovascular risk factors, hemodynamics, sympathetic function, and glucose utilization in man: a controlled study of four levels of activity. Circulation 1986; 73:30–40.

Clear documentation of the multiple benefits of aerobic exercise.

Kaplan NM. Clinical hypertension. 6th ed. Baltimore, Md: Williams & Wilkins, 1994.

The author may be said to be biased, but others seem to agree that this is the best text on all aspects of clinical hypertension. Since written by one author, it is shorter but more complete than most multiauthored mega-texts.

Landin K, Tengborn L, Smith U. Treating insulin resistance in hypertension with metformin reduces both blood pressure and metabolic risk factors. J Intern Med 1991; 229:181–187.
One of the earliest demonstrations of the multiple benefits of metformin. Unfortunately, the lowering of blood pressure noted in this short-term study has not been reconfirmed in most longer studies.

Law MR, Frost CD, Wald NJ. III. Analysis of data from trials of salt reduction. BMJ 1991; 302:819–824.

This meta-analysis shows major antihypertensive effects from moderate sodium restriction. The analysis has been criticized for including numerous poorly controlled studies. Regardless, it documents the need for at least 6 weeks of observation for the antihypertensive effect to be seen.

Lithell HOL. Effect of antihypertensive drugs on insulin, glucose, and lipid metabolism. Diabetes Care 1991; 14:203–209.

A review of the author's extensive work on the effects of various antihypertensive drugs on insulin sensitivity and lipid metabolism.

Modan M, Almog S, Fuchs Z, et al. Obesity, glucose intolerance, hyperinsulinemia, and response to antihypertensive drugs. Hypertension 1991; 17:565–573.

A nicely conducted clinical study demonstrating the relative resistance of obese, glucose-intolerant, and insulin-resistant patients to antihypertensive drugs.

SHEP Cooperative Research Group. Prevention of stroke by antihypertensive drug treatment in older persons with isolated systolic hypertension: Final results of the Systolic Hypertension in the Elderly Program (SHEP). JAMA 1991; 265:3255–3264.

The landmark study of the treatment of systolic hypertension in the elderly, demonstrating even better protection over 3 to 4 years than seen in the trials of younger hypertensive patients.

Silagy CA, Neil AW. A meta-analysis of the effect of garlic on blood pressure. J Hypertens 1994; 12:463–468.

Garlic extract is widely used for many possible benefits. This review supports an antihypertensive effect in a small number of placebo-controlled trials.

Tjoa HI, Kaplan NM. Nonpharmacological treatment of hypertension in diabetes mellitus. Diabetes Care 1991; 14:449–460.

A nice review of the multiple benefits of various nonpharmacologic therapies in hypertensive diabetic patients.

Weidmann P, Ferrari P. Central role of sodium in hypertension in diabetic subjects. Diabetes Care 1991; 14:220–232.

A strong defense of the critical role of excess sodium intake and retention in the pathogenesis of hypertension in diabetic patients.

Wiegmann TB, Herron KG, Chonko AM, et al. Recognition of hypertension and abnormal blood pressure burden with ambulatory blood pressure recordings in type 1 diabetes mellitus. Diabetes 1990; 39:1556–1560.

One of the first demonstrations of the frequent presence of "nondipping" of the nighttime blood pressure in diabetic patients. The lack of dipping may reflect diabetic cardiomyopathy and appears to reflect greater risk status.

SKIN AND SUBCUTANEOUS TISSUES

Jean L. Bolognia, M.D.
Irwin Braverman, M.D.

This chapter discusses the wide range of diseases of the skin and subcutaneous tissue that are related to diabetes mellitus. In disorders such as necrobiosis lipoidica or disseminated granuloma annulare, it is not unusual for the cutaneous lesions to be the initial manifestation of the associated diabetes. In other words, there are specific skin diseases that when diagnosed should precipitate an investigation for the presence of diabetes, even when systemic symptoms are lacking. In contrast, patients with disorders such as bullosis diabeticorum or lipoatrophy are usually known to have diabetes. The range of skin diseases associated with diabetes is wide, but the number of available therapeutic options is somewhat limited. However, the treatments vary depending upon the type of cutaneous disorder; therefore, the therapy of each disorder will be discussed separately.

■ PATHOPHYSIOLOGY

For the majority of cutaneous lesions associated with diabetes mellitus, only a theoretical explanation exists, and it is usually based upon the pathophysiology that has been established in other organs such as the eye and the kidney. Microangiopathy of the dermal vessels is thought to play a primary role in the induction of lesions of necrobiosis lipoidica diabeticorum as well as diabetic dermopathy. The abnormal glycosylation of collagen fibers is most likely a factor in the pathophysiology of scleredema and the waxy skin associated with limited joint mobility. Insulin and related peptides may effect epidermal proliferation through growth factor receptors, resulting in acanthosis nigricans. The only clear-cut underlying mechanism is the hypertriglyceridemia that is responsible for the production of eruptive xanthomas.

■ WAXY SKIN AND STIFF JOINTS

Although both small and large joints can be affected by limited mobility, it is the skin of the hands that becomes thickened and waxy. It is relatively simple to demonstrate involvement of the small joints of the hands because the patient will be unable to appose the palmar surfaces of the hands (Fig. 1). Palpation is usually required however, to appreciate the skin involvement. The joint disease has been observed in up to 40 percent of young type 1 (insulin-dependent) diabetic patients, and one-third of those with moderate to severe joint stiffness have waxy, tight skin on the dorsae of the hands, especially the fingers.

The importance of recognizing these changes lies in their possible correlation with microvascular complications and the necessity of avoiding an incorrect diagnosis such as scleroderma. With regard to treatment, there has been one report of three patients whose skin thickness decreased after their diabetes was brought under better control through the use of an insulin pump. These patients also demonstrated a decrease in their percentage of hemoglobin A1. When evaluating potential therapies for waxy skin in the future, it is important to remember that the natural history of the disease is to progress for a few years and to stabilize by 7 years after its onset.

■ SCLEREDEMA

Scleredema should not be confused with scleroderma, the connective tissue disease. The former is usually asymptomatic and is characterized by induration of the shoulders, posterior neck, and upper back (Fig. 2). Less often, there is involvement of the face, abdomen, and proximal extremities, but the hands are typically spared. Palpation of the skin is usually required to diagnose scleredema, although areas of involvement can have a subtle peau d'orange appearance. Scleredema may be seen in up to 14 percent of patients with diabetes. In biopsy specimens one sees a thickened dermis as well as a deposition of acid mucopolysaccharides, primarily hyaluronic acid. Similar deposits of mucopolysaccharides can occur in the myocardium, skeletal muscle, or serosal surfaces, resulting in congestive heart failure, weakness, and pericarditis.

Patients with scleredema are divided into two major groups based on the presence or absence of diabetes mellitus. The form seen in patients without diabetes may be preceded by trauma or a streptococcal infection, and it can be of limited duration. Unfortunately, the form associated with diabetes is often permanent and is not influenced by the quality of control of the diabetes. Nor does it respond to local injections of insulin into the sites of involvement. Because increased amounts of hyaluronic acid have been demonstrated in areas of scleredema, intralesional injections of hyaluronidase also have been tried, but they have had no effect on the induration. In dermatology, intralesional corticosteroids are often tried in otherwise treatment-resistant diseases, but they also have proved to be an ineffective form of treatment. Lastly, the diabetes-associated form of scleredema may have superimposed erythema, but the erythema represents inflammation, not infection, and should not be mistaken for treatment-resistant cellulitis.

■ DIABETIC DERMOPATHY

Diabetic dermopathy is characterized by brown macules and patches found primarily on the extensor surface of the distal lower extremities (Fig. 3). Associated changes include atrophy and preceding erythema. Pretibial pigmented patches are observed in up to 50 percent of patients with diabetes, and their presence has been correlated with an increased risk of retinopathy (39 percent versus 7 percent in those without diabetic dermopathy). In attempt to explain these lesions Lithner showed that thermal trauma resulted in atrophic circumscribed skin lesions in 16 of 19 patients with diabetic dermopathy. In contrast, none of the controls (n = 25) and only 1 of 16 diabetic patients without dermopathy developed such lesions after thermal trauma. There is no known effective treatment for diabetic dermopathy, and the degree of glycemic control has no effect on disease activity.

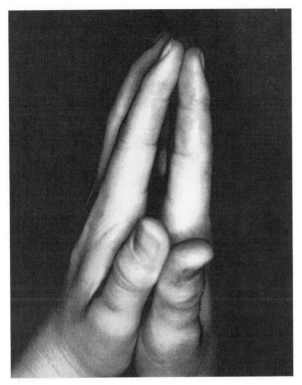

Figure 1
In a patient with stiff joints and waxy skin, the palmar surfaces of the digits fail to approximate. *(From Bolognia JL, Braverman IM. Skin and subcutaneous tissues. In: Lebovitz HE, DeFronzo R, Genuth S, et al, eds. Therapy for diabetes mellitus and related disorders. Alexandria, Va: American Diabetes Association, 1991:204–215; with permission.)*

■ NECROBIOSIS LIPOIDICA DIABETICORUM

Although necrobiosis lipoidica diabeticorum (NLD) is found in only 0.3 percent of diabetic patients, there is a clear-cut association between the two diseases. In one series of 171 patients with NLD, 65 percent had diabetes and 42 percent of the nondiabetics tested had an abnormal glucose tolerance test. The lesions of NLD are found on the distal lower extremities in approximately 85 percent of patients; less common locations include the upper extremities and the face. Although new lesions and the border areas of well-developed lesions can be red to red-brown in color, it is the central area of older lesions that demonstrates the characteristic yellow color, atrophy, and telangiectasias (Fig. 4). The most troublesome complication of NLD is associated ulceration.

The fact that there are multiple therapies for NLD speaks against one consistently successful treatment. Topical corticosteroids have been used for decades, but they usually do not result in resolution of the lesions. More recently, the "superpotent" topical steroids such as clobetasol and halobetasol have become available, and resolution of a large plaque of NLD was observed in a patient treated with topical clobetasol under occlusion for 3 weeks. When small areas of the skin are treated for a limited period of time, the major side effect of the superpotent topical steroids is cutaneous atrophy. Intralesional corticosteroids (e.g., triamcinolone, 5 mg per milliliter) can be injected into the active borders of the lesions to decrease inflammation, but they usually do not have an effect on the central atrophic area. Discussions of intralesional therapy usually contain a warning that it may induce ulcerations within the lesions of NLD, but data to support or refute this statement are lacking. Cessation of disease activity has been reported with 5- to 6-week courses of oral corticosteroids, but given the potential side effects, including hyperglycemia, this would be reserved for severe cases.

Given the histologic evidence of microangiopathy in lesions of NLD plus the observation that platelets from diabetic patients display an increased tendency to aggregate in response to various stimuli, several antithrombotic agents

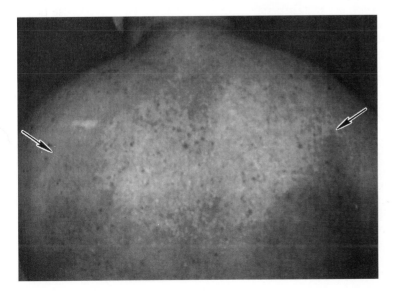

Figure 2
Demarcation of the induration on the back of a patient with scleredema. Arrows point to an area of overlying erythema.

have been tried. In the 1970s uncontrolled reports appeared on the successful use of acetylsalicylic acid (ASA) and dipyridamole, either alone or in combination, for the treatment of NLD. However, when a double-blind, placebo-controlled trial of ASA (325 mg three times a day) plus dipy-

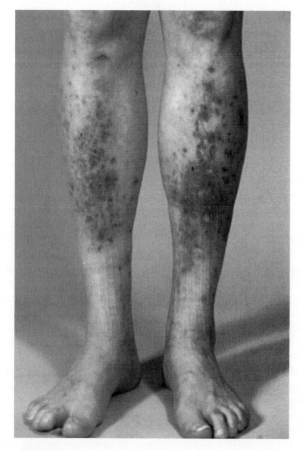

Figure 3
Hyperpigmented patches on the shins of a patient with diabetic dermopathy.

ridamole (75 mg three times a day) was performed in 14 patients with NLD, no therapeutic effect was observed. A randomized, double-blind 6-month trial of low-dose ASA (40 mg a day) also showed no difference between the treatment group and the control group. In spite of the inhibition of platelet aggregation in the ASA group, the lesions became significantly larger in both groups.

Because increased blood viscosity and increased red cell aggregation have been detected in patients with NLD, treatment with pentoxifylline has been tried. A few case reports have been published where extensive ulcerated disease responded to pentoxifylline (400 mg three times a day), but results from a larger series of patients are not available. The reported success of high-dose niacinamide in the treatment of granuloma annulare (see the following page) led to its use in patients with NLD. In an open trial of nicotinamide (500 mg three times a day), which has the same chemical structure as niacin-amide, 8 of 13 patients who took the medication for more than 1 month improved. Their ulcers healed and the associated pain decreased, but the lesional skin did not return to normal. When nicotinamide is used in diabetic patients, glucose levels have to be monitored closely because the dose of insulin may have to be increased or decreased. More recently, 6 of 10 patients reportedly responded to a 6- to 14-month course of clofazimine (200 mg per day). Necrobiosis lipoidica diabeticorum tends to be a chronic disease with only about 15 percent of patients experiencing spontaneous resolution. The degree of control of the hyperglycemia does not affect disease activity.

When ulceration occurs, the oral medications just discussed can be tried, as well as local care such as whirlpool and bio-occlusive dressings. In some patients with recurrent ulcerations, the ulcerations heal more quickly and are less likely to recur if patients lie down and elevate their legs for 1 to 2 hours a day. However, if these therapies are unsuccessful, surgical intervention may be necessary. Plastic surgeons advise excision of the involved area down to fascia and ligation of associated perforating blood vessels followed by split-thickness skin grafts. There is always a possibility of recurrence, but some clinical investigators believe that removal of the entire subcu-

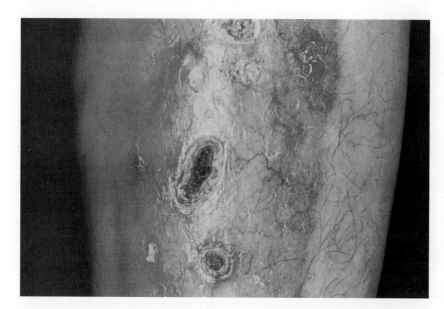

Figure 4
Ulcerated plaque of necrobiosis lipoidica diabeticorum on the shin of a patient with diabetes mellitus. Note the telangiectasias and shiny appearance of the skin; both are a reflection of the associated cutaneous atrophy. (*From Braverman IM. Skin signs of systemic disease, 2nd ed. Philadelphia: WB Saunders, 1981:658; with permission.*)

taneous fat decreases this risk. Ulcerations often begin after minor trauma to the areas of involvement, and for this reason, avoidance of trauma to the lower extermities has to be emphasized to the patient. Some physicians go so far as to have some of their patients wear plastic shin guards.

■ DISSEMINATED GRANULOMA ANNULARE

The skin lesions of disseminated granuloma annulare (GA) range from flesh-colored discrete papules to annular erythematous plaques (Fig. 5). Most clinicians agree that the less common disseminated form of GA is associated with diabetes mellitus. For example, in a group of 100 patients with disseminated GA seen at the Mayo Clinic, 21 percent had diabetes. The debate concerns the relationship of diabetes to the more common localized form of GA. To date, the evidence against an association is stronger than the evidence in its favor. Although the etiology of GA is unknown, explanations for the localized form's predilection for the distal extremities include reactions to trauma and arthropod bites. There is one interesting report of GA developing within puncture sites on the distal fingers in a diabetic patient who was monitoring blood glucose levels.

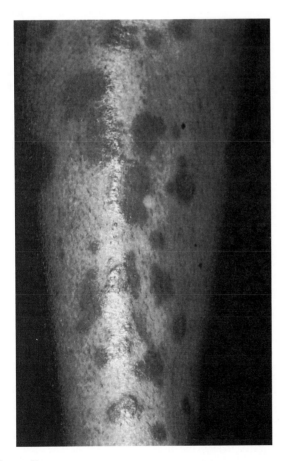

Figure 5
Erythematous plaques of disseminated granuloma annulare. Note the active border in several of the lesions.

Treatment of the localized form of GA consists primarily of potent topical corticosteroids and intralesional corticosteroids (triamcinolone, 5 mg per milliliter). However, these therapies are impractical for the generalized or disseminated form of the disease. Because of its minimal side effects, high-dose niacinamide (500 mg three times a day) is often the initial oral medication tried in patients with disseminated GA. A trial period of several months is given, but it should be emphasized that this treatment protocol is based upon the results obtained in one case report. In our experience with 3 patients, the generalized erythematous plaque form of GA did respond to high-dose niacinamide. Within 4 to 6 weeks a response was seen, and eventually 60 to 80 percent of the lesions cleared completely. When the niacinamide was discontinued or the dosage lowered to 500 mg per day, the GA returned; with reintroduction of the drug or an increase in the dose, the lesions responded again. If niacinamide fails, the available treatment options include psoralens plus UVA (PUVA) and dapsone. In addition, there are scattered reports of the use of antimalarials, retinoids, potassium iodide, and cryotherapy.

In a series of 5 patients with generalized GA, all were completely clear following 21 to 95 treatments with PUVA. The light treatments were given two to three times per week, and improvement was seen by 1 month. To prevent the skin lesions from returning, weekly or biweekly maintenance therapy was required. The potential side effects of PUVA therapy include nausea, phototoxicity, and an increased risk of nonmelanoma skin cancers, especially in fair-skinned individuals. In an open trial, 16 patients with GA (10 with disseminated disease and 6 with localized disease) were given a daily dose of 100 mg of dapsone for 6 to 18 weeks. There was complete remission in 6 patients and a partial response (more than 50 percent of the lesions resolved) in another 7 patients; the response was independent of the type of GA. However, the dapsone was not curative in that all of the adult patients relapsed within 3 months of discontinuating the medication. The side effects of dapsone include hemolysis, leukopenia, and agranulocytosis, the latter having been reported in a patient receiving dapsone for GA. Although other investigators have used cyclosporine and alkylating agents such as chlorambucil to treat GA, we think that the potential risks and side effects of these medications outweigh the seriousness of the cutaneous disease.

■ XANTHOMAS

The cutaneous xanthomas associated with hyperlipidemia are divided into four major groups: planar, tuberous, tendinous, and eruptive. It is the eruptive type of xanthoma that is a manifestation of hypertriglyceridemia in the diabetic patient. When the eruptive xanthomas appear, the diabetes is usually under poor control, and the lesions usually present as a shower of 2 to 3 mm red-yellow papules that favor the elbows, knees, and buttocks (Fig. 6). Treatment of eruptive xanthomas is quite gratifying because the lesions quickly disappear over a few weeks following the administration of insulin. The hypertriglyceridemia seen in diabetic patients is presumably a reflection of the effect of hypoinsulinemia on lipid metabolism. Failure to treat the patient with these lesions can lead to the transformation of eruptive xanthomas into tuberous xanthomas.

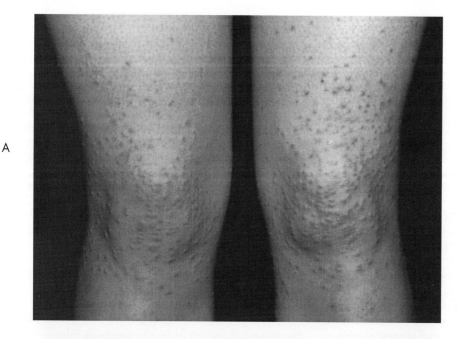

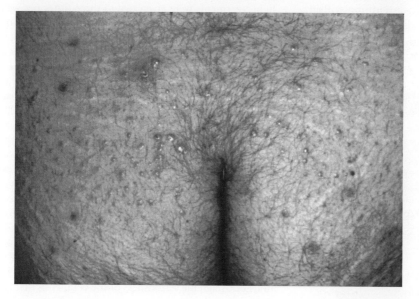

Figure 6
Eruptive xanthomas on the knees (**A**) and buttocks (**B**) of two patients with diabetes and hypertriglyceridemia.

■ LIPODYSTROPHY

The lipodystrophy that is observed in association with diabetes mellitus is primarily in the form of lipoatrophy (i.e., a loss of subcutaneous fat). Patients with lipoatrophy are characteristically insulin resistant, and the loss of subcutaneous fat can be either generalized or partial (e.g., involvement of only the upper half of the body). In the generalized form, the patient may also have hirsutism and acanthosis nigricans, while the partial form is often associated with glomerulonephritis. Unfortunately, there is no known treatment that reverses the lipoatrophy. In patients with localized areas of cutaneous lipoatrophy due to previous inflammation, autologous fat transfers have been attempted, but the areas of involvement in the partial form of lipoatrophy are usually so extensive that this technique does not seem currently feasible. The lipodystrophy that is a complication of insulin therapy is discussed in a later section of this chapter.

■ ACANTHOSIS NIGRICANS

Although acanthosis nigricans is seen most commonly in diabetic patients who are obese (Fig. 7), it also occurs in patients with lipoatrophic diabetes and in those with insulin resistance due to a defect in the insulin receptor or antibodies against the insulin receptor. Several topical agents are available for the treatment of acanthosis nigricans, including 0.1 percent tretinoin cream or gel (Retin-A), and 10 percent to 20 percent alpha hydroxy acids (lactic and glycolic), and 10 percent to 20 percent urea. Following a 2-week course of twice daily topical tretinoin, a decrease in hyperpigmentation and verrucous hyperplasia has been observed, and only a weekly application was required to keep the disease under control. The major side effect of topical tretinoin is irritation, and this may require a reduction in frequency of application. Theoretically, the tretinoin is decreasing the cohesiveness of the keratinocytes and increasing their shedding.

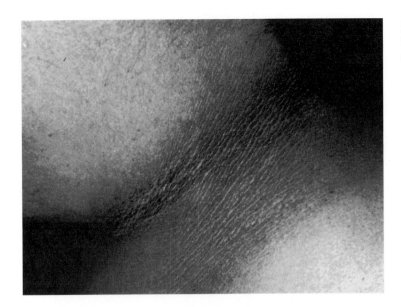

Figure 7
Hyperpigmented, verrucous plaque on the neck of
an obese patient with acanthosis nigricans.

In extensive cases of acanthosis nigricans, two oral vitamin A derivatives, etretinate (50 to 75 mg per day) and isotretinoin (up to 3 mg per kilogram per day), have been tried. However, relatively high doses of these medications were required to control the acanthosis nigricans, and the lesions recurred soon after the drug was discontinued. The multiple side effects of etretinate and isotretinoin, in particular the high risk of fetal abnormalities, have to be weighed against their therapeutic benefit, and we do not recommend their use. Lastly, there is one report of a patient with lipodystrophic diabetes and severe generalized acanthosis nigricans who had a striking improvement when placed on a diet with fat supplementation in the form of ω-3 fatty acid–rich fish oil (10 to 20 g per day).

■ BULLOSIS DIABETICORUM

Diabetic bullae occur on the distal extremities and arise spontaneously on a noninflammatory base (Fig. 8). These lesions can vary in size from 0.5 cm to greater than 8 cm, and the fluid within the bullae is characteristically thicker and more mucoid than the contents of bullae secondary to friction, infection, or edema. The blister formation can be intra- or subepidermal, the latter form sometimes healing with a scar. Other than decompression of the bulla by draining its fluid and allowing the blister roof to remain intact as a protective covering, there is no specific treatment for diabetic bullae. Care must be taken to keep the area clean so that a soft tissue infection does not occur as a secondary complication.

■ NECROLYTIC MIGRATORY ERYTHEMA

The skin lesions in necrolytic migratory erythema (NME) favor the lower extremities and the lower trunk and are characterized by large areas of erythema with evidence of erosions at the border (Fig. 9). Often there is a migration of the areas of erythema, and a biopsy of the skin can aid in the diagnosis if necrosis of the upper third of the epidermis is seen. Associated findings include glossitis, weight loss, diarrhea, abnormal glucose tolerance, and elevated serum glucagon. The vast majority of patients have an associated alpha cell tumor of the pancreas that is secreting glucagon (i.e., a glucagonoma). Although less than 30 percent of glucagonomas are benign, the surgical removal of such tumors results in a complete clearing of the skin and the associated symptoms.

When the tumor is malignant, the primary tumor may be too large to resect completely or there may be liver metastases by the time the clinical diagnosis is made. Clearance of the cutaneous lesions of NME then requires the use of a systemic medication such as somatostatin, the somatostatin analogue SMS 201-995, streptozocin, 5-fluorouracil, and/or dimethyl-triazenoimidazole-carboxamide (DTIC). Following a 36- to 48-hour infusion of somatostatin, clearing of skin lesions for a period of 1 to 2 weeks has been observed. The drawback to the use of intravenous somatostatin is its short half-life (less than 4 minutes), but this problem can be circumvented by the use of the somatostatin analogue SMS 201-995. This analogue was first used in the mid-1980s as a treatment for NME in association with surgically unresectable glucagonomas. It is injected subcutaneously by the patient twice a day and can result in a marked improvement of the lesions within 48 hours. The skin eruption does recur if the analogue is discontinued, but the disease was reportedly kept under control in one patient for a period of 8 months.

Because one explanation for the association of glucagomas and NME is a relative amino acid deficiency, infusions of mixed amino acids (45 g per day for 2 weeks) have also been tried as a treatment for NME, and there are several reports of successful results. Lastly, transcatheter arterial embolization of hepatic metastases of glucagonoma can also lead to amelioration of skin lesions. It should be pointed out that not all cases of NME are due to an underlying glucagonoma; the eruption has also been observed in patients with hepatic cirrhosis, bronchial carcinoma, chronic pancreatitis, and disorders of the small intestine such as malabsorption and celiac disease. In one of the latter cases, the circulating levels of glucagon were only mildly elevated while the levels of enteroglucagon were markedly elevated. Further investigation revealed numerous small intestinal crypt cells that were producing enteroglucagon. Institution of a gluten-free diet

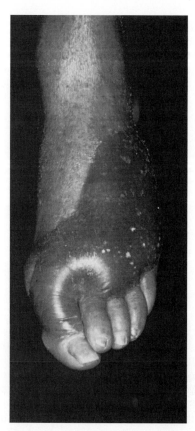

Figure 8
Large tense bulla on the dorsa of the foot is characteristic of bullosis diabeticorum. *(From Braverman IM. Skin signs of systemic disease, 2nd ed. Philadelphia: WB Saunders, 1981:663; with permission.)*

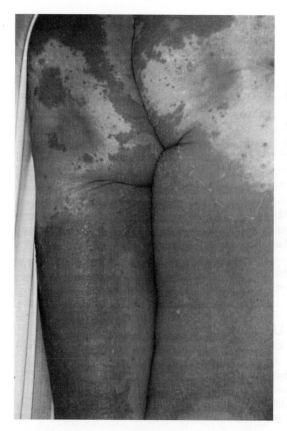

Figure 9
Areas of erythema and superficial desquamation in a patient with necrolytic migratory erythema and an underlying glucagonoma. *(From Braverman IM. Skin signs of systemic disease, 2nd ed. Philadelphia: WB Saunders, 1981:28; with permission.)*

resulted in disappearance of the NME and normalization of the enteroglucagon level.

■ DRUG REACTIONS TO ORAL HYPOGLYCEMIC AGENTS AND INSULIN

Cutaneous reactions to sulfonylureas are similar to those seen with other sulfur-containing medications. They include morbilliform eruptions, urticaria, and erythema multiforme. In addition, both phototoxic (dose-related exaggerated sunburn) and photoallergic (idiosyncratic eczematous dermatitis in a photodistribution) reactions can occur. The most important therapeutic step is to discontinue the offending agent. If the patient is given chlorpropamide, a warning must be given about the possibility of a disulfiram-like reaction following alcohol ingestion.

Allergic reactions to insulin are divided into local and systemic, with the local reactions further subdivided into immediate (urticarial, mediated by immunoglobulin E) and delayed (cell-mediated delayed type hypersensitivity). Local reactions are much more common, and they can usually be prevented by instructing the patient to avoid injections into the dermis and/or switching to a purified, single-component porcine or human insulin. It is also important to consider the possibility that the zinc, protamine, or preservative such as paraben contained in the preparation is responsible. Even with the least antigenic form of insulin, recombinant human insulin, there are occasional reports of allergic reactions. In one case, local reactions were suppressed by the addition of dexamethasone (0.05 mg per injection) to the recombinant human insulin. If the patient progresses to a generalized reaction (often after reintroduction of insulin following a hiatus), then referral to an immunologist for evaluation (e.g., skin testing) and possible desensitization is recommended.

Lipodystrophy as a complication of insulin therapy is seen in up to 30 percent of those patients who require subcutaneous insulin injections. Both lipoatrophy and lipohypertrophy can occur, even in the same patient. In an attempt to prevent lipodystrophy, the patient should rotate injection sites so that no area 3 cm in diameter is injected more than once every 3 to 4 weeks. To aid in this effort, rotation charts can be used with careful recording of injection sites. Because lipoatrophy is thought to result from a local immunologic response to contaminants such as proinsulin in the insulin preparation, the most common treatment for lipoatrophy is a switch from conventional forms of insulin to highly purified, monocomponent forms of porcine or human insulin. These purified insulins can be injected into the atrophic areas, starting at the periphery and progressing toward the center, with successful reversal of the process. The incidence of lipoatrophy has decreased with the increased use of purified forms of insulin, but even recombinant human insulin has been associated with lipoatrophy, albeit infrequently.

In contrast, the chance of developing benign lipohypertrophy is thought to increase when purified, single-component forms of insulin are used. One possible explanation for this lipohypertrophy is the anabolic activity of insulin leading to an increase in the size of adipose cells. There is one report of the use of liposuction to treat lipohypertrophy, but further clinical investigation of this form of therapy is required before it can be endorsed.

Lastly, there are several forms of local reactions to insulin that to date have no known specific or effective therapy. These include localized amyloidosis, zinc granulomas, and acanthosis nigricans–like verrucous plaques.

■ ULCERATIONS OF THE LOWER EXTREMITIES

Although the majority of lower extremity ulcerations are due to venous insufficiency, additional causes such as arterial insufficiency and sensory neuropathy are more common in the diabetic patient than in the nondiabetic patient. Cutaneous clues to the presence of arterial insufficiency are evident on examination of the toes: coolness, loss of hair, and shininess and atrophy of the skin. In addition, arterial ulcers tend to be more painful than venous ulcers, and they are not associated with lymphedema and stasis dermatitis. Arterial ulcers require local care plus a surgical consultation to determine the need for revascularization. Neuropathic ulcers (mal perforans) characteristically occur on the plantar surface of the foot, an unusual location for venous or arterial ulcers. They are a direct result of the sensory neuropathy that accompanies diabetes. Treatment of neuropathic ulcers includes paring of the keratotic rim and application of topical antibiotics, but the most important intervention is to have the patient wear tennis shoes regularly.

Suggested Reading

Braverman IM. Skin signs of systemic disease, 2nd ed. Philadelphia: WB Saunders, 1981.

Reviews the cutaneous manifestations of diabetes mellitus and presents illustrative cases that are accompanied by color photographs.

Huntley AC. The cutaneous manifestations of diabetes mellitus. J Am Acad Dermatol 1982; 7:427–455.

Extensive review of all known associated skin changes in diabetes, with excellent bibliography.

Jelenick JE. The skin in diabetes. Philadelphia: Lea & Febiger, 1986.

Comprehensive review of the author's experience and the literature. Care of the diabetic foot is discussed in detail.

Kerker BJ, Huang CP, Morison WL. Photochemotherapy of generalized granuloma annulare. Arch Dermatol 1990; 126:359–361.

Study of 5 patients with disseminated GA, all of whom were completely clear following 21 to 95 treatments with PUVA.

Lithner F. Cutaneous reactions of the extremities of diabetics to local thermal trauma. Acta Med Scand 1975; 198:319–325.

Examines the pathophysiology of diabetic dermopathy by reproducing the lesions with thermal injury. The latter produced atrophic circumscribed skin lesions in 16 of 19 patients with diabetic dermopathy. In contrast, none of the controls (n = 25) and only 1 of 16 diabetic patients without dermopathy developed such lesions after thermal trauma.

Shelley WB, Shelley ED. Advanced dermatologic therapy. Philadelphia: WB Saunders, 1987.

Therapies, both conventional and nonconventional, are outlined with references for each disease entity.

INFECTIONS AND DIABETES MELLITUS

Merri Pendergrass, M.D., Ph.D.

John Graybill, M.D.

Infection is a frequent, potentially life-threatening complication in patients with diabetes mellitus. Although the specific types of infections that are encountered by diabetic patients usually are not unique to this group, some (e.g., urinary tract infection, tuberculosis, candidiasis, gram-negative pneumonia) occur with a greater frequency. Once established, even common infections in diabetics may be poorly tolerated. This is due to a combination of factors, including alterations in host defense mechanisms and a high prevalence of coexistent disease. Moreover, a vicious cycle may ensue in which the stress of infection complicates management of the diabetes, and worsening metabolic control exacerbates the infection. In addition to the more common infections, there are also a number of unusual infections that occur predominantly in patients with diabetes (Table 1). Many of these can be life-threatening and constitute medical emergencies.

In the following sections, we first review those factors that increase the diabetic patient's susceptibility to infection. Next we discuss several common infections, highlighting special considerations for individuals with diabetes. Lastly, we review some unusual infections that occur principally in diabetics, emphasizing features that are important for prompt diagnosis and treatment.

■ HOST FACTORS PREDISPOSING TO INFECTION

Although the host factors responsible for the diabetic patient's increased susceptibility to infection are incompletely understood, several defects in the immune defense mechanism have been identified (Table 2).

Cutaneous and mucous membrane carriage of potential organisms, including *Staphylococcus aureus,* gram-negative bacilli, and *Candida,* is increased in diabetic patients, which explains in part the frequent occurrence of infections with these pathogens. Subtle alterations in cell-mediated immunity also predispose the diabetic patient to tuberculosis and certain fungal infections, including coccidioidomycosis and cryptococcosis. Abnormalities in monocyte phagocytosis and in polymorphonuclear leukocyte mobilization, chemotaxis, adherence, phagocytosis, and microbicidal function have also been reported. Although the role of hyperglycemia in leukocyte function has been debated, some defects clearly improve with aggressive glycemic control (plasma glucose less than or equal to 200 mg per deciliter) and correction of metabolic acidosis. Therefore, it is critical that metabolic derangements be promptly corrected in all diabetic patients who present with infection or who are at increased risk to develop an infection (e.g., perioperative patients). The diabetic person's abnormal metabolic state also favors the specific nutritional requirements of some microbes. High glucose concentrations in the blood and body fluids promote the overgrowth of certain fungal pathogens, especially *Candida* species and *Zygomycetes. Zygomycetes* also grows more rapidly under conditions of acidosis, making diabetic ketoacidosis a major predisposing condition.

Long-term complications that are frequently associated with diabetes mellitus also predispose to the development of infection. Microvascular and macrovascular complications lead to impaired peripheral circulation, and this reduces the body's ability to provide important nutritional and host defense needs. In addition, the compromised circulation impairs the delivery of antimicrobial agents. Tissue hypoxia can modify the oxygen-dependent function of polymorphonucleocytes and allow the growth of anaerobic organisms. Breaks in the skin, including minor fissures that arise in dystrophic areas, as well as ulcerations due to ischemia or neuropathic trauma, provide a prime avenue for bacterial invasion. Because of these multiple abnormalities in the host defense mechanisms, mixed bacterial infections, especially of the foot, are very common. Autonomic neuropathy causes impaired bladder emptying and fecal incontinence and can lead to urinary tract infections with mixed organisms and cutaneous maceration. Cerebrovascular insults may result in a decreased cough reflex and predispose to pneumonia. In diabetic patients with end-stage renal disease, the institution of hemodialysis, chronic peritoneal dialysis, or renal transplantation further compromises host defense mechnisms and subjects patients to the infectious complications associated with these specific therapeutic interventions. Impaired mobility, resulting from both microvascular and macrovascular complications, predisposes many diabetic patients to the development of decubitus ulcers.

From the above discussion it is clear that many factors conspire to predispose the diabetic patient to infection. Fortunately, many of these predisposing factors are preventable (Table 3). Maintenance of a normal or near-normal metabolic state improves neutrophil function and makes the environment less hospitable to potential fungal pathogens. Maintenance of near-normal blood glucose levels reduces the progression of certain diabetic complications (i.e., neuropathy and nephropathy) that favor the spread of infection. Other strategies to prevent diabetic complications include treatment of other atherosclerotic vascular disease risk factors (e.g., hypertension, tobacco abuse, hyperlipidemia, obesity), proper foot care, and certain specific prophylactic measures (e.g., isoniazid for tuberculin skin-test–positive patients, pneumococcal and influenza vaccines). Finally, it is particularly important that infection be diagnosed and treated aggressively in the diabetic patient. In addition to the conventional indicators of infection, such as fever and elevated levels of white blood cells (WBC), infection should be considered whenever there is a deterioration in metabolic control or the metabolic condition fails to respond to appropriate treatment (e.g., insulin for diabetic ketoacidosis).

■ URINARY TRACT INFECTIONS

The rate of urinary tract infection (UTI) is increased two- to threefold in diabetic women compared to nondiabetic individuals, and the frequency of pyelonephritis is five times higher in diabetic patients. Certain unusual, life-threatening complications, such as emphysematous cystitis, renal papillary necrosis, emphysematous pyelonephritis, and perinephric abscess, occur predominantly in diabetic patients (see Table 1).

Uncomplicated Bacterial Urinary Tract Infections

Bacteriuria is frequently found in diabetic women and is usually associated with upper UTI. Because upper UTI may be asymptomatic, most experts believe that all bacteriuria in diabetic patients should be treated aggressively with a bacteriocidal antibiotic. *Escherichia coli* is the most frequently encountered bacterial pathogen. Other coliforms, such as *Klebsiella pneumoniae* and *Proteus mirabilis,* are also common. *Enterococcus* species and *Pseudomonas aeruginosa* should be considered in diabetic patients who are hospitalized, who have had recent urologic procedures, or who have failed to respond to standard antibiotic regimens. Because of the high likelihood of upper UTI, complicated UTI, and frequent recurrent infections, all UTIs in diabetic patients should be documented by culture, and a follow-up urinalysis should be obtained after completion of antimicrobial therapy. For an uncomplicated lower UTI, a 7- to 14-day oral antimicrobial regimen should be adequate. Suggestions for empiric therapy are given in Table 4. Continuation of therapy should always be guided by culture results. Trimethoprim-sulfamethoxazole usually provides adequate first-line coverage for an uncomplicated UTI. It must be remembered, however, that sulfonamide-containing antibiotics may potentiate the hypoglycemic effects of sulfonylureas.

Fungal Urinary Tract Infections

The most common fungal infections in diabetics are UTIs with *Candida* and *T. glabrata,* a related organism. *Candida* urinary tract colonization is common, and it is especially difficult to distinguish infection from colonization. Predisposing factors that may be associated with invasive pathogens include the presence of a foreign body (e.g., an indwelling catheter), concomitant antibiotic use, and steroid use. Although there are no recognized criteria to differentiate significant infection from colonization, there is probably infection if more than 10^4 *Candida* are present per milliliter of urine. The presence of WBC casts indicates parenchymal renal infection. A major problem is the difficulty in obtaining an uncontaminated specimen from obese diabetic women. A catheterized urine specimen is preferable in this situation. If *Candida* is repeatedly isolated from the urine, consideration should be given to a short course of antifungal therapy (see Table 4). Amphotericin B should be avoided because of nephrotoxicity.

Acute Pyelonephritis

Hospitalization and parenteral antimicrobial therapy (see Table 4) are necessary in all diabetic patients with suspected pyelonephritis. When aminoglycosides are used, the dose should be adjusted for preexisting renal disease. Because aminoglycosides may aggravate renal insufficiency, the serum creatinine concentration should be monitored closely after the institution of therapy. If aminoglycosides are used, they should be given only until in vitro antimicrobial susceptibilities are available. If possible, more specific nonnephrotoxic antibiotics should be instituted. Intravenous therapy is recommended until fever and symptoms resolve, typically within 2 to 3 days after instituting appropriate therapy. An oral regimen with an agent that achieves high serum and tissue levels should be used to complete a 14-day course. Because diabetic patients are at risk for developing emphy-sematous pyelonephritis, a screening plain abdominal radiograph should be obtained in all patients. If fever and symptoms do not resolve after 48 to 72 hours, further evaluation should be initiated to rule out intrarenal or perinephic abscess, papillary necrosis, or urinary tract obstruction.

Table 2 Factors that Increase the Diabetic Patient's Susceptibility to Infection

Increased cutaneous and mucous membrane carriage of potential pathogens
Abnormal phagocyte function
Abnormal cell-mediated immunity
Hyperglycemia and acidosis
Coexisting medical conditions
   Neuropathy
   Angiopathy

Table 1 Infections Associated with Diabetes Mellitus

TYPE OF INFECTION	APPROXIMATE PERCENTAGE OF PATIENTS WITH DIABETES MELLITUS
Malignant otitis externa	90
Emphysematous pyelonephritis	92
Emphysematous cystitis	80
Rhinocerebral mucormycosis	75
Necrotizing fasciitis	75
Papillary necrosis	57
Perinephric abscess	36
Emphysematous cholecystitis	35

Table 3 Measures to Prevent Infection in Diabetic Patients

Normalization of blood glucose
Avoidance of acidosis
Treatment of coexisting atherosclerotic cardiovascular risk factors (hypertension, hyperlipidemia, obesity, smoking)
Proper foot care
Prophylaxis
   Isoniazid for patients with positive tuberculin skin test
   Pneumococcal vaccine
   Influenza vaccine

Table 4 Empiric Antimicrobial Therapy for Diabetic Patients

CLINICAL SITUATION	COMMON CAUSES	TREATMENT	DOSE	DURATION
URINARY TRACT INFECTION				
Uncomplicated bacterial	Enterobacteriaceae (esp. *Escherichia coli, Klebsiella pneumoniae, Proteus mirabilis*)	Trimethoprim-sulfamethoxazole Amoxicillin-clavulanate Ciprofloxacin Norfloxacin	TMP 160 mg–SMX 800 mg PO q.d. 500 mg PO t.i.d. 500 mg PO b.i.d. 400 mg PO b.i.d.	1–2 weeks
Fungal	*Candida* *Torulopsis*	Flucytosine* Fluconazole*	25–35 mg/kg PO q.i.d. 100 mg PO q.d.	2 weeks 2–4 weeks
Acute pyelonephritis	Enterobacteriaceae	Cefotaxime	1–2 g IV q 4–12 hr	2 weeks (uncomplicated)
	Enterococci	Ceftazidime	1–2 g IV q 8–12 hr	2–6 weeks (uncomplicated)
	Pseudomonas aeruginosa	Ticarcillin-clavulanate	500 mg IV q 12 hr	
		Mezlocillin[a] or piperacillin[b] or ticarcillin[c] + Gentamicin*[d] or amikacin*[e] or Tobramycin*[f]	(a) 3 g IV q 4 hr (b) 3–4 g IV q 4–6 hr (c) 3 g IV q 4–6 hr (d) 3–4 mg/kg IV q 12 hr (e) 7.5–10 mg/kg IV q 12 hr (f) 2.5 mg/kg IV q 12 hr	
		Ciprofloxacin	500 mg IV q 12 hr	
		Imipenem	500 mg IV q 8 hr	
SOFT TISSUE INFECTION		**Early or Mild**		
	Streptococci Enterococci *Staphylococcus aureus*	Cephalexin Dicloxacillin Clindamycin Amoxicillin-clavulanate	500 mg PO q 6 hr 500 mg PO q 6 hr 300 mg PO q 6 hr 500 mg PO q 8 hr	10–14 days
		Septic		
	Enterobacteriaceae Anaerobes including *Bacteroides fragilis*	Ampicillin[a] or mezlocillin[b] or piperacillin[c] or ticarcillin[d] + Gentamicin*[e] or amikacin*[f] + Tobramycin*[g] or clindamycin[h]	(a) 500 mg IV q 6 hr (b) 3 g IV q 4 hr (c) 3–4 g IV q 4–6 hr (d) 3–4 g IV q 4–6 hr (e) 3–4 mg/kg IV q 12 hr (f) 7.5–10 mg/kg IV q 12 hr (g) 2.5 mg/kg IV q 12 hr (h) 300 mg IV q 6–8 hr	2–4 weeks

HEAD AND NECK INFECTIONS

Infection	Organism	Therapy	Dose	Duration
Malignant otitis externa	*P. aeruginosa*	Ceftazidime	1–2 g IV q 8–12 hr	4–12 weeks
		Cefotaxime	1–2 g IV q 4–12	
		Ciprofloxacin	750 mg PO b.i.d.	
		Imipenem	500 mg IV q 8 hr	
		Mezlocillin[a] or piperacillin[b] or ticarcillin[c]	(a) 3 g IV q 4 hr (b) 3–4 g IV q 4–6 hr (c) 3 g IV q 4–6 hr	
		+		
		Gentamicin★[d] or amikacin★[e] or tobramycin★[f]	(d) 3–4 mg/kg IV q 12 hr (e) 7.5–10 mg/kg IV q 12 hr (f) 2.5 mg/kg IV q 12 hr	
Rhinocerebral mucormycosis	Fungi of the order *Mucorales*	Amphotericin B★	1–1.5 mg/kg IV q.d.	Total dosage 2–4 g

EMPHYSEMATOUS

Infection	Organism	Therapy	Dose	Duration
Cholecystitis	Enterobacteriaceae, Enterococci, Anaerobes including *Bacteroides*, *Clostridium*	Cefoxtamine[a] or ceftazidime[b] or cefoxitin[c] or mezlocillin[d] or piperacillin[e] or ticarcillin[f]	(a) 1–2 g IV q 4–12 hr (b) 1–2 g IV q 8–12 hr (c) 1–2 g IV q 4–8 hr (d) 3 g IV q 4 hr (e) 3–4 g IV q 4–6 hr (f) 300–600 g IV q 8 hr	2–4 weeks
		+		
		Clindamycin[g] or metronidazole[h]	(g) 7.5 mg/kg q 6 hr	
		Ampicillin[a] or gentamicin[b] or amikacin[c] or tobramycin[d]	(a) 500 mg IV q 6 hr (b) 3–4 mg/kg IV q 12 hr (c) 7.5–10 mg/kg IV q 12 hr (d) 2.5 mg/kg IV q 12 hr	
		+		
		Clindamycin[e]	(e) 300 mg IV q 6–8 hr	
		Ticarcillin–clavulanate	3.1 g IV q 6 hr	
		Ampicillin–sulbactam	1.5–3 g IV q 6 hr	
		Imipenem	500 mg IV q 8 hr	
Pneumonia	*Streptococcus pneumoniae*, Group A streptococci, *Haemophilus influenzae*, Enterobacteriaceae, *Legionella*, *S. aureus*, Anaerobes	Trimethoprim–sulfamethoxazole[a] or amoxicillin–clavulanate[b] or Ticarcillin–clavulanate[c] or Ceftazidime[d] or cefotaxime[e]	(a) TMP 160 mg–SMX 800 mg PO or IV q 12 hr (b) 500 mg PO t.i.d. (c) 3.1 g IV q 6 hr (d) 1–2 g IV q 8–12 hr (e) 1–2 g IV q 4–12 hr	10–14 hr
		+		
		Erythromycin[f]	(f) 250–500 mg PO or IV q 6 hr	

★Reduce dose with impaired renal function.

Complicated Urinary Tract Infections

UTI can result in a number of severe complications, including pyelonephritis, unifocal or multifocal bacterial abscesses, perinephric abscess, xanthogranulomatous pyelonephritis, and papillary necrosis. Some complications, including emphysematous cystitis and emphysematous pyelonephritis, occur almost exclusively in diabetic patients. Others, including renal papillary necrosis and perinephric abscess, occur with markedly increased frequency in diabetic patients (see Table 1). These complications must be sought actively in all patients with evidence of a UTI who fail to respond in a timely fashion to antibiotic therapy. Certain UTIs that occur primarily in diabetic patients are discussed further.

Emphysematous cystitis is an uncommon manifestation of bladder infection that is found primarily in diabetic patients (50 to 80 percent of cases). Gas in the bladder wall is produced by bacterial fermentation. *E. coli* is usually the offending agent, but *Enterobacter aerogenes, Proteus* and *Klebsiella* species, and *Candida* have been described. Symptoms are typically referable to the bladder. Characteristic features suggesting the diagnosis include gross hematuria and pneumaturia. The radiograph shows evidence of air in the bladder wall or lumen. The most important issue becomes to distinguish emphysematous cystitis from other causes of pneumaturia, especially communicating fistulas between the bowel and bladder. In most cases the emphysematous cystitis responds to appropriate parenteral antibiotics.

Renal papillary necrosis is an uncommon but serious condition that has a high predilection for patients with diabetes (approximately 60 percent of cases). Impaired blood flow to the medullary tissues can lead to anoxic damage and eventually to necrosis of the papilla. If the papilla sloughs, it can obstruct the renal pelvis, and the patient will present with a clinical picture similar to that observed with a renal calculus. Upper UTIs can also cause papillary necrosis. This becomes a medical emergency because the infection cannot be eradicated in the presence of urinary tract obstruction. Renal papillary necrosis should be considered in any diabetic patient who presents with symptoms of pyelonephritis and does not respond well to antibiotic therapy or who develops progressive renal insufficiency. A retrograde pyelogram is the diagnostic procedure of choice because it identifies the site of obstruction even if the serum creatinine concentration is very high and it is associated with a lower incidence of acute renal failure than intravenous pyelography. A urinary sediment examination that demonstrates the presence of renal papillary tissue is diagnostic of this condition. The offending urinary pathogens in papillary necrosis are similar to those usually observed in diabetic patients with UTIs. If the patient is afebrile and does not appear toxic, treatment with antibiotics, analgesics, and hydration is usually sufficient for the papilla to be passed and the infection to resolve. If the obstruction persists, surgical intervention may be necessary.

Another fortunately rare form of renal parenchymal infection, emphysematous pyelonephritis, also occurs predominantly in diabetic patients (approximately 90 percent of cases). Gas is present in renal tissue, and the kidney may be destroyed completely unless prompt, specific intravenous antibiotic therapy is instituted. In the majority of cases, *E. coli* is the causative agent. Other gram-negative bacilli, including *K. pneumoniae, E. aerogenes, P. mirabilis,* and *P. aeruginosa,* are responsible for most of the other cases. An infrequent but dramatic physical finding is crepitation over the thigh or flank. The diagnosis of emphysematous pyelonephritis is classically made by demonstrating gas in renal tissue on plain radiographs of the abdomen or by abdominal computed tomography. Prompt treatment with an appropriate antibiotic may be associated with a poor prognosis, and failure to respond to antibiotic therapy may necessitate nephrectomy. Even so, mortality in these patients may be as high as 33 percent.

More than a third of patients with perinephric abscess have diabetes. The most common offending pathogens are *E. coli, Pseudomonas* species, and *S. aureus.* The clinical presentation is insidious, often making the diagnosis elusive. Perinephric abscess should be considered in patients with fever of unknown origin and in diabetics with unexplained peritoneal signs, renal empyema, or pelvic abscess. The diagnosis is usually made by ultrasonography or computed tomography. Drainage of the perinephric abscess is the mainstay of therapy and should be done as soon as possible after the diagnosis is made. Antimicrobial therapy is necessary but adjunctive to surgical drainage. Mortality associated with perinephric abscess ranges from 20 percent to more than 50 percent.

■ SOFT TISSUE INFECTIONS

A wide variety of soft tissue infections, ranging from superficial to deep necrotizing infections, are common in diabetic patients.

Mucocutaneous candidiasis frequently occurs in patients with poorly controlled blood glucose levels. Prior colonization, especially in patients who have previously received antibiotic therapy, is an important contributing factor. These infections can involve the vulva, mouth, skin, and nails and can usually be treated with topical treatment and improved glycemic control. In the presence of high glucose levels, therapy tends to be ineffective.

Superficial soft tissue infections are usually initiated by minor trauma to tissues that are inadequately perfused because of vascular insufficiency. Insensibility to the injury, resulting from peripheral sensory neuropathy, may exacerbate the damage by causing a delay in recognition and institution of appropriate care. The onset of superficial soft tissue infection is insidious, and the serious threat it poses (i.e., limb amputation) must be recognized. Infection may take the form of a cellulitis, draining sinus, or osteomyelitis. The feet are the most common site of these infections, but they also frequently occur in the skin underlying pressure points (decubitus ulcers). Ulceration and infection of the upper extremities are uncommon unless the diabetic patient has renal failure and an arteriovenous fistula that creates a vascular steal syndrome.

Superficial infections are usually caused by a combination of both aerobic and anaerobic organisms, including *E. coli, Proteus* species, a variety of other Enterobacteriaceae, various streptococci, *Staphylococcus, Peptostreptococcus,* and *Bacteroides fragilis.* A higher rate of colonization with *S. aureus* has been observed in diabetic patients. Therefore, even small scratches or blisters are rapidly colonized, with subsequent tissue infection. Patients with diabetes should be treated early with topical antibiotics for abrasions. Several of the organisms that cause superficial infections (i.e., clostridial cellulitis and nonclostridial anaerobic cellulitis) produce gas, probably because of fermentation that occurs in the presence of high glucose levels. This may result in crepitation in the patient with a diabetic foot and must be distinguished from the much less common, and more acutely devastating, gas gangrene. As with any infection, antimicrobial treatment should be directed at organisms identified by culture. However, empiric therapy for the most likely pathogens should be initiated as soon as possible (see Table 4).

Necrotizing soft tissue infections fortunately are rare, but when they do occur, they can be devastating. The terminology for these infections is often confusing because multiple terms (necrotizing fasciitis, necrotizing cellulitis, Meleney's synergistic gangrene, hemolytic streptococcal gangrene, gas gangrene, and others) have been used to describe similar processes. Diabetic patients are particularly susceptible to these infections and account for 75 percent of all cases of necrotizing fasciitis. Necrotizing fasciitis, in the strictest sense, refers to infection of subcutaneous tissues that spreads along fascial planes. When the muscle is involved, it is referred to as "necrotizing cellulitis." The skin itself may initially not be involved, but as the infection in deeper tissues progresses, vessels supplying the cutaneous layer become thrombosed, ultimately resulting in skin necrosis. In other cases, infections that begin on the skin may progress to deeper subcutaneous layers.

Necrotizing soft tissue infections occur most often in the lower extremity or the perianal area and may spread extensively within a few days. Clinical onset is usually acute, with severe systemic toxicity and high fever. Involved skin typically exhibits anesthesia, bullae formation, irregular ulcers with serosanguineous drainage, or various degrees of skin necrosis. Occasionally the overlying skin may appear deceptively normal. Subcutaneous emphysema is commonly present (i.e., gas gangrene). In some cases crepitus may be palpable; in others radiographic films may be necessary to reveal gas in the tissues. Although the diagnosis of necrotizing soft tissue infection is usually clear at its later stages, it is often difficult to distinguish at presentation between cellulitis and necrotizing infections. This distinction is crucial, however, because cellulitis is amenable to antimicrobial therapy whereas necrotizing soft tissue infection requires surgical intervention. Computed tomography or magnetic resonance imaging can be useful in locating the depth of involvement. Ultimately, the extent of involvement can only be determined through surgical exploration.

Although necrotizing fasciitis was originally described with group A streptococci (i.e., streptococcal gangrene), it may occur with a polymicrobial, synergistic mixture of aerobes and anaerobes (i.e., synergistic gangrene), including *Bacteroides* and *Clostridium* species, anaerobic streptococci, *P. aeruginosa,* other gram-negative bacilli, enterococci, and staphylococci. Aggressive surgical debridement of all involved tissue is paramount for therapy. Antimicrobial therapy may be effective in preventing the spread of infections but cannot eradicate microorganisms present in dead tissue. Tenuous vascular supply and poor tissue healing often necessitate amputation more proximally than the obviously infected tissue. Adjunctive antibiotic therapy should consist of a bactericidal agent or agents with a broad spectrum of anaerobic and aerobic coverage (see Table 4). Even with optimal treatment, mortality resulting from these infections may exceed 50 percent.

■ HEAD AND NECK INFECTIONS

Patients with diabetes mellitus are especially susceptible to two severe infections of the head and neck. Malignant otitis externa occurs almost exclusively in diabetic patients, who account for over 90 percent of all cases. Rhinocerebral mucormycosis also predominantly affects diabetics, who account for over 70 percent of all cases.

Malignant otitis externa is an aggressive, locally invasive process that is usually caused by *P. aeruginosa.* Infection begins in the skin and cartilage of the external ear. It may then extend to deeper tissues, leading to osteomyelitis, cranial nerve palsies, and death in up to 20 percent of cases. Unrelenting ear pain, drainage of purulent material, and extensive granulation tissue in the ear canal are characteristically present. Diagnosis is based on the typical constellation of clinical findings. Treatment consists of local debridement of necrotic tissue and adjuvant therapy with prolonged antipseudomonal antibiotics for a period of 4 to 8 weeks (see Table 4).

Rhinocerebral mucormycosis is a rare but potentially lethal infection that occurs predominantly in patients with diabetic ketoacidosis (75 percent of cases). It is an invasive process caused by fungi of the order Mucorales, which includes *Mucor, Rhizopus, Cunninghamella,* and *Absidia.* These fungi, which are nonpathogenic in a normal host, can proliferate rapidly in the presence of hyperglycemia and acidosis. The fungi are able to germinate at the site of infection, usually the nares and the sinuses, and may extend from a small eschar on the nasal septum to involve the paranasal sinuses, orbits, or brain within a matter of days. Necrosis is prominent because of the invasion of blood vessels. Fever, lethargy, headache, facial pain, swelling, bloody nasal discharge, and the development of necrotic black eschars in the nose or palate are the usual clinical features. Orbital invasion causes proptosis, decreased ocular motion, and visual loss. Diagnosis requires prompt surgical biopsy of affected tissues. Treatment requires correction of hyperglycemia and acidosis, vigorous and repeated surgical debridement, and antifungal therapy with high-dose amphotericin B. Even with aggressive therapy, mortality rates in diabetic patients may be as high as 50 percent.

■ EMPHYSEMATOUS CHOLECYSTITIS

Emphysematous cholecystitis is a highly virulent form of acute cholecystitis that is characterized by gas production in or around the gallbladder. Diabetes is present in about one-third of all cases. In contrast to the more common form of acute cholecystitis, emphysematous cholecystitis occurs more commonly in men than women, and gangrene and perforation are more frequent. The usual causative organisms include anaerobes, especially *Clostridium* species, *E. coli,* staphylococci, streptococci, and *P. aeruginosa.* Clinically, patients present with symptoms similar to those with acute cholecystitis. Crepitus on abdominal palpation is an ominous sign. The diagnosis is made radiographically by demonstrating gas in the gallbladder and surrounding tissues on abdominal plain film or CT. Since gas appears over a period of several days, sequential abdominal radiographs in diabetic patients with symptoms of acute cholecystitis will increase the chance of detection at an early stage. Prompt surgical intervention is indicated as soon as the diagnosis is confirmed. Antibiotics must be given but are adjunctive to surgical therapy (see Table 4). There is an associated mortality rate of up to 25 percent.

■ PULMONARY INFECTIONS

There appear to be two patterns of increased susceptibility to pneumonia in the diabetic patient. First, certain types of infections, including those caused by *S. aureus*, gram-negative bacteria, *Mycobacterium tuberculosis*, and certain fungal species, occur with an increased frequency. Second, common pulmonary infections may be poorly tolerated in diabetic patients. Diabetics are thought to be at increased risk for staphylococcal pneumonia because of a high rate of nasal carriage, which is directly related to the degree of glycemic control. Recent hospitalization, most likely related to poor metabolic control and serious debilitating illness, also predisposes the diabetic patient to staphylococcal pulmonary infection. The predisposition of the diabetic patient to the development of gram-negative pneumonia is also attributed to an increased rate of upper-airway colonization with these organisms. Tuberculosis occurs three times more frequently in diabetic patients than in nondiabetic patients, and the susceptibility to tuberculosis is related to the lack of glucose control. Diabetic patients also tend to have more advanced disease at the time of diagnosis and have an increased mortality rate. Although reactivation tuberculosis is classically found in the upper lobes, patients with diabetes more frequently have involvement of the lower lobes. Isoniazid prophylaxis should be considered in all diabetic patients with a positive tuberculin skin test, regardless of age, sex, and the absence of clinical manifestations. Finally, several fungal species can cause primary pneumonia in the diabetic. Predisposition to *Mucor* infection is attributed to the effects of acidosis and defects in macrophage phagocytosis. Although rare, both coccidioidomycosis and cryptococcal pneumonia occur more commonly in diabetic patients than in nondiabetic patients.

Aside from the specific organisms mentioned above, the causative organisms for pneumonia in the diabetic patient are similar to those that affect the general population. Certain of these, however, including *Streptococcus pneumoniae*, *Legionella*, and influenza, may be associated with increased morbidity and mortality in diabetic patients. When a patient presents with pneumonia, aggressive empiric antimicrobial therapy should be initiated as soon as possible (see Table 4). Failure of the infection to respond to conventional therapy should prompt examination for the more unusual pathogens discussed above. Antibody response to influenza and pneumococcal polysaccharide vaccines is not impaired in diabetes. Therefore, all diabetic individuals should be given influenza and pneumococcal vaccinations to provide partial protection against these common infections.

Suggested Reading

Eliopoulous, GM. Infections in diabetes mellitus. Infect Dis Clin North Am 1995; 9(1).

This issue consists of 12 chapters focusing on different aspects of infections in diabetes mellitus. Chapters contain comprehensive discussions concerning pathophysiology, clinical features, diagnostic procedures, and treatment.

File TM Jr, Tan TS. Infectious complications in diabetic patients. Curr Ther Endocrinol Metab 1994; 5:452–457.

This article provides a brief overview of the diagnosis and management of common and unusual infections associated with diabetes mellitus.

Pozolli P, Leslie RDG. Infections and diabetes: Mechanisms and prospects for prevention. Diabetic Med 1994; 11:935–941.

This article focuses on impaired host mechanisms that predispose the diabetic to infection and outlines strategies to minimize risk of infection in these patients.

Smitherman KO, Peacock JE. Infectious emergencies in patients with diabetes mellitus. Med Clin North Am 1995; 79:53–77.

This chapter is an excellent and concise presentation of some of the more unusual and acutely life-threatening infections associated with diabetes mellitus.

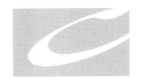

SPECIAL PROBLEMS

GESTATIONAL DIABETES

Marshall W. Carpenter, M.D.

Gestational diabetes mellitus (GDM) is defined as glucose intolerance identified during pregnancy. GDM was originally associated with diabetes subsequent to pregnancy. Increased perinatal mortality was later identified among affected pregnancies (O'Sullivan, 1973). Subsequent clinical investigation has identified an association between GDM and increased risk of perinatal mortality, macrosomia at birth, perinatal polycythemia and hyperinsulinemia, and neonatal hypoglycemia, hypocalcemia, and hyperbilirubinemia. The increase in birth weight and abnormal body composition that is more common among infants of GDM women increases the risk for birth trauma and particularly shoulder dystocia and Erb's palsy (impaction of the fetal shoulder under the maternal symphasis after delivery of the fetal head with occasional subsequent brachial plexus injury) in the infant and operative delivery in the mother.

Gestational diabetes mellitus may be a *forme fruste* of type 2 diabetes. Both diagnoses have been associated with abnormalities of first and second phase insulin response and of insulin sensitivity. The high prevalence of obesity found in GDM is also found in patients with type 2 diabetes. However, only 13 percent of GDM patients have glucose intolerance in the postpartum period, suggesting that GDM is not merely the identification of glucose intolerance present before the affected pregnancy.

■ DIAGNOSIS

The several diagnostic criteria used worldwide are primarily based on oral glucose tolerance tests. The National Diabetes Data Group (NDDG) criteria, in most common use in North America, are based on a 3-hour 100 g oral glucose tolerance test (Table 1). Gestational diabetes mellitus is reliably diagnosed at 24 to 28 weeks of pregnancy, by which time the normal development of insulin resistance, charac-

teristic of pregnancy, has developed. Only a small minority of patients having a normal glucose tolerance test at this gestational age will be found to have GDM later in pregnancy. The use of corticosteroids or betasympathomimetic drugs may suggest later retesting, however, since these drugs predispose to maternal hyperglycemia during pregnancy. We use criteria somewhat lower than those of the NDDG by taking into account both the present use of glucose oxidase methods and the use of plasma rather than the older Somogyi-Nelson method performed with whole blood. These lower thresholds are probably more consistent with O'Sullivan's original data.

■ DIET

Management of GDM is based primarily on dietary modification and standardization. We prescribe a diet consisting of 30 to 40 kcal per kilogram of ideal body weight, depending upon the activity of the individual woman. This is approximately 2,000 to 2,500 kcal per day. We recommend that the diet consist of approximately 100 g of protein per day, with the remaining calories evenly divided between fat and carbohydrate. The diet consists of three small meals and three snacks each day. The reduction in the amount of carbohydrate and calories ingested per meal reduces the glycemic response with each meal and thus reduces the probability that insulin therapy will be required. We find that dietary education and weekly reinforcement is associated with insulin treatment in 20 percent of subjects using weekly surveillance and our treatment thresholds.

■ GLUCOSE MONITORING

Sufficient surveillance of maternal glycemia can usually be accomplished by serial plasma glucose measurements in the laboratory on the day of their weekly outpatient department visit. We obtain fasting, 2-hour after breakfast, and 3:00–4:00 PM glucose concentrations on a whole blood sample run on a glucose analyzer or reflectance meter. Alternative surveillance may be accomplished by use of a glucose reflectance meter provided to the patient, which may be used more frequently as the clinical circumstances demand. Use of home glucose monitoring for diagnostic purposes is probably inappropriate given the wide coefficient of variation of results from most

Table 1 Criteria for 100 G Oral Glucose Tolerance Test in Pregnancy

TIME	MILLIGRAMS PER DECILITER OF GLUCOSE		
	O'SULLIVAN*	NDDG ADAPTION	CARPENTER ADAPTION
Preglucose	90	105	95
1 Hr	165	190	180
2 Hr	145	165	155
3 Hr	125	145	140

*O'Sullivan rounded $\times$ + 2 standard deviation values to nearest 5 mg/dl.
NDDG = National Diabetes Data Group.

meters. However, they have a high utility in patients whose surveillance needs to be more frequent in the home setting, because frequently sampled blood sugars in this environment may be more representative of the patient's usual glycemic control. Fasting levels greater than or equal to 100 mg per deciliter and postprandial values greater than or equal to 120 mg per deciliter measured 2 hours or later after meals require intervention. We generally begin treatment based on as little as one elevated glucose value if glucose tests have been performed only weekly, assuming that the patient's dietary compliance is best when glucose surveillance is taking place. Others have used reflectance meters to obtain multiple whole blood samples daily in GDM. Using the same glucose threshold criteria, approximately 50 percent of patients so monitored meet criteria for insulin therapy. Following this latter management plan, others have found no significant increase in fetal macrosomia incidence compared to nondiabetic pregnancies. Weekly glucose monitoring in our population results in a macrosomia rate of approximately 12 percent.

■ INSULIN

Insulin is begun at 20 U of neutral protamine Hagedorn (NPH) and 10 U of Regular given each morning before breakfast. The dose is increased 10 to 25 percent each day depending on the degree of maternal obesity until a euglycemic response is achieved, requiring daily or every-other-day glucose testing. This usually achieves a euglycemic response within a period of 1 to 2 weeks. Such aggressive management often avoids the need for hospitalization to achieve glycemic control. If the patient is identified as having significant glucose intolerance and hyperglycemia at a time when labor is thought imminent or when induction of labor is planned, hospitalization for glycemic control may be the most efficient method of achieving euglycemia.

We habitually use recombinant human insulin for treatment, but there is no evidence that using beef or pork insulin has any adverse effect on the pregnancy or the mother. An earlier randomized, controlled trial of insulin treatment during pregnancy in GDM suggests that subsequent diabetes, if it occurs, is likely to be less severe in patients treated with beef or pork insulin than in those treated with no insulin at all.

We do not use oral hypoglycemic agents during pregnancy because of the unknown transplacental pharmacokinetics of these agents. Because the sulfonylureas are known to cross the placenta, the potential for fetal hyperinsulinemia may be a contraindication to their use. Fetal hyperinsulinemia is probably the pathogenic mechanism for both fetal macrosomia and fetal hypoxia in diabetic pregnancy.

An alternative therapeutic intervention available for the reduction of fetal macrosomia is that of prophylactic insulin. Clinical trials of insulin prescribed to women with GDM have generally shown a significant reduction in rates of macrosomia compared to untreated and diet-treated groups. Generally, macrosomia rates in prophylactically treated groups of patients are in the 7 to 8 percent range.

Of the various treatment algorithms available, daily surveillance of patients and prophylactic treatment with insulin appear to be the most effective. However, they are complex and burdensome and require a high degree of patient cooperation and effort. Since all of the above treatment plans appear to avoid the incremental perinatal mortality associated with GDM, we consider any of them as adequate treatment during pregnancy. However, all our patients are advised to accept either increased surveillance or prophylactic insulin if this is a treatment option they find desirable, knowing that it will probably result in a modest decrease in their risk of fetal macrosomia and cesarean section.

■ FETAL SURVEILLANCE

Maternal GDM not only predisposes to fetal hyperinsulinemia and growth abnormalities, but may also result in fetal acidosis when associated with acute maternal hyperglycemia. Because absolutely consistent euglycemia cannot be maintained during a diabetic pregnancy, most writers suggest some form of fetal surveillance in addition to observation of maternal glycemia during the last few weeks of gestation. In the past, daily urinary estriol or weekly contraction stress tests were used for fetal surveillance. When these were coupled with careful surveillance of maternal glucose levels, perinatal mortality rates of approximately 19 per 1,000 were observed. Because of the logistical complexities of following urinary estriols and because they have not been shown to add information about the fetus independent from biophysical testing, this type of surveillance has been largely abandoned. Presently, weekly or twice weekly nonstress tests have been advocated as backup fetal surveillance. Neither weekly nor twice weekly fetal biophysical assessment has been adequately demonstrated to improve management of GDM, however. This is due to (1) the exceedingly low rates of perinatal mortality or requirements for acute intervention in these pregnancies when euglycemia is maintained and (2) the problems of segregating

Table 2 Criteria for Inducing Labor in Women with Gestational Diabetes

Poor patient compliance

Elevated maternal glucose concentrations not thought to be amenable to outpatient care

Other pregnancy complications, such as pregnancy-induced hypertension

Pregnancy duration greater than 42 weeks

Elective induction when the cervix is favorable and when fetal pulmonic maturity is assured

GDM from other comorbidities with which it is associated, such as pregnancy-induced or chronic hypertension.

Likewise, there is a limited consensus about the timing of delivery. Most authors do not suggest intervention for delivery until 40 weeks' gestation is reached. Generally we await spontaneous labor in patients with GDM. Aside from spontaneous labor, our criteria for delivering women with GDM are listed in Table 2.

Pregnancies complicated by GDM are often complicated by chronic hypertension. In these circumstances, when the cervix is favorable for induction, amniocentesis is often performed to document fetal pulmonic maturity before induction of labor.

■ MANAGEMENT OF LABOR

Generally during labor an intravenous solution of 5 percent dextrose is infused at 100 to 150 ml per hour. However, lactated Ringer's solution or normal saline should be used for fluid boluses to prevent fetal hyperinsulemia and acidosis. Blood or plasma glucose is monitored on a 1- to 2-hourly basis. Values greater than 100 mg per deciliter are treated with insulin by adding it to the intravenous solution in necessary concentrations while maintaining the same infusion rate. We attempt to maintain maternal glycemia between 80 and 100 mg per deciliter during labor. Often no insulin is needed during labor to maintain euglycemia despite large insulin requirements during the pregnancy. We estimate fetal weight by both the Leopold maneuver and sonographic evaluation within 2 weeks of parturition. Generally, no attempt at vaginal delivery is made if the estimated fetal weight is above

4,500 g because of the risk of fetal shoulder dystocia at the time of birth. There are no prospective data, however, to establish the "safe" threshold for estimated weight. The use of forceps or other means of operative vaginal delivery in mothers with GDM is controversial. Appropriately designed trials of forceps applications in these cases have not been performed. Our practice is generally to avoid all but outlet forceps deliveries in these cases, recognizing that such conservatism may be somewhat arbitrary and may not prevent shoulder dystocia in these clinical circumstances.

Suggested Reading

American Diabetes Association. Principles of nutrition and dietary recommendations for individuals with diabetes mellitus: 1979. Diabetes 1979; 28:1027.

A reference for dietary prescription including recommendations for pregnancy.

Coustan DR, Lewis SB. Insulin therapy for gestational diabetes. Obstet Gynecol 1978; 51:306.

A randomized, controlled trial of insulin therapy during pregnancy complicated by GDM.

O'Sullivan JB, Charles D, Mahan CM, Dandrow RV. Gestational diabetes and perinatal mortality rate. Am J Obstet Gynecol 1973; 116:901.

Early observation of the association between GDM and perinatal mortality. Earlier work referenced.

O'Sullivan JB, Mahan CM, Charles D, Dandrow RV. Medical treatment of the gestational diabetic. Obstet Gynecol 1974; 43:817.

A randomized, controlled trial of insulin therapy during pregnancy complicated by GDM.

Proceedings of the Third International Workshop-Conference on Gestational Diabetes Mellitus. Diabetes 1991; 40 (suppl 2): 1–201.

A synopsis of current information and opinion about the pathogenesis and perinatal effects of GDM.

Reece EA, Coustan DR. Diabetes mellitus in pregnancy: Principles and practice. New York: Churchill Livingstone, 1988.

A general discussion of the management of type 1 and 2 chronic diabetes and GDM during pregnancy.

TYPE 1 DIABETES MELLITUS IN PREGNANCY

Laurence A. Gavin, M.D., F.A.C.P., F.R.C.P.

Lynne Lyons, R.D., M.P.H., C.D.E.

John L. Kitzmiller, M.D.

Management of diabetes before and during pregnancy should be designed to preserve maternal health and secure optimal outcome for the child. The history of the development of such management over the years 1945 to 1990 has been reviewed previously. The major risks to maternal health are ketoacidosis, hypoglycemic coma, proliferative retinopathy, uncontrolled hypertension, and progressive nephropathy. Regarding the fetus, the degree of metabolic control of diabetes is associated with (1) spontaneous abortion, (2) congenital malformation, (3) excessive or insufficient growth, (4) delayed development of the alveolar surfactant system, and (5) hypoxia and asphyxia (stillbirth). The level of control of maternal diabetes is also associated with neonatal biochemical disorders and childhood development marked by obesity and poor performance on intelligence tests. Since perinatal risks of uncontrolled insulin-dependent diabetes mellitus (IDDM) (type 1 diabetes) and non–insulin-dependent diabetes mellitus (NIDDM) (type 2 diabetes) are equivalent, the goals and rationale of therapy for IDDM in pregnancy are the same as for NIDDM. This chapter focuses on the management of IDDM, but we also note the slight modifications of clinical management appropriate for NIDDM.

Since suboptimal control of diabetes at the beginning of pregnancy causes excess rates of spontaneous abortion and major congenital anomalies, intensive preconception care of diabetes is necessary to prevent these poor outcomes. This has been accomplished in several clinical trials. Therefore, we start by reviewing the elements of diabetes management to be applied before pregnancy so that disruptive changes in the treatment plan are not required in early gestation. Then we note adjustments in management appropriate to each stage of pregnancy (Fig. 1).

■ NUTRITIONAL MANAGEMENT

Dietary therapy is the keystone of management to prevent hyper- and hypoglycemia and ketosis. We define euglycemia as a premeal blood glucose of 60 to 100 mg per deciliter and postprandial peak blood glucose of 100 to 130 mg per deciliter. Without a consistent nutritional care plan, blood glucose fluctuations will be erratic despite intensive insulin therapy. The plan must accommodate the woman's food preferences and contain culturally appropriate foods. Recipes may have to be adapted, and the nutrient content of uncommon foods must be clarified, but this will enable the patient to integrate the diet plan into her life-style. Many diabetic women have had prior exposure to counting grams of carbohydrate to match doses of Regular insulin. It is not uncommon for a girl or woman to be given a diabetic diet plan at the time of diagnosis and subsequently receive little education and modification. This diet plan becomes obsolete with her changing needs.

Development of the nutritional care plan must be a collaborative effort between the patient, dietitian, and physicians. It is important that the woman begin the diabetic diet for pregnancy at least 3 months before conception. This allows time to adjust the diet and insulin regimen to achieve BG goals and also to integrate these changes into the life-style. This approach avoids the need to change eating habits in the critical early weeks of gestation, which could disrupt smooth glycemic control.

Some diabetic women seek to lose weight before pregnancy. Many weight loss diets, especially those under 1,200 calories per day, do not meet nutritional needs and may contain food or drinks that disrupt blood glucose control. People following restricted diets are more likely to develop or exacerbate some degree of disordered eating behavior, and women with diabetes are more likely to develop an eating disorder because of their many years of controlled diets and restricted foods. Therefore, it is very important for the diabetic woman to follow a nutritionally appropriate weight loss diet that has been designed specifically to meet her needs. In addition, attention must be given to the psychological issues regarding eating. Frequent medical follow-up is necessary to monitor the rate of weight loss and the need to adjust insulin; weight loss increases insulin sensitivity. Ideally, a woman should attain a weight in the 90 to 120 percent desirable body weight (DBW) range as part of the long-range prepregnancy planning process because underweight and overweight women have more pregnancy-related complications. Weight loss should be discontinued before planned conception.

The principles of the diabetic diet for pregnancy are listed in Table 1. The meal sizes are smaller than usual in an effort to limit carbohydrate and prevent hyperglycemia. It is important to eat meals and snacks at the same time each day because the insulin action is timed to match the effect of the carbohydrate intake. If it is not possible to eat at consistent times, the timed interval between meals and snacks must be maintained and the timing of the insulin must also be modified. Daily food records or a diet diary are essential in determining the cause of erratic blood glucose values, individual responses to certain foods, and reasons for weight changes and for monitoring adherence to the diet plan.

The diet differs from the typical diabetic diet in that it does not include fruit juices or foods that contain sucrose or honey. It is unrealistic to assume that the diet should be devoid of any type of dessert or sweetened food; therefore, foods that contain aspartame can be integrated into the diet plan. Foods with aspartame also contain carbohydrate. Aspartame-sweetened beverages are usually very low calorie and do not contain carbohydrate. Diet sodas can be used as a "free food." The carbohydrate content of the dessert must be substituted for a food with the same carbohydrate content. For example, ½ cup of sugar-free ice cream can be substituted for 1 starch exchange. Although the calorie and nutrients other than carbohydrate are not the same, this substitution should not affect blood glucose. If sugar-free desserts are

Table 1 Ten Principles of the Diabetic Diet for Pregnancy

1. The diet should contain 40–50% carbohydrate (majority complex carbohydrate), 20–25% protein (0.75 g/kg DBW + 10 g for pregnancy or a minimum of 60 g protein), 30–35% fat (majority mono- and polyunsaturated fat).

2. The diet should meet all the RDAs for vitamins and minerals except for iron needs during pregnancy. A 30 mg elemental iron supplement should be given during the second and third trimester or at any time anemia is diagnosed.

3. The daily diet should contain a minimum of the following exchanges: 5 protein, 3 milk, 5 starch, 2 vegetable (at least 1 folate source), 3 fruit (at least 1 vitamin C source), 3 fat.

4. The following food exchanges contain carbohydrate: 1 milk = 12 g, 1 starch = 15 g, 1 fruit = 15 g; 1 vegetable exchange contains 5 g but does not substantially affect glucose rises unless eaten in amounts >1½ cups.

5. Carbohydrate is distributed between 3 meals and at least 3 snacks (necessary to prevent hypoglycemia when insulin doses are targeted for normal BG excursions). Meals should contain 30–55 g, and snacks should contain 7–30 g. Snacks should not exceed 30 g in order to prevent between-meal or premeal hyperglycemia.

6. Meals and snacks are spaced at 2–3 hr intervals during the day. Middle-of-the night snacking is discouraged because it may increase fasting BG.

7. Meals and snacks are eaten at the same time each day to avoid wide variations in BG patterns.

8. The bedtime snack should contain 30 g carbohydrate and 7 g protein to buffer the effect of evening NPH insulin action.

9. If breakfast contains milk or >30 g carbohydrate, extra Regular insulin may be needed.

10. Sucrose, dextrose, purified fructose, honey, and fruit juice should be avoided to prevent hyperglycemia. These foods should only be used to treat hypoglycemia. Highly processed foods, such as cold breakfast cereals (even those without sugar), can contribute to hyperglycemia.

DBW = desirable body weight; *RDA* = recommended daily allowance; *BG* = blood glucose; *NPH* = neutral protamine Hagedorn.

Table 2 Estimating Energy Needs Before and During Pregnancy

DEFINITIONS USED IN THE NUTRITION CALCULATIONS

Basal energy expenditure (BEE) for women = 655 + [9.6 × DBW (kg)] + [1.7 × ht (cm)] − [4.7 × Age (yrs)]

DBW = Desirable body weight based on height according to the 1959 Metropolitan Life Insurance Tables

Activity factor (AF) = Bed rest, 1.2; ambulatory, 1.3; moderate exercise, 1.4

% DBW = (Actual BW ÷ DBW) × 100. If >125% DBW, use adjusted DBW for all calculations

Adjusted DBW = [(Actual BW−DBW) × .25] + DBW kcal = kilocalorie or simply calories

ESTIMATING ENERGY NEEDS BEFORE AND DURING PREGNANCY

1. BEE × AF
   +300 kcal for second and third trimester
   +500 kcal for breast-feeding
2. 25–35 kcal × DBW (kg)
   Range accounts for activity level, %DBW, phase of pregnancy
3. A broad estimate of kcal intake can be determined by use of a 24-hr diet recall or written diet record

eaten on a regular basis, the calories must be compensated for or excess weight gain will result.

Calculation on projected calorie needs can be deceivingly difficult. Refer to Table 2 for three methods of estimating energy needs. Determining the calorie needs of very overweight women (more than 135 percent DBW) can be the most challenging because many of the formulas utilize DBW as a basis for calorie needs. The larger the discrepancy between actual body weight and DBW, the greater the margin of error in the energy calculation. Therefore, it is necessary to modify the calculation by using an adjusted DBW, which increases the weight used in the energy formulas.

■ GLUCOSE MONITORING, CARBOHYDRATE COUNTING, AND INDIVIDUALIZED INSULIN THERAPY

The routine self-monitoring of blood glucose facilitates safe glycemic control. Diabetic women preparing for pregnancy can adjust their insulin dosage based on the pattern of premeal and postmeal blood glucose values observed over a few days. Most women benefit from the use of an individualized algorithm to titrate doses of premeal Regular insulin based on premeal capillary blood glucose values, carbohydrate intake, and anticipated level of activity and stress. By making decisions about diet, exercise, and insulin dosage, the patient assumes the major responsibility for the achievement of tight glucose control at home and in the workplace. In addition to improving perinatal outcome, the associated bonus of this approach is that patients are better educated about their diabetes and highly motivated in regard to good control. Consequently, hospitalization is reduced by avoiding complications, demonstrating the cost-effectiveness of our model of intensive outpatient care, education, and training provided by an integrated multidisciplinary group.

During the preconception period, women are trained to work for blood glucose targets that are important during the subsequent pregnancy. As noted, our targets are premeal values between 60 and 100 mg per deciliter and peak postprandial values between 100 and 130 mg per deciliter. Most women occasionally perform middle-of-the night tests to identify and prevent nocturnal hypoglycemia. Our patients self-test to determine if the peak postmeal blood glucose rise is at 60, 90, or 120 minutes. Targets were selected based on the glycemic thresholds for insufficient or excessive fetal growth and the fact that women using these targets and averaging well under 160 mg per deciliter during organogenesis had no excess spontaneous abortions or congenital malformations.

Basic considerations of glucose metabolism and insulin effects during pregnancy are outlined in Table 3. These serve as the basis for designing guidelines for the insulin treatment plan for pregnancy, including the use of algorithms for self-adjustment of Regular insulin doses. Fasting plasma glucose (FPG) is sustained by the insulin-mediated balance between hepatic glucose production (HGP) and peripheral glucose disposal (GDR). The postprandial blood glucose (PPBG) excursion demonstrates a relationship between the insulin

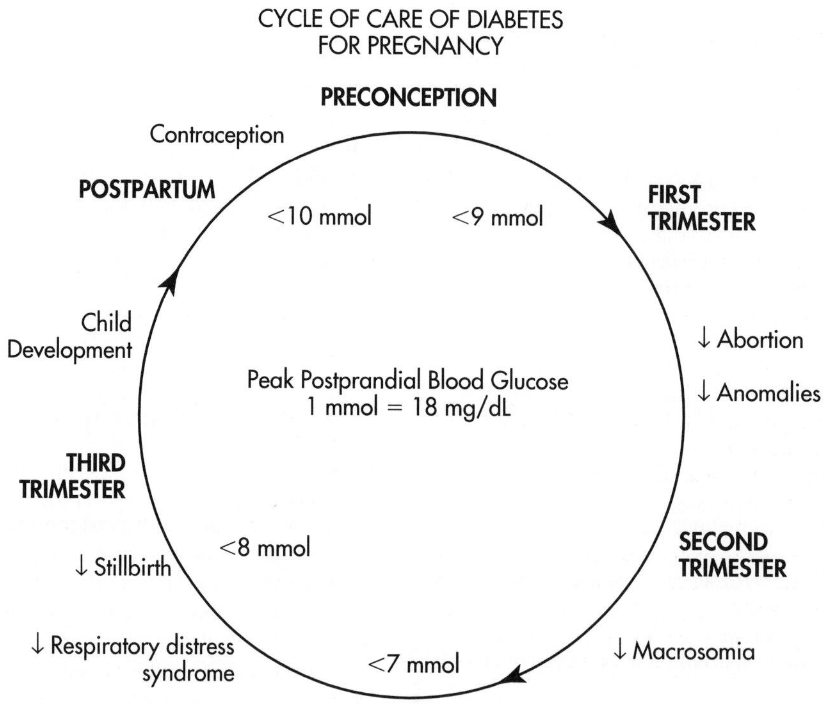

CYCLE OF CARE OF DIABETES
FOR PREGNANCY

PRECONCEPTION

Contraception

POSTPARTUM   **FIRST**
                                                                 TRIMESTER
        <10 mmol   <9 mmol

Child   ↓ Abortion
Development
                                                                ↓ Anomalies
               Peak Postprandial Blood Glucose
                    1 mmol = 18 mg/dL
THIRD
TRIMESTER

                        <8 mmol
↓ Stillbirth   **SECOND**
                                                                TRIMESTER

↓ Respiratory distress
     syndrome   <7 mmol   ↓ Macrosomia

Figure 1
Stages of management of diabetes for pregnancy. Postprandial blood glucose (PPBG) targets within the circle are associated with low risk of the perinatal complications noted outside the circle. Keeping PPBG under 10 mmol in the extended postpartum period allows the diabetic woman to prepare for the next pregnancy safely.

secretory response and the meal carbohydrate load. Generally, under normal fasting and postprandial states 1 U of insulin disposes about 5 to 10 g of blood glucose per hour (see A, B, Table 3). Insulin-sensitive (DBW under 90 percent) and resistant states (DBW over 135 percent, pregnancy, stress, steroids) increase and decrease this ratio, respectively. Applying this knowledge and understanding the glucose flux through a 15 L body glucose pool facilitates the estimation of a premeal bolus dose of Regular insulin, which is based on the meal carbohydrate content and the prevailing blood glucose level (see C, Table 3). However, it is important to individualize these general guidelines appropriately for each patient. Patients are taught how to estimate the carbohydrate content of foods in order to match the premeal doses of Regular insulin (see Table 1, Principle 4).

The total insulin dose may be initially calculated and divided as outlined in Table 4. The larger dose (2/3) is given before breakfast (neutral protamine Hagedorn [NPH] 2: Regular 1), and the smaller dose (approximately 1/3) is allocated before dinner (NPH 1:Regular 1). Many patients can achieve good control on two injections of mixed insulin daily before and during early pregnancy. Patients not controlled by this regimen may need Regular insulin before lunch and a modification of the morning NPH insulin. Should overnight hypoglycemia (from midnight to 4 AM) present a problem, the predinner NPH can be moved to bedtime (10 PM). This maneuver also helps to control fasting glucose in patients showing a significant dawn phenomenon. A great number of our patients progress to a more comprehensive intensive insulin regimen before or during pregnancy (see C,

Table 4). This approach facilitates insulin-food matching and a more effective implementation of the premeal dose adjustment based on an individualized algorithm for the prevailing blood glucose. Subsequent modifications of the bolus dose regimen are determined by the postmeal peak blood glucose and use of the premeal algorithm. In this manner the regimen can be continuously adjusted (usually weekly) as needed in preparation for pregnancy.

To avoid variability of insulin absorption due to exercising muscles, the site of insulin injection should be the abdomen. For timing of injections, patients should test their hypoglycemic response to the selected Regular insulin dosage after reasonable control has been achieved. The time needed to achieve a decrease of 30 mg per deciliter following insulin injection is used to advise the patient on the timing of her insulin dose before meals. In this manner a close matching of the peak of action of Regular insulin and the glycemic response to food intake can generally be achieved.

Follow-up visits to the office should occur frequently to provide the consultation, guidance, and emotional support needed to facilitate adherence to this comprehensive treatment plan. At each office visit the insulin dosage is readjusted according to the supplemental doses that have been required and the blood glucose response. In this manner the supplementary changes are generally small doses of either Regular or intermediate insulin and the control can be continually fine-tuned. This approach is very helpful during progression of the subsequent pregnancy because of the insulin resistance associated with placental hormones.

Table 3 Approximations of Glucose Insulin Metabolism in Pregnancy Used to Determine Regimen of Basal and Supplemented Bolus Insulin Doses

A. Fasting (HGP = 5–10 g/hr = GDR)
    FPG: 60–100 mg/dL
    Basal insulin: 5–10 µU/ml (~ 1 U/hr secretion rate)
    Therefore, 1 U insulin disposes 5–10 g of glucose/hr

B. Postprandial (glucose disposal time 2 hr)
    PPBG: 100–140 mg/dL (60 g glucose load)
    Postprandial insulin: 60–80 µU/ml (~ 6 U/hr
       secretion response)
    Therefore, 1 U insulin disposes 5–10 g of glucose/hr

    Therefore, the premeal bolus dose may be calculated for the
       meal carbohydrate content:
    1 U Regular insulin for every 5 g carbohydrate

C. Body glucose pool: ~ 15 L (VD)
    Total body glucose: ~15 g (FPG 100 mg/dL)
    Addition of 15 g glucose (steady state) would double BG
       (100 $\longrightarrow$ 200 mg/dL)
    However, insulin secretion (~ 3 U) controls BG response.
    Therefore, 1 U insulin modulates BG ~ 30 mg/dL (due to
       ~5 g/U GDR).
    Therefore, bolus dose adjustments as per the premeal BG
       may be calculated from BG actual − desired ÷ 30
       (e.g., 200 − 100 ÷ 30 = 3)
    Insulin algorithms are based on these facts.

HGP = hepatic glucose production; *GDR* = glucose disposal rate; *FPG* = fasting plasma glucose; *PPBG* = postprandial blood glucose; *VD* = volume distribution; *BG* = blood glucose.

Continuous subcutaneous infusion of Regular insulin by an external pump may benefit patients with large deviations from high to low capillary blood glucose despite sincere efforts at intensive conventional therapy. Patients selected for pump therapy are usually admitted for 3 to 4 days for education and blood glucose stabilization. Outpatients starting pump therapy must have daily office visits for training and a knowledgeable person to observe them at home. Assuming prior reasonable blood glucose control, we generally initiate therapy at the previous total insulin dose. Half the total dose is given as the basal rate, and the remainder is divided into 3 main premeal boluses. The basal rate is adjusted depending upon the 2:00 AM fasting, presupper, and 10:00 PM capillary blood glucose values. The premeal and peak postmeal blood glucose levels determine the magnitude of the premeal insulin boluses. The timing of the premeal bolus is tailored for each patient as indicated above. In general, the prebreakfast bolus is greater than for lunch or dinner. Many patients need small bolus doses before snacks, especially before bedtime. The majority of our patients trying pump therapy for pregnancy have been successful. However, any form of intensive insulin therapy is safe only when done by experienced personnel who can provide the necessary supervision and a rapid response to technical problems with the pump and infusion apparatus. Hypoglycemia is always a risk, and the rapid development of severe hyperglycemia and diabetic ketoacidosis with technique malfunctions can be very serious.

■ HYPOGLYCEMIA

Hypoglycemia remains a serious potential complication of tight diabetes control in women preparing for pregnancy. Many practical factors contribute to the increased risk of hypoglycemia in IDDM patients. These include variable meal and snack pattern, irregular and unplanned activity (exercise), infrequent and unreliable blood glucose monitoring, and occasionally excessive alcohol ingestion. In addition, variable absorption of insulin can lead to insulin-food mismatching and consequently hypoglycemia. During pregnancy, placental uptake of glucose also contributes to hypoglycemia in the postabsorptive state.

The potential for severe hypoglycemic episodes is magnified by the development of defective contraregulatory mechanisms with long-established diabetes. The acute phase hormonal response to hypoglycemia is manifested by an increase in serum glucagon and epinephrine. However, after about 5 years of established diabetes, glucagon secretion may be markedly impaired. In addition, many patients develop autonomic neuropathy after about 10 years of diabetes, and this is associated with an impairment of the epinephrine response. Consequently, insulin-induced hypoglycemia can be severe and, in the absence of these contraregulatory hormones, may be fatal. A relative epinephrine deficiency may also develop subsequent to intensive insulin therapy, even in the absence of clinical autonomic neuropathy. Strict diabetes control, especially during pregnancy, leads to a decrease in hypoglycemic warning symptoms. This response, which may develop only after a few weeks of tight control, has been well documented and is a major contributing factor to the development of hypoglycemic unawareness. There is an unfortunate association of strict control and paradoxically places the highly motivated patient at greater risk for severe hypoglycemia.

Because of the multiple factors that predispose a patient to hypoglycemia, prevention has become the fundamental aspect of management. Our team spends a good deal of time with each patient in order to re-emphasize the individual early warning features of impending hypoglycemia. Because many or our IDDM patients have developed autonomic neuropathy, they are devoid of the classic features of hypoglycemia, such as shakiness, diaphoresis, and palpitations. Therefore, it is critical for these patients to recognize the features of neuroglycopenia, such as paresthesias, lethargy, emotional lability, and confusion. In this manner, the patient can take corrective action to prevent a severe hypoglycemic episode. Our patients are advised that should the capillary blood glucose value be 50 mg per deciliter or less they should drink 4 oz of juice and recheck the blood glucose in 15 minutes. More juice may be needed if the blood glucose hasn't risen 20 mg per deciliter. The aim is to avoid overtreatment and rebound hyperglycemia. Table 5 lists the treatment measures we regularly review with all of our patients to reduce the prevalence of hypoglycemia associated with strict control.

As noted earlier, a number of patients in tight control programs may have hypoglycemic unawareness in the absence of autonomic neuropathy. In this potentially dangerous situation, glycemic control should be only moderately stringent. The best defense against hypoglycemia is the implementation

Table 4 Guidelines for Daily Insulin Dose

A. Calculate daily insulin needs

IDDM	Preconception	Pregnancy *
	0.5 U/kg DBW	0.7 U/kg DBW
NIDDM	If body weight >135% DBW (NIDDM and GDM), double calculated insulin dose	

B. Standard dose allocation: [0.7 U/kg DBW $\times$ (60 kg) = 42 U]

Prebreakfast $2/3$	Predinner $1/3$
(NPH:Regular = 2:1)	(NPH:Regular = 1:1)
18 N:9 R	7 N:7R

C. Intensive insulin regimen—bolus doses

B	L	D	HS
9 R	8 R	8 R	17 N

Relationship to meals: (35 kcal/kg = 2,100, 45% carbohydrate = 237 g)

B	(S)	L	(S)	D	(HS)
45 g	(22 g)	55 g	(30 g)	55 g	(30 g)

Carbohydrate:insulin

1:5	1:7	1:7

Bolus Dose Insulin Adjustment (BG algorithm)

Premeal BG	Regular
<60	(−) 3
60–80	(−) 2
81–100	Use bolus dose
101–130	(+) 1
131–160	(+) 2
161–190	(+) 3
191–220	(+) 4
>220	(+) 5

IDDM = insulin-dependent diabetes mellitus; DBW = desirable body weight; NIDDM = non–insulin-dependent diabetes mellitus; GDM = gestational diabetes mellitus; NPH = neutral protamine Hagedorn; Reg = Regular; B = breakfast; L = lunch; D = dinner; HS = bedtime; S = snack; BG = blood glucose.
*Second and third trimester

of a frequent SMBG program, strict attention to diet and exercise patterns, and detailed knowledge regarding the timing of the peak effects of the various insulin preparations.

■ EVALUATION OF COMPLICATIONS OF DIABETES FOR PREGNANCY

Retinopathy

All women should be referred for a diabetic retinal examination before pregnancy. Women with background diabetic retinopathy have a 5 to 10 percent chance of developing proliferative retinopathy during pregnancy. If neovascularization is present before or during early pregnancy, the majority of patients show marked progression during gestation. Therefore, patients with proliferative retinopathy should be stabilized by laser photocoagulation therapy before conception and treated aggressively if diagnosed during pregnancy.

Hypertension

In addition to poor glycemic control, one of the risk factors for progression of retinopathy is the presence of hypertension. Additional hazards of hypertension include worsening of renal function, poor fetal growth, and risk of stillbirth. For all these reasons it is important to evaluate and treat hypertension effectively prior to pregnancy. Patients with systolic or diastolic hypertension (140/90 mm Hg) perform home blood pressure monitoring. It is important to assess blood pressures during normal daily activities rather than just during stressful medical office visits. Data on optimal blood pressures for pregnancy are not so clear as for blood glucose. For nondiabetic pregnant women, diastolic pressures less than 100 mm Hg are thought to be satisfactory. However, studies of nonpregnant diabetic patients indicate that pressures greater than 135/85 mm Hg can be associated with a decline in renal function. Therefore, we use consistent pressures of 140/90 mm Hg as indicating the need for therapy. Methyldopa is the most commonly studied drug for relatively short-term treatment during gestation. Such therapy is not associated with abnormal child development, but it is often not well tolerated and is not effective over the long term. Diuretic therapy is contraindicated during pregnancy because the reduced plasma volume may impair uterine blood flow, so it is reserved for patients with very severe edema or congestive heart failure. Angiotensin converting enzyme therapy is contraindicated for pregnancy because of fetal effects. This is another argument for preconception evaluation and modification of therapy. Beta-blockers are unwise choices for diabetic women because of their effects on glycemic and lipid balance. Of the calcium channel blockers, nifedipine has been the best studied during pregnancy, but this drug increases proteinuria in diabetic patients, so perhaps diltiazem should be employed. Clonidine and the alpha$_2$ blocker prazosin are considered safe and effective during pregnancy.

Table 5 Strategies for Reducing Hypoglycemia

1. All patients must be taught appropriate treatment of hypoglycemia to prevent worsening of hypoglycemia or rebound hyperglycemia.
      If BG ≤ 50 mg/dl, take 4 oz of juice or 15 g of rapidly absorbed glucose (e.g., glucose gel or tablets). Re-test BG in 15 minutes. If BG hasn't risen 20 mg/dl, re-treat with 4 oz of juice or 15 g of glucose.
      If BG = 50–70 mg/dl, drink 8 oz milk or eat 1 fruit. Re-test BG in 15 minutes. If BG hasn't risen 20 mg/dl, re-treat with milk or fruit.
      If BG >70, eat meal or snack at the regularly scheduled time. If feeling of hypoglycemia persists, retest BG and treat accordingly.
2. SMBG pre-postprandial, 10:00 PM and 3:00 AM. Algorithms are provided to each patient with guidelines for premeal bolus dose adjustments.
3. It is critical that each patient have an adequate postprandial BG rise (20–40 mg/dl) and that the 3:00 AM BG be sustained above 60 mg/dl.
4. Educate patients individually to recognize early neuroglycopenic symptoms so that preventive measures can be implemented.
5. Emphasize the delayed effects of both alcohol and aggressive exercise, which may cause a decrease in BG levels, especially overnight and during the subsequent day.
6. Counsel patients regarding the need to always carry rapidly absorbed sugar, such as glucose tablets or gel, especially when driving.
7. Teach family members and colleagues at work the use of glucose gel and parenteral glucagon for the treatment of severe hypoglycemia.

BG = blood glucose; *SMBG* = self monitoring of blood glucose.

Diabetic Nephropathy

Women with diabetes have renal function evaluated prior to pregnancy. Urinary protein excretion, creatinine clearance, and serum creatinine and uric acid are measured, and the urine is cultured for bacteria. Elevated glomerular filtration rate (GFR) (hyperfiltration, creatinine clearance >120 ml per minute) is an indicator to improve glycemic control or reduce dietary protein intake to 1 g per kilogram per day. Diabetic women with microproteinuria (50 to 300 mg per 24 hours) should be informed that this warns of incipient diabetic nephropathy, but data are insufficient to predict the course of pregnancy. In most clinical studies, superimposed preeclampsia occurs in 10 to 20 percent of diabetic women with or without microproteinuria. However, women with macroproteinuria in the absence of urinary tract infection are counseled that (1) there is no evidence that pregnancy permanently worsens renal function unless hypertension is uncontrolled, (2) superimposed preeclampsia is quite common (30 to 50 percent) and can require preterm hospitalization and delivery, (3) severe anemia may require expensive treatment with erythropoitein, (4) hypertension and the degree of reduction of GFR predict the risk of fetal growth delay, hypoxia, and need for preterm delivery, but perinatal survival with diabetic nephropathy should exceed 95 percent, and (5) family members should know that women with clinical diabetic nephropathy are at some risk of renal failure or death from cardiovascular complications in the next 10 to 20 years of life.

Diabetic women with marked azotemia (serum creatinine greater than 2.0 mg per deciliter) are usually counseled to avoid pregnancy until after a successful renal transplant. Subsequent pregnancy does not increase the chance of transplant rejection or renal failure, and perinatal outcome is excellent, although superimposed preeclampsia occurs in 20 to 40 percent.

Planning for Pregnancy

Effective contraception should be used until glycemic excursions are almost all (80 percent) within 60 to 160 mg per deciliter, glycohemoglobin is near normal, and the patient is able to handle the treatment plan without much trouble. Low-dose sequential estrogen-progestin oral contraceptives are acceptable for nonsmoking diabetic women under age 35 because they do not affect carbohydrate and lipid profiles. Barrier methods are chosen by many patients, but recent studies show that new models of small progesterone or copper intrauterine devices are reasonably effective and safe in diabetic women. Subcutaneous implants of progestin are not appropriate for relatively short-term use in the preconception period.

Once the response to intensified diabetes management is acceptable, the diabetic woman and her partner can begin trying for pregnancy. At this point counseling may be useful regarding psychological relaxation for fertility in the face of the intensive, stressful monitoring protocols. Since the accurate timing of tests by gestational age is important during pregnancy, it is helpful if the diabetic woman uses basal body temperature (BBI) charting or other systems to indicate time of ovulation and early testing for urinary human chorionic gonadotrophin to diagnose pregnancy.

■ ADJUSTMENTS OF DIABETES MANAGEMENT DURING PREGNANCY

First Trimester

At present there is no conclusive evidence that pregnancy weight gain recommendations or recommended daily allowances (RDAs) for vitamins and minerals should differ for women with diabetes. Pregnancy weight gain recommendations should follow the National Academy of Sciences, Institute of Medicine guidelines (Table 6), which individualize weight gain based on prepregnant weight status. Excess weight gain can contribute to fetal macrosomia, which can also be the result of persistent hyperglycemia. Very overweight diabetic women who experience frequent hyperglycemia are at the highest risk of delivering a macrosomic infant. The calorie content of the diet should be adequate to promote weight gain in accordance with interval and total weight gain goals. The majority of vitamin and mineral requirements can be met by the diet, if well balanced. The only exception is iron. The RDA for iron in pregnancy is 30 mg. However, 3 oz of beef, one of the best sources of dietary iron, contains only 3 mg of iron. Therefore, 30 oz of meat would have to be eaten daily to meet the RDA for iron. Iron deficiency anemia is the most common anemia in pregnancy. A 30 mg elemental iron supplement is recommended for all pregnant women in the second and third trimesters, or earlier if anemia is diagnosed.

Table 6 Weight Gain Recommendations for Pregnancy

	WEEKS OF GESTATION		
	0–16	17–40	TOTALS
Underweight (<90% DBW)	4–10 lb net	4–5 lb/mo	28–40 lb
	1.8–4.5 kg	1.8–2.3 kg/mo	12.7–18.2 kg
Normal weight (90%–120% DBW)	4–6 lb net	2–5 lb/mo	25–35 lb
	1.8–2.7 kg	0.9–2.3 kg/mo	11–16 kg
Overweight (121%–135% DBW)	0–4 lb net	2–4 lb/mo	15–25 lb
	0–1.8 kg	0.9–1.8 kg/mo	6.8–11 kg
Very overweight (>135% DBW)	0 lb	2–3 lb/mo	15 lb
		0.9–1.4 kg/mo	6.8 kg

*1990 National Academy of Sciences, Institute of Medicine, recommendations.
DBW = desirable body weight.

Protein is a very important nutrient in pregnancy; it is used to build and maintain maternal and fetal tissues. Protein should make up 20 to 25 percent of the diet. Protein content can be adjusted in the case of diminished renal function. Even during moderate renal failure the protein intake is maintained at 0.75 g per kilogram of DBW plus 10 g for pregnancy, or a minimum of 60 g of protein. This should enable the woman to remain in nitrogen balance. The use of a protein catabolic test is most helpful in determining protein needs in a woman with renal failure.

At the very beginning of pregnancy, some well-regulated diabetic women notice a sudden increase in insulin requirements, perhaps related to increasing progesterone levels. During the first trimester, the diet should require only minor adjustment. The calorie level should stay relatively unchanged because only minimal weight gain is needed in the first trimester. There may be a marked tendency toward hypoglycemia at 8 to 14 weeks' gestation (fetal-placental uptake of glucose?), and insulin may need to be reduced. It is especially important to provide dietary carbohydrate every 2 to 3 hours as prevention.

The characteristic nausea and vomiting associated with the first trimester can create problems in maintaining adequate carbohydrate intake and preventing hypoglycemia and ketosis. Women affected by gastroparesis may have particular difficulty with nausea and vomiting throughout pregnancy, and use of metoclopramide during pregnancy may help. Women are instructed on the use of sick day rules for episodes of nausea and vomiting. The diet should continue to provide at least 15 to 30 g of carbohydrate every 2 to 3 hours during the day and adequate fluids to replace losses. Suggested sources of carbohydrate are bread, crackers, noodles, rice, milk, applesauce, and other soft fruit. Simple carbohydrates, such as juice or regular soda, should continue to be avoided unless treating hypoglycemia. Insulin doses may need to be reduced during acute periods of vomiting.

Second Trimester

Calorie intake will need to increase during the second and third trimesters to promote appropriate weight gain. If excess weight gain occurs at any time in pregnancy, the source of extra calories must be identified or the calorie level reduced. The rate of weight gain should be slowed to a minimum of 1 kg per month for the remainder of the pregnancy. It is not recommended that a woman lose weight at any point

during pregnancy or that she just maintain weight for more than 1 month during the last 20 weeks of pregnancy. Inadequate calorie intake or carbohydrate distribution can cause not only weight loss but also ketosis, which also can occur without weight loss.

Insulin requirements usually rise after 12 to 14 weeks' gestation, probably related to postreceptor insulin resistance, which is due to increasing blood levels of progesterone, human placental lactogen, and free cortisol (estrogen reduces its clearance). At the same time the risks of hypoglycemia in the postabsorptive state continue, so timely meals and snacks are still important. The insulin resistance and enhanced lipolysis and ketogenesis of pregnancy make ketoacidosis (DKA) more likely with insufficient or missed insulin doses or intercurrent infections. Rapid diagnosis and treatment of DKA is essential because there is a high possibility of fetal death.

Third Trimester

Many physicians have noted a smoothing of glycemic instability at 24 to 34 weeks' gestation in previously "brittle" diabetic women. It is unclear whether this is due to a "pregnancy-specific buffering effect" or just represents the influence of many weeks of careful attention to diet, exercise, and insulin administration by motivated patients. Late in pregnancy, after 35 weeks' gestation, there is often a substantial, gradual decline in insulin requirements. This should not be interpreted as placental failure.

Although this chapter concerns treatment of diabetes, it is important for physicians and diabetes educators to be well aware of obstetric issues in order to participate in integrated team management. The principles are outlined in Table 7. We must emphasize that aggressive insulin therapy (doubled doses or intravenous infusion of insulin) is necessary to counteract the pronounced hyperglycemic effects of beta adrenergic and corticoid drugs used to treat preterm labor.

Labor and Delivery

During the latent phase of labor, the patient can be maintained on a clear liquid diet (juice, jello, regular soda) that provides 15 to 30 g of simple carbohydrate every 2 to 3 hours. This is an especially important consideration if an insulin infusion is utilized. The additive effects of labor, oxytocin, and insulin can predispose to hypoglycemia. In the active phase of labor, we have found that sudden hyperglycemia associated

Table 7 Suggested Protocol for Laboratory Tests of IDDM and NIDDM During Pregnancy

TIME OF GESTATION	LOW RISK	HIGH RISK*
Baseline	Glycohemoglobin, CBC, TSH and free thyroid index, UA culture, 24-hour urine protein retinal exam	Same plus HDL, ECG
Every 4–8 weeks	Glycohemoglobin	Glycohemoglobin, CrCl, 24-hour protein
16 weeks	Serum alpha fetoprotein	Serum alpha fetoprotein
20 weeks	Fetal survey by ultrasound	Fetal survey by ultrasound
22 weeks		Fetal echocardiogram
25–28 weeks		Fetal growth by ultrasound, tests of fetal wellbeing,† repeated weekly
28–30 weeks	Fetal growth by ultrasound	
32 weeks	Tests of fetal wellbeing,† repeated weekly	
36 weeks		Tests of fetal wellbeing,† repeated daily
Before delivery	Fetal size by ultrasound	Amniocentesis

CBC = Complete blood count; TSH = thyroid-stimulating hormone; UA = Upper airway; CrCl = creatinine clearance; HDL = high-density lipoprotein; ECG = electrocardiogram.
*Definitions of high-risk categories:
    Baseline—Women at risk for coronary artery disease
    Every 4-8 weeks—Women with diabetic nephropathy
    22 weeks—Women with very elevated initial glycohemoglobin
    25–26 weeks—Women with hypertension or diabetic nephropathy
    36 weeks—Women with hyperglycemia or hypertension
†Tests of fetal wellbeing: Nonstress test, backup by contraction stress test and/or biophysical profile. All women should check fetal activity (≥4 movements/hr) three times daily after 26 weeks' gestation.

Table 8 Guidelines for Management of Intrapartum Regular Insulin Infusion

A. Check split specimen blood glucose (fasting or on admission)
B. Begin IV fluids as follows:
    Blood glucose > 130 mg/dL, LR @ 125 ml/hr
    Blood glucose <130 mg/dL, begin D5LR @ 125 ml/hr
C. Diet ("√"activates order)
    — NPO
    — Regular clear liquids (15–30 g CHO q 2–3 hr)/calories:
D. Initiating insulin infusion: Mix 250 U Regular insulin in 250 ml NS (1 U–1 ml)
E. Algorithm:

BLOOD GLUCOSE (MG/DL)	INSULIN (U/HR)	INDIVIDUALIZED DOSE
<70	0.0	
71–90	0.5	
91–110	1.0	
111–130	2.0	
131–150	3.0	
151–170	4.0	
171–190	5.0	
>190	Call MD, check urine ketones	

F. Monitoring insulin infusion:
    Call MD for blood glucose <70 and >110 mg/dL
    Check fingerstick glucose q 30 min × 2, then q 1 hr.

LR = lactated ringer; D5LR = 50% dextrose in lactated ringer; CHO = carbohydrate; NS = normal saline; MD = physician.

with pain or stress can usually be prevented by infusing small maintenance doses of regular insulin when the patient is normoglycemic. Our algorithm for fluid and insulin administration is given in Table 8. Maintaining normoglycemia until delivery decreases the likelihood of fetal hypoxia or neonatal hypoglycemia. If regional anesthesia is to be used for an oper-ative delivery, it is very important that nonglucose solutions be used for preanesthetic volume expansion.

Postpartum

Insulin needs are considerably less postpartum, and we gen-erally halve the pregnancy dose. The aim of therapy is to sustain the following ranges: Fasting blood glucose 80 to 120 and 2-hour postmeal blood glucose 120 to 180 mg per deciliter. Diabetic women generally revert to their prepregnant regimen or a new individualized regimen depending on needs. Following cesarean section these patients remain on the insulin infusion at half previous rates. Many NIDDM patients rapidly achieve blood glucose targets (under 140 mg per deciliter) and the insulin infusion is stopped. IDDM patients remain on the insulin infusion until food tolerance is established and are subsequently converted to a subcutaneous insulin regimen. All patients are seen at 3, 6, and 9 weeks after delivery for further care.

All women should be encouraged to breast-feed. The concentration of glucose in breast milk will rise with maternal hyperglycemia, but the amount is trivial in proportion to lactose. As always, precautions must be taken to avoid hypoglycemia. It continues to be important to eat at least 15 to 30 g of carbohydrate every 2 to 3 hours or after each feeding session. The patient may also require a snack in the middle of the night, after feeding. The nutrient and calorie requirements for breast-feeding women are similar to those of pregnancy; therefore, only minor modifications may be necessary to adapt the diet followed at the end of pregnancy to breast-feeding needs. Calories should be adjusted to promote weight loss to prepregnancy levels within 6 to 12 months. Although rapid postpartum weight loss is discouraged, if the woman is more than 120 percent of DBW, additional weight loss is recommended. The principles learned during pregnancy should provide new skills, enabling the patient to make informed decisions in diabetes management throughout her life.

Contraception for diabetic women was discussed above, under Planning for Pregnancy. During the extended postpartum period the health care team should maintain contact with potentially fertile diabetic women to ensure that glycemic control remains adequate in preparation for the next pregnancy.

Suggested Reading

Combs CA, Gunderson E, Kitzmiller JL, et al. Relation of fetal macrosomia to maternal postprandial glucose control during pregnancy. Diabetes Care, 1992; 15:1251–1257.

Coustan DR, Berkowitz RL, Hobbins JC. Tight metabolic control of overt diabetes in pregnancy. Am J Med 1980; 68:845–852.

Jovanovic L, Druzin M, Peterson C. Effect of euglycemia on the outcome of pregnancy in insulin-dependent diabetic women as compared with normal control subjects. Am J Med 1981; 71:921–927.

Jovanovic-Peterson L, Peterson C, Reed G, Metzger B, Mills J, Knopp R, Aarons J, National Institute of Child Health and Human Development—Diabetes in Early Pregnancy Study. Maternal postprandial glucose levels and infant birth weight: The diabetes in early pregnancy study. Am J Obstet Gynecol 1991; 164:103–111.

Kitzmiller JL. Sweet success with established diabetes: The development of insulin therapy and glycemic control for pregnancy. Diabetes Care, 1993; 16 (suppl 3): 107–121.

Kitzmiller JL, Brown ER, Phillippe M, et al. Diabetic nephropathy and perinatal outcome. Am J Obstet Gynecol 1981; 141:741–751.

Kitzmiller JL, Gavin LA, Gin GD, et al. Pre-conception care of diabetes: Glycemic control prevents congenital anomalies. JAMA 1991; 265:731–736.

Klein BEK, Moss SE, Klein R. Effects of pregnancy on the progression of diabetic retinopathy. Diabetes Care 1990; 13:34–40.

Landon MB, Gabbe SG. Fetal surveillance in the pregnancy complicated by diabetes mellitus. Clin Obstet Gynecol 1991; 34:535–543.

Maternal and Child Health Branch, Dept. of Health Services, State of California. Sweet Success, California diabetes and pregnancy program, guidelines for care. Campbell, CA: Education Program Associates, 1992.

Ney D, Hollingsworth DR: Nutritional management of pregnancy complicated by diabetes: Historical perspective. Diabetes Care 1981; 4:647–655.

Norton M, Buchanan T, Kitzmiller JL. The endocrine pancreas and maternal metabolism. In: Tulchinsky D, Little AB, eds. Maternal-fetal endocrinology. 2nd ed. Philadelphia: WB Saunders, 1994.

Reece EA, Coustan DR, Sherwin RS, et al. Does intensive glycemic control in diabetic pregnancies result in normalization of other metabolic fuels? Am J Obstet Gynecol 1991; 165:126–130.

Rizza R, Mandarino L, Gerich J. Dose response characteristics for effects of insulin production and utilization of glucose in man. Am J Physiol 1981; 240:E630.

Steel JM, Johnstone FD, Hepburn DA, Smith A. Can prepregnancy care of diabetic women reduce the risk of abnormal babies? BMJ 1990; 301:1070–1074.

Tamborlane WV, Amiel SA. Hypoglycemia in the treated diabetic patient. Endocrinol Metab Clin North Am 1992; 21:313–327.

INFANT OF THE DIABETIC MOTHER

Mark A. Sperling, M.D.
Ram K. Menon, M.D.

The fetus of a diabetic mother is provided in utero with a fuel mixture rich in nutrients such as glucose, amino acids, and ketones, whose concentrations may fluctuate widely depending on the mother's degree of metabolic control. With insulin-dependent diabetes, the maternal metabolic abnormalities exist from the time of conception and throughout the period of organogenesis and beyond. In gestational diabetes, maternal metabolism is altered mostly in the last half of gestation, sparing the critical period of organogenesis. Increasingly, evidence indicates that congenital malformations and other formerly classic pathophysiologic features (Table 1) of an infant born to a diabetic mother (IDM) are related to the degree of maternal metabolic control. When compounded by existing maternal vascular complications such as retinopathy, nephropathy, or pelvic vascular calcification, the fetal prognosis generally is worse. The incidence of congenital malformations is proportional to periconceptual maternal glycemic control, and the rate of congenital malformations in infants of diabetic women with meticulous metabolic control approaches that of normal women. Similarly, neonatal hypoglycemia after delivery is more likely to occur if the mother's glucose level remains high during labor, thereby facilitating a dramatic fall after cord cutting. Therefore, therapy of the IDM begins and remains crucially and intimately linked to the therapy of the mother until delivery. All diabetic women in their childbearing years should be advised of the potential impact of metabolic control on fetal outcome and should strive to maintain optimal metabolic control when planning pregnancy. Experience indicates that the best maternal and fetal outcomes occur in centers where teams of collaborating obstetricians, perinatologists, and neonatologists combine to provide care of the diabetic woman and her offspring before, during, and after pregnancy. In such centers, maternal and fetal mortality are similar to those in the general population, and the newborn infant may possess none of the typical stigmata formerly associated with an IDM. Following is an approach to anticipating and managing the common complications of an IDM in the chronologic order in which they are likely to occur (Table 2).

■ FETAL MALFORMATIONS

IDM have a two to three times higher incidence of congenital malformations than the general population. Although a variety of malformations can occur in IDM (Table 3), some,

---

Table 1 Stigmata of the Infant of a Diabetic Mother and Their Possible Causes

PROBLEM	MECHANISM/CAUSE
Fetal demise	Placental insufficiency
	Hyperglycemia
	Hypoxia?
Congenital malformations	Hyperglycemia?
	Genetic linkage?
	Insulin?
	Vascular accident?
Macrosomia	Hyperinsulinism
Hypoglycemia	Hyperinsulinism
	↓ Glucose and fat mobilization
Hyaline membrane disease (RDS type 1)	Insulin antagonism of surfactant synthesis
Wet lung syndrome (RDS type 2)	Cesarean section
Polycythemia	↑ Erythropoietin
	Fetal hypoxia
	HbA_{1c} − ↓ O_2 delivery to fetus?
Renal vein thrombosis	Polycythemia
	Dehydration
Hyperbilirubinemia	↑ Erythropoietic mass
	↑ Bilirubin production
	Immature hepatic conjugation?
	Oxytocin administration
Hypocalcemia	↓ Parathyroid hormone
	Hypomagnesemia
	↑ Calcitonin?
Neonatal small left colon syndrome	Immature GI motility
Cardiomyopathy	Septal hypertrophy

RDS = respiratory distress syndrome; *GI* = gastrointestinal.

like the caudal regression syndrome, are seen almost exclusively in IDM. Cardiomegaly, usually associated with septal hypertrophy and subaortic stenosis, is also common in IDM. The pathogenesis of these malformations is unclear; hyperglycemia, hypoglycemia, hyperinsulinemia, the polyol pathway, prostaglandin metabolism, and genetic factors have been implicated. Good metabolic control of maternal diabetes, however, decreases the incidence of these complications. Hence, meticulous metabolic control of diabetes during the preconception period and during pregnancy remains the primary and most effective mode of prevention. Fetal monitoring via ultrasonography, recommended as part of the management of pregnancy in diabetic women, may identify some of these complications antenatally, thereby alerting the management team to remediable or nonremediable defects in utero and the pediatrician to the need to administer emergency care at delivery. All IDM should be subjected to a meticulous physical examination at birth to detect the presence of any congenital malformations. Additional investigations such as echocardiography, ultrasonography, or radiologic examinations may be also be indicated, depending on the findings at physical examination.

■ MACROSOMIA

The IDM is typically macrosomic (birth weight more than 2 standard deviations above the mean for gestational age). Macrosomia represents the growth-promoting anabolic effects of insulin acting directly or through the genesis of local (autocrine-paracrine) growth factors, principally insulin-like growth factors (IGF) IGF-1 and IGF-II. Macrosomia is also a feature of hyperinsulinemic infants with nesidioblastosis-islet cell hyperplasia in the absence of excessive nutrient transfer stemming from maternal diabetes. Therefore, insulin is the predominantly responsible factor. Poor metabolic control (glycohemoglobin higher than 10 percent of total hemoglobin) during the second half of pregnancy is more likely to result in macrosomia, hence macrosomia may be anticipated and detected by ultrasonography. The consequences of macrosomia are a greater risk of birth trauma and injury from attempted vaginal delivery of a large infant.

■ BIRTH ASPHYXIA AND BIRTH INJURY

IDM have a higher incidence of fetal distress, which may present as birth asphyxia. Antenatal monitoring should identify the fetuses with distress, and the pediatrician should be

Table 2 Management of the Infant of a Diabetic Mother

PROBLEM	MANAGEMENT
DAY 1	
Congenital malformations	Early detection
	Supportive measures
	Specific corrective treatment
Birth asphyxia	Supportive measures (including ventilatory support)
Birth trauma	Early detection (clinical examination, radiographic studies)
	Specific and supportive measures
Macrosomia	Avoid birth trauma
Cardiomyopathy	Confirmation by echocardiography
	Supportive measures
Hypoglycemia	Intravenous glucose
	Rarely glucagon-epinephrine
Respiratory distress syndrome	Prevention (avoid prematurity, corticosteroids, surfactant therapy)
	Supportive and ventilatory therapy
DAYS 2 AND 3	
Hypocalcemia	Calcium and magnesium supplementation
Hyperbilirubinemia	Phototherapy
	Exchange transfusion
Polycythemia	Hydration
	Partial exchange transfusion
Renal vein thrombosis	Supportive measures
	Heparin?
	Nephrectomy?

Table 3 Congenital Malformations Occurring with Greater Than Normal Frequency in Infants of Diabetic Mothers

ANOMALY	RELATIVE RISK	ORGANOGENESIS (WEEK OF GESTATION)
Caudal regression	× 212	3
Situs inversus	× 42	4
Anencephaly	× 6	4
Spina bifida	× 3	4
Renal agenesis	× 5	5
Cystic kidney	× 5	5
Ureter duplex	× 5	5
Heart anomalies		
Transposition of great vessels	× 4	5
Ventricular septal defect	× 4	6
Atrial septal defect	× 4	6
Anal/rectal atresia	× 3	6

Adapted from Mills JL, Baker L, Goldman AS. Malformations in infants of diabetic mothers occur before the seventh gestational week. Implications for treatment. Diabetes 1979; 28:292–293; with permission.

prepared to administer the standard therapy (oxygen, endotracheal intubation) for birth asphyxia at delivery.

Macrosomia predisposes the IDM to birth injuries, especially during vaginal delivery. The use of forceps may compound the problem, even when used during cesarean section. Shoulder dystocia is the most common reason for birth trauma in these deliveries, with injury to the brachial plexus (Erb's palsy) and fractures of the clavicle or humerus being the most common injuries. This sequence of events may be prevented by reducing the chances of macrosomia via maintenance of normoglycemia during pregnancy, electing to deliver via cesarean section, and avoiding excessive traction on the fetus during delivery. Birth injury should be suspected if there is asymmetry of movements of the arms or of Moro's reflex. Clinical (presence of crepitus over the clavicle or humerus) and radiologic studies will confirm bone injuries, and a neurologic examination will confirm nerve injuries. Rarely, injury to the brain may result from a traumatic delivery, and ultrasonography and/or a cranial computed tomographic scan will be needed to diagnose these injuries.

Supportive treatment is the cornerstone of management of birth injuries. Immobilization during the acute period followed by physiotherapy is usually advocated for nerve injuries. Fractures of the upper extremities including the clavicle are treated by immobilization in an elastic binder or splint. Involvement of the central nervous system (CNS) may require evacuation of a subdural hematoma, but most CNS injuries are managed conservatively. Seizures resulting from CNS insult are managed with phenobarbitone and/or benzodiazepines. It should be noted that the absorption of resolving hematomas in the scalp or elsewhere may contribute to the presence of hyperbilirubinemia. When birth trauma and injury are present, consultation with a pediatric neurologist and orthopedic surgeon is recommended.

■ HYPOGLYCEMIA

Neonatal hypoglycemia in IDM results from fetal hyperinsulinism in response to maternal hyperglycemia and hyperaminoacidemia. In the past the consensus was that hypoglycemia should be diagnosed in a newborn if the blood glucose level was less than 30 mg per deciliter or less than 20 mg per deciliter in a preterm infant; corresponding plasma glucose values are 35 to 40 and 25 to 30 mg per deciliter, respectively. Recent studies have questioned the physiologic basis for assigning glucose values in the newborns that are different from those seen in older children and adults. The main concern expressed in these latest studies relates to the long-term neurologic effects of hypoglycemia and the levels of blood glucose at which these effects become manifest in the newborn. It is our opinion that in the absence of evidence to the contrary, it is advisable to accept that normal blood glucose levels in the newborn are the same as those found later in life. Based on this reasoning we recommend that the blood glucose level of 50 mg per deciliter be used as the cutoff between euglycemia and hypoglycemia in the newborn period.

The onset of hypoglycemia is usually 1 to 3 hours after birth. The major clinical manifestations of hypoglycemia are related to neuroglycopenia and include poor feeding, lethargy, jitteriness, and convulsions. However, hypoglycemia in newborns may also be asymptomatic, and it is mandatory that all IDM be monitored by blood-plasma glucose determinations during the first 12 to 24 hours of life. It is important to detect hypoglycemia even if it is asymptomatic because of the possibility of subtle neurologic damage and to avoid progression to frank clinical manifestations of hypoglycemia.

The primary mode of therapy for hypoglycemia is parenteral administration of glucose. Glucose is initially administered at a rate of 6 mg per kilogram per minute. The subsequent rate of infusion is titrated by the response in the rise of blood glucose concentrations. The route of administration is usually a peripheral vein, although in some infants difficulty in venous access may necessitate the administration of glucose via an umbilical venous catheter placed in the ductus venosus or the inferior vena cava. In extreme cases, or when easy venous access is not available, glucagon (50 μg per kilogram IV) and/or epinephrine (0.01 ml of 1:1000 dilution per kilogram per dose SC) have been used to stimulate glycogenolysis and the release of glucose from the glycogen surfeit liver. Rebound hypoglycemia in response to hyperglycemia caused by overenthusiastic treatment should be avoided. In this regard, the use of a continuous infusion of glucose makes it easier to prevent hyperglycemia, whereas the dose of a bolus of either glucagon or epinephrine is empirical and increases the chances of precipitating rebound hypoglycemia. The infant's cardiorespiratory status permitting, oral feeds can be initiated by 4 to 6 hours of age in the form of clear liquids (5 percent to 10 percent glucose in water) followed by formula feeding.

■ RESPIRATORY DISTRESS SYNDROME

Despite the large size of the IDM, many of their organ systems are functionally immature. Pulmonary immaturity predisposes these infants to hyaline membrane disease (type 1 respiratory distress syndrome [RDS]). Fetal hyperglycemia and/or fetal hyperinsulinism results in decreased surfactant phospholipid synthesis, which manifests as hyaline membrane disease. Modern therapy of hyaline membrane disease of IDM is mainly centered on prevention, which encompasses antenatal prediction of fetal lung maturity, pharmacologic acceleration of fetal lung maturation, and surfactant therapy. Antenatal prediction of fetal lung maturity is achieved by estimating the ratio of lecithin (phosphatidyl choline) to sphingomyelin (L:S ratio) in amniotic fluid. As the lung matures, the L:S ratio increases. A ratio greater than 2 predicts fetal lung maturity; a ratio of less than 1.5 is strongly indicative of pulmonary immaturity; and values between 1.5 and 2 are equivocal. However, in a diabetic pregnancy a L:S ratio greater than 2 may not always predict the absence of RDS, because phosphatidyl glycerol (PG) may be low. Testing for the presence of PG will indicate lung maturity in these instances.

Other tests are also of value in predicting fetal lung maturity, especially if used in conjunction with the L:S ratio test. These include measurement of the biparietal diameter of the fetal head by ultrasound examination to determine gestational age, thereby preventing an inadvertent early elective delivery. The knowledge that factors like glucocorticoids, thyroid hormones, epidermal growth factor, and cyclic adenosine monophosphate (AMP) enhance lung maturation has prompted the clinical use of some of these agents to facilitate antenatal fetal lung maturation. Of these, the most commonly used and the most widely studied agents are glucocorticoids. Glucocorticoids (such as dexamethasone or betamethasone) administered to the mother cross to the fetus and by enhancing RNA transcription increase protein synthesis, thereby improving lung maturity. The usual regimen is to administer dexamethasone or betamethasone (6 mg in 4 doses) to the mother at least 24 hours before delivery is anticipated. If parturition does not ensue within 7 days of glucocorticoid administration, the dose should be repeated if premature labor is again threatened. There is still some controversy regarding the efficacy and safety of glucocorticoids when used for this purpose, but we believe that used judiciously and appropriately, these agents can be of use in decreasing the problem of fetal pulmonary immaturity. Recently, surfactant preparations of either bovine or human origin, administered locally into the lung via an endotracheal tube, have been used to either prevent or decrease the severity of RDS. This strategy may become an established mode of treatment after the optimal dosage, timing, and frequency of administration are determined.

In IDM, milder and shorter lasting forms of RDS may occur without hyaline membrane disease. Wet lung syndrome as a result of retention of lung fluids following delivery via cesarean section (type 2 RDS), polycythemia, and hyperviscosity are the common causes of this syndrome.

The IDM at high risk for RDS or manifesting compromise of pulmonary function should be closely monitored by arterial blood gas measurements in addition to routine supportive monitoring. The level of intervention to be instituted depends primarily on the blood gas status and the amount of supplemental oxygen required by the infant to maintain a PaO_2 in the range of 45 to 75 mm Hg and a $PaCO_2$ between 35 and 45 mm Hg. The standard modes of ventilatory support, including continuous positive airway pressure and positive end expiratory pressure, as well as other supportive therapy should be initiated as indicated.

■ POLYCYTHEMIA

The plethoric appearance of the IDM is attributable to polycythemia, itself the result of (1) hyperinsulinemia and relative fetal hypoxia both stimulating fetal erythropoietin production and (2) placental transfusion via the umbilical cord at delivery. The former is influenced by metabolic control, especially in the second half of gestation; the latter is influenced by rapid cord clamping more readily accomplished via cesarean section. The consequences of polycythemia are the hyperviscosity syndrome, hyperbilirubinemia, and renal vein thrombosis. Polycythemia exists when the venous hematocrit is greater than 60 percent. A third of infants born to diabetic mothers may have a hematocrit in excess of 70 percent in the first hours of life. The signs are marked plethora, peripheral cyanosis, occasional pallor due to capillary sludging from hyperviscosity, and tachypnea and tachycardia from right-sided heart failure with evidence of cardiomegaly on chest radiography.

Jitteriness and seizures, sometimes associated with hypoglycemia, can also occur.

Management consists of reducing placental-fetal transfusion at birth by rapid cord clamping. When the signs and symptoms after birth are consistent with polycythemia and the hematocrit is 60 percent, adequate intravenous fluids should be provided. Such management often suffices in the presence of mild polycythemia (i.e., hematocrit no greater than 60 percent and in the presence of minimal symptoms). When the hematocrit exceeds 70 percent, partial exchange transfusion with plasma aiming to reduce the hematocrit to approximately 55 percent is generally recommended. If the infant is totally asymptomatic, exchange transfusion may not be indicated; clinical status rather than a laboratory finding should dictate the therapy. The formula used for partial exchange transfusion is as follows:

Volume of blood to be exchanged =

$$\frac{\text{Hematocrit} - 55}{\text{Hematocrit}} \times \text{Body weight (kg)} \times \text{Blood volume} \atop (80 \text{ ml/kg})$$

■ RENAL VEIN THROMBOSIS

Renal vein thrombosis, along with other organ thromboses, may be a manifestation of the hypercoagulable state resulting from polycythemia. Renal vein thrombosis is rare in infants of diabetic mothers and is usually unilateral, occurring on the second or third day of life. Its manifestations are fever, vomiting, and shock, associated with leucocytosis, thrombocytopenia, hematuria, and albuminuria. An irregularly enlarged kidney mass may be palpable. Modern imaging techniques such as magnetic resonance imaging (MRI) or computed tomography (CT) scan confirm the diagnosis. Formerly, unilateral nephrectomy was almost always recommended in the hope of preventing future renovascular hypertension, or nephrotic syndrome. However, conservative medical management employing the judicious use of fluids and electrolytes (depending on urine output) and antibiotics to avoid infection in the vascularly compromised kidney may result in complete recovery. The use of heparin has been recommended by some. The long-term prognosis is unknown. Re-establishment of the circulation or of collateral channels, documented by MRI, is a favorable prognostic sign. When complete infarction of a kidney has occurred, surgical removal is generally recommended.

■ HYPERBILIRUBINEMIA

Hyperbilirubinemia may represent the convergence of several factors: prematurity and hence incomplete glucuronyl transferase activity, absorption of hematomas, delayed feeding causing increased enterohepatic circulation of unconjugated bilirubin, and increased breakdown of blood resulting from polycythemia itself. Treatment consists of fluids or oral feedings with glucose to decrease enterohepatic circulation and to ensure adequate hydration. As outlined above, partial plasma exchange to decrease the hematocrit level may be helpful to decrease hyperbilirubinemia.

■ HYPOCALCEMIA AND HYPOMAGNESEMIA

Neonatal hypocalcemia with a serum calcium concentration of less than 7 mg per deciliter is common in IDM. The factors responsible include prematurity, birth asphyxia, and maternal magnesium deficiency consequent on excessive urinary magnesium losses in the mother, which are much more likely to occur with poorly controlled diabetes. The resultant magnesium deficiency in the infant may limit the initial parathyroid hormone response observed in normal infants after interruption of the maternal calcium supply. In IDM, serum calcium concentrations are lowest 24 to 72 hours after birth. Total and ionized calcium are both decreased, whereas serum phosphorus levels are increased. Hypomagnesemia may not be apparent from examination of serum magnesium levels, because magnesium is largely an intracellular ion.

Treatment of the newborn with established hypocalcemia involves oral supplements with 10 percent calcium gluconate given three to four times daily to supply 50 to 75 mg of elemental calcium per kilogram per day. Serum calcium levels should be monitored at 24-hour intervals commencing with day 2 of life. Serum calcium should be maintained at 7 mg per deciliter or greater. When serum concentrations of calcium remain at 7 mg per deciliter or higher, supplemental calcium can be halved and eventually discontinued. Intravenous calcium gluconate as a 10 percent solution is also indicated in the symptomatic patient, especially during a hypocalcemic seizure. When administering calcium intravenously, caution should be taken not to give it too rapidly in order to avoid bradycardia. In addition, extreme caution should be taken in administering calcium gluconate intravenously because its extravasation can cause skin sloughing. With a well-established intravenous line, calcium gluconate can be added to a 12-hour infusion. Calcium concentrations tend to stabilize by the third to fourth day of life.

Suggested Reading

Freinkel N. Of pregnancy and progeny: Banting lecture 1980. Diabetes 1980; 29:1023–1035.

Freinkel N, Dooley SL, Metzger BE. Care of the pregnant woman with insulin-dependent diabetes mellitus. N Engl J Med 1985; 313:96–101.

These classic papers encapsulate the elucidation of the hormonal adaptations and resultant metabolic changes of normal pregnancy as well as their predictable impact on the diabetic woman and her offspring, setting the stage for rational therapy.

Infant of the diabetic mother: Report of the Ross Conference on Pediatric Research, Nov 1987.

Thoughts by some leading educators in the field of neonatal research on the causes, prevention, and treatment of the infant of the diabetic mother.

Kitzmiller FL, Gavin LA, Gin GD et al. Preconception care of diabetes: Glycemic control prevents congenital anomalies. JAMA 1991; 265:731–736.

The evidence strongly implicating preconceptual metabolic control and the incidence of congenital malformations is reviewed by leading authorities.

Menon RK, Cohen RM, Sperling MA, et al. Transplacental passage of insulin in pregnant women with insulin dependent diabetes mellitus: Its role in fetal macrosomia. N Engl J Med 1990; 323:309–315.

A current overview of the role of insulin in fetal macrosomia and some other complications in the infant of the diabetic mother.

Metzger BE, Buchanan TA. Diabetes and birth defects: Insights from the 1980's, prevention in the 1990's. Diabetes Spectrum 1990; 3:149–184.

Miodovnik M, Mimouni F, Tsang RC, et al. Management of the insulin dependent diabetic during labor and delivery: Influence on neonatal outcome. Am J Perinatol 1987; 4:106–114.

Reller MD, Tsang RC, Meyer RA, et al. Relationship of prospective diabetes control in pregnancy to neonatal cardiorespiratory function. J Pediatr 1985; 106:86–90.

Weber HS, Copel JA, Reece EA, et al. Cardiac growth in fetuses of diabetic mothers with good metabolic control. J Pediatr 1991; 118:103–107.

The above four articles review the impact of prospective and immediate antenatal maternal management on neonatal outcome measures. They emphasize the intricate relationship between metabolic control of the diabetic mother and reduction of the known complications in her offspring.

GENETIC COUNSELING

Leslie J. Raffel, M.D.
Carrie Garber, M.S.
Jerome I. Rotter, M.D.

It has been appreciated for many years that diabetes mellitus is, to a great extent, caused by inherited susceptibility to glucose intolerance. Until recently, however, the details of this genetic susceptibility have been confusing, making it difficult to apply the information in a clinically useful manner. Over the past two decades, knowledge regarding the interpretation of familial patterns of diabetes has improved significantly, and some of the genes directly involved in diabetes have been identified. Therefore, it is now possible to provide meaningful genetic counseling to patients with diabetes and their families. In this chapter, methods of providing accurate, supportive, and nondirective genetic counseling services are discussed.

■ DIABETES MELLITUS IS GENETICALLY HETEROGENEOUS

One of the reasons it has been difficult to elucidate the role of specific genes in diabetes susceptibility is that diabetes is not a single disorder but rather a group of disorders, all of which result in glucose intolerance. It has therefore been necessary to develop ways of subdividing diabetes into separate categories of disease. This is a process that is by no means complete; much more research is necessary before we know how many discrete genetic entities produce the clinical picture of diabetes. Great progress has been made in this classification, however, and it is now generally accepted that diabetes can be divided into at least three broad categories: (1) insulin-dependent diabetes mellitus (IDDM), type 1 diabetes; (2) non–insulin-dependent diabetes mellitus (NIDDM), type 2 diabetes; and (3) diabetes associated with genetic syndromes and other conditions.

Genetics of Insulin-Dependent Diabetes

Following the appreciation that IDDM was separate from NIDDM, knowledge regarding the genes responsible for susceptibility to IDDM was greatly advanced by the identification of associations between IDDM and alleles of the major histocompatibility region (human leucocyte antigen [HLA]) on chromosome 6. In initial studies of class I loci, associations were found with two B locus alleles, B8 and B15. Subsequently, when typing for the HLA-D region became available, it was found that the association between IDDM and the HLA region was actually stronger with the alleles DR3 and DR4. The explanation for this finding is that the genes in the HLA region are physically very close to each other and tend to be inherited as a unit, a phenomenon called linkage disequilibrium. Therefore, HLA B8 often occurs together with DR3, and B15 often occurs with DR4.

As more has been learned about the molecular genetic organization of the HLA region, questions have been raised about the mechanism by which IDDM predisposition is mediated. The HLA-D region has turned out to be much more complex than originally supposed. This portion of the HLA region encodes a group of membrane-associated proteins known as the class II molecules. The products of this region have been subdivided into at least three different proteins (DR, DQ, and DP), and each of these is encoded by independent loci for an alpha chain and a beta chain. Variations in the sequence of the DQ beta gene seem to be most closely associated with IDDM risk (at least for IDDM associated with DR4), with nucleotide sequences encoding an amino acid other than aspartic acid at position 57 in the DQ beta chain conferring risk. When this finding was initially reported in 1987 to 1988, it was hoped that the actual mutation accounting for IDDM susceptibility had been identified. Numerous exceptions to this relationship have been found, however, indicating that the mechanism by which the HLA region results in IDDM susceptibility is still unclear. There is evidence that in particular haplotypes, other loci (e.g. DQ alpha, DR beta and DP beta) contribute to susceptibility, suggesting that a combination of genes is important.

Given current appreciation of the autoimmune nature of IDDM, the presence of genetic susceptibility loci within the HLA region is not surprising. Importantly, studies of relatives of IDDM patients who are at high risk for developing diabetes have demonstrated that the autoimmune process begins months to years before the development of overt diabetes, as evidenced by the presence of islet cell autoantibodies and/or insulin autoantibodies. As discussed later in more detail, this offers the possibility of attempting to prevent the development of overt diabetes through the use of immunosuppressive therapy in the preclinical phase, assuming that high-risk individuals can be reliably identified.

Evidence has also accumulated in recent years to suggest that other genes, besides those in the HLA region on chromosome 6, also play a role in IDDM susceptibility. The HLA region clearly accounts for the majority of genetic predisposition (possibly as high as 60 to 70 percent), but other genes appear to contribute as well. Several gene regions have been suggested; at present the best evidence exists for the insulin gene region on chromosome 11p, and loci on chromosomes 2q33, 6q25, 6q27, and 11q13. Further work is necessary to elucidate the roles that these loci, as well as other possible genetic regions, have in IDDM.

Genetics of Non–Insulin-Dependent Diabetes

In spite of the fact that NIDDM is clearly inherited, our understanding of the specific genes responsible remains poor. A number of candidate genes have been evaluated, but none have been identified that appear to account for much, if any, of the genetic susceptibility to NIDDM. Specific genetic defects have been found that explain rare cases of NIDDM. For example, point mutations within the insulin gene have been identified in a small number of individuals with severe hyperinsulinemia and/or hyperproinsulinemia. Even within the families of such patients, however, other individuals have been shown to have the same mutation and yet not have diabetes, suggesting that other factors, either genetic or environmental, must be required to generate clinically overt glucose intolerance. The failure to identify the responsible genes in the majority of cases of NIDDM has been extremely frustrating but developments within the last several years suggest that the prospects for the future are better. One subclass of NIDDM, known as maturity onset diabetes of the young as maturity onset diabetes of the young (MODY), has recently been shown to result from mutations in one of three genes; the glucokinase gene on chromosome 7, the hepatocyte nuclear factor-1 alpha gene on chromosome 12, and the hepatocyte nuclear factor-4 alpha gene on chromosome 20. Although results in MODY cannot necessarily be extrapolated to the more typical cases of NIDDM, the success in MODY suggests that susceptibility genes can be found when the clinical disease entity is adequately defined.

Single Gene Disorders Associated with Diabetes

The single gene (Mendelian) disorders that have glucose intolerance as a component account for only a small percentage of diabetes cases (Table 1). It is important to keep these conditions in mind, however, when evaluating a newly diagnosed diabetic patient. Because their inheritance patterns are clearly defined, accurate recurrence risk figures can be provided. Additionally, because these disorders often have other significant complications, accurate diagnosis is important in providing optimal medical care.

■ RECOMMENDATIONS FOR GENETIC COUNSELING AND SCREENING

It is important that diabetic individuals and their families be made aware of the familial nature of glucose intolerance. Unfortunately, this is a topic that is all too often avoided, in part because many physicians fear they will raise anxieties unnecessarily. It has been our experience that families are often already aware that diabetes has a genetic basis, and rather than heightening anxiety by discussing the details, it is frequently possible to allay fears by putting the information in proper perspective.

Process of Genetic Counseling

Genetic counseling is the process by which individuals are given information regarding the inheritance, nature, natural history, and risk of recurrence of a disease entity and are also assisted in understanding the information and coping with their situation. Counseling is often a team effort; physicians, nurses, social workers, and genetic associates all contribute to

Table 1 Examples of Genetic Syndromes Associated with Glucose Intolerance and Diabetes Mellitus

	TYPES OF DIABETES	ASSOCIATED FEATURES
AUTOSOMAL RECESSIVE INHERITANCE		
Cystic fibrosis	IDDM	Chronic respiratory disease, malabsorption
Hemochromatosis	NIDDM	Iron overload producing cirrhosis, cardiac failure, bronze skin, endocrine abnormalities
Isolated growth hormone deficiency	NIDDM	Proportionate dwarfism
Leprechaunism	NIDDM	Failure to thrive, mental retardation, facial dysmorphology, hirsutism, genital hypertrophy
AUTOSOMAL DOMINANT INHERITANCE		
Myotonic dystrophy	NIDDM	Myotonia, cataracts, balding, testicular atrophy
Multiple endocrine neoplasia	IGT → NIDDM	Pituitary, parathyroid, adrenal, pancreatic adenomas; Zollinger-Ellison syndrome
Hereditary relapsing pancreatitis	IGT → IDDM	Abdominal pain, chronic pancreatitis
X-LINKED RECESSIVE INHERITANCE		
Duchenne muscular dystrophy	NIDDM	Progressive muscular weakness, mental retardation
CHROMOSOMAL DISORDERS		
Turner syndrome	NIDDM	Short stature, gonadal dysgenesis, congenital lymphedema, neck webbing
Klinefelter syndrome	NIDDM	Hypogonadism, gynecomastia, tall stature

IDDM = insulin-dependent diabetes mellitus; *NIDDM* = non–insulin-dependent diabetes mellitus; *IGT* = impaired glucose tolerance.

the counseling process. In this chapter, the term "genetic counselor" refers to any health care professional who is providing genetic counseling.

Family History

One of the most important aspects of genetic counseling is obtaining a family history. The easiest way to document the family history is to construct a pedigree using standard symbols, which are shown in Figure 1. Constructing a pedigree is important not only to learn whether other family members are similarly affected, but also to ensure that no other genetic conditions exist. In most instances, asking questions regarding the health of the patient's first-degree (parents, siblings, and children), second-degree (grandparents, grandchildren, aunts, and uncles), and third-degree (first cousins) relatives is sufficient, except when an unusual disorder is clearly being transmitted in a family. Unless you are speaking with a very good family historian, extending the pedigree beyond these individuals is often not very useful, because the information obtained is likely to be inaccurate. For families of diabetic patients, the pertinent information to obtain on each individual is current age and general health status. For any family members who have diabetes, it is also necessary to obtain the age at diagnosis, the initial type of treatment, current therapy, and what complications if any have arisen. Because individuals with IDDM and their relatives are also at increased risk for other autoimmune disorders, such as autoimmune thyroid disease and pernicious anemia, asking specific questions

regarding these conditions is also indicated. Figure 2 gives an example of a pedigree of a child with IDDM.

An accurate diagnosis is essential in order to provide accurate genetic counseling. Whenever possible, it is helpful to confirm information regarding the patient and patient's relatives by obtaining medical records or by examining family members. Useful medical records are those pertaining to diagnostic tests, pathology reports, autopsy reports, and death certificates. Occasionally, obtaining medical records takes herculean effort. However, verifying that a relative was or was not affected with a particular disorder can make a large difference in determining recurrence risks.

Once a diagnosis is made or confirmed, the genetic counselor can assist the patient and/or the family to understand the implications of the disorder. This includes discussion of the inheritance pattern, recurrence risks, prognosis, and the risk of possible complications. The discussion about risks involves the concept of probability, which may be a difficult concept for some individuals. Each person perceives risk uniquely; previous experiences color our views. The genetic counselor's role is to promote an understanding of the probabilities and to present an accurate picture of severity, one that is neither too glum nor too bright.

When the inheritance of a disorder is complex (i.e., non-Mendelian) and our knowledge of the specific genes involved is limited—both of which are true for diabetes—we must rely on empiric data to estimate the risk of recurrence (Table 2). These are risks that have been compiled

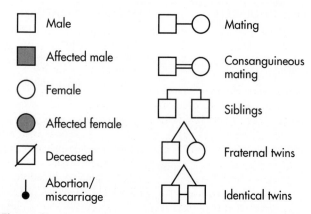

Figure 1
Symbols commonly used in drawing pedigrees.

Table 2 Risks for Developing Diabetes	
INSULIN–DEPENDENT DIABETES (IDDM)	
General population	1/500
Sibling of IDDM patient	1/10–1/20
Offspring of IDDM patient	1/20–1/50
Mother has IDDM	1/30–1/50
Father has IDDM	1/15–1/25
NON–INSULIN-DEPENDENT DIABETES (NIDDM)	
General population	1/20–1/40
First-degree relative of NIDDM	1/7–1/10
MATURITY ONSET DIABETES OF YOUTH (MODY)	
General population	<1/500
First-degree relative of MODY	1/2

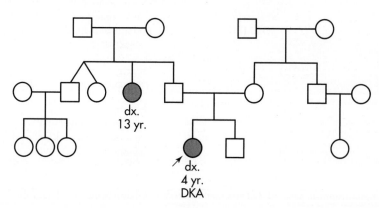

Figure 2
Pedigree of a family with two members who have insulin-dependent diabetes mellitus. The proband (index case) is denoted by the arrow.

from large family population studies. Empiric risks may not be universal in their application but may vary depending upon ethnic background, gender of the affected individual and the individual at risk, and the number of affected family members. In general, the risk is greatest among close relatives and decreases progressively for more distant relatives. The empiric risks may be modified by obtaining additional information, such as HLA typing, for the relatives of an individual with IDDM.

Psychosocial Aspects of Genetic Counseling

Perhaps the most overlooked part of genetic counseling is the psychosocial aspect. Every genetic condition creates a burden for affected individuals and their families. The burden includes practical issues, such as financial problems, but also psychological and social problems. When a child is diagnosed with a genetic disease, the parents often feel guilt for having contributed the "defective" genes to their son or daughter. One parent may feel more responsible; occasionally one parent blames the other. Parents may also grieve the loss of their "normal" child. The needs of the siblings of a child with a genetic condition must also be addressed; the attention focused on the affected child may cause the unaffected siblings to feel neglected. They may also feel guilty for being normal or because they imagine that something they did or thought caused the disorder. The affected individual may have low self-esteem due to feelings of being defective. In the case of a condition such as IDDM, the insulin injections mean that affected individuals are different from most of their peers. This feeling of difference can be especially pronounced during adolescence when the desire to fit in is very strong. Raising such possibilities directly in discussion with the family is important. They often will not tell you of their feelings unless you ask. A sensitive and empathetic genetic counselor can help individuals and their families to recognize and understand their feelings, thereby facilitating the

coping and adaptation processes. When necessary, referrals can be made to outside agencies, such as support groups.

It is widely accepted that genetic counseling should be provided in a nondirective manner, particularly when discussing options related to childbearing. The individual and/or family should be given all the pertinent information, and the various options should be presented to them. The individual and family are then encouraged to make the decisions with which they are most comfortable rather than being told what to do. Help can be provided in a number of ways; for example, by comparing and contrasting different situations and discussing potential short- and long-term consequences of each option. Once it becomes clear that a decision has been reached by the family, the role of the genetic counselor is to support that decision. If health care professionals give patients and their families the impression that they disagree with options chosen by the family, it only serves to alienate the family from the medical profession and to reduce communication and ultimately compliance with other aspects of patient care.

Counseling in Insulin-Dependent Diabetes

The empiric recurrence risk for the siblings of an individual with IDDM is approximately 5 to 10 percent. This risk estimate can be modified by determining HLA haplotypes within a family. Studies of families with two or more children affected with IDDM have demonstrated that the diabetic children are more likely to have inherited the same HLA regions (haplotypes) from their parents than would be expected by chance alone. As is demonstrated in Figure 3, in general any two siblings share both HLA haplotypes 25 percent of the time, one haplotype 50 percent of the time, and neither 25 percent of the time. Diabetic siblings, however, are much more likely to share one or both HLA haplotypes and rarely inherit different haplotypes from both parents. It is therefore possible to determine the siblings' risk of developing IDDM more precisely by comparing their HLA haplotypes with their diabetic sibling's. The general 5 to 10 percent recurrence risk is modified upward to 12 to 24 percent for those who are HLA identical, down to 5 to 7 percent for those sharing one haplotype, and down further to 1 to 2 percent for those sharing neither HLA haplotype. Even further risk refinement can be provided depending upon which HLA DR types the siblings share. If the index diabetic sibling is a DR3/DR4 compound heterozygote (i.e., has both high-risk alleles), his or her HLA-identical sibling may have a risk as high as 25 percent of becoming diabetic as well.

There is some question about whether this information is beneficial to most families. Until recently our group was recommending against HLA typing for clinical counseling purposes (as opposed to research purposes), because of the expense involved and the fact that no intervention was possible. Although HLA typing has the potential to diminish anxiety for those who are found to be at lower risk, those who are HLA identical to a diabetic sibling may have their anxiety level increased without being offered any options for reducing their risk. We have also been concerned about possible stigmatization of the high-risk sibling, with the potential that parents and grandparents may prevent a child from playing normally with other children, fearful that he or she may be exposed to viral infections that could precipitate the onset of

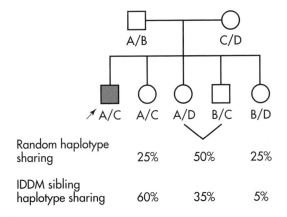

Figure 3

HLA haplotype sharing in siblings with insulin-dependent diabetes mellitus. The random probability of two siblings inheriting 2, 1, or 0 parental haplotypes (A, B, C, D) in common is 25%, 50%, and 25%, respectively. As shown, when two siblings both have insulin-dependent diabetes, they are significantly more likely to have inherited the same parental haplotypes and only rarely do not share either haplotype.

diabetes. It must be emphasized that even in the case of an HLA-identical DR3/DR4 sibling, the chances are still 75 percent against IDDM occurring.

Recent developments suggesting that immunosuppressive therapy may prevent or delay disease onset have led us to consider altering this recommendation against screening. By identifying those siblings at highest risk for development of IDDM, a subset of individuals who should be closely monitored with islet cell autoantibody and anti-insulin autoantibody assays can be identified. Should autoantibodies be present, intravenous glucose tolerance testing can be performed to see if altered first phase insulin secretion, the earliest physiologic abnormality, is present. Prospective studies by several groups have shown that high-risk relatives who have autoantibodies and altered first phase insulin release have a high probability of developing IDDM in the near future (approximately 50 percent within 3 years). Such individuals are the most appropriate candidates for immunosuppressive or immuno-modulating therapy. It must be kept in mind, however, that immunosuppressive therapy has not yet been clearly proved to prevent the development of IDDM and carries with it the potential for serious complications, such as life-threatening infection. Currently, such therapy is also only available experimentally. Therefore, before drawing blood for HLA typing and/or autoantibody studies, the advantages and drawbacks of obtaining such information should be thoroughly discussed with the family. Families must discuss how they will adjust if instead of receiving the reassuring results they are hoping for, they are informed that some family members are at significantly increased risk.

Interestingly, the empiric recurrence risks for the offspring of individuals with IDDM differ depending on which parent has IDDM. When it is the mother, the risk to offspring is 2 to 3 percent. Fathers with IDDM have a greater risk of having diabetic offspring, in the range of 4 to 6 percent. The reasons for this difference are not known. As discussed in the chapter *Insulin-Dependent Diabetes Mellitus in Pregnancy*, women who are diabetic during pregnancy are at increased risk for giving birth to children with congenital malformations, particularly if their diabetes is poorly controlled. It is therefore extremely important that advance planning of pregnancies, with preconceptual optimization of glucose control, and the availability of prenatal diagnostic evaluation, be discussed with all diabetic women of childbearing age. Such a course of action can result in a significant reduction in the frequency of fetal malformations, as well as prenatal detection of many of those malformations that cannot yet be prevented. All too often, and particularly with adolescents, this issue is not discussed until after pregnancy is diagnosed, when it is too late to reduce the risk of malformations.

Screening for Other Autoimmune Diseases

Diabetes is not the only autoimmune disorder for which relatives of an individual with IDDM are at risk. Family members, along with the diabetic patient, are at increased risk for autoimmune thyroid disease, pernicious anemia secondary to autoimmune gastritis, and, to a lesser extent, autoimmune adrenal disease (Addison's disease). Therefore, periodic screening of the individual with IDDM and all first-degree relatives is warranted, particularly for thyroid dysfunction and the vitamin B_{12} deficiency that leads to pernicious anemia. We recommend annual to biannual screening for the presence of thyroid and/or parietal cell autoantibodies in all first-degree relatives, with subsequent thyroid function tests (triiodothyronine, thyroxine, and thyroid-stimulating hormone) for those with thyroid antibodies and vitamin B_{12} levels for those with gastric autoimmunity. Alternatively, if reliable autoantibody studies are difficult to obtain, periodic functional testing alone can be substituted, though in many laboratories this is more expensive.

Counseling in Non–Insulin-Dependent Diabetes

Empiric risk estimates for the relatives of individuals with NIDDM have shown that their risk for diabetes is quantitatively greater than the risk for relatives of individuals with IDDM. First-degree relatives have a 10 to 15 percent risk of developing overt NIDDM and a 20 to 30 percent risk of abnormal glucose tolerance. Periodic screening of relatives with oral glucose tolerance tests is therefore warranted, beginning in the late 30s to early 40s. These relatives should also be carefully tested for lipid abnormalities and hypertension because they are also at increased risk for atherosclerosis, even in the absence of diabetes. We also recommend that first-degree relatives be encouraged to reach their ideal body weight because obesity is clearly an additional (and potentially controllable) risk factor.

It is important to take a careful family history, particularly for relatively early-onset NIDDM patients. As mentioned previously, there is a distinct form of NIDDM known as maturity onset diabetes of the young (MODY), in which affected family members may develop diabetes in adolescence or young adulthood. In most cases, this form of diabetes is inherited as an autosomal dominant disorder. Therefore, the risk to first-degree relatives is 50 percent. As discussed above, the mutations responsible for MODY can now be identified in many families, making DNA-based diagnosis feasible for some families. An important question that will need to be addressed with families is what purpose preclinical diagnosis of MODY will serve. At this point, no intervention is available (with the possible exception of maintaining ideal body weight and exercise) to prevent clinical onset of disease. Similarly, the issue of whether prenatal diagnosis is appropriate also requires careful discussion. As in all forms of genetic counseling, however, it is generally best to have families make these decisions for themselves, with the health care professional providing the information in a nondirective, nonjudgmental fashion.

■ FUTURE DIRECTIONS IN DIABETES COUNSELING

An intriguing development that may be clinically relevant in the near future is the increasing evidence that there is genetic susceptibility not only to diabetes but to specific diabetic complications as well. Several studies have shown, for example, that those IDDM patients who are positive for HLA DR4 are more likely to develop diabetic retinopathy than those who do not have this allele. It has been suggested that insulin gene region plays a role in the risk for nephropathy. Such observations raise the possibility that within the foreseeable future it may be possible to identify which complications an individual is most likely to develop and to provide appropriate counseling and follow-up.

■ COMMENTS

The risk of other family members developing diabetes is of concern to most patients, whether they spontaneously verbalize it or not. Therefore, medical professionals involved in diabetes care have a responsibility to either offer genetic counseling themselves or to refer their patients to a genetics program that can provide these services. Even though there is still more to learn regarding the genes involved in genetic susceptibility, currently available information can be helpful and reassuring to diabetic individuals and their relatives.

Suggested Reading

Enrlich H, Rotter JI, Chang J, et al. HLA class II alleles and susceptibility and resistance to insulin dependent diabetes mellitus in Mexican-American families. Nature Genetics 1993; 3:358–364.

A good review of the immunogenetics of IDDM and the HLA class II region.

Fajans SS, Bell GI, Bowden DW, et al. Maturity-onset diabetes of the young. Life Sciences 1994, 55:413–422.

This article gives an excellent overview of maturity-onset diabetes of the young, discussing its clinical and genetic heterogeneity.

Kelly TE. Clinical genetics and genetic counseling. 2nd ed. Chicago, Year Book Medical Publishers, 1986.

A good introductory genetics text. The chapter on genetic counseling is particularly relevant for professionals with little experience in providing this type of counseling.

Kennedy GC, German MS, Rutter WJ. The minisatellite in the diabetes susceptibility locus IDDM2 regulates insulin transcription. Nature Genetics 1995; 9:293–298.

An article suggesting how the insulin gene region may contribute to IDDM susceptibility.

Luo D-F, Buzzetti R, Rotter JI, et al. Confirmation of three susceptibility genes to insulin-dependent diabetes mellitus: IDDM4, IDDM5 and IDDM8. Human Molecular Genetics 1996; 5:693–698.

An article for those interested in the future directions of gene indentification in IDDM.

Raffel LJ, Scheuner MT, Rotter JI. Genetics of diabetes. In: Ellenberg & Rifkin's diabetes mellitus. D Porte, R Sherwin, eds, Appleton & Lange, 1997.

A comprehensive chapter about the genetics of diabetes.

Riley WJ, Maclaren NK, Krischer J, et al. A prospective study of the development of diabetes in relatives of patients with insulin dependent diabetes. N Engl J Med 1990; 323:1167–1172.

An article for those wanting information about the natural history of IDDM development in high-risk families.

Yamagata K, Furuta H, Oda N, et al. Mutations in the hepatocyte nuclear factor-4 alpha gene in maturity-onset diabetes of the young (MODY1). Nature 1996; 384:458–460.

A recent article about the identification of one of the genes responsible for MODY.

Yamagata K, Oda N, Kaisaki PJ, et al. Mutations in the hepatocyte nuclear factor-1alpha gene in maturity-onset diabetes of the young (MODY3). Nature 1996; 384:455–458.

A recent article about the identification of one of the genes responsible for MODY.

SURGERY AND DIABETES MELLITUS

Jennifer B. Marks, M.D.
Irl B. Hirsch, M.D.

Diabetic patients who require surgery present problems in perioperative management which should be familiar to those involved in their care. In addition to surgery required for the same indications as in nondiabetic patients, certain procedures are performed more commonly in diabetic patients; that is, cardiovascular and ophthalmologic procedures. Surgical intervention may also be necessary for conditions specifically associated with diabetes, that is, kidney and/or pancreatic transplantation, penile prosthesis implantation, ulcer debridement, and limb amputation. The presence of diabetes and its associated complications may place the patient at increased risk for a variety of complications, including acute renal failure and cardiovascular events. Patients with diabetes have higher rates of surgical morbidity and mortality than those without diabetes, in large part because of the presence of underlying atherosclerotic cardiovascular disease and acquired derangements in metabolic control.

■ MAINTENANCE OF METABOLIC HOMEOSTASIS

In simplest terms, the regulation of metabolic homeostasis is the result of a balance between the primary anabolic hormone, insulin, and those counter-regulatory hormones that have chiefly catabolic effects, including epinephrine, glucagon, cortisol, and growth hormone. Insulin stimulates glucose utilization in peripheral tissues and suppresses endogenous hepatic glucose production from both glycogenolysis and gluconeogenesis. Therefore, in the absence of other intervening factors, an increase in plasma insulin concentration lowers the plasma glucose level. Insulin also exerts important anabolic effects on protein and lipid metabolism. Insulin promotes protein anabolism by increasing tissue uptake of amino acids, stimulating protein synthesis, and decreasing proteolysis and oxidation of amino acids. With regard to fat metabolism, insulin stimulates fatty acid synthesis in the liver, inhibits lipolysis and the breakdown of stored triglycerides, and accelerates the removal of circulating triglycerides by stimulating lipoprotein lipase activity in adipose tissue. Insulin effectively suppresses ketosis by inhibiting oxidation and mobilization of free fatty acids from adipose tissue and by increasing the utilization of ketones by peripheral tissues. Insulin also enhances renal sodium and fluid reabsorption, contributing to the prevention of volume depletion.

The anabolic effects of insulin are antagonized by an increase in the levels of counter-regulatory hormones: epinephrine, glucagon, cortisol, and growth hormone.

Epinephrine increases the blood glucose level by stimulating hepatic glucose production (both gluconeogenesis and glycogenolysis) and by inhibiting glucose utilization by peripheral tissues, primarily muscle. The catecholamine indirectly causes hyperglycemia by stimulating glucagon and inhibiting insulin secretion. Other deleterious metabolic effects of epinephrine include stimulation of lipolysis and ketogenesis and promotion of negative nitrogen balance. Glucagon produces a rise in plasma glucose concentration by stimulating hepatic glycogenolysis and gluconeogenesis and by inhibiting the action of insulin on peripheral tissues. Glucagon also exerts a powerful effect to increase hepatic ketogenesis; it is probably the primary signal regulating this process. Both cortisol and growth hormone decrease glucose utilization by muscle, potentiate the stimulatory effects of epinephrine and glucagon on hepatic glucose production, and increase lipolysis and ketogenesis. Cortisol also enhances proteolysis.

■ EFFECTS OF SURGERY ON METABOLIC CONTROL

Anesthesia elicits a complex neuroendocrine stress response with release of cortisol, growth hormone, catecholamines, and to varying degrees, glucagon. Activation of the sympathetic nervous system and increased circulating epinephrine levels impair insulin secretion and cause insulin resistance, while the increase in counter-regulatory hormone levels produces hyperglycemia (increased glycogenolysis and gluconeogenesis; decreased glucose utilization) and excess catabolism (increased lipolysis and proteolysis). The magnitude of the catabolic response is related to the severity of the surgery and postsurgical complications, including sepsis, hypotension, hypovolemia, acidosis, and others.

■ EFFECTS OF SURGERY ON METABOLIC CONTROL IN THE DIABETIC PATIENT

Although the stress response to surgery does not usually present a problem for the nondiabetic patient, high levels of counter-regulatory hormones can contribute to serious metabolic disturbances in diabetic individuals. In addition

to the presence of insulin deficiency (relative or absolute) and excess counter-regulatory hormone release, two other factors predispose the diabetic patient to metabolic decompensation: prolonged fasting and volume contraction. It is important to note that ketoacidosis in type 1 diabetic patients can occur without extreme plasma glucose elevations. Although ketoacidosis is not likely to develop in the type 2 patient, surgery-induced hyperglycemia is common, and if the surgical stress is severe enough, diabetic ketoacidosis (DKA) can ensue. Hyperosmolar hyperglycemic nonketotic coma (HHNC) is a well-described complication of patients with type 2 diabetes who undergo surgery. This syndrome, characterized by marked hyperglycemia, hyperosmolarity, volume depletion, and mental status changes, results from inadequate insulinization and osmotic diuresis, often compounded by inadequate fluid replacement or the injudicious perioperative use of diuretics.

In addition to the prevention of severe hyperglycemia and ketoacidosis, there are other important reasons to maintain near-normal metabolic control before and during the perioperative period. Hyperglycemia inhibits normal leukocyte function and impairs wound healing. Studies have shown that hyperglycemia impairs collagen formation and causes a decrease in the tensile strength of surgical wounds. These defects can be prevented by correction of hyperglycemia with insulin. The maintenance of glucose levels below 200 mg per deciliter has been shown to improve granulocyte adherence and phagocytosis, important components of the defense against bacterial infection, especially against common gram-positive organisms such as pneumococci and staphylococci. Acidemia also impairs leukocyte chemotactic and phagocytic responses. Finally, studies in both animals and humans suggest that hyperglycemia may exacerbate ischemic brain damage, a factor of potential importance in the elderly diabetic patient with cerebrovascular disease.

The overall goal of perioperative management of the surgical diabetic patient is to avoid the excess morbidity and mortality that is associated with metabolic decompensation and/or associated diabetic complications. This involves prevention of hypoglycemia, excessive hyperglycemia, unwarranted protein catabolism, ketoacidosis, and hyperosmolarity, which may result in excessive fluid losses and potentially serious electrolyte disturbances. The prevention of these metabolic catastrophes is best achieved by providing adequate insulin and fluids to counterbalance the catabolic responses to the stress of surgery. This means that all patients with type 1 diabetes and many patients with type 2 diabetes require insulin perioperatively.

■ PREOPERATIVE MANAGEMENT

Evaluation for Elective Surgery

Preoperative evaluation is separated into two categories: (1) assessment of the level of metabolic control, and (2) appraisal of chronic diabetic complications that may affect the surgical outcome. It is essential to restore normoglycemia or near-normoglycemia prior to surgery and to correct any existing electrolyte or fluid abnormalities in all diabetic patients. Preoperative plasma glucose and electrolyte concentrations and urinary ketones should be measured on the day of surgery.

Complete assessment of the various chronic complications should be completed before admission. It is essential that underlying cardiovascular disease be identified. The optimum preoperative cardiovascular assessment is controversial, in part because of the high frequency of asymptomatic myocardial ischemia in this population. All diabetic patients should have a complete history and physical examination with emphasis on the cardiovascular system. Special attention should be focused on the presence of orthostatic hypotension and diabetic cardiovascular autonomic neuropathy (see the chapter *Autonomic Neuropathy*) because these abnormalities are strongly correlated with the presence of coronary artery disease. The presence of hypertension is not a contraindication to surgery as long as the blood pressure is well controlled. Beta-blockers may be associated with the development of hypoglycemia in the postoperative period. All diabetic patients should have a resting electrocardiogram (ECG) and consideration given to the performance of a stress ECG depending upon the physician's suspicion of underlying coronary artery disease.

Preoperative evaluation also requires assessment of renal function. A serum creatinine concentration is not a reliable indicator of renal disease in diabetic patients, because its level usually remains normal until the nephropathy is advanced. Because the first harbinger of diabetic nephropathy is proteinuria, dipstick for urinary protein should be included in the minimum assessment of renal disease. A more complete assessment would include a 24-hour urine collection for proteinuria (or microalbuminuria) and creatinine clearance. The preoperative assessment of proteinuria is important for several reasons: (1) diabetic patients with heavy proteinuria or elevated serum creatinine are at increased risk to develop acute renal failure; (2) potential nephrotoxic agents should be avoided in patients with proteinuria; (3) proteinuria is a predictor of mortality (mainly cardiovascular) in patients with type 2 diabetes.

The presence of autonomic neuropathy should also be assessed prior to surgery because diabetic autonomic neuropathy predisposes to perioperative hypotension. In such patients, careful monitoring of blood pressure and volume status during the entire perioperative period is essential. In addition to routine questioning about the typical symptoms of autonomic dysfunction, the physician may wish to carry out formal autonomic testing (see the chapter *Autonomic Neuropathy*).

Evaluation for Emergency Surgery

As many as 5 percent of all diabetic patients require emergency surgery at some time during their lives. The most common procedures are appendectomy, lower extremity incision and drainage, and/or amputation. A large percentage of these patients are admitted with poor metabolic control (blood glucose greater than 200 mg per deciliter) and some may even have DKA. The key points of preparing the diabetic patient for emergency surgery are summarized in Table 1. The first priority is to assess glycemic, acid-base, electrolyte, and volume status. A saline infusion should be started while awaiting results of these laboratory tests. If ketoacidosis is present, surgery should be delayed, if possible, while the patient receives treatment for this metabolic emergency. It is imperative that volume deficits and electrolyte abnormalities, especially hyperkalemia, by corrected prior to surgery.

Patient with Type 1 Diabetes

Ideally, the patient with type 1 diabetes should be admitted to the hospital 1 to 2 days prior to surgery in order to maximize metabolic control. Unfortunately, this is rarely possible with the cost constraints of today's medical climate. Early admission in a controlled environment allows the physician to achieve good glycemic control and to correct pre-existing acid-base, electrolyte, and fluid disturbances. Most diabetic patients, however, are admitted on the morning of surgery. Fortunately, the widespread use of home blood glucose monitoring makes the outpatient correction of derangements in glycemic control possible prior to admission.

Traditionally, long-acting (e.g., Ultralente) insulin is stopped 2 to 3 days before surgery, and the patient is stabilized on a regimen of intermediate (neutral protamine Hagedorn [NPH] or Lente) and short-acting (Regular) insulin twice a day, or Regular insulin before meals and intermediate-acting insulin at bedtime. However, if the patient's daily regimen includes long-acting insulin and metabolic control is good, it is acceptable to continue this regimen through the day prior to surgery. On the morning of surgery, patients maintained on long-acting insulin should either be given their usual morning insulin dose or receive the more traditional insulin regimen intraoperatively (see discussion of Intraoperative Management below). During the week before surgery, home blood glucose monitoring should be performed routinely before each meal and at bedtime, with adjustments in the regimen made with the advice of a physician or diabetes nurse specialist.

Patient with Type 2 Diabetes

In both absolute numbers and percentages, type 2 diabetics represent the largest group of patients undergoing surgery. These individuals have the most macrovascular complications, including peripheral vascular, coronary, and renovascular disease. In preparing type 2 patients for major surgical procedures (greater than 1 hour of general anesthesia), the same guidelines should be followed as for patients with type 1 diabetes (see above), keeping in mind the following special management problems. Sulfonylureas should be discontinued 1 day prior to surgery (longer, 48 to 72 hours for chlorpropamide and metformin), and an insulin regimen begun on the day of surgery (see Intraoperative Management). Cessation of short-acting sulfonylureas for 24 hours or chlorpropamide or metformin for 48 hours has no significant

---

Table 1 Diabetes and Emergency Surgery

Emergent determination of plasma glucose, urea, and electrolyte concentrations and blood pH

Assess status of intravascular volume by measuring blood pressure/pulse lying and standing

If diabetic ketoacidosis is present, immediate treatment is indicated and surgery should be delayed, if possible, until metabolic control is reestablished

Begin insulin infusion at appropriate rate

Begin glucose and potassium (if appropriate) infusion

Infuse saline (if appropriate) to correct volume loss

Check blood glucose concentration at bedside hourly and plasma potassium concentration every 4 hours

Note: Insulin requirements may be increased

impact on glycemic control. Because of the concern about lactic acidosis, cessation of metformin is mandatory. In patients with good metabolic control, particularly if they require only local anesthesia, many diabetologists prefer to maintain oral agent therapy (excluding patients on metformin) up to the day of surgery and not start them on insulin (see Intraoperative Management).

Choice of Anesthesia

No anesthetic agent is specifically contraindicated or specifically beneficial for the diabetic patient. All general anesthetic agents trigger the release of counter-regulatory hormones and have the potential to cause significant hyperglycemia. The choice of anesthetic agent should depend entirely on the experience and preferences of the anesthesiologist, the type of surgery, the medical status of the patient, and the surgical risk. Local anesthesia has no appreciable effect on carbohydrate metabolism. Field block and spinal or epidural anesthesia usually do exert a major adverse on glycemic control.

Asymptomatic hypoglycemia is a common event in diabetic patients, especially in type 1 individuals. Any type of sedation may impair the recognition of symptoms of hypoglycemia. There are few published data for patients receiving central nervous system depressants, but one review found a 13 percent incidence of perioperative hypoglycemia in a group of 85 patients with type 1 diabetes. Therefore, any patients receiving a glucose-lowering agent and any sedation requires regular blood glucose monitoring.

■ INTRAOPERATIVE MANAGEMENT

Type 1 Diabetic Patients Requiring General Anesthesia

The two essential therapeutic interventions that must be considered in the perioperative care of the patient with type 1 diabetes are insulin and glucose administration. Infusion of non–glucose-containing fluids to maintain the intravascular volume and, in some cases, provision of potassium are also very important considerations.

Insulin

Considerable controversy exists about the route of insulin administration during surgery. Several successful treatment regimens have been published. However, there are no data that clearly demonstrate superiority of any therapeutic approach over another, either in morbidity or mortality. Whatever regimen is used, it should fulfill the following criteria: (1) maintain good glycemic control and prevent other metabolic disturbances, (2) be easily understood, (3) be associated with a low possibility of iatrogenic mistakes, and (4) be applicable to a variety of situations, including busy operating suites, recovery rooms, and surgical wards. Absolutely critical to the success of any regimen is careful monitoring to detect early metabolic decompensation and appropriate adjustment of the intervention as needed.

The use of intravenous (IV) insulin infusion during surgery in diabetic patients was popularized in the late 1970s. Initially, intermittent IV boluses of insulin were given every 2 hours. However, significant deterioration in glycemic control was common. This was not unexpected, because the biologic half-life of Regular insulin is less than 20 minutes. For this reason we do not advocate the use of intermittent IV boluses of insulin in ketosis-prone diabetic patients. Subsequently, the simultaneous infusion of glucose, insulin, and potassium was reported to be effective. The major problem associated with this approach is the inability to adjust the rates of insulin and glucose delivery independently, as may be required by fluctuations in the plasma glucose concentration.

The variable rate IV insulin infusion technique has been demonstrated to be both safe and highly effective in perioperative diabetic management. Most recent reviews and studies support its use because of its simplicity, the predictability of insulin absorption, its titrability in response to fluctuating insulin requirements, and its flexibility in unexpected situa-

---

Table 2 Variable-Rate Intravenous Insulin Infusion

Add 25 units of Regular human insulin to 250 ml of normal saline (0.1 U/ml).
Flush 50 ml of the infusion mixture through the intravenous tubing.
Do not start the insulin infusion until the blood glucose concentration is above 120 mg/dl.
General guidelines for initial dose for patients with type 1 diabetes: men—1.0 U/hr, women 0.5 U/hr; for patients with type 2 diabetes: 1.0 U/hr for all patients.
Blood glucose should be measured hourly during and immediately after surgery.
After starting the insulin infusion, use the algorithm below to adjust the insulin infusion rate.
The insulin algorithm may need to be altered depending on level of glycemic control.
Do not stop the insulin infusion until patient is able to tolerate foods. At that time, give the usual dose of premeal Regular insulin (may give 4–8 U of subcutaneous Regular insulin for lunch meal if insulin is not usually given at this time).

BLOOD GLUCOSE (MG/DL)	INSULIN INFUSION
<70	Turn infusion off for 15 min and administer 10 g glucose*
70–120	Decrease infusion by 3 ml/hr (0.3 U/hr)
121–180	No change in infusion rate
181–240	Increase infusion by 3 ml/hr (0.3 U/hr)
241–300	Increase infusion by 6 ml/hr (0.6 U/hr)
>300	Increase infusion by 10 ml/hr (1.0 U/hr)

*Blood glucose should be remeasured 15 min after turning off insulin infusion. If it is still less than 100 mg/dl, wait another 15 min (repeat procedure as necessary). Restart insulin infusion at 3 ml/hr (0.3 U/hr) after blood glucose is greater than 100 mg/dl.

tions (e.g., a delay of surgery). It allows reaction to a wide range of insulin requirements according to a simple algorithm and results in improved stability of glycemic control throughout the perioperative period.

In a type 1 diabetic patient who has a blood glucose level reflecting good control (e.g., 120 to 180 mg per deciliter), the insulin infusion is begun at a rate of 0.5 to 1 U per hour and is adjusted according to a glucose-feedback formula (Table 2) to maintain the plasma glucose concentration within that target range. Fingerstick capillary (or venous) blood glucose values are obtained at the bedside (or in the operating room) using one of many available glucose meters. The nurse or physician who is making the measurement should be familiar with the use of the meter. One or more plasma samples, drawn simultaneously with the sample for the meter test, should be sent to the laboratory for confirmation of accuracy.

Many authors suggest initiating the variable rate insulin infusion at 1.0 U per hour. However, in very thin women (who tend to be particularly sensitive to insulin) we start at 0.5 U per hour. Insulin requirements may be markedly increased in the poorly controlled patient, and it may be necessary to begin the insulin infusion at a higher than usual initial rate (i.e., 2–3 U per hour). To avoid problems with insulin absorption to plastic, 50 ml of the infusion mixture should be flushed through the tubing before connecting it to the patient. The algorithm in Table 2 represents a simple guide that we have found to be quite effective. However, extremely high or low blood glucose levels require close monitoring and frequent adjustments.

The desirable frequency of glucose monitoring has been debated. All authors agree that with general anesthesia, blood glucose and electrolyte levels should be measured just before and immediately after surgery. While the patient is receiving the IV insulin infusion, we obtain bedside glucose determinations every hour during and immediately after surgery. Every 2 hours thereafter is usually sufficient if there are no problems. Others feel that it is safe to monitor less frequently. There are no studies that have examined the optimum frequency of perioperative blood glucose monitoring.

We strive for blood glucose levels between 120 and 180 mg per deciliter, but slightly higher targets (150 to 200 mg per deciliter) have been recommended by some diabetologists. These values are chosen to minimize the risk of hypoglycemia while at the same time preventing the excessive catabolism that is associated with hyperglycemia and impaired insulin action. Maintaining the blood glucose level below 200 mg per deciliter also prevents the deleterious effect of hyperglycemia on wound healing, tensile collagen strength, phagocytic function, and the exacerbation of

---

Table 3 Conditions Associated with Increased Insulin Requirements
Liver disease
Obesity
Severe infection
Steroid therapy
Cardiopulmonary bypass
Hypotension
Poor glycemic control
Recent ketoacidosis

---

ischemic brain damage. If this goal is strictly adhered to, hyperosmolarity and DKA do not develop.

As a general guideline, most patients with type 1 diabetes require between 0.3 and 0.4 U of insulin per gram of glucose per hour to achieve targeted glucose goals. Septic patients often require 0.6 to 0.8 U per gram of glucose per hour, while those undergoing coronary artery bypass surgery often need 0.9 to 1.2 U per gram of glucose per hour. Some conditions associated with increased insulin requirements are listed in Table 3. With the variable-rate insulin infusion approach, there is sufficient flexibility to increase or decrease the rate in order to achieve targeted blood glucose levels rapidly.

Subcutaneous (SC) insulin is often used for perioperative management in the diabetic surgical patient. However, a number of problems can develop with this regimen, and we do not recommend its use. Unpredictable absorption, which often occurs with SC insulin injection, is made worse by changes in tissue perfusion that occur in the perioperative period. The SC insulin approach advocates the injection of one-half of the usual dose of intermediate-acting insulin on the morning of surgery. This can present a major problem if there is a delay or prolongation of the surgical procedure because the insulin reserve is then exhausted before or during the procedure, leading to a deterioration in glycemic control.

Patients using continuous subcutaneous insulin infusion (CSII) via a pump receive only Regular insulin, and are therefore easily converted to IV infusion just before surgery. Although its intraoperative use has not been evaluated, continuation of CSII during this period should probably be avoided because of potential problems with insulin absorption. However, CSII is an acceptable regimen for procedures utilizing local anesthesia.

If frequent (hourly), reliable blood glucose monitoring cannot be performed during surgery and the immediate postoperative period, we recommend giving half of the patient's usual morning dose of long-acting (NPH or Lente) insulin SC. The patient's blood sugar level should be checked immediately after surgery is completed and an IV insulin infusion initiated as described above and in Table 2. Glucose monitoring devices should be available in all surgical recovery rooms.

Glucose and Fluids

The nondiabetic adult needs a minimum of 100 to 125 g (400 to 500 calories) of glucose per day to prevent protein catabolism and the development of ketosis. Therefore, diabetic patients should be given at least 5 to 10 g per hour (1.2 to 2.4 mg per kilogram per minute in a 70 kg person) to provide basal energy requirements and prevent hypoglycemia during surgery. The dextrose concentration of the IV solution can be adjusted based upon the anticipated length of time the patient will be receiving it. For a relatively short, minor operation, 5 percent dextrose in water or 0.45 percent saline can be given. For longer intraabdominal or intrathoracic procedures, 10 percent dextrose should be used to avoid excessive fluid administration. A 20 percent or 50 percent dextrose solution can be infused through a central venous catheter if fluid restriction is critical. If additional fluids are required (e.g., to replace intraoperative blood loss), they should be given as non–glucose containing solutions. Lactated Ringer's solution should be avoided. If the patient needs alkali, it should be given as sodium bicarbonate.

Potassium

A normal serum potassium level does not necessarily imply a normal total body potassium content, because only 2 percent of total body potassium stores are extracellular. Moreover, a number of metabolic factors, which can change rapidly in diabetic patients, influence the serum potassium level: (1) insulin, which stimulates potassium uptake by cells, (2) hyperosmolarity, which causes a translocation of potassium and fluid from the intracellular to extracellular compartment, (3) acidemia, which causes hyperkalemia due to the exchange of intracellular potassium for extracellular hydrogen ions, and (4) epinephrine, which stimulates potassium uptake by cells. In the diabetic patient with normal renal function and a normal serum potassium concentration, 10 to 20 mEq of potassium chloride should be added to each liter of dextrose-containing fluid. More potassium is required in patients with hypokalemia. For the patient with an elevated serum potassium concentration (more than 5.5 mEq per liter), potassium should be withheld from the IV fluids and the serum level monitored closely.

Type 1 Diabetic Patients Requiring Local Anesthesia

For short procedures done under local anesthesia it may be acceptable to utilize the SC route of insulin administration in a patient with type 1 diabetes. If, for example, the patient is on a regimen of intermediate (NPH) and short-acting (Regular) insulin, if metabolic control is good, and if the procedure is scheduled early in the day, 50 to 60 percent of the usual AM dose can be given in the morning, with elimination of the Regular insulin if there is normoglycemia or hypoglycemia (i.e., blood glucose less than or equal to 90 mg per deciliter). Higher blood glucose concentrations can be managed with small doses of Regular insulin. Obviously, additional guesswork is introduced with this approach. The lower dose of intermediate-acting insulin reduces the risk of patient's developing hypoglycemia later in the day, particularly if the procedure is delayed. As with general anesthesia, the patient should receive a glucose infusion, and the blood glucose concentration should be monitored by fingerstick or venous blood before, during (hourly), and immediately after surgery. If required, supplemental Regular insulin can be administered SC every 4 hours in doses of 0.05 to 0.1 U per kilogram. Similarly, if the patient's daily regimen includes long-acting (e.g., Ultralente) insulin and if metabolic control is good, it is acceptable to give the usual morning dose of Ultralente on the morning of surgery, with fingerstick monitoring as outlined above. Again, Regular insulin should be given only as a supplemental SC injection or as a low variable-rate IV insulin infusion, as required by fluctuations in blood glucose levels. With either of these strategies, SC Regular insulin injection should be restarted 30 minutes before resuming the usual diet. For patients who use CSII via pump as their daily regimen, this method of insulin delivery may be an acceptable regimen for a procedure requiring only local anesthesia. With any of the strategies that utilize the SC route of insulin administration, the patient's preoperative metabolic status, timing of the surgical procedure, and careful glucose monitoring are the key elements to ensure success.

Type 2 Diabetic Patients Requiring General Anesthesia

For procedures that require general anesthesia, specific treatment, other than hourly blood glucose monitoring, is not required for type 2 diabetic patients who are well controlled on diet therapy alone (fasting blood glucose less than 125 mg per deciliter). Because of the hyperglycemic response that occurs during surgery, many of these patients will require insulin. The insulin should be administered as a variable-rate IV insulin infusion, as outlined in Table 2. Targeted blood glucose concentrations are identical to those of patients with type 1 diabetes. In type 2 patients who are treated with diet alone but who are poorly controlled (fasting blood glucose greater than 180 mg per deciliter), we initiate an insulin infusion before surgery and employ the same strategy outlined in Table 2. A fasting glucose above 180 mg per deciliter is chosen as the cutoff value because this reflects absolute deficiency with respect to insulin secretion. We also treat type 2 diabetic patients with a fasting glucose between 140 and 180 mg per deciliter with an IV insulin infusion. If the procedure is of short duration and straightforward and the physician decides not to initiate insulin in this group (fasting glucose 140 to 180 mg per deciliter), it is imperative to monitor the blood sugar closely (hourly) during surgery.

There is some disagreement regarding management strategies for patients who require general anesthesia and who are well controlled with sulfonylureas. Some recommend withholding the sulfonylurea on the morning of surgery for procedures requiring either general or local anesthesia because with general anesthesia an insulin infusion will probably be required to control the hyperglycemia that occurs during surgery. Administration of oral agents is potentially dangerous in the well-controlled patient because of its stimulatory effects on endogenous insulin secretion if enough calories are not provided. If insulin is not instituted at the beginning of the procedure, it should be initiated when the blood glucose exceeds 200 mg per deciliter. As a general rule, SC insulin should not be used for any type 2 patient receiving general anesthesia. This is particularly true for obese type 2 diabetic patients, in whom absorption of insulin from the subcutaneous adipose tissue is likely to be quite variable. Any patient who is taking metformin should have the drug discontinued 48 hours prior to surgery. This is done prophylactically in case lactic acidosis develops secondary to hypotension, septic shock, or myocardial infarction, complicating the surgical procedure. Since the action of metformin lasts for several days, the physician does not have to be concerned with the development of acute hyperglycemia after stopping metformin. Cessation of acarbose does not present a problem because the drug works only when there is food (starch) in the gastrointestinal tract.

Increased insulin requirements may be encountered in the patient undergoing coronary artery bypass surgery, because of the metabolic stress response invoked by the surgery, the use of hypothermia, and the infusion of glucose-containing cardioplegic solutions. These factors exacerbate the hyperglycemic response of surgery and should be anticipated and prevented with higher insulin infusion rates. Frequent intraoperative blood glucose measurements are imperative to avoid metabolic decompensation.

Type 2 Diabetic Patients Requiring Local Anesthesia

Treatment decisions for type 2 diabetes patients receiving local anesthesia are similar to those described above. Well-controlled patients, who are treated with diet alone or diet plus oral agents, most likely will not require insulin therapy. One study showed that 93 percent of patients with type 2 diabetes achieved acceptable blood glucose control during local anesthesia without insulin. Therefore, unless blood glucose levels rise above the targeted values, no further specific therapy is required and the sulfonylurea can be safely omitted on the day of surgery. Metformin should be withheld for 48 hours prior to surgery. If insulin is required, there is no particular advantage of IV over SC insulin in this population. If SC insulin is used, we suggest starting with 0.05 to 0.075 U per kilogram of Regular insulin every 4 hours.

Patients who are poorly controlled prior to admission on sulfonylureas or metformin will require insulin to achieve the targeted blood glucose goals outlined in Table 2. Therefore, there is no situation in which it would be appropriate to administer the oral hypoglycemic agent before surgery with either general or local anesthesia.

The decision to begin an insulin infusion versus using SC insulin in patients receiving local anesthesia should be based on: (1) most importantly, the patient's current metabolic status; (2) how soon the patient will be resuming a diet after the procedure; (3) the type of insulin regimen (or oral hypoglycemic regimen) the patient usually receives; and (4) timing of the procedure during the day. Insulin-requiring patients with type 2 diabetes receiving local anesthesia should be managed similarly to patients with type 1 diabetes. Many of these patients are insulinopenic and behave metabolically like those with type 1 diabetes. Therefore, use of the variable-rate insulin infusion is appropriate for this population.

■ POSTOPERATIVE MANAGEMENT OF DIABETIC PATIENTS RECEIVING INSULIN

Continuation of the variable-rate IV insulin infusion into the postoperative period is a simple and flexible approach to management. Although there are no prospective studies, it affords the same advantages as during the earlier perioperative period. Capillary glucose is monitored every 1 to 2 hours at the bedside, and the variable insulin infusion is adjusted as outlined in Table 2 to achieve targeted blood glucose levels. Serum electrolytes should be measured immediately after surgery in all diabetic patients and, at a minimum, on a daily basis for those receiving an insulin infusion for a prolonged period of time. Hyper- and hypokalemia are common in the postoperative period and should be treated promptly, based upon the presumed cause of the electrolyte disorder. The presence of a widened anion gap suggests the development of DKA or lactic acidosis secondary to unsuspected sepsis or tissue hypoperfusion. If food is not tolerated for more than 24 hours, urinary ketones should be measured daily in all patients because the presence of ketonuria in the existence of well-controlled glycemia indicates the need for greater quantities of glucose

(starvation ketosis) or, in patients with type 1 diabetes, may identify early DKA, which may be exacerbated by starvation.

We have found it easiest to continue the insulin infusion until solid food is tolerated. Therefore, if nausea and vomiting are present, there is no interruption of the glucose and insulin infusions. If solid food is permitted for the lunch or supper meal on the day of surgery, the regular home dose of insulin may be administered 20 to 30 minutes before the meal and the insulin (and glucose) infusion stopped 15 to 20 minutes after the meal. If Regular insulin is not usually given before the lunch meal, 4 to 6 U of Regular insulin (SC) should be administered, because the onset of NPH or Lente insulin is delayed for 2 to 4 hours. It should be noted that the insulin infusion is discontinued only *after* the SC insulin regimen is started to avoid leaving gaps in insulin coverage that might lead to the loss of metabolic control. If the patient will be spending the night in the hospital, it is sometimes easier to continue with the insulin infusion until the next morning to ensure that the morning meal is well tolerated.

The use of a sliding scale SC insulin infusion during the postoperative period has been advocated by some individuals, who cite its simplicity and general familiarity with its use. However, there are several problems with this approach. It represents a retrospective treatment for hyperglycemia and as such tends to create swings in glucose levels, in some cases to extreme degrees. In addition to the risk of creating hypoglycemia with excessive doses of insulin, the use of the sliding scale regimen can predispose to the development of DKA in the insulin-deficient patient before significant hyperglycemia is identified.

■ OUTPATIENT SURGERY

In recent years, there has been a major trend toward performing many operations that previously required hospital admission on an outpatient basis in patients with or without diabetes. However, if general anesthesia is used, major changes in counter-regulatory hormones can occur even during minor procedures. Additionally, the stress and associated pain of an outpatient procedure may contribute to the development of metabolic decompensation. There are no definitive studies comparing treatment alternatives for patients with type 1 diabetes who are undergoing outpatient surgery. Acceptable management may include either a variable-rate insulin infusion or one of several strategies using SC insulin injection, as previously discussed.

For diabetic patients taking oral hypoglycemic agents, the same management guidelines should be followed as described under elective surgery in the patient with type 2 diabetes. Metformin should be discontinued 48 hours prior to surgery.

With the increasing emphasis on outpatient procedures, it is imperative that patients with diabetes be instructed about how to manage their diabetes after discharge. Blood glucose monitoring should be continued every 1 to 2 hours after returning home. For patients receiving insulin, a predetermined plan for insulin supplements should be created before discharge from the hospital. Patients who are controlled by diet or oral agents should be instructed to contact the health care provider if the blood glucose concentration exceeds a certain level or if urine ketones become positive. Patients with type 1 diabetes should be instructed to measure urinary ketones at home, and any diabetic patient with nausea and vomiting should be screened for ketonuria. If postoperative nausea and vomiting develop after discharge, patients should call their health care provider for further instructions. Metformin therapy should not be reinstated until 48 hours after surgery and when the diabetic patient is eating normally. This means that an interim insulin regimen must be designed and reviewed with the patient before discharge from the hospital or outpatient surgical unit. Most importantly, all patients should have specific guidelines for when their health care providers should be contacted.

Suggested Reading

Alberti KG, Marshall SM. Diabetes and surgery. In Alberti KG, Krall LP, eds. Diabetes annual. vol 4. Amsterdam: Elsevier Science Publishers, 1988:248.

A thorough review of diabetes management during surgery with an emphasis on the glucose-insulin-potassium infusion.

Burgos LG, Ebert TJ, Asiddao C, et al. Increased intraoperative cardiovascular morbidity in diabetics with autonomic neuropathy. Anesthesiology 1989; 70:591–597.

Heart rate and blood pressure declined to a greater degree during induction of anesthesia in diabetic patients with autonomic neuropathy (as identified by respiratory sinus arrhythmia, heart rate responses to Valsalva's maneuver, tilt and cold pressor tests) than in nondiabetic surgical patients.

Elwyn DH. Nutritional requirements of adult surgical patients. Crit Care Med 1980; 8:9–20.

A comprehensive review of nutritional requirements in surgical patients.

Hirsch IB, McGill JB. Role of insulin in management of surgical patients with diabetes mellitus. Diabetes Care 1990; 13:980–981.

Surgery produces a diabetogenic response involving elevation of counter-regulatory hormones and suppression of endogenous insulin. A complete review including discussion of methods of providing insulin during the surgical period.

Hirsch IB, Paauw DS, Brunzell J. Inpatient management of adults with diabetes. Diabetes Care 1995; 18:870–879.

A review of diabetes management for nonsurgical patients.

Lavie CJ, Khandheria BK, Ballard DJ, Palumbo PJ. Diabetes and cardiovascular disease. In: Bergman M, Sicard GA, eds. Surgical management of the diabetic patient. New York: Raven Press, 1991:69.

An excellent review of diabetes and heart disease with a special emphasis on the preoperative cardiac evaluation for this population.

Marhoffer W, Stein M, Maeser E, Federlin K. Impairment of polymorphonuclear leukocyte function and metabolic control of diabetes. Diabetes Care 1992; 15:256–260.

The authors observed impaired polymorphonuclear leukocyte functions in diabetic patients compared with normal control patients. The defect in leukocyte function correlated with the elevation in HbA_{1c} levels. The observation suggests a possible role for protein glycosylation in the impairment in leukocyte function and altered host defense mechanism.

McMurry JF Jr. Wound healing with diabetes mellitus: Better glucose control for better wound healing in diabetes. Surg Clin North Am 1984; 64:769–777.

This study presents experimental and epidemiologic data on wound infections and healing in diabetic patients and suggestions for the control of hyperglycemia.

Schade DS. Surgery and diabetes. Med Clin North Am 1988; 72:1531–1543.

A comprehensive review of the pathophysiology of metabolic decompensation in the diabetic surgical patient and suggestions for perioperative management, including insulin delivery.

Werb MR, Zinman B, Teasdale SJ, et al. Hormonal and metabolic responses during coronary artery bypass surgery: Role of infused glucose. J Clin Endocrinol Metab 1987; 69:1010–1018.

The metabolic and hormonal responses of two groups of nondiabetic patients undergoing coronary artery bypass surgery were compared: half of the patients received glucose-containing cardioplegic solutions, and the other half, receiving standard therapy, served as the control. Implications for diabetic patients undergoing this type of surgery are reviewed.

GERIATRICS AND DIABETES MELLITUS

Jacqueline A. Pugh, M.D.
Michael S. Katz, M.D.

The elderly population (defined as persons 65 years of age and older) is the fastest growing segment of the U.S. population, currently representing close to 13 percent of the population and projected to rise to 22 percent by the year 2050. The most dramatic changes will occur in the age group 85 and older, predicted to increase from 2.2 million in 1990 to 16 million in 2050 in the United States. By the year 2000, the group over age 65 is expected to account for 41 percent of health care dollars spent by the U.S. government. In 1990 the cost of health care services provided to elderly persons with diabetes was estimated to be $5.16 billion, 80 percent of which was attributed to hospital costs.

The prevalence of diabetes rises dramatically with age (Fig. 1): 44 percent of persons with diabetes are 65 years of age or older. As with all geriatric care, the risk versus benefit of treatment must be carefully weighed, resisting the temptation to dismiss the elderly as "too old to change." In this chapter we answer the following questions:

1. When do the physiologic changes in glucose metabolism that occur with aging become disease in need of treatment?

2. Is there an altered presentation of hyperglycemia and hypoglycemia in the elderly?
3. Do elderly persons with diabetes experience complications, and are the complications different from those in younger persons with diabetes?
4. Should diabetes be treated vigorously in the elderly, and what should the treatment goals be?
5. What is the best choice of treatment in the elderly?
6. What is the role of patient education and home glucose monitoring in the elderly?
7. Should the elderly be screened for complications in the same way as younger persons with diabetes?

■ WHEN DO THE PHYSIOLOGIC CHANGES IN GLUCOSE METABOLISM THAT OCCUR WITH AGING BECOME DISEASE IN NEED OF TREATMENT?

Glucose intolerance increases with age: fasting plasma glucose increases by 1 to 2 mg per deciliter and 2-hour postprandial plasma glucose level by 8 to 20 mg per deciliter per decade of age after the age of 30 to 40 years. Although insulin secretion may decline with age, the primary defect underlying age-related glucose intolerance appears to be a decrease in insulin-mediated peripheral glucose metabolism. Insulin responsiveness, as measured by the euglycemic insulin clamp, declines to a similar degree. Insulin receptors have not been shown to decrease with advancing age. Changes in body composition, physical activity, and diet composition probably contribute to, but do not fully explain the loss of insulin sensitivity with aging (Table 1). The principal age-related defect may be a postreceptor defect in insulin action with a decreased maximum velocity of glucose transport, due to a decreased number of glucose transporters, although each transporter functions

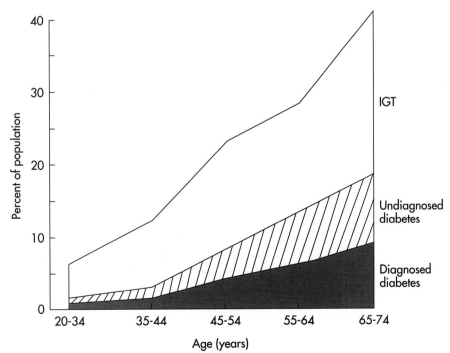

Figure 1
Prevalence of diagnosed diabetes, undiagnosed diabetes, and impaired glucose tolerance (IGT) by age decade in the United States, 1976–1980. (*From Harris MI. Epidemiology of diabetes mellitus among the elderly in the United States. Clin Geriatr Med 1990; 6:703–719; with permission.*)

Table 1 Factors Responsible for the Hyperglycemia of Aging

MOST LIKELY CANDIDATE
Decreased insulin-mediated peripheral glucose utilization due to decreased intracellular glucose transporter pool or other postreceptor defects
POSSIBLE CONTRIBUTORS
Decreased second phase insulin response
Decreased lean body mass and increased adiposity
Decreased physical activity
Changes in diet composition
Raised fasting free fatty acid levels

Table 2 Drugs That Cause or Worsen Hyperglycemia

Diuretics, especially thiazides
Glucocorticoids
Estrogens
Nicotinic acid
Phenothiazines
Phenytoin
Sympathomimetic agents
Lithium
Growth hormone
Isoniazid
Sugar-containing medications

From Goldberg AP, Coon, PJ et al. Diabetes mellitus and glucose metabolism in the elderly. In:Hazard WR, et al, eds. Principles of geriatric medicine and gerontology, New York: McGraw-Hill, 1994; with permission.

normally (Jackson, 1990). What is not clear is whether there is a depletion of the intracellular pool of transporters or a defect in their insulin-mediated translocation to the plasma membrane. There may also be an impairment of the intracellular glucose metabolism beyond the defect in transporters.

If increased glucose levels are a natural result of aging, is there a point at which hyperglycemia becomes a disease in need of treatment? The cutoff levels for the diagnosis of diabetes were chosen with two pieces of biologic evidence in mind. The first was that in populations with high rates of diabetes, bimodality exists in the distributions of glucose levels between those with and without diabetes. The nadir between these two distributions is very close to the current cutoff point. To date there is no specific evidence confirming or denying bimodality in the elderly population. The second reason for the chosen glucose cutoff points is that the bulk of evidence regarding occurrence of complications suggests that the minimum level of glucose required for complications to occur is around 140 to 150 mg per deciliter. Although bimodality has not been demonstrated in the elderly, older persons do develop complications of hyperglycemia. Therefore, the same National Diabetes Data Group or World Health Organization criteria used to make the diagnosis of diabetes in younger individuals should be used in the elderly.

Once an elderly individual meets the criteria for diabetes, precipitating or aggravating factors must be carefully evaluated before starting pharmacologic treatment. Because the elderly are more likely to have multisystem disease, they are also more likely to be on drugs that cause hyperglycemia. Table 2 lists drugs that should, if possible, be replaced by other medication in an effort to improve hyperglycemia and prevent need for treatment.

■ IS THERE AN ALTERED PRESENTATION OF HYPERGLYCEMIA AND HYPOGLYCEMIA IN THE ELDERLY?

Presenting complaints for symptomatic elderly persons with diabetes may be significantly altered from the classic triad of polyuria, polydipsia, and weight loss. Many elderly patients have a diminished thirst perception and do not develop polydipsia. This lack of thirst is one of the reasons for the increased frequency of hyperosmolar states in the elderly. Polyuria may be manifest by urinary incontinence rather than a complaint of frequent urination. With concomitant symptoms of prostatic hypertrophy, elderly men may assume that their symptoms are secondary to their prostate. Altered cognition may be a presenting symptom not usually seen in a younger population. A number of studies have shown subtle alterations of learning, reasoning, and complex psychomotor performance with hyperglycemia in the elderly. In many different community surveys of diabetes, 50 percent of those who meet the criteria for diabetes do not know they have diabetes and are asymptomatic. In Rancho Bernardo, California, 56 percent of diabetic men and 74 percent of diabetic women aged 50 to 89 were unaware of having diabetes at the time of screening. Given both the increased prevalence of diabetes and the diminished presence of classic symptoms in the elderly, case finding or screening in the clinical setting is recommended in this age group.

For management of the elderly person with diabetes, knowledge of the altered presentation of hypoglycemia is also important. The symptoms of hypoglycemia can be broken into two categories: adrenergic and neuroglycopenic. The adrenergic symptoms are those classically associated with hypoglycemia: sweating, nervousness, tremor. Neuroglycopenic symptoms, usually manifest by confusion, are due to the inability of the brain to use any fuel other than glucose. Elderly individuals tend to lose the adrenergic symptoms, due in part to loss of autonomic nerve function, but can have more pronounced neuroglycopenic symptoms than younger individuals. In the extreme case, symptoms such as reversible hemiparesis have been described. Altered perception of hypoglycemia in the elderly can cause a profound clinical problem. The neuroglycopenic symptoms occur late in the course of hypoglycemia, and the confusion prevents the individual from responding appropriately to reverse the hypoglycemia. Further, many elderly individuals, especially those institutionalized and severely disabled, do not have ready access to food. In the past, many physicians preferred not to treat asymptomatic hyperglycemia in the elderly, assuming that hypoglycemia was a worse risk than hyperglycemia. However, hyperglycemia can lead to important symptoms as well, such as urinary incontinence, altered cognition, and hyperosmolar states. Although hypoglycemia should be a concern in the choice and goals of treatment, it should not be used as an excuse to let hyperglycemia go untreated.

■ DO ELDERLY PERSONS WITH DIABETES EXPERIENCE COMPLICATIONS, AND ARE THE COMPLICATIONS DIFFERENT FROM THOSE IN YOUNGER PERSONS WITH DIABETES?

Just 10 years ago, many textbooks of medicine and endocrinology stated that persons with non–insulin-dependent diabetes mellitus (NIDDM) were unlikely to progress to diabetic end-stage renal disease and had much less risk than persons with insulin-dependent diabetes mellitus (IDDM) of developing other complications such as blindness or amputations. With the aging of the population, the decline in mortality from coronary artery disease, and a continuing improvement in tracking of complications, persons with NIDDM have been documented to acquire all complications, often at close to the same rates as those with IDDM. Diabetic complications in the elderly are compounded by the fact that many of the organ systems affected by diabetes (kidneys, eyes, blood vessels, nerves) are also affected by aging itself. In the older individual, diabetes increases the chance of renal disease or blindness by 25 times, gangrene or vascular insufficiency by 20 times, hypertension by 3 times, myocardial infarction by 2.5 times, and stroke by 2 times. (See Figure 2 for contrast of the risk of retinopathy in IDDM versus NIDDM.)

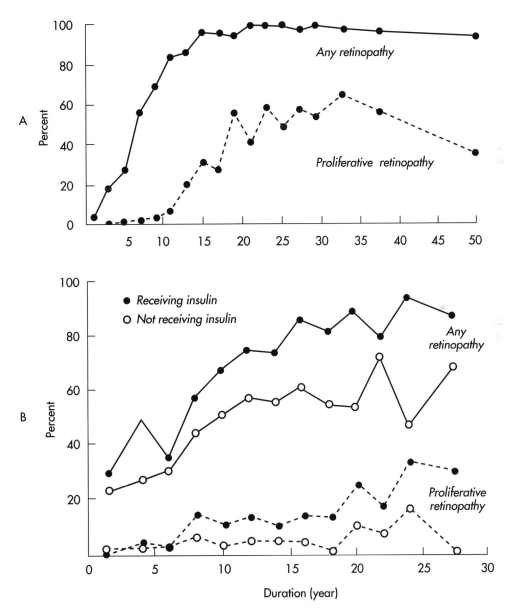

Figure 2
A, Prevalence of any retinopathy and of proliferative retinopathy in patients with younger-onset diabetes (under 30 years of age at diagnosis and taking insulin). **B**, Prevalence of any retinopathy and of proliferative retinopathy in patients with older-onset diabetes (over 30 years of age at diagnosis and either taking or not taking insulin). (*From Wisconsin Epidemiologic Study of Diabetic Retinopathy, Arch Ophthalmol 1984; 102:527–532; with permission.*)

In addition to the burden of illness to the individual, the burden to society is also large. NIDDM-related end-stage renal disease (ESRD) accounts for 50 to 60 percent of diabetic ESRD incident cases and in some minority groups, such as Mexican-Americans and African-Americans, as many as 85 to 90 percent of cases. Diabetes is the second leading cause of blindness in individuals over 65 years of age. The rate of nontraumatic lower extremity amputation is threefold higher in persons with diabetes over the age of 64 than for those aged 45 to 64.

While older individuals have similar and, for some complications, even elevated risk for chronic complications, the pattern of acute complications is different. Individuals with NIDDM are much less likely than IDDM patients to have diabetic ketoacidosis (DKA), although DKA is by no means rare in NIDDM. The rate of DKA among persons with diabetes aged 65 years or older is one-tenth that of those under age 44. In our own Veterans Affairs Hospital, which primarily serves an older population, 56 percent of the admissions with DKA as a discharge diagnosis are associated with NIDDM. While DKA is more likely to be precipitated by a severe illness such as acute myocardial infarction or infection, it can occasionally be the presenting complaint for new-onset NIDDM. (See the chapter *Diabetic Ketoacidosis in Adults* for a more in-depth discussion of DKA in adults.)

Older individuals with diabetes often present with hyperosmolar states. In Rhode Island over a 3-year period, for individuals over the age of 60, 62 percent presented with a hyperosmolar state, 21 percent with a mixed hyperosmolar-DKA, and 11 percent with DKA. Although older studies reported mortality rates of 50 percent with hyperosmolar states, newer studies place the rate at 15 percent, still a high in-hospital mortality. The risk factors for development of hyperosmolar states include dementia, decreased thirst perception, limited access to fluids (as in nursing home residents or disabled elderly living alone), acute illness, new-onset diabetes, and undertreatment or noncompliance with treatment of diabetes. Risk factors for mortality include advanced age, nursing home residence, level of consciousness at admission, degree of hyperosmolarity, and higher serum sodium and blood urea nitrogen at admission. (See the chapter *Hyperglycemic Hyperosmolar Nonketotic Coma* for a discussion of hyperosmolar states.)

■ SHOULD DIABETES BE TREATED VIGOROUSLY IN THE ELDERLY, AND WHAT SHOULD THE TREATMENT GOALS BE?

Both the chronic and acute complications provide a rationale for undertaking treatment of diabetes in the elderly. The most important single principle by which treatment should be guided is to tailor the treatment to the individual. For the "physiologically young" individual, the same rationale for glycemic control as in the younger age groups should apply. This is the individual who despite being 65 years of age or older has no known complications of the disease, looks younger than his or her stated age, is physically active, and is likely to survive the 5 to 15 years necessary to begin to have microvascular complications. Microvascular complications may appear after a shorter duration of diabetes in NIDDM

than in IDDM because there is often a period of time in which the disease is present but the individual is not yet symptomatic enough to seek treatment. The Diabetes Control and Complications Trial data conclusively show that achieving tight control decreases complications without severe risk in the IDDM patient. A similar study is under way looking at the risk:benefit ratio of tight glucose control in NIDDM patients (UK Prospective Diabetes Study).

For those individuals in whom chronic complications have already developed or who have other life-threatening illnesses, higher glycemic goals may be appropriate. Table 3 lists some of the contraindications to tight control (defined as an attempt to normalize the serum glucose) that occur frequently in the elderly. Dementia is a particularly important contraindication to tight control because it prevents the individual from taking appropriate action should hypoglycemia occur. Therefore, the goal in dementia should be control of symptoms and prevention of hyperosmolar states but not tight glucose control. In chronic renal insufficiency, the half-life of both endogenous and exogenous insulin is prolonged. As renal failure progresses, many persons with NIDDM will need their insulin or oral agents reduced or even discontinued. In cirrhosis, the liver is damaged to the point that the normal glycogen stores are depressed or absent, significantly decreasing the ability of the individual to respond to hypoglycemia. Autonomic nerve dysfunction leads to an inability to sense and respond to hypoglycemia. Patients with orthostatic hypotension, gastroparesis, or moderate to severe peripheral neuropathy should be suspected of also having significant autonomic neuropathy. Active alcoholism can lead to severe hypoglycemia because normal food intake is often neglected and gluconeogenesis is inhibited. Severe physical disability is a relative contraindication to tight glycemic control if food and drink are not readily available to the individual. Without access to food, one cannot respond to hypoglycemia even when symptoms are appropriately perceived. Although this seems obvious, many physicians fail to inquire about their patients' living situations and eating habits. These questions should be a central concern in treating the elderly diabetic patient. Goals for all of these individuals should be aimed at decreasing hyperglycemic symptoms and decreasing the chance of developing a hyperosmolar state.

■ WHAT IS THE BEST CHOICE OF TREATMENT IN THE ELDERLY?

As with treatment goals, choice of treatment should be tailored to the individual's needs. The absence of hyperglycemic symptoms allows an initial trial of diet alone, while the pres-

Table 3 Common Contraindications to Tight Glucose Control in the Elderly
Dementia
Chronic renal insufficiency
Cirrhosis
Active alcoholism
Autonomic nerve dysfunction
Physical disability combined with social isolation or food restriction

ence of symptoms suggests a need for pharmacologic treatment. Diet should continue to be the mainstay of treatment in the elderly. Reducing total calories is the most effective therapy because the majority of persons with NIDDM are overweight and relatively small amounts of weight loss in these individuals can lead to large improvements in glucose tolerance. Dietary change is difficult to achieve in all individuals, but there is no good evidence that dietary change is more difficult to achieve in elderly individuals. Exercise is also an important part of therapy. In this age group the aim is a mild to moderate increase in activity; for example, walking, yard and house work, stationary bicycling. The exercise will reduce insulin resistance and may allow for less or no pharmacologic treatment.

When caloric restriction and exercise fail, sulfonylureas or metformin are the next line of therapy. The second-generation sulfonylureas glyburide, and glipizide are preferred agents because of the substantially reduced dosage and total body stores of drug that accumulate at steady state. These drugs do not require renal function for metabolism, because both are metabolized in the liver. Glipizide also has the theoretical advantage of having inactive metabolites and therefore no accumulation of active metabolites in renal failure. All three drugs must be used with caution in patients with hepatic disease. Chlorpropamide is specifically discouraged because its half-life and duration of action are so long (35 and up to 72 hours, respectively). If chlorpropamide-induced hypoglycemia does occur, it can be profound and prolonged, even requiring hospitalization. However, recent data from the United Kingdom Prospective Diabetes Study show that chlorpropamide and glyburide cause hypoglycemia at equivalent rates. Chlorpropramide is also more likely than the other sulfonylureas to cause hyponatremia. Since many elderly patients are also taking diuretics for hypertension or congestive heart failure, their risk of developing hyponatremia may be increased. Although all of the sulfonylureas are highly (more than 90 percent) protein bound, glyburide and glipizide have a single binding site on albumin, while chlorpropamide and tolbutamide have multiple binding sites. The second-generation agents show less displacement by warfarin, salicylate, and phenylbutazone in vitro and may have less potential for hypoglycemia secondary to drug-drug interaction. (See the chapter *Sulfonylureas.*)

Metformin is an alternative to sulfonylureas but should not be used in the presence of renal insufficiency or congestive heart failure, because of an increased risk of lactic acidosis. Since renal insufficiency is common with advancing age, renal function should be evaluated before starting metformin. In elderly persons with decreased lean body mass, determination of serum creatinine may not adequately substitute for measurement of creatinine clearance in the assessment of renal function. Theoretically, metformin alone might be safer than sulfonylureas in older obese individuals with normal renal and cardiac function because it does not cause hypoglycemia but only corrects to euglycemia. In combining metformin with either sulfonylureas or insulin, however, hypoglycemia would be a risk. (See the chapter *Metformin.*)

Insulin therapy may be necessary to control symptoms, but one needs to be aware of the barriers to insulin therapy, which include decreased manual dexterity due to arthritis or stroke, poor visual acuity leading to inappropriate dosing, and impaired cognition leading to problems in remembering both the appropriate dose and the technique of administration. These problems, once identified, can be overcome through the use of a caretaker or visiting home nurse (who draws insulin up ahead of schedule for later administration by the patient).

■ WHAT IS THE ROLE OF PATIENT EDUCATION AND HOME GLUCOSE MONITORING IN THE ELDERLY?

Studies have shown that learning capacity continues throughout life and that the elderly are capable of learning both new knowledge and new skills. The three domains of learning include cognitive, affective, and psychomotor. Many of the consequences of aging affect both the content of diabetic education and the ability of the patient to participate fully. Table 4 lists age-related and diabetes-associated changes that affect the ability of the elderly person with diabetes to learn and to comply with prescribed treatment regimens. It is crucial to include relatives or caregivers in the educational process, especially if these individuals control food and/or medication dispensation.

Is home glucose monitoring efficacious in the elderly? Despite the knowledge that blood glucose monitoring is significantly more accurate than urine glucose monitoring, the barriers to home glucose monitoring are similar to those for insulin administration. Manual dexterity, visual acuity, and cognition often make home glucose monitoring problematic in the elderly. One study in England showed that among a sample of 57 elderly individuals who required insulin, 53 percent incorrectly performed either urine or blood home tests. At least one trial has suggested that for achieving good control in the elderly, urine monitoring may be just as effective a motivational tool as home glucose monitoring. Others have shown that urine testing has poor correlation with glycosylated hemoglobin. If monitoring is being used primarily as a feedback tool rather than for changing the insulin titration, either method may be successful in the elderly. If the patient is being asked to change insulin doses in accordance with monitoring, then blood rather than urine monitoring is preferred.

■ SHOULD THE ELDERLY BE SCREENED FOR COMPLICATIONS IN THE SAME WAY AS YOUNGER PERSONS WITH DIABETES?

The answer to this question depends on the complication. Recently published guidelines for retinopathy state that all persons with NIDDM should be screened at diagnosis. If patients require insulin, they should be screened annually thereafter because their risk of developing retinopathy in need of laser therapy is significant although not as high as in IDDM. For individuals with NIDDM who do not require insulin, the risk is much decreased. If the initial screening is performed with seven standard field stereoscopic photography and there is no retinopathy present, screening can be deferred for 4 years.

Persons with NIDDM, especially Native Americans, African-Americans, and Mexican-Americans, may have a

Table 4 Age-Related and Diabetes-Associated Changes That Affect Learning

SYSTEM CHANGED	EFFECT
COGNITION	
Memory	May need repetition or caretaker help
Complex psychomotor tasks	May have difficulty with insulin and home glucose monitoring
SENSORY	
Visual acuity	Decreased ability to read syringes
Lens clarity	Decreased perception of blue-tone colors
Night vision	Decreased ability to interpret home blood glucose monitoring strips
Hearing	Impaired communication leading to possible nonadherence
CUTANEOUS	
Vibratory and thermal sensitivity	Impaired ability to discern temperature and pressure
Tactile sensitivity	Potential for burns and ischemia
	Decreased manual dexterity for injections and home blood glucose monitoring
VESTIBULAR-PROPRIOCEPTIVE	
Equilibrium	Vertigo and imbalance
Sense of bodily orientation	Potential for falls
	Decreased motivation for exercise and other activity
GUSTATORY, OLFACTORY	
Taste, smell	Reduced dietary adherence
GASTROINTESTINAL	
Thirst mechanism	Altered dietary intake
Motility	Potential for hypoglycemia
Delayed gastric emptying	Potential for dehydration
URINARY	
Decreased renal function	Potential for hypoglycemia, increased drug half-life
Altered renal threshold for glucose	Decreased utility of urine testing

Adapted from education and counseling for diabetes self-care. In: Gambert SR, ed. Diabetes mellitus in the elderly. New York: Raven Press, 1990; with permission.

risk similar to those with IDDM for developing nephropathy, justifying the need to screen in NIDDM. However, screening in the elderly is problematic in that proteinuria increases with age even in the absence of diabetes. The current Health and Nutrition Survey (HANES3) is obtaining age-specific norms for microalbuminuria and should be helpful in the future. Even if microalbuminuria is not as good a predictor of progression to end-stage renal disease in NIDDM as in IDDM, it is a predictor of higher cardiovascular mortality. The presence or absence of albuminuria may therefore help the clinician decide the target level of hypertension and perhaps even lipid control. Recent studies suggest that albuminuria (both micro and macro) benefits from treatment with ACE inhibitors, although no trials have been conducted specifically in elderly subjects.

Screening and education for diabetic foot problems should be undertaken more vigorously in the elderly than in the young person with diabetes because the elderly are at higher risk due to the combination of vascular and neuropathic disease. Education has been shown to reduce amputations.

Cholesterol screening is controversial in elderly nondiabetic patients because of decreased benefit from intervention. However, in diabetic patients who are already at high risk of vascular disease, lipids should be screened early in the course of disease and treated independently of glycemic control.

The prevalence of diabetes is high in the elderly. Diabetic complications, both acute and chronic, do occur at rates compared in some cases comparable to IDDM. Treatment goals should be tailored to the individual to maximize quality of life and well-being. This means that "physiologically young" individuals over the age of 65 may be treated vigorously, while "physiologically old" individuals may be treated only to prevent symptoms or hospitalization from hyperglycemia. The patient must be an active participant in the assessment of risk and benefit and the choice of treatment.

Suggested Reading

Am J Med 1986; 80 (suppl 5A):1–63. Diabetes Care 1990; 13(suppl 2):1–92.

Two journal supplements on diabetes mellitus in the elderly.

Clin Geriatr Med 1990; 6:693–991.

This issue is devoted to diabetes in the elderly.

DeFronzo RA. Glucose intolerance and aging. Diabetes Care 1981; 4:493–501.

A review article on the mechanisms of glucose intolerance with aging.

Diabetes in America. NIH Publication No. 95–1468. Bethesda, Md: U.S. Department of Health and Human Services, 1995.

Current information on the prevalence of diabetes.

Gambert SR, ed. Diabetes mellitus in the elderly: A practical guide. New York: Raven Press, 1990.

A monograph on the subject of diabetes mellitus in the elderly.

Jackson RA. Mechanisms of age-related glucose intolerance. Diabetes Care 1990; 13(suppl 2):9–19.

A review article on glucose intolerance in the elderly.

Minaker KL. What diabetologists should know about elderly patients. Diabetes Care 1990; 13(suppl 2):34–46.

A review of geriatrics for the diabetologist.

Pegg A, Fitzgerald F, Wise D, et al. A community-based study of diabetes-related skills and knowledge in elderly people with insulin-requiring diabetes. Diabetic Med 1991; 8:778–781.

An article concerning knowledge of diabetes and diabetes education in the elderly.

Singer DE, Nathan DM, Fogel HA, Schachat AP. Screening for diabetic retinopathy. Ann Intern Med 1992; 116:660–671.

Wachtel TJ, Tetu-Mouradjian LM, Goldman DL, et al. Hyperosmolarity and acidosis in diabetes mellitus: A three year experience in Rhode Island. J Gen Intern Med 1991; 6:495–502.

The two preceding journal articles deal with complications of diabetes.

Wingard DL, Sinsheimer P, Barrett-Connor EL, McPhillips JB. Community-based study of prevalence of NIDDM in older adults. Diabetes Care 1990; 13(suppl 2):3–8.

An article on the prevalence of diabetes and glucose intolerance in the elderly.

Index